PRIMARY CARE OF THE NEWBORN

fourth
EDITION

PRIMARY CARE OF THE NEWBORN

EDITORS

Seidel, MD
Professor Emeritus of Pediatrics
The Johns Hopkins University School of Medicine
Attending Physician, Department of Pediatrics
The Johns Hopkins Hospital
Baltimore, Maryland

Beryl J. Rosenstein, MD
Professor of Pediatrics
The Johns Hopkins University School of Medicine
Attending Physician, Department of Pediatrics
The Johns Hopkins Hospital
Baltimore, Maryland

Ambadas Pathak, MD
Assistant Professor Emeritus of Pediatrics
The Johns Hopkins University School of Medicine
Clinical Associate Professor of Pediatrics
University of Maryland School of Medicine
Distinguished Emeritus Staff, Department of Pediatrics
Greater Baltimore Medical Center
Baltimore, Maryland

Wendell H. McKay, MD
Community Pediatrician, Department of Pediatrics
The Johns Hopkins Hospital
Baltimore, Maryland
Department of Pediatrics
Howard County General Hospital
Columbia, Maryland

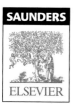

SAUNDERS

ELSEVIER

SAUNDERS
ELSEVIER

1600 John F. Kennedy Blvd.
Ste 1800
Philadelphia, PA 19103-2899

PRIMARY CARE OF THE NEWBORN

ISBN-13: 978-0-323-03724-2
ISBN-10: 0-323-03724-0

Notice

Knowledge and best practice in this field are constantly changing. As new research and experience broaden our knowledge, changes in practice, treatment, and drug therapy may become necessary or appropriate. Readers are advised to check the most current information provided (i) on procedures featured or (ii) by the manufacturer of each product to be administered, to verify the recommended dose or formula, the method and duration of administration, and contraindications. It is the responsibility of the practitioner, relying on their own experience and knowledge of the patient, to make diagnoses, to determine dosages and the best treatment for each individual patient, and to take all appropriate safety precautions. To the fullest extent of the law, neither the Publisher nor the Editors assume any liability for any injury and/or damage to persons or property arising out of or related to any use of the material contained in this book.

Previous editions copyrighted 2001, 1997, 1993

Library of Congress Cataloging-in-Publication Data

Primary care of the newborn / [edited by] Henry M. Seidel ... [et al.] — 4th ed.
    p. ; cm.
  Includes bibliographical references and index.
  ISBN 0-323-03724-0
    1. Infants (Newborn)—Medical care. 2. Neonatology. I. Seidel, Henry M.
    [DNLM: 1. Infant Care—Outlines. 2. Infant, Newborn—Outlines. 3. Infant, Newborn, Diseases—Outlines. WS 18.2 P952 2006]
  RJ253.P74 2006
  618.92'01—dc22   2005056176

Acquisitions Editor: James Merritt
Publishing Services Manager: Frank Polizzano
Project Manager: Jeff Gunning
Design Direction: Karen O'Keefe-Owens

Printed in the United States of America

Last digit is the print number: 9 8 7 6 5 4 3 2 1

Working together to grow
libraries in developing countries
www.elsevier.com | www.bookaid.org | www.sabre.org

ELSEVIER   BOOK AID International   Sabre Foundation

To our children and grandchildren, who are also our teachers;
to the pediatricians, nurse practitioners, and
residents with whom we have worked.

Contributors

Max M. April, MD, FAAP, FACS
Co-Director of Pediatric Otolaryngology
Department of Otolaryngology
Lenox Hill Hospital
New York, New York

Joel I. Brenner, MD
Associate Professor
Department of Pediatrics, Division of Cardiology
The Johns Hopkins University School of Medicine
Baltimore, Maryland

Michael D. Cabana, MD, MPH
Associate Professor of Pediatrics
Chief, Division of General Pediatrics
University of California, San Francisco

James F. Casella, MD
Rainey Professor of Pediatric Hematology
Department of Pediatrics, Division of Hematology
The Johns Hopkins University School of Medicine
Chief, Pediatric Hematology
The Johns Hopkins Hospital
Baltimore, Maryland

Bernard A. Cohen, MD
Professor of Pediatrics and Dermatology
The Johns Hopkins University School of Medicine
Director of Pediatric Dermatology
The Johns Hopkins Children's Center
Baltimore, Maryland

David W. Cooke, MD
Associate Professor
Department of Pediatrics, Division of Endocrinology
The Johns Hopkins University School of Medicine
Baltimore, Maryland

John P. Gearhart, MD
Professor of Pediatric Urology and Pediatrics
The Johns Hopkins University School of Medicine
Director of Pediatric Urology
The Johns Hopkins Hospital
Baltimore, Maryland

Ada Hamosh, MD, MPH
Associate Professor of Pediatrics
Institute of Genetic Medicine
The Johns Hopkins University School of Medicine
Attending Physician
The Johns Hopkins Hospital
Baltimore, Maryland

Rebecca N. Ichord, MD
Assistant Professor of Pediatric Neurology and Pediatrics
University of Pennsylvania School of Medicine
Director, Pediatric Stroke Program
The Children's Hospital of Philadelphia
Philadelphia, Pennsylvania

Timothy R.B. Johnson, MD
Bates Professor of Diseases of Women and Children
Chair, Department of Obstetrics and Gynecology
University of Michigan Medical Center
Ann Arbor, Michigan

Gregory J. Kato, MD
Associate Professor of Pediatrics and Oncology
Department of Pediatrics, Division of Hematology
The Johns Hopkins University School of Medicine
Attending Physician, Department of Pediatrics
The Johns Hopkins Hospital
Baltimore, Maryland

Robert M. Naclerio, MD
Professor and Chief
Section of Otolaryngology–Head and Neck Surgery
The University of Chicago Pritzker School of Medicine
Chicago, Illinois

Ambadas Pathak, MD
Assistant Professor Emeritus of Pediatrics
The Johns Hopkins University School of Medicine
Clinical Associate Professor of Pediatrics
University of Maryland School of Medicine
Distinguished Emeritus Staff, Department of Pediatrics
Greater Baltimore Medical Center
Baltimore, Maryland

Michael X. Repka, MD
Professor, Department of Ophthalmology
Associate Professor, Department of Pediatrics
The Johns Hopkins University School of Medicine
Attending Physician, Department of Ophthalmology
The Johns Hopkins Hospital
Baltimore, Maryland

Beryl J. Rosenstein, MD
Professor, Department of Pediatrics
The Johns Hopkins University School of Medicine
Attending Physician, Department of Pediatrics
The Johns Hopkins Hospital
Baltimore, Maryland

Jose M. Saavedra, MD
Attending Physician, Department of Pediatrics
Division of Gastroenterology and Nutrition
The Johns Hopkins Hospital
Baltimore, Maryland

Henry M. Seidel, MD
Professor Emeritus of Pediatrics
The Johns Hopkins University School of Medicine
Attending Physician, Department of Pediatrics
The Johns Hopkins Hospital
Baltimore, Maryland

Patricia H. Smouse, MSN, CRNP
Nurse Practitioner
Department of Gynecology and Obstetrics
The Johns Hopkins Hospital
Baltimore, Maryland

Paul D. Sponseller, MD
Professor, Department of Orthopedic Surgery
The Johns Hopkins University School of Medicine
Head, Division of Pediatric Orthopedics
The Johns Hopkins Hospital
Baltimore, Maryland

Timothy Townsend, MD
Associate Professor, Department of Pediatrics
The Johns Hopkins University School of Medicine
Attending Physician, Department of Pediatrics
The Johns Hopkins Hospital
Baltimore, Maryland

Judith W. Vogelhut, RN, BS, CRNP, IBCLC
Nurse Coordinator, Breastfeeding Center
Department of General Pediatrics and Adolescent Medicine
The Johns Hopkins Hospital
Baltimore, Maryland

Jean S. Wheeler, BSN, CPNP
Assistant in Pediatrics, Department of Pediatrics
The Johns Hopkins University School of Medicine
Baltimore, Maryland

Siew-Jyu Wong, MD
Instructor, Department of Pediatrics
The Johns Hopkins University School of Medicine
Attending Neonatologist
St. Agnes Hospital
Baltimore, Maryland

Preface

The editors of this fourth edition of *Primary Care of the Newborn* span at least three generations in medicine, each of us with a somewhat different experience but all committed to the care of newborn infants. We long ago—for one of us, more than half a century!—took up *The Harriet Lane Handbook* as a ready, pocket-sized volume for those who care for children during a busy day. *Primary Care of the Newborn* initially was prepared because we believed that there was still room in our pockets for a companion volume devoted solely to the care of the newborn in the first hours and days of life—the newborn who is *not* a resident in an intensive care nursery.

A new feature in this edition is introductory sections for select chapters that highlight considerations especially relevant to the primary care of the newborn. These introductions were written by Wendell H. McKay, the newest member of our team and an active primary care pediatrician. Each introduction includes material on three specific topics:

- *Immediate Issues in the Nursery*
- *Important Reminders after Discharge*
- *Helpful Information for Parents*

These introductory sections should be especially helpful to those community practitioners who may not have ready and immediate access to pediatric subspecialists at their local institutions. The highlighted information also is meant to provide a focus on key elements of comprehensive newborn care and to remind the practitioner about some of the sensitivities and fears experienced by parents during this joyous yet stressful time.

It is our hope that this compact volume will be an important resource for those who care for newborns and for the infants and their families.

Henry M. Seidel
Beryl J. Rosenstein
Ambadas Pathak
Wendell H. McKay

Acknowledgments

We owe a great debt to the many men and women who have helped us realize this fourth edition of *Primary Care of the Newborn*. Certainly, we are grateful for the expertise and efforts of the authors of the individual chapters and for their timely response to our needs. The contributions of others are perhaps less apparent but nevertheless important. These include Nancy Barnett, Francine Cheese Wethersby, Tuvia Blechman, George Dover, Edward E. Lawson, Sujay Pathak, Wayne Reisig—and, indeed, our families, who allowed us the time to do this, too often carved out of evening and weekend hours, without complaint and with good humor.

There are also those in the past—teachers, mentors, and colleagues—who enriched our experience in the care of babies: Harry Gordon and Alexander Schaffer when three of us were still tyros and, later, Billy Andrews, Mary Ellen Avery, Stephen Ludwig, Jeffrey Maisels, Nicholas Nelson, and Beth Rezet.

No book is born without the skill, patience, and dedication of those who work effectively and quietly behind the scenes to ensure a positive outcome. They, too, teach us and are patient with us. In this regard, initially, Dolores Meloni and Anna Solomon were the midwives for our effort; subsequently, Joanne Husovski and Jeff Gunning made certain that our effort was presented in a form that ensures the reader excellent accessibility and the opportunity to learn. They are true professionals, and we thank them for adding pleasure as well as competence as we went about our task.

Contents

Contents

Prenatal Visit

Henry M. Seidel

I. GENERAL

Prenatal visits are invaluable, particularly during a first pregnancy, when practitioner and patient are strangers. These visits provide an opportunity to learn much about each other (e.g., history relevant to the pregnancy, practice habits of the practitioner) and to begin to build the foundation of trust and mutual respect that are essential in continuity care and in moments of great stress, e.g., in the event of unanticipated congenital defect in the neonate. There is much to discuss, ideally with both mother and father or other possible caretakers, to assure active family participation in decision-making and to initiate counseling about the experience of living with an infant. A partnership is formed with the goal of serving the parents as well as the baby. Importantly, such a visit enables you to gather basic information, provide information and advice, increase the potential of parenting skills and, particularly, identify high-risk situations, e.g., family disequilibrium, guns in the house, history of genetic abnormality.

1

Note: *Among mothers whose first infant has a birth defect, the risk of the same defect in a second infant is notably increased and the risk of a different defect in that second infant is slightly increased. There is a genetic causation often demonstrable and, as well, an environmental effect.*

Note: *If there has not been opportunity for a prenatal visit, everything discussed in this chapter is relevant to the time of first introduction to the baby and family (see Chapter 5). Also, in lieu of this basic visit if it is not possible, a brief "get to know you" visit may at least facilitate future interactions. Even a telephone call can acquaint the parents with the rudiments of the practitioner's office practices and give you some sense of the approaches of the parents.*

II. TIMING

By early in the third trimester much of the *history* of the pregnancy is available and parents have time to seek other resources if they are dissatisfied with the practitioner for any reason.

III. DETAILS OF THE HISTORY

A. FAMILY.

1. Consanguineous marriage.
2. Development of a chart of genetic lineage, essential to the third generation when counseling in this regard is necessary.
3. Particular disease concerns: Questions regarding heritable and contagious illnesses; effect of major illness in parents or in others in family of the expected child.
4. Status of siblings.

5. Specific topics, at the least, that should be addressed include the following:
   a. Allergy.
   b. Blood dyscrasias.
   c. Cardiovascular conditions (e.g., congenital disorders, rheumatic fever).
   d. Pulmonary conditions.
   e. Renal conditions.
   f. Contagion (e.g., tuberculosis, syphilis, hepatitis, herpes, acquired immunodeficiency syndrome [AIDS], rubella, and much more).

B. PREGNANCY.

1. Previous pregnancies; results.
2. Intercurrent illness.
   a. Infection of any kind (e.g., hepatitis, tuberculosis, sexually transmitted disease, herpes).
   b. Vaginal bleeding.
   c. Toxemia (pretoxic states).
3. Chronic illness (e.g., lupus erythematosus, diabetes, thyroid disease).
4. Weight gain (excessive or insufficient).
5. Time and intensity of fetal movement.
6. Care of animals (e.g., cats and the possibility of toxoplasmosis).
7. Drugs.
   a. Prescribed (e.g., anticonvulsants, anticoagulants).
   b. Over-the-counter (OTC), e.g., vitamin, folic acid supplements.
   c. Illicit (in some areas, illicit drug use is virtually an epidemic),
   d. Tobacco and/or alcohol intake.

C. PRENATAL SCREENING.

1. Amniocentesis.
2. Sonography.
3. Chorionic villus sampling (CVS).
4. Rh sensitization and setup.
5. Maternal and paternal blood types.
6. Serologic studies for sexually transmitted disease (rapid plasma reagin [RPR] for syphilis; hepatitis B surface antigen, and human immunodeficiency virus [HIV] status).
7. Tuberculin test.
8. Alpha-fetoprotein.
9. X-rays.
10. Serologic studies for cytomegalovirus (CMV) or toxoplasmosis.

D. SOCIAL.

1. Family constellation.
   a. Members of household.
   b. Intergenerational relationships: Grandparents, aunts and uncles, close family friends.

c. Sources of child care: Relatives, paid helpers.
d. Sources of income.
e. Attitudes on discipline.
2. Physical setting.
3. Religious preferences (e.g., question of blood transfusion, mandate for circumcision).
4. Ethnic preferences, background.

IV. ANTICIPATORY GUIDANCE

A. FEEDING OPTIONS; MOTHER'S PREFERENCE; FATHER'S SUPPORT.
B. ROOMING IN AND THE MEANING OF BONDING.
C. CIRCUMCISION, YES OR NO?
D. NECESSARY HOME FURNISHINGS AND EQUIPMENT; TYPE OF DIAPERS.
E. THE FIRST RIDE HOME. APPROPRIATE AUTOMOBILE RESTRAINTS.
F. PREPARING SIBLINGS FOR THE BABY'S ARRIVAL.
G. PRACTITIONER'S PRACTICE RULES, PREFERENCES, AND STYLE.
1. Call arrangements.
2. Appointment schedules.
3. Fees and billing.
4. Hospital affiliations.

H. OPEN-ENDED DISCUSSION.
1. Explore potential of expressed or unexpressed concerns (e.g., What do I do when I want to "flush the baby down the toilet?").
2. Handouts.

V. ADOLESCENT PREGNANCY

A. THE TEENAGER.
These very young women are subject to all the pleasures and problems of pregnancy and delivery. In addition, as with all patients, the practitioner should be aware of the particular circumstances and characteristics of the adolescent, including the following:
1. Level of education.
2. Communication skills.
3. Family structure.
4. Relationship with putative father when he does not join in the discussion.

B. THE PRACTITIONER SHOULD ALSO
1. Adjust his or her language and style of presentation to the needs of the patient without limiting the range of issues for discussion.
   The information does not have to be communicated in one session.
2. Involve family if at all possible.
3. Involve father of the child if at all possible.

Note: *Be sure to discuss and provide for follow-up contraception.*

VI. CULTURAL CONSIDERATIONS

The prenatal interview and *any* ensuing interactions require insight into the culture of the family and an understanding of what it is that differentiates individuals and groups if all patient needs are to be appropriately served (see Chapter 6). Any individual may, and most often does, belong to more than one group or subgroup. These multiple classifications can be the result of any combination of ethnic origin, religion, gender, social network, occupation, or profession.

A. SOME GUIDELINES TO CULTURAL UNDERSTANDING.

1. Respect individuals as unique, with the cultural group as but one determinant.
2. Respect the unfamiliar and try to understand it.
3. Identify and examine personal cultural beliefs.
4. Recognize that different cultural groups have varying practices that attempt to promote health and cure illness. If the cultural view is "scientific" in that a precise cause can be determined for every problem, the family is more apt to be comfortable with Western approaches to care. A more naturalistic or "holistic" approach views life as part of a harmonious greater whole. If the balance is disturbed, illness can result, and the goal then is to retrieve balance or harmony. Aspects of these concepts are evident among many persons of Hispanic, Native American, Asian, and Arab cultures, and they are increasingly evident in the United States today. There are also beliefs in the "supernatural," forces for good and evil which determine individual fate. In such a context, illness may be believed to be a punishment for wrongdoing.
5. Be prepared to adapt care in keeping with the patient's cultural values; appreciate that these values are often deep seated and possibly difficult or undesirable to change.
6. Do not confuse the physical with the cultural or allow the physical to symbolize the cultural. This does not deny their interdependence. Skin color, for example, precedes most of the experience of life and the subsequent obvious interweaving of color with cultural experience.
7. Do not assume homogeneity in any group. The stereotype is to be rejected. People within groups can and do respond differently to the same stimuli.
8. The health care worker and the newborn's caretaker(s) must understand one another fully and clearly. Ask if not sure. Do not make assumptions without validation from the family.

B. FAMILY RELATIONSHIPS.

Family structure and the social organizations to which a family belongs (e.g., churches, clubs, and schools) are among the many imprinting and constraining cultural forces, particularly with the shift toward dual-income families, single-parent families, an increasing number of teenage pregnancies, the prevalence of divorce, and the increasing involvement of fathers in child care.

Note: *One type of behavior may predict another type (e.g., mothers who take advantage of appropriate prenatal care will generally provide appropriate infant care regardless of educational level, marital status, family relationships, or illicit drug use).*

C. QUESTIONS THAT CAN PROVIDE CULTURAL INSIGHTS.
1. Health beliefs and practices.
a. How does the family define health and illness?
b. What is the attitude toward preventive health measures?
c. Are there health topics that may be particularly sensitive or that are considered taboo?
d. What are the attitudes toward pain, handicapping conditions, chronic disease, death, and dying?
2. Religious influences and special rituals.
a. Is the family adherent to a religion? To what degree?
b. Are there special religious practices or beliefs that may affect health care?
c. What events, rituals, and ceremonies are considered important within the life cycle, such as birth and baptism?
3. Language and communication.
a. What language is spoken in the home?
b. How well is English understood, both spoken and written?
c. Are there special behaviors for demonstrating respect or disrespect?
4. Parenting styles and role of family.
a. Who makes the decisions in the family?
b. What is the composition of the family and the number of generations involved? Which relatives compose the family unit?
c. What is the role of and attitude toward children in the family?
d. Are there special beliefs and practices surrounding conception, pregnancy, childbirth, lactation, and child rearing?

VII. ETHICAL CONSIDERATIONS
The ethical context to the relationship with the newborn and the family has been better defined in recent years. Ethics does not provide answers; rather, it offers a disciplined approach to understanding and to determining ultimate behavior and decision-making. Given a problem (e.g., a perceived necessary violation of confidentiality), several concepts must be considered.

A. AUTONOMY.
The need for self-determination: with a newborn, parents, family, and other significant persons must each have the boundaries of their autonomy clearly set. The core question: Who shall speak for the baby? For example,

the decisions regarding continuation of treatment in supposedly futile circumstances demands that the pediatrician feel sufficiently certain that what is proposed is in the best interest of the child.

B. BENEFICENCE.
Beneficence is the mandate to do good for the patient. There is always a concern that doing good may be too eagerly pursued and may result in a paternalism that might smother the family's autonomy.

C. NONMALEFICENCE.
Nonmaleficence is the mandate to do no harm to the patient; *primum non nocere.*

D. UTILITARIANISM.
Utilitarianism is the practical need to consider the allocation of resources for the greater good of the larger community (distributive justice).

E. FAIRNESS AND JUSTICE.
Fairness and justice enable recognition of the often precarious balance between the competing interests of the individual and the community.

F. DEONTOLOGIC IMPERATIVES.
Deontologic imperatives are the duties of caregivers established by tradition and in a cultural context.

These principles often come into conflict (e.g., the use of limited resources in situations believed to be futile, the difficulties in end-of-life decisions). Consideration of each with the baby in mind can, however, lead to helpful outcomes. Respect for all involved and flexibility in attitudes are key ingredients in the search for answers.

Note: *Although what we outline is obviously more than enough for an hour's conversation, the prenatal visit is important to the development of sound, ongoing relationships. No one approach or style is best. There is much room for individual variation in length, frequency, and content of discussion. Content may certainly be shared with the first postpartum and subsequent visits as you and the baby and the parents (caretakers) get to know each other. First time parents may be the neediest but multiple parenthood should not lead to the inappropriate assumption that past experience has been a good teacher. That should be determined and, in any event, there is still much that you, new to a family, must learn.*

BIBLIOGRAPHY

Charney E: Counseling of parents around the birth of a baby. Pediatric Review 4:167, 1982.

Committee on Bioethics: Appropriate boundaries in the pediatrician-family-patient relationship. Pediatrics 104:334, 1999.

Committee on Psychosocial Aspects of Child and Family Health: The prenatal visit. Pediatrics 107:1456, 2001.

van der Heide A, van der Maas PJ, van der Wal G, et al: The role of parents in end-of-life decisions in neonatology: Physicians' views and practices. Pediatrics 101:413, 1998.

Wessel MA: The prenatal pediatric visit. Pediatrics 32:926, 1963.

High-Risk Pregnancy

Timothy R.B. Johnson

I. DEFINITION OF HIGH-RISK PREGNANCY

A. VARIES DEPENDING ON PATIENT POPULATION.

B. THE MOST COMMON HIGH-RISK CONDITIONS
include age >35, age <17, post-term pregnancy, associated medical complications, previous preterm labor, multiple pregnancy, and socioeconomic problems. Some maternal medical problems can be associated with specific neonatal conditions (**Box 2-1**).

C. RISK ASSESSMENT IS USEFUL.
An attempt is made to identify the 20% of patients that account for 60% or more of perinatal morbidity and mortality.

D. VARIOUS RISK ASSESSMENT SCORES
have been developed for perinatal morbidity and mortality. Generally, risk is assessed at registration, in middle to late pregnancy, and again in labor. Obstetric preconception assessment is recommended, analogous to a prenatal pediatric visit. Risk assessment has been developed for preterm labor and includes historical assessment and clinical tools such as sonographic cervical length measurement and maternal vaginal fetal fibronectin (FFN) measurement.

BOX 2-1	
NEONATAL COMPLICATIONS OF MATERNAL DISEASE	
DIABETES MELLITUS	TOXEMIA/PREECLAMPSIA
Congenital malformation (especially caudal regression)	IUGR
Macrosomia	Magnesium sulfate exposure
Birth trauma	Acidosis/decreased fetal reserve
Intrauterine growth retardation (IUGR)	BLOOD DISORDERS
Fetal death	Rh and atypical antibodies/ABO incompatibility
Cardiomyopathy	Hyperbilirubinemia and kernicterus
Hypoglycemia	Alloimmune thrombocytopenia
Respiratory distress syndrome	Fetal thrombocytopenia
Hyperbilirubinemia	Isoimmune thrombocytopenia*
Polycythemia	? Neonatal thrombocytopenia
Hypocalcemia	
Hypomagnesemia	

*Many other specific conditions can cause similar or associated fetal complications (myasthenia gravis/neonatal myasthenia, lupus/neonatal lupus syndrome, myotonic dystrophy).

E. THE TERM *HIGH-RISK PREGNANCY* CAN HAVE MEDICOLEGAL IMPLICATIONS.

As with the term *asphyxia,* the term *high-risk pregnancy* must be used carefully. Depending on the degree of risk, referral to perinatal specialists or neonatal specialists prenatally is indicated.

F. GROUP B STREPTOCOCCUS SCREENING

and treatment protocols exist; the pediatrician should be aware of what protocols are in use (**Figs. 2-1 and 2-2**).

G. HUMAN IMMUNODEFICIENCY VIRUS (HIV).

Retroviral therapy has been shown to decrease vertical transmission of HIV. Therapy should follow the most current recommendation. Cesarean section is recommended for delivery.

II. PRENATAL RECORD

A. ONE ADVANTAGE OF PRENATAL CARE IS THE IDENTIFICATION OF RISK FACTORS.

B. MANY RISK FACTORS ARE ASSOCIATED WITH A COMMONLY DERIVED MEDICAL OBSTETRIC HISTORY. MAJOR FACTORS INCLUDE THE FOLLOWING:

1. Previous history of preterm labor, illicit drug use, alcohol consumption, smoking, low socioeconomic status, and problematic genetic background.
2. Previous history of stillbirth or miscarriage.
3. Associated medical complications, such as hypertension or diabetes.

C. LABORATORY STUDIES (FIG. 2-3) CAN IDENTIFY RISK AND SHOULD INCLUDE THE FOLLOWING:

(See also **Chapter 3**)
1. Blood type, Rh status, and antibody status.
2. Syphilis serology.
3. Hematocrit.
4. Hepatitis B screen.
5. HIV test.
6. Gonococcus culture.
7. Glucose screen at 26 to 28 weeks.
8. Group B streptococcus (GBS) screen at approximately 36 weeks.

D. THE PRENATAL RECORD

should clearly indicate high-risk conditions that have been identified and should detail the management plan. Example: "Partner of intravenous (IV) drug user-HIV infection. Plan: Screening for HIV status."

FIG. 2-1

Intrapartum antimicrobial prophylaxis (IAP) for group B streptococcus (GBS). ROM, rupture of membranes.

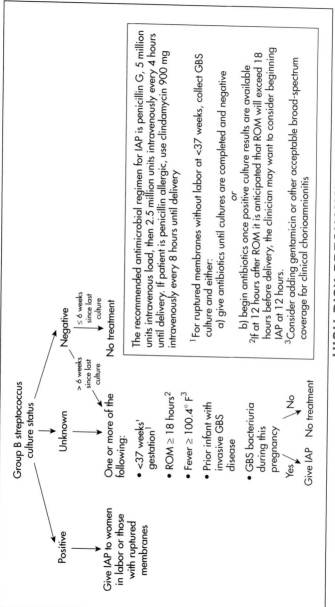

Group B streptococcus culture status

Positive → Give IAP to women in labor or those with ruptured membranes

Unknown → One or more of the following:
- <37 weeks' gestation[1]
- ROM ≥ 18 hours[2]
- Fever ≥ 100.4° F[3]
- Prior infant with invasive GBS disease
- GBS bacteriuria during this pregnancy

Yes → Give IAP No → No treatment

Negative
- >6 weeks since last culture → (One or more of the following)
- ≤ 6 weeks since last culture → No treatment

The recommended antimicrobial regimen for IAP is penicillin G, 5 million units intravenous load, then 2.5 million units intravenously every 4 hours until delivery. If patient is penicillin allergic, use clindamycin 900 mg intravenously every 8 hours until delivery

[1] For ruptured membranes without labor at <37 weeks, collect GBS culture and either:
a) give antibiotics until cultures are completed and negative
or
b) begin antibiotics once positive culture results are available

[2] If at 12 hours after ROM it is anticipated that ROM will exceed 18 hours before delivery, the clinician may want to consider beginning IAP at 12 hours.

[3] Consider adding gentamicin or other acceptable broad-spectrum coverage for clinical chorioamnionitis

HIGH-RISK PREGNANCY 2

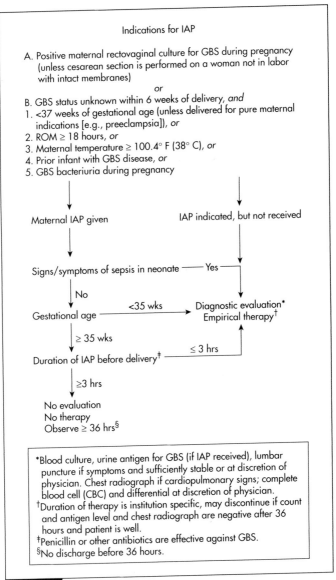

Indications for IAP

A. Positive maternal rectovaginal culture for GBS during pregnancy (unless cesarean section is performed on a woman not in labor with intact membranes)

or

B. GBS status unknown within 6 weeks of delivery, *and*
1. <37 weeks of gestational age (unless delivered for pure maternal indications [e.g., preeclampsia]), *or*
2. ROM ≥ 18 hours, *or*
3. Maternal temperature ≥ 100.4° F (38° C), *or*
4. Prior infant with GBS disease, *or*
5. GBS bacteriuria during pregnancy

Maternal IAP given   IAP indicated, but not received

Signs/symptoms of sepsis in neonate ——— Yes ———

No

Gestational age ——— <35 wks ———→ Diagnostic evaluation*
                                    Empirical therapy†

≥ 35 wks   ≤ 3 hrs

Duration of IAP before delivery‡ ———

≥3 hrs

No evaluation
No therapy
Observe ≥ 36 hrs§

*Blood culture, urine antigen for GBS (if IAP received), lumbar puncture if symptoms and sufficiently stable or at discretion of physician. Chest radiograph if cardiopulmonary signs; complete blood cell (CBC) and differential at discretion of physician.
†Duration of therapy is institution specific, may discontinue if count and antigen level and chest radiograph are negative after 36 hours and patient is well.
‡Penicillin or other antibiotics are effective against GBS.
§No discharge before 36 hours.

FIG. 2-2

Guidelines for management of the neonate born to a mother who is a candidate for intrapartum antimicrobial prophylaxis (IAP). GBS, group B streptococcus; ROM, rupture of membranes.

	Preconception or 1st visit	6-8*	14-16	24-28	32	36	38	39	40	41
History										
Medical, including genetic	X									
Psychosocial	X									
Update medical & psychosocial		X	X	X	X	X	X	X	X	X
Physical examination										
General	X									
Blood pressure	X	X	X	X	X	X	X	X	X	X
Height	X									
Weight	X	X	X	X	X	X	X	X	X	X
Height & weight profile	X									
Pelvic examination & pelvimetry	X	X								
Breast examination	X	X								
Fundal height			X	X	X	X	X	X	X	X
Fetal position & heart rate			X	X	X	X	X	X	X	X
Cervical examination	X									
Laboratory tests										
Hemoglobin or hematocrit	X	X		X		X				
Rh factor	X									
Pap smear	X									
Diabetic screen				X						
MSAFP			X							
Urine										
Dipstick (protein, sugar)	X	X	X	X	X	X	X	X	X	X
Culture		X								
Infections										
Rubella titer	X									
Syphilis test	X			X						
Gonococcal culture	X	X				X				
Hepatitis B	X									
HIV (offered)	X	X								
Illicit drug screen (offered)	X									
Genetic screen	X									

*If preconception care has preceded.

FIG. 2-3

Medical components of prenatal care. Note that screens for syphilis, hepatitis B, HIV, and illicit drugs may need to be repeated at delivery in high-risk situations. MSAFP, maternal serum alpha-fetoprotein.

HIGH-RISK PREGNANCY

2

III. RISK-SCORING FORMS

A. VARIOUS RISK-SCORING FORMS

have been developed, both freestanding and associated with the prenatal record. Example: The Hollister record (Hollister Inc., Libertyville, Ill.), a computer-based record; genetic risk-scoring systems; preterm labor risk-scoring systems.

B. THERE IS NO WELL-DEFINED PRENATAL RECORD THAT IS USED THROUGHOUT THE UNITED STATES.

Generally used forms include those of the American College of Obstetricians and Gynecologists **(Fig. 2-4)**, the Hollister record, and various other forms.

Patient Addressograph

DATE _____

NAME _____ FIRST _____ MIDDLE _____
LAST

ID # _____ HOSPITAL OF DELIVERY _____

NEWBORN'S PHYSICIAN _____ REFERRED BY _____

PRIMARY PROVIDER/GROUP _____

FINAL EDD _____

BIRTH DATE	AGE	RACE	MARITAL STATUS	ADDRESS:
MONTH DAY YEAR			S M W D SEP	
OCCUPATION			EDUCATION	ZIP: PHONE: (H) (O)
☐ HOMEMAKER			(LAST GRADE COMPLETED)	INSURANCE CARRIER/MEDICAID #
☐ OUTSIDE WORK				
☐ STUDENT Type of Work				EMERGENCY CONTACT: PHONE:
HUSBAND/FATHER OF BABY:		PHONE:		

TOTAL PREG	FULL TERM	PREMATURE	AB. INDUCED	AB. SPONTANEOUS	ECTOPICS	MULTIPLE BIRTHS	LIVING

MENSTRUAL HISTORY

LMP ☐ DEFINITE ☐ APPROXIMATE (MONTH KNOWN) MENSES MONTHLY ☐ YES ☐ NO FREQUENCY: Q ____ DAYS MENARCHE ____ (AGE ONSET)
☐ UNKNOWN ☐ NORMAL AMOUNT/DURATION PRIOR MENSES ____ DATE ON BCP AT CONCEPT ☐ YES ☐ NO hCG + ____ / ____ / ____
☐ FINAL ____

PAST PREGNANCIES (LAST SIX)

DATE MONTH / YEAR	GA WEEKS	LENGTH OF LABOR	BIRTH WEIGHT	SEX M/F	TYPE DELIVERY	ANES.	PLACE OF DELIVERY	PRETERM LABOR YES / NO	COMMENTS / COMPLICATIONS

PAST MEDICAL HISTORY

	O Neg + Pos.	DETAIL POSITIVE REMARKS INCLUDE DATE & TREATMENT		O Neg + Pos.	DETAIL POSITIVE REMARKS INCLUDE DATE & TREATMENT
1. DIABETES			16. D (Rh) SENSITIZED		
2. HYPERTENSION			17. PULMONARY (TB, ASTHMA)		
3. HEART DISEASE			18. ALLERGIES (DRUGS)		
4. AUTOIMMUNE DISORDER			19. BREAST		
5. KIDNEY DISEASE / UTI			20. GYN SURGERY		
6. NEUROLOGIC/EPILEPSY					
7. PSYCHIATRIC			21. OPERATIONS / HOSPITALIZATIONS (YEAR & REASON)		
8. HEPATITIS / LIVER DISEASE					
9. VARICOSITIES / PHLEBITIS					
10. THYROID DYSFUNCTION			22. ANESTHETIC COMPLICATIONS		
11. TRAUMA/DOMESTIC VIOLENCE			23. HISTORY OF ABNORMAL PAP		
12. HISTORY OF BLOOD TRANSFUS.	AMT/DAY PREPREG	AMT/DAY PREG	#YEARS USE	24. UTERINE ANOMALY/DES	
				25. INFERTILITY	
13. TOBACCO				26. RELEVANT FAMILY HISTORY	
14. ALCOHOL					
15. STREET DRUGS				27. OTHER	

COMMENTS: _____

The American College of Obstetricians and Gynecologists, 409 12th Street, SW, PO Box 96920, Washington, DC 20090-6920

Copyright © 1997 (Version 4)

ACOG ANTEPARTUM RECORD (FORM A)

FIG. 2-4

Antepartum record of the American College of Obstetricians and Gynecologists (ACOG). *(Copyright 1997, ACOG.)*

Patient Addressograph

SYMPTOMS SINCE LMP

GENETIC SCREENING/TERATOLOGY COUNSELING
INCLUDES PATIENT, BABY'S FATHER, OR ANYONE IN EITHER FAMILY WITH:

	YES	NO		YES	NO
1. PATIENT'S AGE ≥ 35 YEARS			12. MENTAL RETARDATION/AUTISM		
2. THALASSEMIA (ITALIAN, GREEK, MEDITERRANEAN, OR ASIAN BACKGROUND); MCV < 80			IF YES, WAS PERSON TESTED FOR FRAGILE X?		
3. NEURAL TUBE DEFECT (MENINGOMYELOCELE, SPINA BIFIDA, OR ANENCEPHALY)			13. OTHER INHERITED GENETIC OR CHROMOSOMAL DISORDER		
4. CONGENITAL HEART DEFECT			14. MATERNAL METABOLIC DISORDER (EG. INSULIN-DEPENDENT DIABETES, PKU)		
5. DOWN SYNDROME			15. PATIENT OR BABY'S FATHER HAD A CHILD WITH BIRTH DEFECTS NOT LISTED ABOVE		
6. TAY-SACHS (EG. JEWISH, CAJUN, FRENCH CANADIAN)			16. RECURRENT PREGNANCY LOSS, OR A STILLBIRTH		
7. SICKLE CELL DISEASE OR TRAIT (AFRICAN)			17. MEDICATIONS/STREET DRUGS/ALCOHOL SINCE LAST MENSTRUAL PERIOD?		
8. HEMOPHILIA			IF YES, AGENT(S):		
9. MUSCULAR DYSTROPHY					
10. CYSTIC FIBROSIS			18. ANY OTHER		
11. HUNTINGTON CHOREA					

COMMENTS/COUNSELING: _____
_____
_____

INFECTION HISTORY	YES	NO		YES	NO
1. HIGH RISK HEPATITIS B/IMMUNIZED?			4. RASH OR VIRAL ILLNESS SINCE LAST MENSTRUAL PERIOD		
2. LIVE WITH SOMEONE WITH TB OR EXPOSED TO TB			5. HISTORY OF STD, GC, CHLAMYDIA, HPV, SYPHILIS		
3. PATIENT OR PARTNER HAS HISTORY OF GENITAL HERPES			6. OTHER (SEE COMMENTS)		

COMMENTS: _____
_____
_____ INTERVIEWER'S SIGNATURE _____

INITIAL PHYSICAL EXAMINATION

DATE ____ / ____ / ____   PREPREGNANCY WEIGHT _____   HEIGHT _____   BP _____

1. HEENT	☐ NORMAL	☐ ABNORMAL	12. VULVA	☐ NORMAL	☐ CONDYLOMA	☐ LESIONS
2. FUNDI	☐ NORMAL	☐ ABNORMAL	13. VAGINA	☐ NORMAL	☐ INFLAMMATION	☐ DISCHARGE
3. TEETH	☐ NORMAL	☐ ABNORMAL	14. CERVIX	☐ NORMAL	☐ INFLAMMATION	☐ LESIONS
4. THYROID	☐ NORMAL	☐ ABNORMAL	15. UTERUS SIZE	_____ WEEKS		☐ FIBROIDS
5. BREASTS	☐ NORMAL	☐ ABNORMAL	16. ADNEXA	☐ NORMAL	☐ MASS	
6. LUNGS	☐ NORMAL	☐ ABNORMAL	17. RECTUM	☐ NORMAL	☐ ABNORMAL	
7. HEART	☐ NORMAL	☐ ABNORMAL	18. DIAGONAL CONJUGATE	☐ REACHED	☐ NO	_____ CM
8. ABDOMEN	☐ NORMAL	☐ ABNORMAL	19. SPINES	☐ AVERAGE	☐ PROMINENT	☐ BLUNT
9. EXTREMITIES	☐ NORMAL	☐ ABNORMAL	20. SACRUM	☐ CONCAVE	☐ STRAIGHT	☐ ANTERIOR
10. SKIN	☐ NORMAL	☐ ABNORMAL	21. SUBPUBIC ARCH	☐ NORMAL	☐ WIDE	☐ NARROW
11. LYMPH NODES	☐ NORMAL	☐ ABNORMAL	22. GYNECOID PELVIC TYPE	☐ YES	☐ NO	

COMMENTS (Number and explain abnormals): _____
_____
_____ EXAM BY _____

2

FIG. 2-4—cont'd

HIGH-RISK PREGNANCY

ACOG ANTEPARTUM RECORD (FORM B)

NAME _____
　　　　LAST　　　　　　　　　FIRST　　　　　　　MIDDLE

DRUG ALLERGY:

RELIGIOUS/CULTURAL CONSIDERATIONS _____ | ANESTHESIA CONSULT PLANNED ☐ YES ☐ NO

PROBLEMS/PLANS	MEDICATION LIST:	Start date	Stop date
1.	1.		
2.	2.		
3.	3.		
4.	4.		
5.	5.		
6.	6.		

EDD CONFIRMATION

INITIAL EDD:

LMP _____ / _____ / _____ = EDD _____ / _____ / _____

INITIAL EXAM _____ / _____ / _____ = _____ WKS = EDD _____ / _____ / _____

ULTRASOUND _____ / _____ / _____ = _____ WKS = EDD _____ / _____ / _____

INITIAL EDD _____ / _____ / _____ INITIALED BY _____

18-20-WEEK EDD UPDATE:

QUICKENING _____ / _____ / _____ +22 WKS = _____ / _____ / _____

FUNDAL HT. AT UMBIL. _____ / _____ / _____ +20 WKS = _____ / _____ / _____

FHT W/FETOSCOPE _____ / _____ / _____ +20 WKS = _____ / _____ / _____

ULTRASOUND _____ / _____ / _____ = _____ WKS = _____ / _____ / _____

FINAL EDD _____ / _____ / _____ INITIALED BY _____

VISIT DATE (YEAR)	WEEKS GEST (BEST EST.)	FUNDAL HEIGHT (CM)	PRESENTATION	FHR	FETAL MOVEMENT	PRETERM LABOR SIGNS/SYMPTOMS • PRESENT O=ABSENT	CERVIX EXAM (DIL/EFF/STA.)	BLOOD PRESSURE	EDEMA	WEIGHT	URINE (GLUCOSE/ALBUMIN)	NEXT APPOINTMENT	PROVIDER (INITIALS)	COMMENTS:

PROBLEMS: _____

COMMENTS: _____

ACOG ANTEPARTUM RECORD (FORM C)

FIG. 2-4—cont'd

LABORATORY AND EDUCATION

Patient Addressograph

INITIAL LABS	DATE	RESULT	REVIEWED
BLOOD TYPE	/ /	A B AB O	
D (Rh) TYPE	/ /		
ANTIBODY SCREEN	/ /		
HCT/HGB	/ /	_____ % _____ g/dL	
PAP TEST	/ /	NORMAL / ABNORMAL / ____	
RUBELLA	/ /		
VDRL	/ /		
URINE CULTURE/SCREEN	/ /		
HBsAg	/ /		
HIV COUNSELING/TESTING	/ /	☐ POS. ☐ NEG. ☐ DECLINED	

OPTIONAL LABS	DATE	RESULT	
HGB ELECTROPHORESIS	/ /	AA AS SS AC SC AF TA₂	
PPD	/ /		
CHLAMYDIA	/ /		
GC	/ /		
TAY-SACHS	/ /		
OTHER			

8-18-WEEK LABS (WHEN INDICATED/ELECTED)	DATE	RESULT	
ULTRASOUND	/ /		
MSAFP/MULTIPLE MARKERS	/ /		
AMNIO/CVS	/ /		
KARYOTYPE	/ /	46, XX OR 46, XY / OTHER____	
AMNIOTIC FLUID (AFP)	/ /	NORMAL____ ABNORMAL____	

24-28-WEEK LABS (WHEN INDICATED)	DATE	RESULT	
HCT/HGB	/ /	_____ % _____ g/dL	
DIABETES SCREEN	/ /	1 HOUR_____	
GTT (IF SCREEN ABNORMAL)	/ /	____FBS ____1 HOUR	
		____2 HOUR ____3 HOUR	
D (Rh) ANTIBODY SCREEN	/ /		
D IMMUNE GLOBULIN (RhIG) GIVEN (28 WKS)	/ /	SIGNATURE _____	

32-36-WEEK LABS (WHEN INDICATED)	DATE	RESULT	
HCT/HGB (RECOMMENDED)	/ /	_____ % _____ g/dL	
ULTRASOUND	/ /		
VDRL	/ /		
GC	/ /		
CHLAMYDIA	/ /		
GROUP B STREP (35-37 WKS)	/ /		

COMMENTS/ADDITIONAL LABS

PLANS/EDUCATION (COUNSELED ☐)

☐ ANESTHESIA PLANS _____
☐ TOXOPLASMOSIS PRECAUTIONS (CATS/RAW MEAT) _____
☐ CHILDBIRTH CLASSES _____
☐ PHYSICAL/SEXUAL ACTIVITY _____
☐ LABOR SIGNS _____
☐ NUTRITION COUNSELING _____
☐ BREAST OR BOTTLE FEEDING _____
☐ NEWBORN CAR SEAT _____
☐ POSTPARTUM BIRTH CONTROL _____
☐ ENVIRONMENTAL/WORK HAZARDS _____

☐ TUBAL STERILIZATION _____
☐ VBAC COUNSELING _____
☐ CIRCUMCISION _____
☐ TRAVEL _____
☐ LIFESTYLE, TOBACCO, ALCOHOL _____

REQUESTS _____
_____

TUBAL STERILIZATION	DATE	INITIALS
CONSENT SIGNED	___/___/___	

PROVIDER SIGNATURE (AS REQUIRED) _____

AA201   12345/10567

2

HIGH-RISK PREGNANCY

ACOG ANTEPARTUM RECORD (FORM D)

FIG. 2-4—cont'd

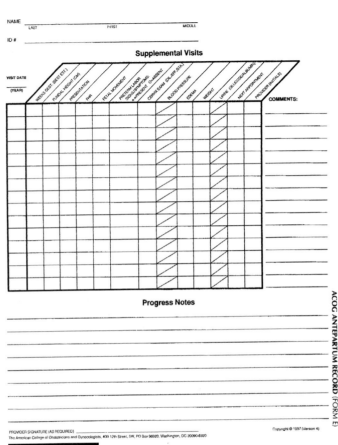

FIG. 2-4—cont'd

The prenatal and hospital obstetric forms contain much important risk-assessment information for appropriate newborn care.

BIBLIOGRAPHY

American College of Obstetricians and Gynecologists: Scheduled cesarean delivery and the prevention of vertical transmission of HIV infection, ACOG Committee opinion #219, August 1999.

Centers for Disease Control and Prevention: Prevention of perinatal group B streptococcal disease: A public health perspective. MMWR 51[RR-11]:1, 2002.

Creasy RK, Gummer BA, Liggins GC: System for predicting spontaneous preterm birth. Obstet Gynecol 55:692, 1980.

Gabbe SG, Niebyl JR, Simpson JL (eds): Obstetrics: Normal and Problem Pregnancies, ed 4, New York, Harcourt Brace, 2001.

Perinatal Monitoring

Timothy R.B. Johnson

I. GENETIC SCREENING AND PRENATAL DIAGNOSIS

A. FIRST TRIMESTER SCREENING (FTS)

has been designed to identify pregnancies at risk for Down syndrome between 11 and 14 weeks' gestation. It involves a special ultrasound examination for nuchal thickness/translucency (NT) and maternal serum free beta-human chorionic gonadotropin (β-HCG) and pregnancy-associated plasma protein A (PAPP-A).

B. THE "QUAD" TEST

3

is a maternal serum test performed between 15 and 21 weeks' gestation that combines the alpha-fetoprotein (AFP), β-HCG, unconjugated estriol and inhibin A values to more precisely identify the risk of fetal chromosomal anomalies.

C. CHORIONIC VILLUS SAMPLING (CVS)

can be performed from 11 to 14 weeks' gestation; amniocentesis can be performed from 15 to 20 weeks' gestation. Genetic probes are available for many disorders (e.g., cystic fibrosis [CF], sickle cell disease). Prenatal screening for many of these disorders is becoming more wide spread. Prenatal genetic centers have access to the most current tests, are reliable, and offer counseling. Karyotype or fluorescence in situ hybridization (FISH) techniques are available.

II. ULTRASOUND

Most pregnant women undergo one or more ultrasound survey examinations during which measurements can be made to assess gestational age. Fetal survey screening between 17 and 20 weeks' gestation is common. The most accurate measurements are those obtained before 28 weeks. At least two measurements (e.g., biparietal diameter and femur length) are used. Late intrauterine growth retardation (IUGR) can be recognized by ultrasound. Targeted ultrasound scans (formally called *level II*) direct attention to suspicious areas of fetal development. Fetal echocardiography at 18 to 22 weeks is available for at-risk pregnancies or when cardiac abnormalities are suspected.

III. ASSESSMENT OF THE HIGH-RISK NEONATE (FETAL ASSESSMENT)

A. FETAL MOVEMENT COUNTING

can begin as early as 28 weeks; the mother is asked to count fetal movements on a daily basis. Although randomized clinical trials have not documented efficacy of routine fetal movement counting, it is often used in high-risk pregnancies and can be used routinely.

B. SHARP DIMINUTION OF FETAL MOVEMENT

or no fetal movement in a 24-hour period is an alarm for further evaluation of the fetus.

IV. NON-STRESS TESTING

The non-stress test (NST) uses the electronic fetal monitor to assess fetal well-being.

A. EVIDENCE OF FETAL WELL-BEING

during an NST consists of two fetal heart rate accelerations of 20 beats per minute lasting for 20 seconds. Generally, this test is done twice weekly.

B. THE SENSITIVITY OF THE NST

is fair and the specificity is poor. The incidence of stillbirth within 1 week of a reassuring test result is approximately 3:1000. More frequent testing (two to three times per week) may increase the sensitivity of the test.

C. THE POSITIVE (NON-REASSURING, NON-REACTIVE) TEST RESULT

can lead to further testing or delivery, depending on clinical circumstances.

V. CONTRACTION STRESS TESTS

The contraction stress test consists of similarly derived electronic fetal heart rate strips and the induction of contractions either by intravenous oxytocin or nipple stimulation to see whether decelerations of the heart rate occur.

A. A POSITIVE TEST RESULT

is one in which there are late decelerations after contractions, or variable decelerations, which can be indications of cord compression or oligohydramnios. The incidence of death within one week of a reassuring test result is 0.6:1000.

B. A POSITIVE TEST RESULT

can lead to further testing or delivery, although care must be taken because of a high rate of false-positive test results.

VI. BIOPHYSICAL PROFILE

The biophysical profile includes electronic fetal heart rate testing (NST) and ultrasound examination to evaluate fetal movement, breathing, and tone and to measure amniotic fluid volume. Two points are assigned for each reassuring result. Testing is generally done on a weekly basis or more often. Test scores <4 generally indicate need for delivery.

A. A HIGH SCORE OF 10 IS ASSOCIATED WITH A GOOD OUTCOME.

Some add placental grading (with a "mature" placenta suggesting adverse outcome) to their scoring system.

B. SCORES OF <4 ARE ASSOCIATED WITH INCREASED PERINATAL RISK.

C. THE INCIDENCE OF DEATH WITHIN 1 WEEK OF A REASSURING TEST RESULT IS APPROXIMATELY 0.5:1000.

The positive predictive value is high at about 80%.

VII. OLIGOHYDRAMNIOS/POLYHYDRAMNIOS/AMNIOTIC FLUID INDEX

Oligohydramnios and polyhydramnios can be clinically diagnosed using ultrasound techniques. The amniotic fluid index (AFI) **(Figs. 3-1 and 3-2)**

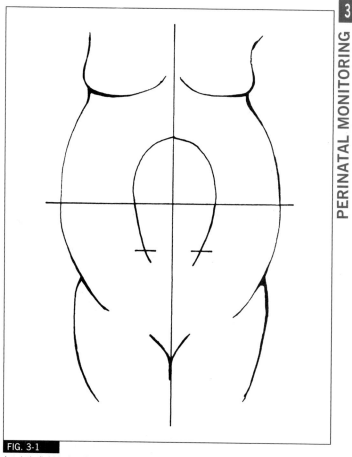

FIG. 3-1

Amniotic fluid index. Quadrant boundaries for amniotic fluid index after 20 weeks.

3

PERINATAL MONITORING

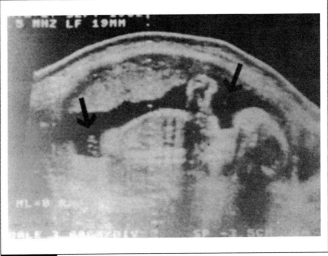

FIG. 3-2
Amniotic fluid (arrows) is easily identified sonographically.

is the most widely used technique and combines measurements of the deepest vertical pocket in each of four quadrants to give an aggregate AFI score. Values <5 = oligohydramnios; >18 = polyhydramnios. The AFI has recently been combined with the NST in a two-test strategy known as the *modified biophysical profile*. Evidence of oligohydramnios should lead to a search for congenital anomalies such as renal agenesis and other conditions associated with oligohydramnios. In cases of polyhydramnios, consider tracheoesophageal (TE) fistula, anencephaly, hydranencephaly, and neural tube defects.

VIII. DOPPLER

Umbilical arterial Doppler studies and other Doppler studies that assess placental function and uteroplacental blood flow can be used. These studies are occasionally useful in cases associated with hypertensive disease and IUGR. Monitoring too early and therapy with aspirin may delay appreciation of such problems, although work on this topic is still investigational. At present, routine Doppler study is not indicated and the modality is useful only as an adjunct in the evaluation of a high-risk pregnancy and only in the aforementioned cases. A systolic/diastolic (S/D) ratio of 3 or greater, as measured by continuous or pulsed Doppler and displayed on a spectrum analyzer, is associated with increased placental resistance and increased perinatal mortality and morbidity.

IX. ELECTRONIC FETAL MONITORING

Intrapartum monitoring generally consists of electronic fetal monitoring (EFM), which measures heart rate and uterine contractions. Internal modes consist of a scalp electrode, which has a minimal risk of infection, or an intrauterine pressure catheter, which is associated with risk of chorioamnionitis. External devices use Doppler and tocodynamometry.

A. FETAL HEART RATE.

The areas assessed include the following:

1. Baseline rate, the normal rate being 120 to 160 beats per minute (**Fig. 3-3**).
2. Baseline variability; decrease in beat-to-beat variability is an ominous sign.
3. Periodic changes. The presence of accelerations (**Fig. 3-4**) is reassuring (see NST, earlier); the presence of decelerations (**Fig. 3-5**) or late decelerations suggests uteroplacental insufficiency; variable decelerations suggest cord compression. Variable decelerations are unusual in the absence of ruptured membranes or oligohydramnios.

B. EFM IS SENSITIVE BUT HAS LOW SPECIFICITY.

This is often backed up with scalp pH sampling. Randomized controlled trials have not shown that EFM improves perinatal outcome or has any effect on long-term neurodevelopment (e.g., cerebral palsy), even in preterm infants.

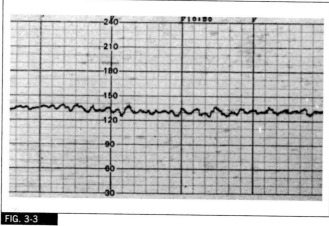

FIG. 3-3

Normal heart rate and variability.

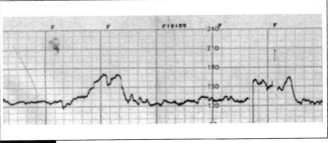

FIG. 3-4
Normal rate variability and fetal heart rate accelerations.

C. RISKS OF SCALP ELECTRODE PLACEMENT INCLUDE SCALP ABSCESS.
With internal monitoring, there is an increasing risk of ascending infection because the membranes are ruptured.

D. SCALP PH SAMPLING VALUE OF >7.25 IS NORMAL;
7.2 to 7.25 is borderline; <7.2 indicates acidosis.

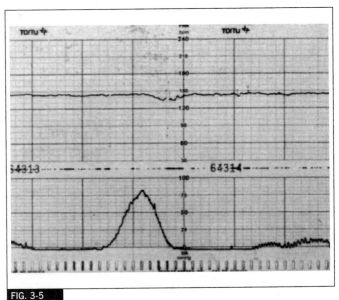

FIG. 3-5
Decreased beat-to-beat variability and late deceleration of fetal heart rate after contraction.

E. FETAL PULSE OXIMETRY
has been introduced experimentally as a method to evaluate intrapartum fetal status.

F. OCCASIONALLY, METHODS ARE USED TO STIMULATE FETAL REACTIVITY IN LABOR.
These include pinching the scalp, scratching the scalp, scalp blood sampling, and vibroacoustic stimulation to induce fetal heart-rate accelerations.

X. LUNG MATURITY
Pulmonary maturity is a major predictor of good neonatal outcome and usually can be assessed by amniotic fluid characteristics.

A. A LECITHIN/SPHINGOMYELIN (L/S) RATIO >2 GENERALLY SUGGESTS MATURITY.
When phosphatidylglycerol (PG) is present, there is a very low risk of respiratory distress syndrome. The PG level is seldom mature at <36 weeks of gestation.

B. THE SHAKE TEST IS A FOAM STABILITY TEST.
It is more rapid than the L/S ratio and it has comparable sensitivity and specificity with the L/S.

C. RAPID FOAM STABILITY TESTS THAT ALSO ASSESS FETAL LUNG MATURITY ARE CLINICALLY AVAILABLE.
Rapid tests of L/S can be performed on amniotic fluid obtained transabdominally in sterile fashion, by vaginal collection of fluid, or from gastric aspirate from the newborn.

XI. PRETERM LABOR/PREMATURE RUPTURE OF MEMBRANES
Prematurity is a major cause of infant morbidity and mortality. Preterm labor is diagnosed by regular uterine contractions associated with cervical change. Cervical change without contractions is termed *cervical incompetence* and generally occurs before 20 weeks. Sonographic measurement of cervical length and vaginal fetal fibronectin (FFN) measurements are used clinically.

A. PRETERM LABOR, WHEN DIAGNOSED, IS GENERALLY TREATED AGGRESSIVELY.
with betamimetics, magnesium sulfate, or indomethacin. Potential side effects of each include the following:
1. Betamimetics: Fetal tachycardia.
2. Magnesium sulfate: Pharmacologic impact on the fetus.
3. Indomethacin: Premature closure of the ductus, decreased amniotic fluid.

3

PERINATAL MONITORING

B. PREMATURE RUPTURE OF MEMBRANES IS A COMMON CAUSE OF PREMATURITY.

There is an association with vaginal infection and cervical infection, although the exact mechanisms and etiologic organisms are unknown. Premature rupture of membranes is managed by various protocols, including the following:

1. Patients are often hospitalized until delivery occurs.
2. Patients may be discharged if risk of ascending infection is found to be low.
3. Antibiotic coverage for prevention of group B streptococcus and corticosteroids should be considered. Antibiotic treatment for a short course also appears to improve fetal outcome. Broad-spectrum antibiotics are reserved for clinical evidence of infection.
4. Preterm labor and premature ruptured membranes not associated with evidence of chorioamnionitis can be treated with tocolytic therapy and other agents. Culture for pathogens can be useful; infection with group B streptococci and *Neisseria gonorrhoeae* should be eradicated.

XII. FEVER

Fever in the obstetric patient must be evaluated in a rigorous fashion. Common causes include the following:

A. PYELONEPHRITIS.
B. VIRAL SYNDROME.
C. CHORIOAMNIONITIS

is often associated with fever, leukocytosis, maternal/fetal tachycardia, purulent vaginal discharge, or premature rupture of membranes. The diagnosis of chorioamnionitis is often clinical, with positive evidence from Gram stain if *organisms* (but not leukocytes) are present; a positive leukocyte esterase test is often useful.

XIII. APGAR SCORE

The Apgar score was developed to identify those infants needing resuscitation.

A. APGAR SCORING

is generally performed at 1 minute and 5 minutes after birth, although if the score is depressed at 5 minutes, the test should be repeated at 10 minutes.

B. THE APGAR SCORE DEPENDS ON GESTATIONAL AGE.

Many preterm infants have decreased Apgar scores (**Table 3-1**) purely representative of low gestational age.

C. THE APGAR SCORE IS NOT PREDICTIVE OF LONG-TERM NEUROLOGIC OUTCOME OR DEVELOPMENT OF CEREBRAL PALSY AND IS NOT A GOOD INDICATOR OF PERINATAL ASPHYXIA.

The diagnosis of perinatal asphyxia should be restricted to those infants with a low 10-minute Apgar score, early neonatal seizures, and early hypotonia.

TABLE 3-1

APGAR SCORE

Sign	0	1	2
Heart rate	Absent	Under 100 beats/min	Over 100 beats/min
Respiratory effort	Absent	Slow (irregular)	Good crying
Muscle tone	Limp	Some flexion of extremities	Active motion
Reflex irritability	No response	Grimace	Cough or sneeze
Color	Blue, pale	Pink body, blue extremities	All pink

BIBLIOGRAPHY

American Academy of Pediatrics: Use and abuse of the Apgar score. Pediatrics 78:1148, 1986.

Gabbe SG, Niebyl JR, Simpson JL (eds): Obstetrics: Normal and Problem Pregnancies, ed 3, New York, 2001, Harcourt Brace.

Neonatal Encephalopathy and Cerebral Palsy: Defining the pathogenesis and pathophysiology. American College of Obstetricians and Gynecologists, 2003.

3

PERINATAL MONITORING

Neonatal Resuscitation

Siew-Jyu Wong

Every hospital (level 1, 2, or 3) with delivery services should have skilled personnel immediately available for neonatal resuscitation, and appropriate equipment should be present at all deliveries. Although the percentage of anticipated high-risk deliveries has been increasing steadily, there are still unavoidable, unanticipated high-risk deliveries that require the presence of skilled personnel in house at all times. Such personnel include trained registered nurses, neonatal nurse practitioners, respiratory therapists, physician assistants, and physicians skilled in neonatal resuscitation.

There are numerous causes of an unanticipated compromise of the newborn at delivery. Examples include precipitous delivery; prenatally undiagnosed congenital malformations, such as bilateral choanal atresia or congenital diaphragmatic hernia; and cord accidents, such as short cord, rupture of cord, true knot, tight nuchal cord, or prolapsed cord.

4

I. CONDITIONS COMMONLY ASSOCIATED WITH ANTICIPATED MODERATE-RISK AND HIGH-RISK DELIVERIES

A. PREMATURITY (<37 WEEKS).

B. CESAREAN SECTION (EXCEPT FOR ELECTIVE REPEAT CESAREAN SECTION).

C. PREGNANCY-INDUCED HYPERTENSION.

D. MULTIPLE GESTATION.

E. INTRAUTERINE GROWTH RETARDATION (IUGR).

F. OLIGOHYDRAMNIOS OR POLYHYDRAMNIOS.

G. SIGNIFICANT VAGINAL BLEEDING.

H. POST-TERM GESTATION.

I. MECONIUM STAINING.

J. ABNORMAL FETAL MONITORING PATTERN.

K. ADMINISTRATION OF NARCOTICS WITHIN 4 HOURS OF DELIVERY.

L. ABNORMAL PRESENTATION.

M. MATERNAL DIABETES.

N. IN UTERO DRUG OR ALCOHOL EXPOSURE.

O. RH SENSITIZATION.

P. PROLONGED LABOR, RUPTURE OF MEMBRANES (ROM) >24 HR OR MATERNAL FEVER/CHORIOAMNIONITIS.

Note: *The American Academy of Pediatrics (AAP) and the American Heart Association (AHA) have developed an excellent neonatal resuscitation program, referred to as the NRP. Encourage your hospital to provide training programs for* **all** *personnel involved in the care of the pregnant mother and the newborn. Details of resuscitation as outlined in the aforementioned program include the following:*

1. Resuscitation supplies and equipment list.
2. Overview of resuscitation in the delivery room. This is an easy-to-follow algorithm to determine the specific intervention needed.

3. Medications for neonatal resuscitation. This is a comprehensive and updated list of indicated medications.

II. NEONATAL RESUSCITATION SUPPLIES AND EQUIPMENT

A. SUCTION EQUIPMENT.
1. Bulb syringe.
2. DeLee mucus trap with a 10F catheter or mechanical suction.
3. Suction catheters: 3F, 6F, 8F, and 10F.
4. An 8F feeding tube and 20-ml syringe.
5. Meconium aspirator.

B. BAG-AND-MASK EQUIPMENT.
1. Infant resuscitation bag with a pressure-release valve or pressure manometer; the bag must be capable of delivering 90% to 100% oxygen.
2. Face masks: Newborn and premature sizes (cushioned-rim masks preferred).
3. Oxygen with flowmeter and tubing.

C. INTUBATION EQUIPMENT.
1. Laryngoscope with straight blades, No. 0 (premature)* and No. 1 (newborn).
2. Extra bulbs and batteries for laryngoscope.
3. Endotracheal tubes, sizes 2.5, 3.0, 3.5, and 4.0 mm.
4. Stylet.
5. Scissors.
6. Tape and/or other securing device for endotracheal tube.
7. Alcohol sponges.
8. CO_2 detector.
9. Laryngeal mask airway (optional).

D. MEDICATIONS.
1. Epinephrine 1:10,000, 3-ml or 10-ml ampules.
2. Naloxone hydrochloride (1 mg/ml).
3. Isotonic crystalloid for volume expansion, 100 or 250 ml.
a. Normal saline.
b. Ringer's lactate.
4. Sodium bicarbonate 4.2% (5 mEq/10 ml), 10-ml ampules.
5. Dextrose 10%, 250 ml.
6. Normal saline, 30 ml for flushes.

---

*Laryngoscope blade No. 00 is available for extremely-low-birth-weight (ELBW) infants.

E. MISCELLANEOUS.
1. Radiant warmer.*
2. Stethoscope.
3. Warm linens.
4. Clock.
5. Oropharyngeal airways (0, 00, and 000 sizes or 30-, 40-, and 50-mm lengths).
6. Monitors: Cardiotachometer with electrocardiograph (ECG) oscilloscope (desirable). Pulse oximeter.
7. Adhesive tape, $1/2$-inch or $3/4$-inch width.
8. Syringes, 1, 3, 5, 10, 20, and 50 ml.
9. Needles, 25, 21, and 18 gauge.
10. Alcohol, povidone-iodine sponges.
11. Gloves (sterile and nonsterile) and other appropriate personal blood and body fluid protection equipment.
12. Umbilical artery catheterization tray.
13. Umbilical tape.
14. Umbilical catheters, $3^1/2$F and 5F.
15. Three-way stopcocks.
16. A 5F feeding tube.

III. OVERVIEW OF RESUSCITATION IN THE DELIVERY ROOM (FIG. 4-1)

IV. MEDICATION FOR NEONATAL RESUSCITATION (TABLE 4-1)

V. SPECIAL PROBLEMS
A. MECONIUM.
All infants who have meconium-stained fluid should undergo thorough oral, nasal, and pharyngeal suctioning at the delivery of the head. If the infant is not vigorous at birth, with depressed respirations, low tone and/or a heart rate of 100 beats per minute, tracheal suctioning should be done immediately after delivery.

B. DIAPHRAGMATIC HERNIA.
If diagnosed prenatally or suspected in a non-IUGR newborn with scaphoid abdomen and respiratory distress, do not use face-mask ventilation; proceed immediately to tracheal intubation to provide intermittent positive-pressure breathing (IPPB).

C. AIRWAY OBSTRUCTION (E.G., BILATERAL CHOANAL ATRESIA, NECK MASSES).
Proceed immediately to endotracheal intubation.

---

*Polyethylene occlusive skin wrapping for <28 weeks' gestation to decrease heat loss; it is difficult to keep these neonates warm because of very little body fat and high surface area for conductive, evaporative, and radiation heat loss.

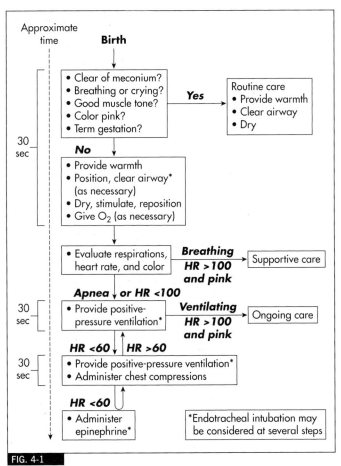

FIG. 4-1

Algorithm for resuscitation of the newly born infant. HR, heart rate. *(Modified from Kattwinkel J (ed): Textbook of Neonatal Resuscitation, ed 4, Chicago, American Heart Association and American Academy of Pediatrics, 2000.)*

D. EXTREMELY-LOW-BIRTH-WEIGHT (ELBW) INFANTS WHO REQUIRE RESUSCITATION

Should have early tracheal intubation; administration of surfactant should be done after stabilization. Premature infants have fragile germinal matrix and immature cerebrovascular autoregulation that may be further impaired by asphyxia, so volume expanders (normal saline) and sodium bicarbonate, which is hyperosmolar, should be given slowly.

TABLE 4-1

MEDICATIONS FOR NEONATAL RESUSCITATION

Drug	Indication	Concentration and Dose	Route	Precaution
Epinephrine	Heart rate <60 after 30 sec of **adequate** ventilation and Chest Compression	1:10,000; 0.1-0.3 ml/kg every 3-5 min	Endotracheal Intravenous Intraosseous	Do not give intra-arterially
Volume expanders (normal saline or Ringer's lactate)	*Hypovolemia suspected:* Shocked infant with history of blood loss, such as maternal vaginal bleeding, or infant who has not responded to other resuscitative measures	10 ml/kg slowly over 5-10 min; may repeat dose after clinical assessment and observation of response	Intravenous Intraosseous	Give slowly over 5-10 min and observe response before repeating dose
Sodium bicarbonate	Insufficient data for recommendation; if using, give only during prolonged cardiac arrest unresponsive to other resuscitative measures	0.5 mEq/ml; 1-2 mEq/kg very slowly over 2 min	Intravenous Intraosseous	Give very slowly over at least 2 min; do not give intra-arterially
Naloxone	Respiratory depression with history of maternal narcotic administration within 4 hours of delivery	1 mg/ml; 0.1 mg/kg	Endotracheal Intravenous Subcutaneous or intramuscular if circulation is good	Do not give to infants whose mothers have or are suspected of recent narcotic drug abuse; provide ventilatory support before and during administration until adequate response is observed; continue to observe for hypopnea or apnea because repeat dosing might be necessary

NEONATAL RESUSCITATION 4

E. INFANTS WITH SEVERE MALFORMATIONS.
Resuscitate first if there has been no prior prenatal discussion with parents. If resuscitation is successful, establish diagnosis, to be followed by compassionate supportive discussion with parents regarding management and continuation of life support.

F. EXTREMELY IMMATURE INFANTS.
In a high-risk pregnancy, prepartum discussions with the couple regarding prognosis and resuscitation should be done on an ongoing basis if possible. In case of uncertainty, after a rapid assessment of the infant after birth, resuscitative options include non-initiation of efforts, initiation and discontinuation, initiation and trial of therapy. All will include parental involvement and support of family.

G. PLEURAL EFFUSION AND PNEUMOTHORACES.
Hydropic newborns may need thoracentesis and paracentesis at birth and transfusion for severe anemia. Pneumothoraces at birth associated with pulmonary hypoplasia may complicate resuscitation and require thoracentesis.

H. SEVERE HYPOVOLEMIA.
Hypovolemia should be suspected in a newborn not responding to adequate ventilation. History of labor and delivery events may help in establishing the diagnosis, and volume replacement with normal saline should be provided.

VI. SPECIAL PRECAUTIONS
A. AVOID USING EXCESSIVE PRESSURE IN RESUSCITATION.
B. BE GENTLE WITH SUCTIONING.
C. ALWAYS MAKE SURE ADEQUATE VENTILATION IS ESTABLISHED. MEDICATION IS NOT A SUBSTITUTE FOR VENTILATION.
D. CONTINUE MONITORING AND SUPPORT IN A SPECIAL CARE UNIT UNTIL TRANSITION TO A NORMAL POSTNATAL STATUS IS ESTABLISHED.
Watch blood pressure and perfusion, respirations, and oxygen saturation. Check blood glucose. Guidelines should be established for the continuing care of this newborn as to whether the care should be in the "normal newborn unit" or in the "special care unit."

E. DISCONTINUATION OF RESUSCITATIVE EFFORT MAY BE APPROPRIATE IF THERE IS NO SPONTANEOUS CIRCULATION AFTER 15 MINUTES.
The following are controversial issues regarding newborn resuscitation addressed in September 1999 at the Evidence Evaluation (E2) conference and the recommendations discussed in February 2000 by the Emergency Cardiovascular Care (ECC) Committee by the Neonatal Program

Resuscitation Steering Committee, American Academy of Pediatrics and American Heart Association:

1. Tracheal suctioning when meconium-stained amniotic fluid is present.
2. Room air versus 100% oxygen for resuscitation.
3. Cerebral hypothermia after perinatal asphyxia (which has since been shown to be beneficial).
4. Fluids for volume replacement.
5. Discontinuation and noninitiation of resuscitation in the delivery room.

BIBLIOGRAPHY

Goldsmith JP, Spitzer AR: Controversies in neonatal pulmonary care. Clin Perinatol 25:39-45,203-214,228-229, 1998.

Jain L, Keenan W: Resuscitation of the fetus and newborn. Clin Perinatol 26:641, 731, 1999.

Kattwinkel J (ed): Textbook of Neonatal Resuscitation, ed 4, Chicago, American Heart Association and American Academy of Pediatrics, 2000.

Taeusch HW, Ballard RA: Avery's Diseases of the Newborn, ed 7, Philadelphia, WB Saunders, 1998.

4

NEONATAL RESUSCITATION

Physical Examination of the Newborn

Henry M. Seidel

Ideally, the full-term newborn should be examined at least two and preferably three times between birth and discharge: in the delivery room immediately at birth (particularly in the event of a high-risk pregnancy or delivery), in the nursery within 12 hours at most, and at discharge from the hospital. On one of the latter two occasions, it is important to examine the infant in the presence of the mother and, if possible, the father. This is a marvelous means for education, for observing their interaction with the baby, and for reinforcing your ongoing relationship with the parents. Some examiners prefer to do the first nursery physical alone in case there are unanticipated findings. A premature, sick, or congenitally compromised infant's particular needs will mandate changes in approach.

This, however, is not a perfect world. A short hospital stay (obviously now more the rule than the exception) compresses these steps. The guidelines for perinatal care acknowledge this by suggesting that one examination no later than 24 hours after birth and within 24 hours before discharge from the hospital will be satisfactory. This recommendation confronts the reality of medicine today. The American Academy of Pediatrics (AAP), in an important policy statement, "Hospital Stay for Healthy Term Newborns," also recommends that infants discharged in less than 48 hours be seen within 48 hours of discharge, and breast-fed infants also at 48 to 72 hours after discharge for the necessary assessment and, particularly, for breast-feeding evaluation and support (see **Chapter 30**). If discharge is to be considered before 48 hours, the preferable conditions are a singleton birth with an uncomplicated pregnancy, vaginal delivery, postpartum experience for both mother and baby, at least 38 to 42 weeks' gestation, and a birth weight appropriate for gestational age.

We agree with the AAP that the decision for discharge should be made by the physician caring for the infant, that an arbitrary policy established by third-party payers cannot prevail, and that the following requirements should first be fulfilled:

- Vital signs documented and stable within appropriate ranges for the 12 hours before discharge: respirations <60/minute; heart rate at 100-160/minute; axillary temperature 36.5° C to 37.4° C
- The infant has voided with a good stream and passed one spontaneous stool
- There have been two successful, well-documented feedings
- Physical examination has not revealed a need for further hospitalization
- No excessive bleeding at a circumcision site

- Appropriate management plans have been made for any existent jaundice
- There is assurance that the mother and her supports are prepared to provide the required infant care; any discovered family, environmental, and social risk factors have been assessed and necessary safeguards put in place to protect the infant; barriers to continuing care are overcome, e.g., transportation, language, and medical insurance difficulties (See **Chapter 30**)
- All laboratory tests have been reviewed and needed follow-up care arranged
- Necessary hepatitis B vaccine has been administered
- Hearing screening has been done according to state regulations and hospital protocol
- A physician-directed source of care has been identified and the necessary appointment arranged. There should be at that follow-up visit the necessary weighing and physical examination; an assessment of the findings and of the mother-infant interaction; continuing education for the mother and other caretakers; review of laboratory tests taken in the hospital and additional necessary testing, e.g., serum bilirubin in the presence of jaundice; and verification of the plans for management of perceived problems and continuing well-baby and emergency care.

Note: *If there has not been an opportunity for a prenatal visit, everything discussed in **Chapter 1** is relevant to the time of first introduction to baby and family. No physical examination is complete without a thorough, well-understood family, maternal, and fetal history. Given a healthy infant after an uncomplicated delivery, there are transitional stages that set the context of the examination.*

I. THE CONTEXT OF THE EXAMINATIONS: PATTERNS OF ACTIVITY
A. FIRST 15 TO 30 MINUTES.
1. Immediate tachycardia to 160 to 180 beats per minute, with a gradual drop to 100 to 120 beats per minute.
2. Irregular respirations, tachypnea to 60 to 80 respirations per minute, brief moments of apnea.
3. Moist-sounding lung fields, transient grunting and retraction.
4. Awake, moving, alert, easily startled, crying, transient tremors.

B. NEXT 60 TO 90 MINUTES.
1. Sleepy or sleeping, somewhat unresponsive.
2. Heart rate 100 to 120 beats per minute, transient tachycardia.
3. Respiratory rate 50 to 60 respirations per minute, transient tachypnea.
4. Usually, passage of meconium.

C. THE NEXT 10 MINUTES TO SEVERAL HOURS.
Again, awake, alert, easily startled, crying, easily stimulated, and reactive.

D. AT LAST, BEHAVING LIKE A BABY.

"Over" being born, eager for feeding and the world, and eager, at times, for sleep.

II. DELIVERY-ROOM EXAMINATION

Remember that inspection is as important as touching and listening. The baby should be nude and under a warmer, and the Apgar 1-minute score (**Table 5-1**) should be determined. Immediate concerns include assessment of pulmonary, cardiovascular, and central nervous system (CNS) function. If a pediatrician is not called to the delivery room, these observations become the responsibility of those in attendance, and the nursery examination should then be performed as soon as possible. The list of observations noted can be altered depending on the particular circumstance. The full list is probably achievable only in a perfect world (**Box 5-1**).

Note: *Whenever you observe something that violates your sense of the expected— the "normal"—pay attention. It may be a clue to something obvious or something obscure, one of many hidden anomalies or infrequently detected syndromes.*

A. PARTICULAR ATTENTION SHOULD BE GIVEN TO THE FOLLOWING:

1. Apgar scores at 1 and 5 minutes: A 5-minute score >8 is reassuring; a 1-minute score <7 suggests the possibility of CNS difficulty; a score of <4 indicates a need for resuscitation.
2. Placenta: Look for infarction, separation at margin, velamentous insertion of vessels, meconium staining, foul odor.
3. Umbilical cord: The cord should have two arteries and one vein; only one artery (<1:100 births) suggests associated congenital defects. The cord should be examined early before drying obscures findings. The average cord length at term is 50 to 60 cm (a shortened cord may be associated with in utero hypotonia).
4. Perinatal events: Consider the possibility of delivery trauma (e.g., shoulder dystocia, evidence of asphyxia, cord around neck) (see **Table 5-1**).
5. Obvious and unexpected abnormalities (e.g., meningomyelocele, club feet, cleft lip, nevi, hemangiomas).
6. Weight: If baby weighs >4 kg, think of maternal diabetes and baby's potential for hypoglycemia.
7. Using a small catheter, probe the nares (for suction and to judge patency) and, if indicated, the stomach (for aspiration and to judge esophageal continuity); excessive stomach contents, as little as 30 ml, suggests intestinal obstruction.
8. Possible voiding and passage of meconium: Note vigor of urinary stream and ensure patency of relevant orifices. (Catheter in rectum is not routine; it can help ensure patency if there is a question.)

5

PHYSICAL EXAMINATION OF THE NEWBORN

TABLE 5-1

OBSTETRIC SITUATIONS IN WHICH DELIVERY TRAUMA MAY OCCUR

Type of Injury	Normal Vertex	Cesarean	Premature	Precipitate	Breech Extraction	Difficulty	
						Large Infant	High Midforceps
HEMORRHAGE							
Cerebral							
Subdural							X
Subarachnoid				X			
Intraventricular			X		X	X	X
Abdominal							
Liver					X	X	
Spleen					X	X	
Adrenal gland					X	X	
Cutaneous, presenting part	X				X		
Conjunctival	X						
FRACTURE OR DISLOCATION							
Clavicle							
Humerus					X	X	
Femur					X		
Skull							X
NERVE INJURY							
Brachial plexus							
Spinal cord					X	X	
Facial	X				X		
LACERATION	X						

From Nelson NM: Neonatal adaptations. In Hoekelman RA, Friedman SB, Nelson NM, et al (eds): Primary Pediatric Care, St. Louis, Mosby, 2001.

BOX 5-1

DELIVERY ROOM ASSESSMENT

A. GENERAL

1. Whole
   Proportions
   Symmetry
   Facies
   Gestational age (approximate)
2. Skin: color, subcutaneous tissue, and imperfections (bands and birthmarks)
3. Neuromuscular
   Movements
   Responses
   Tone (flexor)

B. HEAD AND NECK

1. Head
   Shape
   Circumference
   Molding
   Swellings
   Depressions
   Occipital overhang
2. Fontanelles, sutures
   Size
   Tension
3. Eyes
   Size
   Separation
   Cataracts
   Colobomas
4. Ears
   Placement
   Complexity
   Preauricular tags or sinuses
5. Mouth
   Symmetry
   Size
   Clefts
6. Neck
   Swellings
   Fistula(s)

C. LUNGS AND RESPIRATION

1. Retraction
2. Grunt
3. Air entry (breath sounds)

5

PHYSICAL EXAMINATION OF THE NEWBORN

Continued

BOX 5-1 —Cont'd

DELIVERY ROOM ASSESSMENT

D. HEART AND CIRCULATION
1. Rate
2. Rhythm
3. Murmurs
4. Sounds

E. ABDOMEN
1. Musculature
2. Bowel sounds
3. Cord vessels
4. Distention
5. Scaphoid shape
6. Masses

F. GENITALIA AND ANUS
1. Placement
2. Testes
3. Labia
4. Phallus

G. EXTREMITIES
1. Bands
2. Digits (number and overlapping)

H. SPINE
1. Symmetry
2. Scoliosis
3. Sinuses

From Nelson NM: Neonatal adaptations. In Hoekelman RA, Friedman SB, Nelson NM, et al (eds): Primary Pediatric Care, St Louis, Mosby, 2001.

Note: *Atresia higher up in the rectum can sometimes be difficult to detect. The baby must ultimately pass a stool.*

9. Mouth: Cleft palate, teeth.
10. Color: Generalized cyanosis turns to pink as respirations are established.
   a. Persistent generalized central cyanosis: Cardiac abnormality, pulmonary compromise, sepsis.
   b. Pallor: Asphyxiation, anemia, acute blood loss.
   c. Meconium staining: Asphyxiation, other causes of fetal distress; stained fingernails suggest prolonged distress.
11. Respiratory pattern: Tachypnea; grunts; flaring alae nasi; intercostal retractions of more than momentary duration, particularly after suctioning; stridor; presence or absence of abnormal breath sounds of any sort.
12. Cardiac auscultation: murmurs, quality of heart sounds, arrhythmia.

13. Pulses: Strength, palpability. **Do not forget to assess the femoral pulses.**
14. Abdomen: Prominence (masses), concave (diaphragmatic hernia), auscultation (presence or absence of borborygmi).
15. Genitalia: Rule out ambiguity, undescended testes, hypospadias.
16. Reactivity: Compatible with expected neuromuscular behavior for the first few minutes of life.

B. IN ADDITION, MEASURE WEIGHT AND ASSESS GESTATIONAL AGE.

It is vital to assess the appropriateness of growth and development to gestational age. The date of the last menstrual period (LMP) is a helpful indicator even if compromised at times by fickle memory or the many variables in contraception and previous pregnancies. The sonographic record can also help, completing the triad of LMP, sonogram, and physical examination (PE). The key designations are AGA, appropriate for gestational age; SGA, small for gestational age; and LGA, large for gestational age.

1. Birth weight and length alone are insufficient for determining gestational age, although the infant can be placed in an appropriate percentile for these measures using standardized charts. Using a variety of physical and neuromuscular characteristics, there are standardized criteria necessary for making a more accurate assessment of gestational age (**Fig. 5-1**).
2. Vascularity of the anterior capsule of the lens can be an additional guide. Direct ophthalmoscopy during the second day of life can indicate the degree of vascularity from major involvement of the entire capsule before 28 weeks of gestational age to only peripheral fringe involvement, if that, after 34 weeks. This is most helpful in the very premature baby (see **Fig. 5-1**).
3. SGA: Weight below the 10th percentile for gestational age may be related to a variety of factors, including the following:
a. Maternal.
   (1) Chronic disease (e.g., cardiovascular, renal, diabetes, hemoglobinopathies).
   (2) Habits (e.g., drugs [legal and illegal], cigarettes, diet preferences).
   (3) Obstetric (e.g., placental infarct, separation, velamentous vessel insertion).
b. Neonate.
   (1) Severe congenital anomalies.
   (2) Congenital infection.
   (3) Inborn errors of metabolism.
   (4) Twin-to-twin competitions (e.g., for blood).

Note: *Mortality and morbidity are increased when birth weight for an infant born at term is equal to or below the third percentile relative to gestational age.*

5

PHYSICAL EXAMINATION OF THE NEWBORN

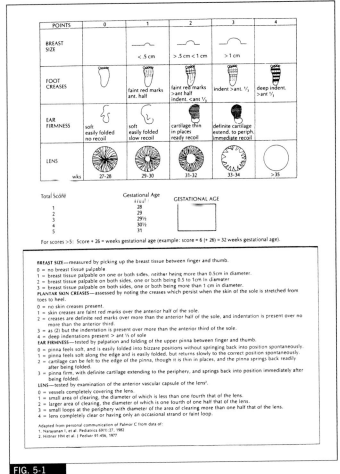

POINTS	0	1	2	3	4
BREAST SIZE		< .5 cm	> .5 cm < 1 cm	>1 cm	
FOOT CREASES		faint red marks ant. half	faint red marks >ant half indent. <ant ⅓	indent >ant. ⅓	deep indent. >ant ⅓
EAR FIRMNESS	soft easily folded no recoil	soft easily folded slow recoil	cartilage thin in places ready recoil	definite cartilage extend. to periph. immediate recoil	
LENS					
wks	27-28	29-30	31-32	33-34	>35

Total Score	Gestational Age (wks)	GESTATIONAL AGE
1	28	
2	29	
3	29½	
4	30½	
5	31	

For scores >5: Score + 26 = weeks gestational age (example: score = 6 (+ 26) = 32 weeks gestational age).

BREAST SIZE—measured by picking up the breast tissue between finger and thumb.
0 = no breast tissue palpable
1 = breast tissue palpable on one or both sides, neither being more than 0.5cm in diameter.
2 = breast tissue palpable on both sides, one or both being 0.5 to 1cm in diameter.
3 = breast tissue palpable on both sides, one or both being more than 1 cm in diameter.
PLANTAR SKIN CREASES—assessed by noting the creases which persist when the skin of the sole is stretched from toes to heel.
0 = no skin creases present.
1 = skin creases are faint red marks over the anterior half of the sole.
2 = creases are definite red marks over more than the anterior half of the sole, and indentation is present over no more than the anterior third.
3 = as (2) but the indentation is present over more than the anterior third of the sole.
4 = deep indentations present > ant ⅓ of sole
EAR FIRMNESS—tested by palpation and folding of the upper pinna between finger and thumb.
0 = pinna feels soft, and is easily folded into bizzare positions without springing back into position spontaneously.
1 = pinna feels soft along the edge and is easily folded, but returns slowly to the correct position spontaneously.
2 = cartilage can be felt to the edge of the pinna, though it is thin in places, and the pinna springs back readily after being folded.
3 = pinna firm, with definite cartilage extending to the periphery, and springs back into position immediately after being folded.
LENS—tested by examination of the anterior vascular capsule of the lens².
0 = vessels completely covering the lens.
1 = small area of clearing, the diameter of which is less than one fourth that of the lens.
2 = larger area of clearing, the diameter of which is one fourth of one half that of the lens.
3 = small loops at the periphery with diameter of the area of clearing more than one half that of the lens.
4 = lens completely clear or having only an occasional strand or faint loop.

Adapted from personal communication of Palmor C from data of:
1. Narayanan I, et al. Pediatrics 69(1):27, 1982
2. Hittner HM et al. J Pediatr 91:456, 1977

FIG. 5-1

Rapid assessment of gestational age. *(From Nelson NM: Neonatal adaptations. In Hoekelman RA, Friedman SB, Nelson NM, et al (eds): Primary Pediatric Care, St. Louis, Mosby, 2001.)*

4. **LGA (weight beyond the 90th percentile for gestational age, or weighing >4000 g) may be related to a variety of factors, including the following:**
   a. Maternal: Chronic disease, most commonly diabetes.
   b. Parental (e.g., body habitus, race, gestational weight gain).

c. Neonate: Congenital growth disorders.
   (1) Beckwith-Wiedemann syndrome (e.g., macrosomia, macroglossia, omphalocele, occasional hypoglycemia).
   (2) Sotos syndrome (e.g., big head, big hands, hypertelorism, big jaw).
d. A compelling obstetric concern pits baby size against pelvic outlet; judgment often must be made before delivery with examination, sonogram, and pelvic measurements to guide management and mode of delivery.

III. NURSERY EXAMINATION

A. FIRST STEPS.

Best done within 12 hours of delivery. The purpose is assessment of the baby's stability after the rush of perinatal and immediate postnatal events and of continuing respiratory, cardiovascular, and neurologic competence. The baby should be nude, warmed, and offered a pacifier (or gloved finger). The strength and eagerness of sucking give a first, important message about "competence." Begin gently with inspection, proceeding to auscultation, gentle and then deeper palpation, and finally the more stimulating experiences of abduction of the hips, examination of the mouth, and elicitation of Moro and other neurologic reflexes. If the baby is particularly reactive and crying, note the intensity and pitch—how shrill or how stridorous the cry may be.

B. THE SETTING.

Most examiners welcome parental presence at this point. Watching the mother hold and react to the baby offers clues to her feelings, from warmth and tenderness, to tension, and much between. The father's behavior indicates his approach and attitudes toward mother and baby, ranging from wholehearted to tentative or noninvolvement. The length of stay is probably too brief these days to count on a third (discharge) examination for this opportunity.

C. THE CONCLUSION.

Minute attention is then given to each aspect of the full examination. Adopt a comfortable sequence and style; remember that a fixed routine, whatever it might be, helps prevent missed observations, and in the long run, no specific sequence, so long as it is inclusive, offers better outcomes. Be ready, however, to be flexible given the demands of the baby's condition. Among the myriad possible findings on both history and physical examination, the information in **Tables 5-2 to 5-11** suggests the range of those that require parental reassurance, at most, to those suggesting genuine alarm. There may be disagreement about some of the listings (e.g., rupture of the membranes at <36 weeks might alarm some and alert others; yawning might alert some to drug exposure; and polydactyly might alert rather than alarm others).

PHYSICAL EXAMINATION OF THE NEWBORN

5

TABLE 5-2

LEVELS OF SURVEILLANCE OF THE NEWBORN BASED ON THE
OBSTETRIC HISTORY

History	Level of Surveillance		
	Normal	Alert	Alarm
Pregnancy surveillance	Registered during first trimester	Unregistered during second trimester	Unregistered and in labor
Genetic disease	None known	In family	In sibling of fetus
Uterine volume		Polyhydramnios	Oligohydramnios
Fetal movement		Increased	Decreased
Biochemical		Decreased estriol levels	
Biophysical		Positive oxytocin challenge test	Uterine ultrasound abnormality
Maternal disease		Diabetes and hypertension	Active tuberculosis
Rupture of membranes		<36 weeks	
Labor	36-42 weeks	<36, >42 weeks	<34 weeks
Delivery Vaginal Cesarean	Elective (repeat)	"Difficult" breech Elective (initial)	Emergency
Fetus	Apgar 8-10	Apgar 4-7, visible congenital anomaly	Asphyxia and hydrops fetalis

From Nelson NM: Neonatal adaptations. In Hoekelman RA, Friedman SB, Nelson NM, et al (eds): Primary Pediatric Care, St. Louis, Mosby, 2001.

IV. GENERALIZATIONS

A. SKIN.

Inspection should be followed by gentle palpation of affected areas to judge the feel of the skin and to discover associated underlying findings.

1. Acrocyanosis is common, particularly if the baby is insufficiently warmed; mottling is also common, particularly peripherally.
2. Vernix caseosa—cheesy, greasy, and white—covers large areas of skin, more so in premature infants.
3. Lanugo, fine hair covering much of the body, is common, particularly in premature infants; it disappears after several weeks. Scalp hair, ordinarily dark at birth, usually falls out in several weeks and often changes color.
4. The longer the fingernails, the more mature the baby.
5. Breaks in skin, or sinuses, defects, and tags are surface clues to underlying cysts and masses, particularly those that are preauricular, along the sternocleidomastoid area, and midline from the nose over the head and down to the coccyx.
6. The fatter the baby, the lesser the redness.

TABLE 5-3

LEVELS OF SURVEILLANCE OF THE NEWBORN BASED ON VITAL FUNCTIONS

Vital Function	Level of Surveillance		
	Normal	Alert	Alarm
Respiration	Paradoxical	Periodic tachypnea or retractions	Apnea, bradycardia, grunting, or gasping
Circulation	Acrocyanosis and heart rate rate 110-165 beats/min	Tachycardia, or cardiac murmur	Central cyanosis, hypertension, bradycardia, hypotension, enlarged heart, or pallor
Metabolism	Body temperature of 95.9° F to 99.5° F (36.5° C to 37.5° C)	Hyperthermia	Hypothermia
Digestion	Drooling or "transitional" stools	Spitting	Vomiting or diarrhea
Excretion		No voiding (>24 hr) and no stooling (>24 hr)	Dribbling stream
Behavior	Alert, responsive, reactive, startle, or sneeze	Hyperactive, jittery, or yawning	Coma or convulsions

From Nelson NM: Neonatal adaptations. In Hoekelman RA, Friedman SB, Nelson NM, et al (eds): Primary Pediatric Care, St. Louis, 2001, Mosby.

7. Color: Pallor, plethora, cyanosis, and clinically apparent jaundice suggest a variety of illnesses described more completely in sections devoted to hematology, cardiology, pulmonary system, and gastroenterology.

8. Jaundice is common (**See Chapter 21**)—perhaps half of all neonates are jaundiced; the earlier the onset, the more acute the problem. Intensity can be measured by descent on the body—the lower and the more peripheral the appearance of jaundice, the higher the bilirubin level. Use daylight preferably for making the judgment; applying pressure with a finger on the infant's forehead or other area, which empties the capillary bed, provides the best opportunity to evaluate the color change. Clinically apparent jaundice indicates a bilirubin level of >6 mg/dl.

9. Melanin is not always fully apparent at birth. It often takes a while to appear, and pigmentation below the nails and on the scrotum or vulva provides an early clue to later skin color.

10. Spots, blotches, plugs, and growths are common; the presence of vesicles is always of concern (e.g., may indicate herpes).

11. Yellow-green meconium staining of vernix or fingernails suggests possible fetal distress.

5

PHYSICAL EXAMINATION OF THE NEWBORN

TABLE 5-4

LEVELS OF SURVEILLANCE OF THE NEWBORN BASED ON EXAMINATION OF THE APPENDAGES AND THE SKIN

Characteristic	Level of Surveillance		
	Normal	Alert	Alarm
Color (age of occurrence)	Acrocyanosis (<12 hr)	Central (<1 hr)	Central (>1 hr)
Jaundice	>24 hr	18-24 hr	<18 hr
Pallor			<3 min
Epidermis	Dermatoglyphics	Excoriations	Sloughing
Hair	Lanugo	Lumbosacral tuft and scalp defect	
Texture	Soft and moist	Dry and scaling	Thickened and crusting
Vascular pattern	Harlequin, mottling (cold)	Persistent mottling	
Cysts	Milia and Epstein pearls		
Papules	Acne and miliaria		
Desquamation	Delicate scaling (>2 days)	Peeling (<2 days)	Denuded sheets (anytime)
Hemangiomas	Telangiectatic (forehead, lids, lips, and nape)	Telangiectatic (trigeminal) and angiomatous (few)	Angiomatous (multiple)
Hemorrhage	Petechiae (head or upper body)	Petechiae (elsewhere)	Ecchymoses and purpura
Macules	Mongolian spots	Café au lait spots (<6 spots)	Café au lait spots (>5 spots) and "mountain ash" leaf
Pustules	Erythema toxicum		Large and dermal
Vesicles			Any
Nodules		Subcutaneous fat necrosis	Sclerema

From Nelson NM: Neonatal adaptations. In Hoekelman RA, Friedman SB, Nelson NM, et al (eds): Primary Pediatric Care, St. Louis, 2001, Mosby.

B. HEAD AND NECK (SEE CHAPTER 9).

1. Caput succedaneum is more common than cephalhematoma; caput can cross suture lines, but a cephalhematoma is limited by them. Differentiation at first examination may be difficult.
2. A subgaleal hemorrhage, not common, crosses suture lines.
3. Molding is common and appropriate in vaginal deliveries, not so in cesarean. The molding will often obscure the fontanel, but the head returns to its expected shape in a few days.
4. Intracranial bruits will not be heard unless they are listened for.

TABLE 5-5

LEVELS OF SURVEILLANCE OF THE NEWBORN BASED ON THE HEAD AND NECK EXAMINATION

Location	Level of Surveillance		
	Normal	Alert	Alarm
Skull	Caput succedaneum molding, or occipital overhang	Cephalhematoma, craniotabes, large fontanel, or forceps mark	Craniosynostosis, transillumination, or bruit
Facies		Hypoplasia or palsy	
Eyes		Mongoloid slant	Aniridia and enlarged cornea
Nose		Nasal obstruction	
Mouth		High-arched palate or macroglossia	Cleft palate and/or lip or micrognathia
Ears		"Simple" structure or low set	
Neck	Rotation ± 90°	Dimple or webbing	

From Nelson NM: Neonatal adaptations. In Hoekelman RA, Friedman SB, Nelson NM, et al (eds): Primary Pediatric Care, St. Louis, 2001, Mosby.

5. Hydrocephalus may not be found unless the skull is transilluminated.
6. Low-set or "funny-looking" ears: Look for other anomalies, particularly renal, and hearing loss; ears are often floppy and may be folded on themselves.
7. Dimples in the neck or about the ears: Look for cysts; dimples in this area occur in 1:100 infants and most often are no problem.
8. Nose may be distorted and flat after delivery; it should recover to the expected shape in a few days.
9. A large, potentially obstructive, tongue suggests concern (e.g., hypothyroidism); watch the baby feed to be sure that it is not a problem.
10. An apparent tongue tie is common; time, use, and stretching almost always take care of it.
11. Teeth at birth are unusual; 10% are extra, usually unrooted teeth and may need removal by a dentist; 90% are prematurely erupted and should be left in unless extremely loose. Natal teeth may be a clue to a variety of syndromes.
12. Extremely wide sutures and a huge fontanel deserve sonographic study; rarely, absence of the corpus callosum (e.g., as seen in Aicardi syndrome) may be found.

C. CHEST.

1. Paradoxical respirations may or may not be a problem; retractions or grunting intensify the concern.

TABLE 5-6

LEVELS OF SURVEILLANCE OF THE NEWBORN BASED ON THE CHEST EXAMINATION

	Level of Surveillance		
Characteristic	Normal	Alert	Alarm
Respiration		Paradoxical, periodic, or retractions	Apnea, expiratory grunt, or flaring alae nasi
Auscultation		Decreased air entry	Bowel sounds
Chest X-ray		Enlarged heart	Oligemia or plethora
Cardiac			
Impulse	Tapping	Heaving, lifting	
Pulses	Full	Decreased	Absent (femoral) and lag (cardiac-radial)
Rate and rhythm	110-165, sinus arrhythmia	Sinus bradycardia	Persistent sinus tachycardia
Sounds	"Tic-tock"	S_2 widely split	S_2 fixed split
Murmurs	Systolic (<24 hr)	Systolic (>24 hr)	Diastolic
Electrocardiograph (QRS)			
Vector	+35° to +180°		0° to −90°; −90° to −180°
Amplitude			
V_1	Rs	Rs	Rs
V_6	qrS	qrS	qrS

From Nelson NM: Neonatal Adaptations. In Hoekelman RA, Friedman SB, Nelson NM, et al (eds): Primary Pediatric Care, St. Louis, 2001, Mosby.

TABLE 5-7

LEVELS OF SURVEILLANCE OF THE NEWBORN BASED ON EXAMINATION OF THE ABDOMEN

	Level of Surveillance		
Characteristic	Normal	Alert	Alarm
Shape	Cylindrical	Scaphoid	Distended
Muscular wall	Diastasis recti		Absent
Umbilicus	Amniotic navel or cutaneous navel	Exudation or leakage, granuloma, hernia, inflammation, or less than three cord vessels	Gastroschisis, omphalitis, or omphalocele
Liver	Smooth edge		Enlarged
Spleen	Nonpalpable	Palpable	Enlarged
Kidneys	Lobulated or palpable (lower poles)	Horseshoe	Enlarged

From Nelson NM: Neonatal adaptations. In Hoekelman RA, Friedman SB, Nelson NM, et al (eds): Primary Pediatric Care, St. Louis, 2001, Mosby.

TABLE 5-8

LEVELS OF SURVEILLANCE OF THE NEWBORN BASED ON EXAMINATION OF
THE PERINEUM

		Level of Surveillance	
Location	Normal	Alert	Alarm
Anus		Coccygeal dimple	Imperforate, fistula, patulous
Female			
Clitoris		Enlarged, hooded	
Vulva	Bloody secretion, edema, gaping labia, or hymenal tags		Hydrometrocolpos
Male			
Gonad	Edema, hydrocele	Bifid scrotum, cryptorchidism, inguinal hernia	
Phallus	Phimosis	Chordee, hypospadias	Microphallus

From Nelson NM: Neonatal adaptations. In Hoekelman RA, Friedman SB, Nelson NM, et al (eds): Primary Pediatric Care, St. Louis, 2001, Mosby.

TABLE 5-9

LEVELS OF SURVEILLANCE OF THE NEWBORN BASED ON EXAMINATION OF
THE MUSCULOSKELETAL SYSTEM

		Level of Surveillance	
Characteristic	Normal	Alert	Alarm
Fetal posture	Flexor, position of comfort	Frank breech	Extensor
Hand	Webbing	Cortical thumb, overlapping fingers, short, incurved little finger	Polydactyly, syndactyly
Foot	Dorsiflex 90°, plantarflex 90°, abduct or adduct forefoot 45°, invert or evert ankle 45°	Decreased range of motion	Fixed
Extremities	Tibial bowing		Constriction bands, amputations
Neck	Rotate ±90°		
Joints		Reluctance to use	Subluxation (hips), contracture

From Nelson NM: Neonatal adaptations. In Hoekelman RA, Friedman SB, Nelson NM, et al (eds): Primary Pediatric Care, St. Louis, 2001, Mosby.

TABLE 5-10

LEVELS OF SURVEILLANCE OF THE NEWBORN BASED ON EXAMINATION OF THE NERVOUS SYSTEM

Characteristic	Level of Surveillance		
	Normal	Alert	Alarm
State	*Awake*: crying, active, quiet alert *Asleep*: active, indeterminate, quiet	Hyperalert, lethargic	Stupor, coma
Motor			
Posture	Flexor, symmetrical	Extensor, asymmetrical	Obligatory, decerebrate
Tone	Obtuse popliteal angle	Limp in upright suspension	Limp in ventral suspension
Movement	All extremities, non-repetitive, random, symmetrical	Jitteriness, tremor	Seizures
Reflexes	Deep tendon, grasp, Moro, placing and stepping, sucking, tonic neck	Asymmetrical, do not habituate	Absent
Sensory	Pinprick response slow (2-3 sec)	Pinprick response equivocal	No response

From Nelson NM: Neonatal adaptations. In Hoekelman RA, Friedman SB, Nelson NM, et al (eds): Primary Pediatric Care, St. Louis, 2001, Mosby.

TABLE 5-11

LEVELS OF SURVEILLANCE OF THE NEWBORN BASED ON EXAMINATION OF THE CRANIAL NERVES

Cranial nerves	Level of Surveillance		
	Normal	Alert	Alarm
Forebrain: 2	Fix and follow (visual-evoked potential)	Equivocal (arc <60 degrees)	No response
Midbrain: 3, 4, 6, and 8	Pupillary response, doll's eye response	Unequal, discon-jugate, nystagmus	Absent, fixed position
Hindbrain: 8	Crib-O-Gram (auditory-evoked potentials)	Diminished	No response
5, 7, and 12	Sucking	Weak	Unequal
9 and 10	Swallowing	Uncoordinated	
11	Sternocleidomastoid muscles	Weak	

From Nelson NM: Neonatal adaptations. In Hoekelman RA, Friedman SB, Nelson NM, et al (eds): Primary Pediatric Care, St. Louis, 2001, Mosby.

2. Bowel sounds in the chest usually mean trouble (e.g., diaphragmatic hernia).
3. Swollen breasts in a boy or girl—the result of passively transferred maternal hormones—are ordinarily no problem and will subside. There may even be a discharge, called "witch's milk" by some.
4. A chest X-ray should be a quick resort if physical examination is worrisome.
5. Diminished peripheral pulses are a concern (e.g., coarctation of the aorta); an echocardiogram and cardiology consult should be a quick resort if findings are worrisome.

D. ABDOMEN.
1. A draining umbilicus should *not* be ignored.
2. Triple dye confuses an umbilical examination.
3. A single cord artery mandates concern about a congenital anomaly, particularly renal.
4. Enlargement of the liver cannot be judged by palpation alone; percuss the upper border.
5. Many physicians believe newborn kidneys are easy to palpate; others, equally adept, dispute this. The sonogram is a valuable tool for this or other worrisome abdominal findings.

E. PERINEUM.
Be careful: assigning the wrong sex in the presence of ambiguous genitalia confuses the infant's and the family's lives, sometimes irreparably.

Note: *Babies have been shown to void prenatally on ultrasonography. Postnatally, most will void by 12 hours, almost all by 24. Be sure—an obstruction or absent kidneys can occur. Swollen labia and hymenal tags are common and will shrink, usually within 1 month.*

F. MUSCULOSKELETAL SYSTEM.
1. Gently press on the infant's soles; the fetal position and quiet can often be restored.
2. Worry about persistent extension of the extremities, particularly in the full-term (and even in the premature) infant.
3. Syndactyly and polydactyly should alert a practitioner to the possibility of other anomalies; a second toe longer than the great toe is not unusual among those from the Mediterranean.
Clinodactyly might indicate other anomalies.
4. "Fisting" (clenching) might mean neurologic difficulty, but not always.
5. Do *not* miss dislocated hips (dysplasia).
6. Any persistent rigidity or resistance to passive motion should be a source of concern.

5

PHYSICAL EXAMINATION OF THE NEWBORN

G. NERVOUS SYSTEM.

1. Newborns are sensate individuals aware of their environment.
2. Early depression suggests asphyxia, sepsis, trauma, or drugs; later depression (once feeding is well established) suggests an inborn error of metabolism.
3. Extension and asymmetry in posture are causes for concern, particularly when persistent.
4. Floppiness is hard to judge; this often calls for a second observer for confirmation.
5. Real seizures are hard to define; degrees of cortical inhibition are hard to define; jitteriness is common; if a finger gently applied to a shaking limb quiets it, it is probably not a seizure.

V. NEONATAL BEHAVIORAL AND DEVELOPMENTAL ASSESSMENTS

The newborn period represents a moment in a developmental process already 9 months along and moving forward rapidly, abetted by an already well-developed CNS housed in a not nearly so mature body. The infant is from the start an interactive being with a sophisticated sensory apparatus and a not as well developed motor ability. Genetic and environmental factors contribute to the potential (or constraint) of these abilities. An undesirable outcome can sometimes be traced to a single risk factor, but most often the hazards are multiple and individual causes are obscured. It is necessary to evaluate the newborn's behavioral developmental status and to anticipate (and perhaps forestall) risk.

Note: *A single assessment is but a "snapshot"; a sequence of assessments is usually needed to get the full story.*

A. PRENATAL AND PERINATAL RISK FACTORS.

1. Maternal.
   a. Anatomic.
      (1) Structural malformations of the uterus and birth canal.
      (2) Inadequate pelvic outlet.
   b. Disease.
      (1) Infection (e.g., genitourinary tract): Viral (e.g., rubella, herpes, severe flu), bacterial (e.g., group B streptococcus, tuberculosis), sexually transmitted infection.
      (2) Mild to severe anemia from any cause (e.g., sickle cell anemia).
      (3) Chronic systemic disease (e.g., renal, cardiovascular, pulmonary).
      (4) Metabolic abnormality (e.g., diabetes, thyroid).
   c. Variables of pregnancy.
      (1) Maternal age: Increasing risk with decreasing or increasing age (e.g., ages <20 and >35 years).
      (2) Birth weight: Increasing risk if underweight or overweight.
      (3) Gestational age: Increasing risk with degree of prematurity, small size for gestational age (SGA), or large size for gestational age (LGA).

(4) Birth status: Increasing risk with diminished Apgar score, especially if prolonged.

Note: *Diagnosis of asphyxia should never be based solely on Apgar scores at 1 and 5 minutes.*

    (5) Complications.
- (a) Eclampsia, milder toxemia.
- (b) Abnormal fetal position.
- (c) Polyhydramnios.
- (d) History of prematurity, spontaneous and elective abortions, cesarean section, multiparity, prior fetal anomaly.

d. Other risk factors.
- (1) Alcohol.
- (2) Smoking.
- (3) Drugs (prescribed, over the counter, or illicit).
- (4) Adequacy of prenatal care.

2. OTHER GESTATIONAL INFLUENCES:

Malnutrition for any reason (e.g., underweight for length); baby *may* be neurologically compromised.

$$\text{Ponderal index} = \text{weight (g)}/(\text{length [cm]})^3 \times 100$$

Malnutrition is indicated by a score of 2 or less.

B. PERINATAL RISK FACTORS.

Complications of delivery include the following:
1. Premature rupture of membranes.
2. Evidence of fetal distress (e.g., bradycardia, tachycardia).
3. Sluggish labor.
4. Inappropriate anesthesia: The heavier the medication, the greater the likelihood of compromise.

Note: *An effort has been made to score these factors. Scoring is not yet a necessarily fruitful quantitative step, therefore I suggest being alert to the potential risks.*

C. QUANTITATIVE ASSESSMENT OF A NEWBORN'S DEVELOPMENT AND BEHAVIORAL STATE HAS BEEN ATTEMPTED IN A VARIETY OF WAYS. I SUGGEST THE FOLLOWING AS BEST SUITED TO THE NEED:

Note: *These scales measure a point in time; they are best used repetitively, or confusion may result. Remember that a score will vary if taken during the "alert period" right after delivery or during the subsequent "depressed period" and then the "recovery."*

BOX 5-2

BRAZELTON BEHAVIORAL SCALE

Environmental interactions
Alertness
Consolability
Cuddliness
Orientation
Stress responses
Skin color lability
Startle reaction
Tremulousness
Motor processes
Activity
Defensive reactions
Hand-to-mouth movement
Maturity
Reflex
Tone
Physiologic state
Habituating to stimuli
Self-quieting

From Nelson NM: Neonatal adaptations. In Hoekelman RA, Friedman SB, Nelson NM, et al (eds): Primary Pediatric Care. St. Louis, Mosby, 2001.

1. Apgar score: Already in universal use.
2. Brazelton behavioral scale, or neonatal behavioral assessment scale (NBAS) (**Box 5-2**). This scale takes advantage of the full-term neonate's ability to react and participate in the environment (e.g., selecting the human face over inanimate objects for intense gazing, responding to variations in speech, and to cuddling in the fetal position). The findings vary with the baby's level of sleep or alertness and the age in hours; the most fruitful observations are made when the infant is quiet but alert. Notably, an infant's neurologic and organizational competency is better judged by the Brazelton behavioral scale performed by someone experienced with it and a competent neurologic examination (**Box 5-3**) than by the neurologic examination alone.
3. Neuromuscular competency: Neuromuscular assessment (see **Box 5-3**) can complement the NBAS observations in judging the effect of known risk factors for an individual neonate.

VI. NEONATAL PAIN ASSESSMENT (See Chapter 7)

Note: The potential of pain in the newborn should never be ignored. (**Table 5-12**).

TABLE 5-12
INFANT PAIN SCORE

Indicator	Behavior Scale			Score*
	0	1	2	
Sleep during preceding hour	None	Short naps (5-10 min)	Longer naps	
Facial expression: brow bulge, open mouth, chin quiver, stretch mouth horizontal, nasolabial furrow, eye squeeze	Marked	Less marked	Calm	
Quality of cry	Screaming, pain, high pitched	Modulated, infant can be distracted	No cry	
Spontaneous motor activity	Thrashing, incessant agitation	Moderate	Normal	
Excitability and responsiveness to stimulation	Tremulous, clonic movement, spontaneous Moro reflex	Excessive reactivity to nay stimulation	Quiet	
Flexion of fingers and toes	Pronounced and constant	Less marked, intermittent	Absent	
Sucking	Absent or disorganized	Intermittent (3 or 4), stops with crying	Strong, rhythmic, pacifies	
Overall tone	Strong, hypertonicity	Moderate hypertonicity	Normal	
Consolability	None after 2 minutes of comforting	Quiet after 1 minute of effort	Quiet within 1 minute	
Sociability (eye contact) in response to voice, smile, or face	Absent	Difficult to obtain	Easy and prolonged	
				Total:

*0 = severe pain, 20 = comfort.

From Strauss SG, Lynn AM, Spear RM. Contemp Pediatr 19:80, 1995.

PHYSICAL EXAMINATION OF THE NEWBORN 5

BOX 5-3

TECHNIQUES FOR ASSESSMENT OF NEUROMUSCULAR MATURITY

POSTURE

With the infant supine and quiet, score as follows:

Arms and legs extended = 0

Slight or moderate flexion of hips and knees = 1

Moderate to strong flexion of hips and knees = 2

Legs flexed and abducted, arms slightly flexed = 3

Full flexion of arms and legs = 4

POPLITEAL ANGLE

With the infant supine and the pelvis flat on the examining surface, the leg is flexed on the thigh and the thigh is fully flexed with the use of one hand. With the other hand the leg is then extended, and the angle attained is scored as in **Fig. 5-1**.

SQUARE WINDOW

Flex the hand to the wrist; exert pressure sufficient to get as much flexion as possible. The angle between the hypothenar eminence and the anterior aspect of the forearm is measured and scored according to **Fig. 5-1**. Do not rotate the wrist.

ARM RECOIL

With the infant supine, fully flex the forearm for 5 seconds, then fully extend by pulling the hands and releasing. Score the reaction according to the following:

Remains extended or random movements = 0

Incomplete or partial flexion = 1

Brisk return to full flexion = 2

SCARF SIGN

With the infant supine, take the infant's hand and draw it across the neck and as far across the opposite shoulder as possible. Assistance to the elbow is permissible by lifting it across the body. Score according to the location of the elbow:

Elbow reaches beyond the opposite anterior axillary line = 0

Elbow reaches to the opposite anterior axillary line = 1

Elbow is between opposite anterior axillary line and midline of thorax = 2

Elbow is at midline of thorax = 3

Elbow does not reach midline of thorax = 4

HEEL-TO-EAR MANEUVER

With the infant supine, hold the infant's foot with one hand and move it as near to the head as possible without forcing it. Keep the pelvis flat on the examining surface. Score as in **Fig. 5-1**.

Modified from Amiel-Tison C: Arch Dis Child 43:89, 1968 and Dubowitz LMS, et al: Clinical assessment of gestational age in the newborn infant. J Pediatr 77:1, 1970.

VII. DISCHARGE EXAMINATION

The compression of time spent in the hospital often precludes separate first, nursery, and discharge examinations. Regardless, the effort should be made if at all possible, for the baby's sake, for parental education and reassurance, for the family dynamic, and for reinforcement of the continuity relationship with the practitioner (**see Chapter 30**).

BIBLIOGRAPHY

American Academy of Pediatrics and American College of Obstetricians and Gynecologists: Guidelines for Prenatal Care, ed 4. Elk Grove Village, IIII and Washington, DC, AAP and ACOG, 1997.

American Academy of Pediatrics Policy Statement: Breastfeeding and the Use of Human Milk. Pediatrics 100:1035, 1997.

American Academy of Pediatrics Policy Statement: Hospital Stay for Healthy Term Newborns. Pediatrics 113:1434, 2004.

Amiel-Tison C: Neurological evaluation of the maturity of newborn infants. Arch Dis Child 43:89, 1968.

Ballard JL, Novak KK, Driver M: A simplified score for assessment of fetal maturation of newly born infants. J Pediatr 95:769, 1979.

Dubowitz LMS, Dubowitz V, Goldberg C: Clinical assessment of gestational age in the newborn infant. J Pediatr 77:1, 1970.

Eisen LN, Field TN, Bandstra ES, et al: Perinatal cocaine effects on neonatal stress behavior and performance on the Brazelton scale. Pediatrics 88:477, 1991.

Hittner HM, Hirsch NJ, Rudolph AJ: Assessment of gestational age by examination of the anterior capsule of the lens. J Pediatr 94:455, 1977.

McIntire DD, Bloom SL, Casey BM, Leveno KG: Birth weight in relation to morbidity and mortality among newborn infants. N Engl J Med 340:1234, 1999.

Naeye RL: Umbilical cord length: Clinical significance. J Pediatr 107:278, 1985.

Nelson NM: Neonatal adaptations. In Hoekelman RA, Friedman SB, Nelson NM, et al (eds): Primary Pediatric Care, St. Louis, Mosby, 2001.

Oh W, Merenstein G: Fourth edition of the Guidelines for Perinatal Care: Summary of changes, Pediatrics 100:1021, 1997.

Sanders M, Allen M, Alexander GR, et al: Gestational age assessment in preterm neonates weighing less than 1500 grams. Pediatrics 88:542, 1991.

Strauss SG, Lynn AM, Spear RM: Progress in pain control for very young infants. Contemp Pediatr 12:80, 1995.

5

PHYSICAL EXAMINATION OF THE NEWBORN

Cultural Considerations

Henry M. Seidel

Cultures reflect the whole of human behavior, what we think, how we act, how we relate to one another, how we speak; and, too, the results of our ingenuity, imagination and physical effort, and how we put our ideas into useful practice. Race, for example, is not a cultural characteristic. How we react to differences in skin color is. If we are to serve our infant patients well, we must understand that each baby is born into a group that may have cultural characteristics that vary in small or large extent from ours and, also, that individuals within a group cannot be assumed to accept the practice of that group in its entirety. We cannot rely on stereotypical notions to characterize individuals. Tables 6-1 and 6-2, too rigidly interpreted, can suggest the stereotype. Back away from too easy assumptions; use them as guides and make sure of the cultural behaviors and attitudes of the particular infant and family you are serving. You will be helped in this by keeping in mind the questions related to culture suggested in **Chapter 1**.

6

TABLE 6-1

SOME RELIGIOUS BELIEFS THAT AFFECT NEWBORN CARE

Religion	Beliefs about Birth		Beliefs Regarding Medical Care
Adventist (Seventh Day Adventist; Church of God)	**Birth:**	Opposed to infant baptism Baptism in adulthood	Some believe in divine healing and practice anointing with oil and use of prayer May desire communion or baptism when ill Believe in man's choice and God's sovereignty
Baptist (27 groups)	**Birth:**	Opposed to infant baptism Believers baptized by immersion as adults	May encounter some resistance to some therapies, such as abortion Believe God functions through physician Some believe in predestination; may respond passively to care
	Death:	Counsel and prayer with clergy, family, patient	
Buddhist Churches of America	**Birth:**	No infant baptism Infant presentation	Illness believed to be a trial to aid development of soul; illness is due to karmic causes May be reluctant to have surgery or certain treatments on holy days Cleanliness believed to be of great importance Family may require Buddhist priest for counseling
	Death:	Last rites chanting often practiced at bedside soon after death Priest should be contacted	
Church of Christ Scientist (Christian Science)	**Birth:** **Death:**	No baptism No last rites	Deny the existence of health crisis; see sickness and sin as errors of mind that can be altered by prayer Oppose human intervention with drugs or other therapies; however, most accept legally required immunizations Many adhere to belief that disease is a human mental concept that can be dispelled by "spiritual truth" to extent that they refuse all medical treatment

Church of Jesus Christ of Latter Day Saints (Mormon)	**Birth:**	No baptism at birth Infant is "blessed" by church official at first opportunity after birth (in church) Baptism by immersion at 8 years	Devout adherents believe in divine healing through anointment with oil and "laying on of hands" by church official (elder) Medical therapy not prohibited
	Death:	No special rites	
Eastern Orthodox (e.g., Turkey, Egypt, Syria, Romania, Bulgaria, Cyprus, Albania)	**Birth:**	Most believe in infant baptism by immersion 8 to 40 days after birth	Anointment of the sick No conflict with medical science
	Death:	Last rites obligatory for impending death	
Episcopal (Anglican)	**Birth:**	Infant baptism mandatory; urgent if poor prognosis	Some believe in spiritual healing Rite for anointing sick available but not mandatory
	Death:	Last rites available but not mandatory	
Friends (Quarkers)	**Birth:**	No baptism Infant's name recorded in official book	No special rites or restrictions
Greek Orthodox	**Birth:**	Baptism considered important Performed 40 days after birth If not possible to baptize by sprinkling or immersion, church allows child baptism "in the air" by moving the child in the form of a cross as appropriate words are said	Each health crisis handled by ordained priest; deacon may also serve in some cases Holy Communion administered in hospital Some may desire Sacrament of the Holy Unction performed by priest
	Death:	Last rites, administration of Sacrament of Holy Communion; should be performed while dying person is still conscious	

Continued

CULTURAL CONSIDERATIONS

6

TABLE 6-1

SOME RELIGIOUS BELIEFS THAT AFFECT NEWBORN CARE—cont'd

Religion	Beliefs about Birth	Beliefs Regarding Medical Care
Hindu	**Birth:** No ritual **Death:** Special prescribed rites Priest pours water into the mouth of dead child, ties a thread around neck or wrist to signify blessing (should not be removed) Family washes body and is particular about who touches body	Illness or injury believed to represent sins committed in previous life Accept most modern medical practices
Islam (Muslim/Moslem)	**Birth:** No baptism **Death:** Family should be present Family washes and prepares body, then turns it to face Mecca Only relatives and friends may touch body	Faith healing not acceptable unless psychological condition of patient is deteriorating; performed for morale Ritual washing after prayer; prayer takes place five times daily (on rising, midday, afternoon, early evening, and before bed); during prayer, face Mecca and kneel on prayer rug
Jehovah's Witness	**Birth:** No baptism **Death:** No last rites	Adherents are generally absolutely opposed to blood transfusions, including banking of own blood; individuals can sometimes be persuaded in emergencies
Judaism (Orthodox and Conservative)	**Birth:** No baptism Ritual circumcision of male infants on eighth day; performed by Mohel (ritual cimcumciser familiar with Jewish law and aseptic technique) Reform Jews favor ritual circumcision, but not as a religious imperative	May resist surgical procedures during Sabbath, which extends from sundown Friday until sundown Saturday

TABLE 6-2

CULTURAL CHARACTERISTICS RELATED TO NEWBORN CARE

Cultural Group	Health Beliefs	Health and Diet Practices	Family Relationships	Communication	Comments
Asian Americans					
Chinese	A health body is viewed as a gift from parents and ancestors and must be cared for Health is one of the results of balance between the forces of *yin* (cold) and *yang* (hot), energy forces that rule the world Illness is caused by imbalance Believe blood is source of life and is not regenerated *Chi* is innate energy Lack of *chi* and blood result in deficiency that produces poor constitution and long illness	Goal of therapy is to restore balance of *yin* and *yang* Wide use of medicinal herbs procured and applied in prescribed ways Folk healers are herbalist, spiritual healer, temple healer, fortune healer	Extended family pattern common Strong concept of loyalty of young to old Family and individual honor and "face" important Self-reliance and self-restraint highly valued; self-expression repressed Males valued more highly than females; women submissive to men in family	Open expression of emotions unacceptable Often smile when do not comprehend	Are especially upset by drawing of blood Deep respect for their bodies and believe it best to die with bodies intact; therefore may refuse surgery May believe in reincarnation Children sometimes breast-fed for up to 4 or 5 years*

Continued

CULTURAL CONSIDERATIONS

TABLE 6-2

CULTURAL CHARACTERISTICS RELATED TO NEWBORN CARE—cont'd

Cultural Group	Health Beliefs	Health and Diet Practices	Family Relationships	Communication	Comments
Japanese	Three major belief systems: *Shinto*—religious influence, human inherently good, evil caused by contact with polluting agents (e.g., blood, corpses, skin disease); *Chinese and Korean influences*—health achieved through harmony and balance between self and society, disease caused by disharmony with society and not caring for body; *Portuguese influence*—upholds germ theory of disease	Believe evil removed by purification *Kampo medicine*—use of natural herbs Believe in removal of diseased parts Trend is to use both Western and Eastern healing methods Care for disabled viewed as family's responsibility Take pride in child's good health Seek preventive care, medical care for illness	Close intergenerational relationships Family provides anchor Family tends to keep problems to self Value self-control and self-sufficiency Many adopt practices of contemporary middle class Co-sleeping of infants with parents is common	*Issei*—born in Japan; usually speak Japanese only *Nisei, Sansei, and Yonsei* have few language difficulties New immigrants able to read and write English better than to speak or understand it Make significant use of nonverbal communication with subtle gestures and facial expressions Tend to suppress emotions Will often wait silently	Generational categories: *Issei*—first generation to live in United States *Nisei*—second generation *Sansei*—third generation *Yonsei*—fourth generation Cleanliness highly valued Time considered valuable, to be used wisely Tendency to practice emotional control may make assessment of situation more difficult
Vietnamese	Good health considered to be balance between *yin* (cold) and *yang* (hot)	Fortune-tellers determine event that caused disturbance May visit temple to procure	Family is revered institution Multigenerational families Family is chief social	Many immigrants are not proficient in speaking and understanding English	Consider status more important than money Time concept more relaxed—consider

	Believe person's life has been predisposed toward certain phenomena by cosmic forces	divine instruction	network	May hesitate to ask questions	punctuality less significant than other values (e.g., propriety)
	Health believed to be result of harmony with existing universal order; harmony attained by pleasing good spirits and avoiding evil ones	Regard health as family responsibility; outside aid sought when resources run out	Children highly valued	Questioning authority is sign of disrespect; asking questions considered impolite	Place high value on social harmony
	Belief in *am duc*, the amount of good deeds accumulated by ancestors	Certain illnesses considered only temporary (such as pustules, open wounds) and ignored	Individual needs and interests are subordinate to those of family group	Use indirectness rather than forthrightness in expressing disagreement	
	Many use rituals to prevent illness	Seek generalist health healers	Father is main decision maker	May avoid eye contact with health professionals as a sign of respect	
	Practice some restrictions to prevent incurring wrath of evil spirits		Women taught submission to men		
Filipino	Believe God's will and supernatural forces govern universe	Some use amulets as a shield from witchcraft or as good luck pieces	Family is highly valued, with strong family ties	Immigrants and older persons may not be able to speak or understand English	Tend to have a fatalistic outlook on life
	Illness, accidents, and other misfortunes are	Catholics substitute religious medals and other items	Multigenerational family structure common, often with collateral members as well		Believe time and providence will solve all

Continued

TABLE 6-2

CULTURAL CHARACTERISTICS RELATED TO NEWBORN CARE—cont'd

Cultural Group	Health Beliefs	Health and Diet Practices	Family Relationships	Communication	Comments
African American	Illness classified as *natural*—affected by forces of nature without adequate protection (e.g., cold air, pollution, food and water); *unnatural*—evil influences (e.g., witchcraft, voodoo, hoodoo, hex, fix, rootwork); symptoms often associated with eating Believe serious illness sent by God as punishment God's punishment for violations of his will Widely accept "hot" and "cold" balance and imbalance as causes of health and illness	Self-care and folk medicine prevalent Folk therapies usually religious in origin Attempt home remedies first; poorer people do not seek help until illness is serious Prayer is common means for prevention and treatment	Strong kinship bonds in extended family; members come to aid others in crisis Less likely to view illness as a burden Sex-role sharing among parents Personal interests are subordinate to family interests and needs Members avoid any behavior that would bring shame on the family	Alert to any evidence of discrimination Place importance on nonverbal behavior May use nonstandard English or "Black English" Use "testing" behaviors to assess personnel in health care situations before seeking active care	High levels of caution and distrust of majority group Social anxiety related to tradition of humiliation, oppression, and loss of dignity Will elect to retain dignity rather than seek care if values are compromised Strong sense of peoplehood Minister a strong influence in African-American community

	(e.g., parents punished by illness or death of child) Believe serious illness can be avoided May resist health care because illness is "will of God"			Visits by family minister are sought, expected, and valued in helping to cope with illness and suffering
Haitian	Illness has supernatural or natural origin Supernatural illnesses are caused by angry voodoo spirits, enemies, or the dead, especially ancestors Natural illnesses based on conceptions of natural causes: Irregularities in blood Movement and consistency of mother's milk Hot/cold imbalance in the body Health is maintained by good dietary and hygienic habits	Health is a personal responsibility Food has properties of "hot"/"cold" and "light"/"heavy" and must be in harmony with one's life cycle and bodily states Natural illnesses are treated by home remedies first Supernatural illnesses are treated by healers: voodoo priest (*houngan*) or priestess (*mambo*), midwife (*fam saj*), and herbalist or leaf doctor (*dokte fey*)	Maintenance of family reputation is paramount Lineal authority supreme; children in a subordinate position in family hierarchy Children valued for parental social security in old age and expected to contribute to family welfare at an early age Children viewed as "gifts from god" and treated with indulgence and affection	Recent immigrants and older persons may speak only Haitian Creole May prefer family/friends to act as translators and confidants Often smile and nod in agreement when do not understand Quiet and gentle communication style and lack of assertiveness may lead health care providers to believe wrongly that they comprehend health teaching and are compliant	Will use biomedical and ethnomedical (folk) systems simultaneously Adherence to prescribed treatments directly related to perceived severity of illness

Continued

CULTURAL CONSIDERATIONS

6

TABLE 6-2

CULTURAL CHARACTERISTICS RELATED TO NEWBORN CARE—cont'd

Cultural Group	Health Beliefs	Health and Diet Practices	Family Relationships	Communication	Comments
Hispanic-American Mexican-American (Latino, Chicano, Raza-Latino)	Health beliefs have strong religious association Believe in body imbalance as a cause of illness, especially imbalance between *callente* (hot) and *frio* (cold) or "wet" and "dry" Some maintain good health is a result of "good luck"—a reward for good behavior Illness is a punishment from God for wrongdoing, forces of nature, and the supernatural	Amulets and prayer used to protect against illness caused by curses or willed by evil people Treatments involve use of herbs, rituals, and religious artifacts; visit shrines, offer medals and candles, offer prayers Adhere to "hot" and "cold" food prescriptions and prohibitions for prevention and treatment of illness	Traditionally men considered breadwinners, women homemakers Males are considered big and strong (*macho*) Strong kinship; extended families include *compadres* (godparents) established by ritual kinship Children valued highly and desired	Will not ask questions if health care provider is busy or rushed May use nonstandard English Most bilingual; may speak only Spanish May have a strong preference for native language and revert to it in times of stress	High degree of modesty—often a deterrent to seeking medical care Magicoreligious practices common

Puerto Rican	Subscribe to the "hot-cold" theory of causation of illness Believe some illness caused by evil spirits and forces	Infrequent use of health care systems Seek folk healers—use of herbs, rituals Treatment classified as "hot" or "cold"	Family usually large and home centered—the core of existence Father has complete authority in family—family provider and decision maker Wife and children subordinate to father Children valued—seen as a gift from God Strong family ties with mother and father kinship	May use nonstandard English Spanish speaking or bilingual Strong sense of family privacy—may view questions regarding family as impudent	Relaxed sense of time Pay little attention to exact time of day Suspicious and fearful of the hospital
Cuban American	Prevention and good nutrition are related to good health	Diligent users of the medical model Eclectic health-seeking practices, including preventive measures and, in some instances, folk medicine of both religious and nonreligious origins; in many instances seek assistance of *santeros* (Afro-Cuban healers) and spiritualists to complement medical treatment		Most are bilingual (English/Spanish) except for segments of the senior population	In less than 30 years Cubans have been able to obtain a higher standard of living than other Hispanic groups in the United States Have been able to retain many of their former social institutions Many do not feel discriminated against or harbor feelings of inferiority with respect to Anglo-Americans or the "mainstream" population

Continued

CULTURAL CONSIDERATIONS

TABLE 6-2

CULTURAL CHARACTERISTICS RELATED TO NEWBORN CARE—cont'd

Cultural Group	Health Beliefs	Health and Diet Practices	Family Relationships	Communication	Comments
Native American (numerous tribes)	Believe health is state of harmony with nature and universe Respect of bodies through proper management All disorders believed to have aspects of the supernatural Violation of a restriction or prohibition believed to cause illness Fear of witchcraft May carry objects believed to guard against witchcraft	Nutrition is important; parents show over-concern with eating habits of their children Medicine persons: altruistic persons who must use powers in purely positive ways Persons capable of both good and evil—perform negative acts against enemies Diviner-diagnosticians—diagnose but do not have powers or skills to implement medical treatment Specialist—use herbs and curative but nonsacred medical procedures	Extended family structure—usually includes relatives from both sides of family Elder members assume leadership roles	Most speak both their own language and English Nonverbal communication important	Time orientation—present Respect for age Going to hospital associated with illness or disease; therefore may not seek prenatal care because pregnancy viewed as natural process

Theology and medicine
strongly interwoven

Medicine persons—
use herbs and ritual

Singers—cure by the
power of their song
obtained from
supernatural beings,
effect cures by laying
on of hands

Modified from Wong DL: *Whaley & Wong's Nursing Care of Infants and Children*, ed 3. St Louis, Mosby, 1995.

*Most Asian cultures consider the child 1 year old at the time of birth. Traditional Chinese custom adds 1 year on January 1 regardless of the birthday—a child born in December is 2 years old the following January.

CULTURAL CONSIDERATIONS

6

Pain and the Control of Pain

Henry M. Seidel

7

Pain, a reaction to some degree of actual or anticipated damage to tissue (and, many would argue, to the psyche), is unpleasant emotionally and physically. It is no longer disputed that newborns are exquisitely sensate creatures. Their potential for pain should never be ignored and it is no longer acceptable to subject them to a painful experience without conscientious attempts to ameliorate it.

The nervous system is competent to perceive pain by 26 weeks of gestation and probably sooner. There is also evidence that painful experience is remembered even by infants. Berde and Sethna in one study and Taddio and her colleagues in an earlier one, for example, reported that infant boys circumcised without analgesia react more distressfully to their routine immunizations than those who have had the advantage of a topical local anesthetic.

Circumcision is but one of the following painful experiences imposed on healthy—as well as sick—newborns by regulatory requirement, the need to evaluate suspected illness, the advice of physicians, or religious practice:

- Venipuncture
- Heel sticks
- Lumbar puncture
- Necessary surgical procedures
- A variety of other possible manipulations

Newborns have visible, easily observed reactions to pain as manifested by

- Facial expression (tightly shut eyes, wide open mouth, wrinkled brow, quivering chin)
- Crying (often high-pitched and shrill)
- Bodily activity (hypertonicity)
- Wakefulness (disturbed sleep, fussy, even thrashing)
- Consolability (not so easy)
- Feeding difficulty (unable to suck well or at all)

Many investigators have used these observations to develop pain scales so that a permanent record might be available. Such efforts have value but there is a caveat in the subjective quality of individual assessments. Nevertheless, we offer one example for your consideration (see **Table 5-12**). Approaches to the alleviation of pain:

- Regional anesthesia with nerve block and local infiltration (e.g., with 1% or 2% lidocaine or 0.25% or 0.5% bupivacaine, without epinephrine)—the preferred approach with circumcision
- Local anesthesia with a eutectic cream (e.g., such as EMLA)—helpful, not as good as regional block with circumcision; probably helpful with less invasive procedures but not as helpful as sucrose pacifiers
- Acetaminophen—effective, perhaps, postoperatively, not so effective during circumcision; questionable at best for heel sticks, lumbar puncture, and similar procedures

- Oral sucrose pacifiers (25% sucrose; 12% no more effective than water)—helpful but no substitute for regional anesthesia with circumcision; a safe and effective intervention for heel sticks and similar invasions.

Note: The pacifier must be sucked; sugar by nasogastric tube is ineffective.

A variety of other approaches to pain relief have been studied, some of them time honored, e.g., maternal cuddling and rocking, breast-feeding, pacifiers; some of them more recently employed are music therapy, padded circumcision chairs; the use of various approaches in tandem. They may be helpful but we see no evidence to support their use in preference to regional anesthesia for circumcision or for sucrose pacifiers for heel sticks, etc. There is no objection to using them as supplements.

BIBLIOGRAPHY

Berde CB, Sethna NF: Analgesics for the treatment of pain in children. N Engl J Med 347:1094, 2002.

Hebry PR, Haubold K, Dobrzykowski TM: Pain in the healthy full-term neonate: Efficacy and safety of interventions. Newborn and Infant Nursing Reviews 4(2):106, 2004.

Porter FL, Wolf CM, Gold J, et al: Pain and pain management in newborn infants: A survey of physicians and nurses. Pediatrics 100:626, 1997.

Porter FL, Wolf CM, Miller JP: The effect of handling and immobilization on the response to acute pain in newborn infants. Pediatrics 102:1383, 1998.

Ramenghi LA, Evans DJ, Levene MI: Sucrose analgesia: Absorptive mechanism or taste perception. Arch Dis Child Neonatal Ed 80:F146, 1999.

Solodiuk J, Curley MAQ: Pain assessment in nonverbal children: The individualized numeric rating scale (INRS). J Pediatr Nursing 18:295, 2003.

Stevens B, Johnson CC: Pain in the infant: Theoretical and conceptual issues. Maternal-Child Nursing J 21:3, 1993.

Stevens B, Johnson CC, Tadio A: Premature infant pain profile: Development and initial validation. Clin J Pain 12:13, 1996.

Strauss SG, Lynn AM, Spear RM: Progress in pain control for very young infants. Contemp Pediatr 12:80, 1995.

Tadio A, Katz J, Hersich AL, Koren G: Effect of neonatal circumcision on pain response during routine vaccination. Lancet 349:599, 1997.

Wolf AR: Pain, nociception and the developing infant. Paediatr Anaesth 9:7, 1999.

Transitional Period: The First 6 Hours of Adaptation from Intrauterine to Extrauterine Life

Patricia H. Smouse

8

I. DEFINITION

A. COMPLEX PROCESS OF PHYSIOLOGIC ADJUSTMENTS.

1. Changes in function of organ systems.
a. Onset of respiration.
b. Change from fetal to neonatal circulation.
c. Change of hepatic and renal function.
d. Clearance of meconium from bowel.
2. Reorganization of metabolic processes.

B. PATTERNS OF ACTIVITY.

1. Normal transition (Fig. 8-1).
a. Period of reactivity: Initial 15 minutes of life.
   (1) Spontaneous startle reactions.
   (2) Tremors.
   (3) Crying.
   (4) Increased motor activity.
   (5) Excellent time for initial feeding and bonding.
b. Second stage: Next 60 to 90 minutes of life.
   (1) Marked decrease in motor activity.
   (2) Neurologic component of maturation assessments examination may be affected by marked hypotonia.
c. Second period of reactivity: Approximately 2 to 6 hours after birth, lasting 10 minutes to several hours.
2. **Abnormal transition: Although variability may be seen in aforementioned stages, certain findings require further evaluation, workup, and possibly treatment.**
a. Respiratory: Rule out pneumonia, respiratory distress syndrome, transient tachypnea of the newborn, sepsis, pneumothorax, congenital heart disease, polycythemia.
   (1) Respiratory rate >100, or >70 after the first 8 hours (placing infant in prone position may cause mild respiratory distress).
   (2) Respirations accompanied by grunting, flaring, retractions after first 2 hours of life.
   (3) Central cyanosis after first 5 minutes.

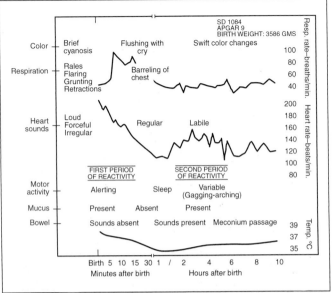

FIG. 8-1

A summary of the physical findings noted during the first 10 hours of extrauterine life in a representative infant with high Apgar score delivered under spinal anesthesia without prior medications. *(From Desmond MM, Rudolf AJ, Phitaksphraiwan P: Pediatr Clin North Am 13:656, 1966.)*

   b. Neurologic: Rule out sepsis, maternal drug abuse, maternal medication administration during labor or pregnancy (including magnesium sulfate), neuromuscular disorder, chromosomal anomaly, hypoglycemia, polycythemia.

     (1) Inability of a term infant to suck.

     (2) Extreme or persistent jitteriness or hypertonia.

     (3) Extreme or persistent hypotonia.

II. NEWBORN ASSESSMENT

A. EVALUATION IN DELIVERY ROOM.

1. Brief assessment of condition of newborn.
2. Determine appropriate level of care.
3. Communicate with parents.

B. CLASSIFICATION BY GESTATIONAL AGE AND INTRAUTERINE GROWTH.

1. Recommended by the American Academy of Pediatrics (AAP) for all newborns.

2. Used to anticipate needs, clinical course, and outcome.
3. Terms.
a. Appropriate for gestational age (AGA).
b. Small for gestational age (SGA).
c. Large for gestational age (LGA).
d. Preterm (<37 weeks).
e. Term (37 to 42 weeks).
f. Post-term (>42 weeks).
4. Methods of newborn gestational age assessment (used to confirm or supplement obstetric dating).
a. Performed on every neonate soon after birth.
b. Scoring systems.
   (1) New Ballard Score (**Fig. 8-2**). Revised to include extremely preterm infants based on six neuromuscular and six physical criteria which when added correspond to a gestational age. Accurate within 2 weeks.
   (2) Rapid assessment. (**Fig. 8-3**). Accuracy in descending order of significance: creases on sole of foot, size of breast nodule, consistency of scalp hair, firmness of ear cartilage, scrotal rugae, and testicular descent.
c. Determine relationship of birth weight to gestational age by plotting on a birth weight-gestational age chart appropriate to the population (**Fig. 8-4**).

C. SGA INFANT. WEIGHT <10TH PERCENTILE FOR ESTIMATED GESTATIONAL AGE.

1. Associated with a higher morbidity and mortality rate than a preterm infant of comparable weight.
2. Symmetrical growth retardation versus asymmetrical growth retardation.
a. Symmetrical growth retardation.
   (1) Proportionately small infant (head, weight, and length <10th percentile).
   (2) Represents slow growth rate beginning early in the pregnancy.
   (3) More likely to represent severe genetic constraints on growth, a dysmorphic syndrome, or congenital infection (e.g., TORCH syndrome).
   (4) Constitutionally small infant.
b. Asymmetrical growth retardation.
   (1) Greatest reductions are in weight and length with relative sparing of head circumference.
   (2) Newborn appears wasted and malnourished.
   (3) Usually the result of an extrinsic influence on the fetus later in gestation when growth is usually rapid.
   (4) Seen with multiple-gestation pregnancies, pregnancy-induced hypertension, placental insufficiency, in utero drug exposure (including tobacco).

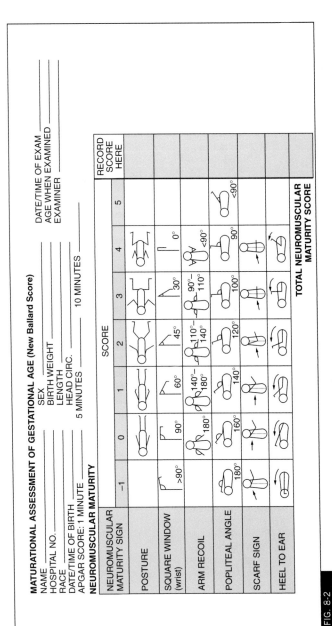

FIG. 8-2

Maturational assessment of gestational age (New Ballard Score).

PHYSICAL MATURITY

PHYSICAL MATURITY SIGN	-1	0	1	2	3	4	5	RECORD SCORE HERE
SKIN	sticky friable transparent	gelatinous red translucent	smooth pink visible veins	superficial peeling and/or rash, few veins	cracking pale areas rare veins	parchment deep cracking no vessels	leathery cracked wrinkled	
LANUGO	none	sparse	abundant	thinning	bald areas	mostly bald		
PLANTAR SURFACE	heel-toe 40–50 mm−1 <40 mm−2	>50 mm no crease	faint red marks	anterior transverse crease only	crease ant. 2/3	creases over entire sole		
BREAST	imperceptible	barely perceptible	flat areola no bud	stippled areola 1–2 mm bud	raised areola 3–4 mm bud	full areola 5–10 mm bud		
EYE-EAR	lids fused loosely −1 tightly −2	lids open pinna flat stays folded	st. curved pinna; soft slow recoil	well-curved pinna; soft but ready recoil	formed and firm instant recoil	thick cartilage ear stiff		
GENITALS (Male)	scrotum flat smooth	scrotum empty faint rugae	testes in upper canal rare rugae	testes descending few rugae	testes down good rugae	testes pendulous deep rugae		
GENITALS (Female)	clitoris prominent and labia flat	prominent clitoris and small labia minora	prominent clitoris and enlarging minora	majora and minora equally prominent	majora large minora small	majora cover clitoris and minora		

TOTAL PHYSICAL MATURITY SCORE

SCORE
Neuromuscular _____
Physical _____
Total _____

MATURITY RATING

Score	Weeks
-10	20
-5	22
0	24
5	26
10	28
15	30
20	32
25	34
30	36
35	38
40	40
45	42
50	44

GESTATIONAL AGE (weeks)
By dates _____
By ultrasound _____
By exam _____

FIG. 8-2—cont'd

8

TRANSITIONAL PERIOD

Evaluation		Approximate week of gestation when findings appear							
Evaluation		24	28	30	32	34	36	38	40
Head circumference in cm ± 2 SD		Clinical	23–28.3	25–30.4	26.8–32.4	28.6–34	30.5–35.5	32–36.5	33–37
Clinical	Sole creases		Anterior transverse crease only →				Occasional creases anterior two thirds →		Sole covered with creases →
Clinical	Breast nodule diameter		Not palpable – absent →				2 mm →	4 mm →	7 mm →
Clinical	Scalp hair	Fine and fuzzy → Hard to distinguish individual strands						Thick and silky → Appears as individual strands	
Clinical	Earlobe		Pliable – no cartilage →				Some cartilage →		Stiffened by thick cartilage →
Clinical	Testes and scrotum		Testes in lower canal Scrotum small – few rugae →				Interme-diate →	Testes pendulous, scrotum full, extensive rugae →	

From Behrman RE, et al.: Adv Pediatr 17:13F55, 1970.

FIG. 8-3
Estimation of gestational age.

CLASSIFICATION OF NEWBORNS (BOTH SEXES)
BY INTRAUTERINE GROWTH AND GESTATIONAL AGE

NAME _____ DATE OF EXAM _____ LENGTH _____

HOSPITAL NO. _____ SEX _____ HEAD CIRC. _____

RACE _____ BIRTH WEIGHT _____ GESTATIONAL AGE _____

DATE OF BIRTH _____

Continued

FIG. 8-4
Classification of newborns (both sexes) by intrauterine growth and gestational age.

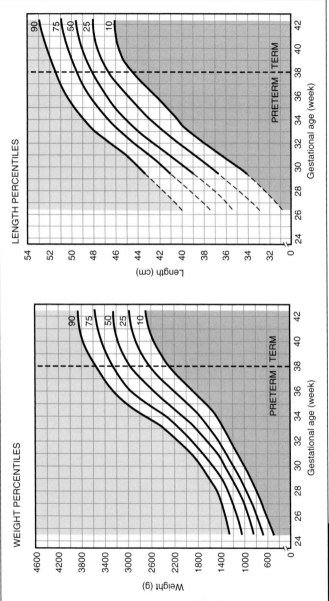

FIG. 8-4—cont'd

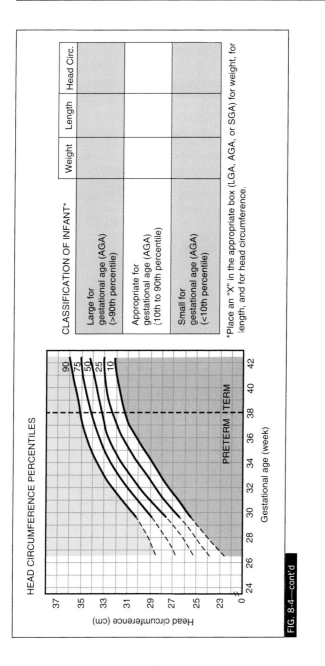

FIG. 8-4—cont'd

3. Clinical problems associated with SGA.
a. Asphyxia and intrauterine distress.
b. Respiratory distress.
c. Persistent fetal circulation.
d. Hypoglycemia.
e. Hypothermia.
f. Polycythemia.
g. Congenital malformations.

D. LGA INFANT. WEIGHT >90TH PERCENTILE FOR ESTIMATED GESTATIONAL AGE.
1. Etiology.
a. Infants of diabetic mothers (except mothers with advanced disease).
b. Genetic predisposition (large parents).
c. Beckwith-Wiedemann syndrome.
d. Constitutionally large infants.
2. Clinical problems associated with LGA.
a. Birth injuries.
   (1) Fractured clavicle.
   (2) Brachial plexus injury.
   (3) Facial palsy.
b. Hypoglycemia.
c. Polycythemia.

III. INITIAL MANAGEMENT

A. AVOID SEPARATION OF MOTHER AND NEWBORN WHENEVER POSSIBLE.
B. TEMPERATURE HOMEOSTASIS: ESSENTIAL FOR STABILIZATION AFTER DELIVERY (ESPECIALLY IN PRETERM AND SGA INFANTS).
1. Importance of heat balance.
a. Decrease metabolic and oxygen requirements.
b. Essential for stabilization after delivery.
2. Monitoring temperature in the newborn.
a. Rectal temperature should be checked within first hour of life (normal is 36.5° to 37.5° C).
b. Axillary temperature should be monitored thereafter (normal is 36.5° to 37.4° C).
c. If axillary temperature is subsequently abnormal, rectal temperature should be taken to confirm temperature.
d. Infant should be maintained, until stable, under a radiant warmer with the servo control mode set at 36.5° to 37.0° C.
e. An abnormal body temperature may not be an indicator of thermal stress but of the inability of the baby to adequately compensate.
3. Hypothermia (assists in the initiation of neonatal breathing but if prolonged is dangerous).
a. Etiology.
   (1) Large amounts of evaporative heat loss.

      (2) Increased surface area/body mass ratio.

      (3) Decreased subcutaneous tissue.

      (4) Sepsis.

  b. Risk situations.

      (1) Preterm and SGA infants.

      (2) Air-conditioned labor and recovery rooms.

      (3) Inadequate or delayed drying and warming after delivery.

  c. Neonatal response.

      (1) Nonshivering thermogenesis.

      (2) Hypoxemia.

      (3) Metabolic acidosis.

      (4) Depletion of glycogen stores.

      (5) Reduction of blood glucose levels.

      (6) Increased oxygen consumption.

  d. Prevention and treatment.

      (1) Placing under preheated radiant warmer.

      (2) Rapid drying with prewarmed towels.

      (3) Covering the head with a cap.

      (4) Maintain rectal temperature between $36.5°$ and $37.0°$ C.

      (5) Skin-to-skin contact with the mother or wrapping in prewarmed towels and holding by mother may be substituted in a term infant if infant and mother are stable.

      (6) After initial stability is determined, the infant may be bathed and then closely monitored for temperature instability for another hour.

      (7) Normal newborn may then be dressed, swaddled, and placed in an open bassinet.

      (8) Preterm, SGA, and unstable infants should be maintained undressed in a radiant warmer with temperature servoregulation (see **Appendix G**).

4. Hyperthermia.

  a. Etiology.

      (1) Impaired ability to sweat in response to environmental temperatures.

      (2) Sepsis.

      (3) Maternal fever at delivery.

      (4) Over bundling or over warming.

  b. Risk situations.

      (1) Maternal fever.

      (2) Prolonged resuscitation under warmer.

      (3) Lack of proper probe placement while infant is under radiant warmer or in isolette.

  c. Neonatal response.

      (1) Hypernatremia.

      (2) Volume depletion.

      (3) Increased metabolic demands.

      (4) Apnea.

  d. Prevention and treatment.

      (1) Tape the thermometer probe securely to the anterior abdominal wall with the infant in the supine position.

(2) Treat hyperthermia (skin temperature 37.5° to 39.0° C) by undressing the neonate and exposing to room temperature.

C. MONITORING.

1. Temperature, pulse, and respirations every 15 minutes for first hour or until stable.
2. Measurement of temperature, pulse, and respirations should continue every hour for 4 hours, then every 8 hours if stable.
3. Note changes in respiratory status, color, tone, mucus production, meconium passage (see Appendix G), first void (see Table G-1).

D. SCREENING TESTS.

1. Hematocrit/hemoglobin.
   a. Normal range for a hematocrit level in a full-term neonate is 45% to 65%.
   b. Normal range for a hemoglobin level in a full-term neonate is 15 to 22 g/dl.
   c. If obtaining a heel-stick measurement and infant is stable, obtain blood at about 4 hours of age when peripheral blood flow is improved (capillary hemoglobin exceeds venous level by about 3.6 g in the first week of life).
   d. Indications for testing: Perinatal asphyxia, respiratory distress, pallor, plethora, twins, infant of diabetic mother, SGA, uncontrolled delivery.
2. Blood glucose.
   a. Normal range is 40 to 130 mg/dl.
   b. Indications for screening: SGA, LGA, prematurity, infant of diabetic mother, twins, perinatal asphyxia, poor feeding, plethora.
3. Blood type and Coombs test should be considered under the following circumstances:
   a. If mother is Rh negative, to determine the need for maternal RhoGAM administration.
   b. If mother is O, to rule out ABO incompatibility; this is especially important in conjunction with early discharge policy.
   c. If the maternal blood type is unknown, to rule out Rh incompatibility.
4. Rapid plasma reagin (RPR) or serologic test for syphilis (STS) of mother at delivery.
   a. Most accurate screen for congenital syphilis is serial testing of mother prenatally and again at delivery.
   b. Cord blood and neonatal serum may not be as sensitive as maternal serum.
5. Human immunodeficiency virus (HIV).
   a. AAP recommends routine counseling and testing for all pregnant women in the U.S.
   b. If not determined prenatally, mother should be informed of the potential benefits of HIV testing for the newborn and immediate HIV testing is recommended.

c. Should be performed on a baby to be placed for adoption when maternal status is unknown.

6. Urine toxicology test on first available void.

a. Unregistered or high-risk pregnancy.

b. To confirm clinical suggestion of in utero drug exposure.

E. PROPHYLAXIS.

1. Eye prophylaxis.

a. Purpose is prevention of neonatal gonococcal infection.

b. Current recommendation is routine administration of one of the following to all newborns within the first hour of life:

   (1) Erythromycin, 0.5% ophthalmic ointment or drops in single-dose tube or ampule instilled in each eye.

   (2) 1% silver nitrate solution in single-dose ampule (associated with high incidence of chemical conjunctivitis).

   (3) Tetracycline, 1% ophthalmic ointment or drops in single-dose ampule.

   Note: *All of the aforementioned agents are equally effective in the prevention of gonococcal infection but do not prevent chlamydial eye infection.*

c. Infant born to mother with known gonococcal infection.

   (1) When prophylaxis is administered correctly infant should be adequately protected.

   (2) Current recommendation, however, is to administer a single dose of ceftriaxone, 125 mg intravenously or intramuscularly; for low-birth-weight infants, the dose is 25 to 50 mg/kg.

2. Vitamin K_1 administration.

a. Purpose of prophylaxis: To prevent hemorrhagic disease of the newborn.

   (1) Infants develop vitamin K deficiency by day 2 to 3 of life if supplement is not given at birth.

   (2) Maternal drugs that interfere with vitamin K synthesis: Phenytoin (Dilantin), phenobarbital, salicylates.

   (3) One recommended policy is to double the dose of vitamin K_1 for infants of mothers on anticonvulsant therapy.

b. Standard recommended dose: Single intramuscular dose of 0.5 to 1.0 mg phytonadione (vitamin K_1) in the anterolateral thigh to all newborns within one hour of birth.

3. Hepatitis B vaccine and hepatitis B immunoglobulin (see Chapter 22 and Table 22-3).

F. INITIAL FEEDING.

1. Timing.

a. Healthy term and near term infants should be breast- or bottle-fed within 1 hour after delivery.

b. Benefits of early feeding.

   (1) Maintain normal metabolism during transition to extrauterine life.

   (2) Decrease incidence of hyperbilirubinemia in breast-fed infants.

(3) Decrease incidence of hypoglycemia.

(4) Decrease incidence of dehydration.

(5) Early onset of breast-feeding may contribute to breast-feeding success.

2. What to feed?

a. Breast milk (preferred feeding choice for term, preterm, and sick infants).

b. Standard infant formula with iron.

c. Premature formula <36 weeks (lower osmolality, higher vitamin and mineral concentrations). Promotes growth at intrauterine rates.

d. Sterile water, 5% dextrose water and 10% dextrose water should be avoided as initial feeds.

3. Technique.

a. Breast-feed or bottle feed.

(1) Stable respiratory status.

(2) >34 weeks with good suck-swallow coordination.

b. Gavage.

(1) Poor suck-swallow coordination.

(2) Severe SGA.

(3) <34 weeks.

(4) Respiratory rate 60-80/minute (gavage contraindicated if respiratory rate >80/minute).

4. Frequency/amount.

a. Healthy full-term infant.

(1) Breast-fed infants should nurse within an hour after birth and then on demand (avoid rigid feeding schedules); frequent feedings, 8 to 12 feedings per day, should be encouraged to help establish maternal milk supply, prevent engorgement, and decrease neonatal jaundice.

(2) Formula-fed infants should also feed within an hour after birth and then on demand every 3 to 5 hours and should progress rapidly from about 30 ml every feed to full feeds (120 kcal/kg per day) by 3 to 5 days of life.

b. Slightly preterm and near term breast-fed infants may require formula supplementation to maintain adequate glucose levels.

c. Infants <2500 grams require more careful consideration of fluid and caloric requirements based on weight, stability, and risk for necrotizing enterocolitis (NEC) which would preclude early enteral feeds.

G. SKIN CARE.

1. Bathing.

a. After stabilization.

b. Nonmedicated soap may be used to remove blood and meconium.

c. Vernix caseosa need not be removed.

d. Cleanse skin abrasions (including scalp electrode sites) carefully with an antiseptic such as Betadine.

2. Cord care.

a. No single procedure is recommended to prevent colonization or subsequent infection.

b. Currently acceptable method is initial application of triple dye or antibiotic ointment followed by regular application of alcohol with every diaper change.

c. An alternative is to leave the cord dry and to spot clean the periumbilical area whenever it becomes soiled.

H. INDICATIONS FOR ISOLETTE USE.

1. Temperature regulation of the preterm or cold-stressed infant.
2. Reverse isolation for infant.
3. Facilitate observation of the high-risk or unstable infant.
4. Kangaroo Mother Care (KMC): Safe alternative to isolette for small, stable infants.

a. Mothers are used as "incubators" and main source of food and stimulation.

b. Babies are kept 24 hours a day in strict upright position, skin-skin contact, firmly attached to mother's chest.

c. Advantages include mother-infant bonding and reduction in number of hospital days without compromising growth of infant.

BIBLIOGRAPHY

American Academy of Pediatrics and American College of Obstetricians and Gynecologists; Guidelines for Perinatal Care, ed 5, Elk Grove Village, Ill and Washington, DC, 2002, AAP and ACOG.

American Academy of Pediatrics: 2003 Redbook: Report of the Committee on Infectious Diseases, ed 25, Elk Grove Village, Ill, American Academy of Pediatrics.

Ballard JL, Khoury JC, Wedig K, et al: New Ballard score, expanded to include extremely premature infants. J Pediatr 119:417, 1991.

Charpak N, Ruiz-Pelacz JR: Kangaroo mother versus traditional care for new infants ≤2000 grams: A randomized, controlled trial, Pediatrics 100:682, 1997.

Cheng TL, Partridge JC: Effect of bundling and high environmental temperature on neonatal body temperature. Pediatrics 92:238, 1993.

Chhabra RS, Brion LP, Castro M, et al: Comparison of maternal sera, cord blood, and neonatal sera for detecting presumptive congenital syphilis: Relationship with maternal treatment. Pediatrics 91:88, 1993.

Donn SM: The Michigan Manual. Mount Kisco, NY, Futura, 1992.

Gomella TL: Neonatology: Management, procedures, on-call problems, diseases and drugs, ed 5, McGraw-Hill, 2004.

Klaus MH, Fanaroff AA: Care of the high-risk neonate. Philadelphia, WB Saunders, 2001.

Lubchenco LO: Classification of high risk infants by birth weight and gestational age: An overview. Major Probl Clin Pediatr 14:1, 1976.

Lubchenco LO, Hansman C, Boyd E: Intrauterine growth in length and head circumference as estimated from live births at gestational ages 26 to 42 weeks. Pediatrics 37:403, 1966.

The Head

Beryl J. Rosenstein

FAST FACTS

Immediate Issues in the Nursery

- For infants born with head circumference above the 98th percentile, immediate attention should focus on looking for evidence of bleeding (external or internal from birth trauma), hydrocephalus (congenital lesions), or phenotypic dysmorphisms (suggestive of an associated syndrome).
- A head circumference below the third percentile is almost always associated with delayed brain growth and development.
- Defects of the sagittal suture are the most common type of craniosynostosis and occur in a 4:1 male to female predominance.
- Serial measurement of head circumference is vital in determining the cause and clinical significance of macrocephaly.
- Signs of increased intracranial pressure include distended scalp veins, widened cranial sutures, large/bulging fontanels, vomiting, irritability, and lethargy.

Important Reminders After Discharge

- Unless increased intracranial pressure exists, the optimal time to repair craniosynostosis is between 3 and 6 months of age.
- Natal teeth should be evaluated by x-rays to assess root development and to differentiate supernumerary from prematurely erupted deciduous teeth.
- A third "fontanel" is seen occasionally just in front of the posterior fontanel. It is more common in preterm infants. It may be associated with Down syndrome or minor congenital anomalies.

Helpful Information for Parents

- Surgical treatment of craniosynostosis is mainly cosmetic, except if multiple suture lines are involved or if there is increased intracranial pressure.
- Microcephaly (head circumference less than the third percentile) is correlated with low IQ scores.
- In most cases, the size and shape of a newborn's head are determined by birth-related factors and genetics. Family history is important in the assessment of head appearance.
- The "Back to Sleep" campaign has resulted in more babies with flattening of the occiput and positional plagiocephaly. Parents should be instructed to turn their infant's heads to the side for sleeping. Alternating of head position (e.g., head to the left on odd dates and to the right on even dates) along with encouraged belly time while awake can help reduce the degree to which the head is flattened.

I. EVALUATION

A. ATTENTION SHOULD BE PAID TO THE SIZE AND CONFIGURATION OF THE HEAD.

Look for ridging or separation of sutures, size of the fontanels, skull defects, asymmetry, and softening. Head size, measured by maximum occipitofrontal head circumference, and the size of the fontanels should be compared with appropriate standards. Serial head circumference measurements are more important than any single value.

Note: *Occipitofrontal circumference may not be a valid measure in a newborn with an abnormally shaped head (e.g., craniosynostosis).*

B. EXAMINATION SHOULD INCLUDE THE FOLLOWING:

1. Percussion: A hollow or "cracked-pot" sound will be heard over dilated ventricles.
2. Auscultation: A bruit can be heard with vascular lesions.
3. Transillumination: Will be positive with subdural hematoma, cortical atrophy, porencephaly, hydranencephaly.

C. IN A PATIENT WITH A LARGE OR ASYMMETRICAL HEAD, IT IS IMPORTANT TO LOOK FOR EVIDENCE OF INCREASED INTRACRANIAL PRESSURE, WHICH MAY INCLUDE THE FOLLOWING:

1. Distention of scalp veins.
2. Separation of cranial sutures (especially squamosal).
3. Enlargement and distention of fontanels.
4. Sixth-nerve palsy (rarely seen in the newborn period).
5. "Setting sun" eye findings.
6. Vomiting, irritability, lethargy.

Note: *Because of open sutures, however, signs of increased intracranial pressure, such as papilledema, are rarely seen in the newborn period.*

D. DIAGNOSTIC PROCEDURES THAT MAY BE HELPFUL

include skull x-rays, ultrasound, computed tomography (CT) with and without contrast medium, magnetic resonance imaging (MRI), cerebral angiography (rarely), and radionuclide bone scans.

II. FONTANELS

A. SIZE.

1. At birth, the anterior fontanel is highly variable in size and shape. Mean size (average of length plus width) is 2.1 cm; range is 0.6 to 3.6 cm in white newborns and 1.4 to 4.7 cm in African Americans. The average size of the posterior fontanel is 0.5 cm in white newborns and 0.7 cm in African Americans. The anterior fontanel tends to enlarge during the first postnatal month.

2. In otherwise normal infants, there is no correlation between the initial size of the anterior fontanel and the time of closure and head circumference.
3. In the upright position, there may be a slight pulsation of the fontanel.

B. LARGE ANTERIOR FONTANEL.

1. A nonbulging, large anterior fontanel may be seen in the following disorders:
   a. Achondroplasia.
   b. Apert syndrome.
   c. Cleidocranial dysostosis.
   d. Hypophosphatasia.
   e. Osteogenesis imperfecta.
   f. Pyknodysostosis (osteopetrosis, cranial and digital anomalies, dwarfism, frontal and occipital bossing).
   g. Kenny syndrome.
   h. Down syndrome.
   i. Trisomies 13 and 18.
   j. Hypothyroidism.
   k. Rubella syndrome.
   l. Russell-Silver syndrome.
   m. Intrauterine malnutrition.
   n. Hydrocephalus.
2. A large anterior fontanel with widened sutures (>1 cm) may be seen in normal newborns.
3. A large anterior fontanel may be associated with poor calcification of the cranium or delayed closure of the anterior fontanel, but normal head growth.
4. A bulging fontanel may be seen with infection, hydrocephalus, space-occupying lesions, and hypoxic-ischemic brain injury.

C. SMALL ANTERIOR FONTANEL.

1. A small or closed anterior fontanel does not always correlate with small head circumference.
2. With a cranium of normal size and shape and without ridging along sutures, a small anterior fontanel is usually of no significance.
3. A small anterior fontanel may be a normal variant or may be secondary to one of the following disorders:
   a. Primary microcephaly.
   b. Craniosynostosis (sagittal or coronal sutures).
   c. Hyperthyroidism.
   d. A wormian bone in the anterior fontanel.

D. THIRD FONTANEL.

1. A third fontanel is not a true fontanel, but is a bony defect of variable size situated along the sagittal suture, 2 cm anterior to the posterior fontanel. It ranges in size from 0.7 to 3.5 cm.

9

THE HEAD

2. A third fontanel is present in approximately 6% of neonates and occurs more often in preterm than in full-term infants.
3. A large third fontanel (>13 mm) is associated with minor congenital anomalies and is a common finding in infants with Down syndrome.

III. SKULL SOFTENING

Skull softening may be seen in a variety of conditions, including the following:

A. CLEIDOCRANIAL DYSOSTOSIS.
Complete or partial absence of the clavicles; large head with defective ossification.

B. CRANIOTABES.
1. Reduction in bone mineralization of the skull.
2. Most often occurs in the occipital and parietal bones along the lambdoidal sutures.
3. Usually of no clinical significance.

C. LACUNAR SKULL.
1. Defects in the inner table of the cranial vault.
2. Skull x-ray shows decreased densities described as "soap bubble" rarefactions.
3. May be associated with spina bifida or other central nervous system (CNS) abnormalities.

D. OSTEOGENESIS IMPERFECTA.

E. MULTIPLE WORMIAN BONES.
Small multiple bones that occur within sutures.

IV. LARGE HEAD

A large head is defined as an occipitofrontal circumference greater than 3 standard deviations above the mean or above the 98th percentile. Differential diagnosis includes the following:

A. BIRTH TRAUMA.
A large head may be secondary to cephalhematoma, subgaleal effusion, or caput succedaneum. These are usually obvious on physical examination and resolve spontaneously over days to weeks.

B. BENIGN FAMILIAL MACROCEPHALY.
1. The absolute head circumference is large, but serial measurements demonstrate a proportionate rate of growth; sutures and fontanels are normal; neurologic examination is normal.

2. This condition is often familial and inherited as an autosomal dominant trait. Determination of the head circumference of other family members (physical examination, photographs, hat size) may be helpful. Diagnosis may be suggested by prenatal ultrasound in association with appropriate family history.
3. May rarely be associated with underlying CNS structural or storage disease (megalocephaly), such as the following:
   a. Retardation, hypotonia, convulsions.
   b. Achondroplasia (may be associated with mildly to moderately dilated ventricles).
   c. Cerebral gigantism (Sotos syndrome).
   d. Beckwith-Wiedemann syndrome.
4. A normal CT scan is the definitive diagnostic test.

C. HYDROCEPHALUS.

1. Hydrocephalus is the most common cause of head enlargement in the newborn period (0.39 to 0.87 cases per 1000 births); congenital cases are more common than acquired cases (3:1).
2. Etiology.
   a. Congenital.
      (1) Aqueductal stenosis is the most common cause.
      (2) Dandy-Walker syndrome: Cystic dilation of the fourth ventricle, with defective development of the cerebellum. Associated malformations include capillary angioma, cardiac malformations, ophthalmic anomalies, agenesis of the corpus callosum, and occipital meningocele.
      (3) Arnold-Chiari malformation: Downward displacement of the cerebellar tonsils through the foramen magnum; downward displacement of the cervical cord; often seen with meningomyelocele.
      (4) Vein of Galen malformation: Dilated vein compresses aqueduct; a bruit can be heard over the vertex; cardiac failure.
      (5) Choroid plexus papilloma: Overproduction of cerebrospinal fluid (CSF).
      (6) Holoprosencephaly.
      (7) Hydranencephaly.
   b. Acquired.
      (1) Posthemorrhagic; usually secondary to intraventricular bleed or temporal lobe hematoma.
      (2) Inflammatory or postinflammatory; secondary to meningitis.
      (3) Toxoplasmosis.
   c. Syndromic.
      (1) Trisomies.
      (2) Craniosynostosis.
      (3) VACTERL association.
      (4) [illegible]
      (5) [illegible]

9

THE HEAD

3. Clinical manifestations.

a. There may be obvious head enlargement at birth or gradual enlargement; this may be the only manifestation in the newborn period.

b. Anorexia, vomiting, lethargy, hyperirritability.

c. Signs of increased intracranial pressure (rare in the newborn).

d. "Cracked-pot" sign on percussion over dilated ventricle.

4. Diagnosis.

a. Confirmed by CT studies with and without contrast medium.

b. MRI may help define anatomic abnormalities.

c. Ultrasound useful for serial assessment of ventricular size.

d. Cerebral angiography may be helpful in delineation of vascular lesions.

e. Transillumination is usually negative unless cerebral mantle is <1 cm.

f. Antenatal diagnosis can be made by ultrasound. If the fetus has progressive hydrocephalus and the biparietal diameter is >100 mm, delivery should be by elective cesarean section.

Note: *Fetal hydrocephalus occurs in 1 of 2000 pregnancies. Polyhydramnios occurs in about 30% of those pregnancies and is frequently the only sign of hydrocephalus. The presence of additional malformations is a poor prognostic sign. Prenatal cytogenetic studies are indicated, especially when there are associated abnormalities. The overall outcome is not good. Prenatal shunting procedures have shown no improvement over that expected from the natural history.*

5. Treatment.

a. Direct operative procedure (e.g., removal of congenital cyst).

b. Ventricular shunting procedure.

c. The role of acetazolamide and furosemide in neonatal posthemorrhagic ventricular dilation remains highly controversial.

d. Prognosis depends on the underlying etiology.

D. SUBDURAL COLLECTIONS.

1. Etiology.

a. Hematoma secondary to birth trauma or bleeding disorder.

b. Hygroma secondary to traumatic laceration of piarachnoid.

c. Effusion secondary to meningitis.

2. Clinical features.

a. Head enlargement with boxlike configuration and biparietal bossing.

b. Signs of increased intracranial pressure.

c. Positive transillumination.

d. Retinal hemorrhages with traumatic hematoma.

3. Diagnosis is by CT scan or ultrasound.

4. Treatment may include evacuation of blood and subdural shunting.

5. Prognosis depends on the following:

a. Nature and severity of the underlying problem.

b. Size, location, and duration of the lesion.

c. Success or failure of interventions.

E. INTRACRANIAL CYSTS AND TUMORS.

1. Tumors are exceedingly rare.
   a. Most commonly teratomas, followed by astrocytomas, neuroectodermal and choroid plexus tumors.
   b. Usually present with macrocephaly, signs of increased intracranial pressure or specific neurologic findings related to type and site of lesion.
   c. Some grow enormously in utero and can lead to fetal hydrops, polyhydramnios, dystocia, or stillbirth.
   d. Diagnosis can be made in utero or in the neonatal period by sonography, CT scan, or MRI.
   e. Outcome is related to size, location, type, and resectability, but is generally poor.

2. Hydranencephaly.
   a. Absence of cerebral hemispheres with intact dura, skull, and scalp.
   b. Large head, spasticity, seizures, lack of eye fusion.
   c. Diagnosis is by ultrasound or CT scan; on transillumination, islands of preserved cortical tissue are seen as small opacities.

3. Porencephaly.
   a. Abnormal CSF cavities within the cerebral hemispheres.
   b. Seizures, focal neurologic deficit, hydrocephalus, overlying cranial defects.
   c. Diagnosis is by ultrasound or CT scan; transillumination is locally positive.
   d. Treatment includes surgical removal or shunting of the cyst.

4. Miscellaneous.
   a. Neurofibromatosis.
   b. Bannayan syndrome (lipomatosis, angiomatosis, macrocephaly).

V. SMALL HEAD

A. A SMALL HEAD IS DEFINED AS AN OCCIPITOFRONTAL CIRCUMFERENCE GREATER THAN 3 STANDARD DEVIATIONS BELOW THE MEAN OR LESS THAN THE THIRD PERCENTILE.

1. It is always secondary to delayed brain growth and development.
2. Although microcephaly is significantly correlated with low IQ scores, the relationship is not absolute.

B. ETIOLOGY.

1. Intrauterine infection (rubella, cytomegalovirus [CMV], toxoplasmosis).
2. Chromosomal abnormalities: Trisomies 13, 18, 21; deletion syndromes (4, 5, 13).
3. Familial (Primary).
   a. Autosomal recessive
   b. Furrowed brow, backward sloping of the forehead, and small cranial volume.
4. In utero drug exposure (e.g., cocaine, tobacco, alcohol).
5. Intrauterine growth retardation (IUGR) secondary to malnutrition, hypertension, placental insufficiency.
6. Poorly controlled maternal phenylketonuria; aminoacidurias.

9

THE HEAD

7. Component of >500 syndromes, including the following:
   a. Rubinstein-Taybi.
   b. Smith-Lemli-Opitz.
   c. de Lange.
   d. Prader-Willi.
8. Perinatal infection (e.g., herpes simplex).
9. Intrapartum or neonatal hypoxic-ischemic insults.

C. DIAGNOSIS

is based on physical examination, serologic studies, family history, skull x-rays, neuroimaging studies, amino acid screening, and chromosome analysis.

D. THERE IS NO SPECIFIC THERAPY; PROGNOSIS DEPENDS ON THE UNDERLYING ETIOLOGY.

VI. ABNORMAL HEAD CONFIGURATION

A. FRONTAL BOSSING.

May be seen in achondroplasia, osteopetrosis, GM_1 gangliosidosis, and I-cell disease (lysosomal storage disease).

B. MOLDING.

1. Molding is a common finding secondary to the fetal head passing through the birth canal.
2. Molding usually consists of lengthening in the occipitofrontal diameter, flattening of the forehead, narrowing of the biparietal diameter, and protuberance of the occiput.
3. The configuration steadily improves over a period of several days.

C. CRANIOSYNOSTOSIS.

1. Premature closure of one or more of the cranial sutures. Because this usually occurs prenatally, a diagnosis can be made in the neonatal period. Affects approximately 1 in 2000 newborns. A single suture is involved in 80% of cases; multiple sutures are involved in 20%. There may be an increased incidence with breech positioning and with twins.
2. At birth, the cranial bones tend to override one another. Within hours to days the bones no longer override, definite sutures are established, and the edges of the flat bones are separated by fibrous tissue.
3. Growth normally occurs perpendicular to the line of the suture but is inhibited by the premature closure of the suture. The skull is forced to grow parallel to the fused suture, but additional growth abnormalities can occur throughout the calvarium. In infants with nonsyndromic craniosynostosis, there is no reduction in intracranial volume.
4. The final configuration of the head depends on the sutures involved. The deformity is greatest in the axial direction of the affected suture. Closure of one of the paired sutures results in flattening of the skull on that side.

5. Single-suture synostosis usually results only in cosmetic defect and does not impair brain growth; hydrocephalus is a rare event in cases of nonsyndromic craniosynostosis and never occurs in cases of single-suture synostosis other than by coincidence; in contrast, it is a relatively frequent finding in cases of syndromic craniosynostosis.

6. Etiology.
   a. Often unknown.
   b. May be secondary to developmental, mechanical, teratogenic (fetal hydantoin syndrome), metabolic, or genetic factors; a number of mutations in the fibroblast growth factor receptor family of genes have been identified.
   c. Is not related to abnormalities of brain growth, but may occur in association with CNS malformations.
   d. May occur as an isolated defect or (when multiple sutures are involved) as a component of a syndrome (e.g., Apert, Crouzon, Pfeiffer, Saethre-Chotzen).

7. Diagnosis.
   a. Physical findings: Irregular or asymmetrical skull; detection of an area where overriding sutures cannot be felt; inability to move the cranial bones in relation to one another; palpation of a bony ridge along the suture line; hypertelorism; difference in level or position of the eyes and ears.
   b. Careful funduscopic examination is needed to rule out optic atrophy, papilledema.

Note: *An open anterior fontanel does not rule out craniosynostosis.*

   c. Skull x-rays.
   d. Three-dimensional CT scan is useful in cases of complicated suture pathology, when the diagnosis is in question, to evaluate underlying brain abnormalities, and to rule out increased intracranial pressure.
   e. Affected neonates should be referred to a craniofacial center for a multidisciplinary evaluation.

8. Specific defects.
   a. Sagittal.
      (1) Sagittal defects are the most common type of defect seen (50% of cases); they occur in males more often than females (4:1); they may be familial and are rarely associated with other abnormalities.
      (2) Scaphocephaly, or "boat shaped"; increased anteroposterior length and decreased cranial width; neurologic examination and development are normal. The suture is usually ridged and quite long.
      (3) Plain-film x-rays confirm the diagnosis.
      (4) The head may assume a more normal shape over time without treatment.

Note: *Some cases occur in premature infants laid with their heads turned to the side ("NICUcephaly").*

9

THE HEAD

b. Coronal.
   (1) Coronal defects occur in females more often than males; unilateral and bilateral types occur with equal frequency; there is a familial incidence in 8% of cases.
   (2) Unilateral synostosis leads to flattening of the forehead on the side of the involved suture and contralateral forehead bossing (anterior plagiocephaly); there may be associated abnormalities in binocular eye movement.
   (3) Bilateral synostosis causes brachycephaly—a short head with expansion of the vertex and lateral aspects of the skull. It may be associated with retardation, developmental abnormalities, proptosis, and strabismus.
c. Metopic.
   (1) Trigonocephaly: Bullet-shaped configuration of the forehead with a prominent ridge in the midforehead region (frontal keel), narrow forehead, close-set eyes. A palpable, and often visible, ridge is present along part or all of the suture.
   (2) Plain-film x-rays confirm the diagnosis.
   (3) Most often an isolated finding, but may be associated with related anomalies of the limbs/digits, cleft palate, coloboma, genitourinary and cardiac anomalies, and holoprosencephaly; 5% of cases are familial.
   (4) May be associated with mental retardation, which is most likely related to associated CNS abnormalities.
d. Lambdoid.
   (1) True lambdoid synostosis is relatively rare (2% to 4% of all cases of craniosynostosis); occurs in males more often than in females.
   (2) Manifests as flattening of the occipital bone with compensatory bossing of the ipsilateral frontal region. In severe cases, the head may be shaped like a parallelogram.
   (3) Diagnosis is based on perisutural ridging and x-ray evidence of bony fusion.
   (4) In later infancy, it needs to be differentiated from positional (deformational) flattening, seen with increased frequency after the recommendation for supine sleeping position.
   (5) Most children with true lambdoid synostosis benefit from surgical correction.
e. Multiple synostoses.
   (1) Oxycephaly: The skull expands toward the vertex, resulting in a pointed, tower-shaped head.
   (2) May be associated with increased intracranial pressure, mental retardation, and neurologic complications.
   (3) Early surgery is almost always indicated.
9. Treatment.
a. Indications for treatment are cosmetic only, except when multiple sutures are involved or there is evidence of increased intracranial pressure or interference with binocular vision.
b. Optimum timing of surgery is 3 to 6 months of age; the only indication for surgical intervention in the neonatal period is to relieve intracranial pressure, which occurs in only a small percentage of affected children.

VII. ENCEPHALOCELE/MENINGOCELE

A. AN ENCEPHALOCELE REPRESENTS THE PROTRUSION OF A PORTION OF THE BRAIN AND MENINGES THROUGH A SKULL DEFECT.

B. IF ONLY THE MENINGES HERNIATE, THE LESION DEVELOPS INTO A MENINGOCELE.

The incidence is 1:5000 births; 75% occur in the occipital area, 25% in the frontal area. They are often associated with other congenital defects or associated CNS abnormalities. Hydrocephalus is a common problem in patients with large occipital encephaloceles.

C. AN ENCEPHALOCELE CAUSES A SOFT, FLUCTUANT, BALLOON-LIKE MASS THAT PROTRUDES FROM THE CRANIUM.

It may pulsate and may be covered by erythematous translucent or opaque material, or by normal skin; it may vary in size from 1 cm to two to three times the infant's head circumference.

D. DIAGNOSIS.

1. Plain-film x-rays show the associated skull defect.
2. Transillumination may be helpful.
3. CT scan, MRI, and ultrasound can define the anatomic defect and provide information on associated cerebral anomalies.
4. In many cases, the presence of a large convexity encephalocele is diagnosed prenatally based on an elevated alpha-fetoprotein level or abnormalities seen on in utero ultrasonograms.
5. A basal encephalocele may not be directly visible but may cause upper airway obstruction.

E. TREATMENT. WHENEVER POSSIBLE, SURGICAL REPAIR EARLY IN LIFE SHOULD BE PERFORMED.

F. PROGNOSIS.

1. The size of the sac is not a reliable predictor of functional outcome.
2. Meningoceles have a substantially better prognosis than encephaloceles. With encephaloceles, there may be significant mortality in the first day of life.
3. The finding of substantial brain tissue in the sac or association with an underlying syndrome (e.g., Meckel syndrome) is a poor prognostic sign.

VIII. CONGENITAL SCALP DEFECT (APLASIA CUTIS CONGENITA)

A. LOCALIZED AREA OF CONGENITAL ABSENCE OF SKIN, USUALLY AT THE VERTEX.

At birth, it usually manifests as a noninflammatory, sharply marginated hairless area, but it may appear ulcerated and crusted. There may be a surrounding area of hypertrichosis ("hair collar" sign). Over time the area epithelializes but remains devoid of hair. The underlying skull is usually intact, but the lesion may extend to the dura or meninges.

B. ETIOLOGY.

1. It may be inherited as an autosomal dominant (sometimes in association with limb abnormalities) or may occur sporadically; a detailed family history is important.
2. The defect may be isolated or may occur with other cerebral or extracranial anomalies, such as those associated with the following:

a. Johanson-Blizzard syndrome (mental retardation, congenital deafness, hypothyroidism).

b. Chromosome 4 deletion.

c. Cleft lip or palate; tracheoesophageal fistula; renal and cardiac anomalies.

d. Trisomy 13.

e. Epidermal nevus syndrome.

f. Vascular malformations.

C. TREATMENT.

Treatment is usually conservative, but plastic surgical repair may be indicated in select cases.

IX. NATAL TEETH

A. CLINICAL FEATURES.

1. Natal teeth are defined as teeth present at the time of birth; neonatal teeth, which are less common, erupt from birth to 30 days of age.
2. Natal teeth may be fully erupted or partially covered by gingival tissue; they are almost always the lower central incisors and often occur in pairs. Most represent premature eruption of deciduous teeth, but occasionally they represent supernumerary teeth.
3. Incidence is 1:2000 births; natal teeth may occur as early as 26 weeks' gestation.
4. Most natal teeth occur as isolated events, but there is a positive family history in 15% to 25% of cases (may be autosomal dominant). There is an increased incidence in cases involving cleft lip and palate. Natal teeth may also be seen with several syndromes (e.g., Ellis-van Creveld [chondroectodermal dysplasia], Hallermann-Streiff [oculomandibulofacial syndrome], Jadassohn-Lewandowsky [pachyonychia congenita], Pfeiffer and Teebi [hypertelorism]).
5. Complications include the following:

a. Discomfort during feeding.

b. Trauma to the mother's nipple during feeding.

c. Ulceration of the adjacent lip or tongue.

d. Aspiration of a loose tooth (always mentioned but rarely documented).

B. MANAGEMENT.

1. X-rays are always indicated to differentiate premature eruption of deciduous teeth from supernumerary teeth and to provide information about tooth root development and the relationship of the tooth to adjacent teeth.

2. Extraction is indicated if the tooth is supernumerary or very loose; this is best done by a dentist who must be alert to the possibility of excessive bleeding.
3. If the tooth is not causing any difficulty it should be left in place.
 a. Early mobility often resolves within a month.
 b. Early extraction may lead to overcrowding of the permanent teeth or loss of the permanent tooth bud.

BIBLIOGRAPHY

Aviv RI, Rodger E, Hall CM: Craniosynostosis. Clinical Radiology 57:93, 2002.

Brann AW Jr, Schwartz JF: Developmental anomalies and neuromuscular disorders. In Fanaroff AA, Martin RJ (eds): Neonatal-Perinatal Medicine, ed 4. St. Louis, Mosby, 1987.

Chemke J, Robinson A: The third fontanelle. J Pediatr 75:617, 1969.

Cohen MM Jr: Sutural biology and the correlates of craniosynostosis. Am J Med Genet 47:581, 1993.

Duc G, Largo RH: Anterior fontanel: Size and closure in term and preterm infants. Pediatrics 78:904, 1986.

Frieden IJ: Aplasia cutis congenita: A clinical review and proposal for classification. J Am Acad Dermatol 14:646, 1986.

Jacobson RI: Congenital structural defects. In Swaiman KF (ed): Pediatric Neurology: Principles and Practice, St. Louis, Mosby, 1989.

Kiesler J, Ricer R: The Abnormal Fontanel. Am Fam Physician 67:2547, 2003.

Leung AKC: Natal teeth. Am J Dis Child 140:249, 1986.

Menkes JH: Malformation of the central nervous system. In Taeusch HW, Ballard RA, Avery ME (eds): Schaffer and Avery's diseases of the newborn, ed 6, Philadelphia, WB Saunders, 1991.

Popich GA, Smith DW: Fontanels: Range of normal size. J Pediatr 130:386, 1972.

Shilito J Jr, Matson DD: Craniosynostosis: A review of 519 surgical patients. Pediatrics 41:829, 1986.

Suri M: What's new in neurogenetics? Focus on "primary microcephaly." Euro J Paediatr Neurol 7:389, 2003.

Tan KL: Wide sutures and large fontanels in the newborn. Am J Dis Child 130:386, 1976.

9

THE HEAD

Otolaryngology

Max M. April and Robert M. Naclerio

FAST FACTS

Immediate Issues in the Nursery

- Airway obstruction at or above the supraglottic region is associated with inspiratory stridor. Obstruction at the glottic and subglottic areas manifests as biphasic stridor. Tracheal obstruction results in expiratory stridor.
- Nasal septal dislocation can cause airway obstruction and occurs at a higher incidence (1% to 3%) than choanal atresia.
- Laryngomalacia is the most common congenital anomaly resulting in airway obstruction, followed by vocal cord paralysis.
- A vascular malformation should be suspected in an infant with skin hemangiomata and a neck mass.

Important Reminders After Discharge

- Facial paralysis that has not resolved after 14 days is an indication for electromyography and referral to a neurologist.
- If an infant has failed the initial evoked otoacoustic emissions (EOAE) or the auditory brainstem response (ABR) testing, check to make sure the tympanic membrane is visible indicating a patent external auditory canal (EAC). Dried blood and amniotic fluid often settle in the EAC making it difficult to visualize the entire length of the canal.
- Muscular torticollis can occur anytime in the first month of life. Treatment involves massage, positioning, and stretching.

Helpful Information for Parents

- There is a fair amount of variability in symptoms of airway obstruction. Parents should be reassured that when "noisy breathing" exists in the presence of normal feeding, sleeping, and disposition, the prognosis is generally good, and observation is all that is needed.
- Laryngomalacia usually resolves by 12 to 24 months of age.
- Because cleft lip and palate is a significant congenital deformity (the most common congenital anomaly of the head and neck), it is best treated by a team including cosmetic surgeons, dentists and orthodontists, speech therapists, and ear-nose-throat specialists. Surgical correction and postsurgical treatment by a multi-specialty team usually result in normal eating, drinking, and speech development.

I. AIRWAY OBSTRUCTION

A. STRIDOR.

1. Harsh sound produced by turbulent airflow through a partial obstruction. Stridor is a description, not a disease entity. Symptoms associated with the site of airway obstruction are listed in **Table 10-1**. There are three types of stridor:

a. Inspiratory.

TABLE 10-1

SYMPTOMS ASSOCIATED WITH SITE OF AIRWAY OBSTRUCTION

Site of Obstruction	Inspiratory Stridor	Expiratory Stridor	Feeding Problems	Abnormal Cry
Nose	++		++	+
Oropharynx	++		++	
Supraglottis	++		++	++
Glottis/subglottis	++	++	+	++
Trachea		++		

+, mild symptoms; ++, moderate-to-severe symptoms.

   b. Expiratory.
   c. Biphasic.
2. Stridor may be associated with abnormalities of feeding (nasal, oropharyngeal, supraglottic) or crying (glottic).
3. If there is stridor with severe airway compromise the first step in treatment is establishment of a stable airway with endotracheal intubation.

B. NASAL OBSTRUCTION.
1. Choanal atresia.
   a. Newborn infants are obligate nasal breathers.
      (1) Bilateral atresia is recognized at birth (respiratory distress) when the infant has paradoxical cyanosis (cyanotic with mouth closed but not with crying).
      (2) Unilateral atresia is usually not recognized clinically until the infant is older, when the unilateral nasal obstruction is complicated by purulent rhinorrhea.
   b. Incidence is 1:8000 births.
   c. Unilateral to bilateral ratio is 2:1.
   d. Ninety percent of nasal obstructions involve the bony plates; 10% are membranous.
   e. Up to 50% of infants with choanal atresia have associated anomalies (CHARGE association: coloboma, heart disease, atresia choanae, retarded central nervous system [CNS], genital hypoplasia, ear anomalies).
   f. Diagnosis: Diagnosis is suspected when a 6F catheter cannot be passed through the nasal airway (make sure catheter is seen in mouth, not curled in nose); diagnosis can be confirmed by computed tomography (CT) scan.
   g. Treatment:
      (1) Establish an oral airway using a McGovern nipple (a large nipple modified with its end cut off and ties attached to secure it in place, acting like an oral airway).
      (2) Surgical repair (transnasal [endoscopic] versus transpalatal) may be required. A tracheotomy should be performed for obstruction related to CHARGE association.

2. Congenital nasal masses (intranasal or extranasal) can be caused by the following:
a. Encephalocele: Herniation of brain.
   (1) An encephalocele is compressible and pulsates.
   (2) An encephalocele enlarges with crying.
b. Glioma: Glial tissue that has lost a CNS connection (80% of cases) or has an intracranial extension (20%). Gliomas are noncompressible and nonpulsatile.
c. Dermoid: Contains ectodermal and mesodermal elements; often contains hair follicles in a dimple.
d. Diagnosis: CT scan or magnetic resonance imaging (MRI).
e. Treatment: Surgical excision.

3. Nasal septal dislocation.
a. Related to passage through birth canal.
b. Incidence is 1% to 3% of newborns (higher in primiparas).
c. Diagnosis: External nose twisted, with poor tip and dorsal support on vertical pressure (compression test).
d. Treatment: Reduction (mechanical repositioning by otolaryngologist) with local anesthesia in nursery.

4. Craniofacial anomalies.
a. Crouzon disease (craniofacial dysostosis): Craniostenosis, midface hypoplasia, and bulging eyes.
b. Apert syndrome (acrocephalosyndactyly): Crouzon disease with syndactyly.

10

OTOLARYNGOLOGY

C. OROPHARYNGEAL OBSTRUCTION.

1. Macroglossia.
a. Down syndrome.
b. Hypothyroidism.
c. Beckwith-Wiedemann syndrome (exomphalos, macroglossia, gigantism), often with visceromegaly.

2. Glossoptosis: Pierre Robin sequence (micrognathia, cleft palate).

D. SUPRAGLOTTIC LARYNX.

1. Laryngomalacia.
a. Laryngomalacia is the most common congenital anomaly.
b. Inspiratory stridor is present; it is worse when the infant is supine, excited, or feeding.
c. Stridor may improve when the infant is prone or resting.
d. The infant has a normal cry, and cyanosis is absent.
e. Diagnosis: Confirmed by fiberoptic laryngoscopy.
f. Treatment: Usually self-limited (12 to 24 months); rarely, laser excision of the aryepiglottic fold or a portion of the epiglottis is needed for failure-to-thrive infants or those in extreme distress (1% to 4%).

2. Laryngeal cleft.
a. A laryngeal cleft causes respiratory distress during feeding.

b. Diagnosis: Confirmed by barium swallow and endoscopy.

c. Treatment: Surgical repair.

3. Laryngocele.

a. A laryngocele is a cystic lesion in the larynx.

b. It presents in the newborn as stridor or airway obstruction.

c. Diagnosis: Confirmed by endoscopy with or without plain-film x-rays.

d. Treatment: Endoscopic marsupialization.

E. GLOTTIC OBSTRUCTION.

1. Web-type obstruction.

a. Poor cry is an indication.

b. Airway symptoms depend on size of obstruction.

c. Diagnosis: Confirmed by endoscopy.

d. Treatment: Endoscopic division, with possible intraluminal stent placement.

2. Vocal cord paralysis: Second most common anomaly.

a. Bilateral.

   (1) Causes acute respiratory distress.

   (2) Infant may have normal cry.

   (3) Seen in Arnold-Chiari malformation, hydrocephalus, and meningocele.

   (4) Diagnosis: Confirmed by fiberoptic nasolaryngoscopy.

   (5) Treatment: Tracheotomy is needed in 50% of cases. If CNS-related problem is treated, many infants do not need tracheotomy.

b. Unilateral.

   (1) Infants with unilateral vocal cord paralysis are often asymptomatic.

   (2) Indications are a hoarse cry, possible aspiration.

   (3) Diagnosis: Confirmed by fiberoptic nasolaryngoscopy.

   (4) Treatment: Observation.

3. Atresia.

a. Rare.

b. Incompatible with life unless tracheoesophageal fistula is also present.

F. SUBGLOTTIC OBSTRUCTION.

1. Congenital subglottic stenosis.

a. Congenital subglottic stenosis usually causes recurrent croup or stridor after a few months.

b. Diagnosis: Endoscopy reveals a lumen <3.5 mm in diameter.

c. Treatment: Depends on extent of obstruction; it may respond to endoscopic treatment or the patient may need tracheotomy with subsequent laryngotracheal reconstruction.

2. Subglottic hemangioma.

a. A subglottic hemangioma usually appears as stridor at 1 to 6 months of age but can appear in neonates.

b. Fifty percent have associated skin hemangiomata.

c. Diagnosis: Endoscopy.

d. Treatment: CO_2 laser, steroids, tracheotomy, interferon-α.

G. TRACHEOBRONCHIAL OBSTRUCTION.
The following entities are associated with varied signs and symptoms ranging from mild expiratory stridor and no distress to tachypnea and acute distress necessitating immediate intervention.

1. **Stenosis.**
   a. Diagnosis: Endoscopy, fluoroscopy.
   b. Treatment is based on severity of the stenosis (i.e., endoscopic versus open surgical management).

2. **Tracheomalacia.**
   a. Indication is collapse of the lower airway.
   b. Diagnosis: Confirmed by endoscopy or fluoroscopy.
   c. Treatment: Condition often improves with time, but tracheotomy may be necessary.

3. **Vascular ring.**
   a. Double aortic arch.
   b. Right aortic arch.
   c. Innominate artery compression.
   d. Pulmonary artery sling.
   e. Diagnosis: Confirmed by endoscopy, barium swallow, or MRI.
   f. Treatment depends on severity of the obstruction; may need open thoracic repair.

4. **Tracheoesophageal fistula (TEF). Presentation may be immediate, with first feed not tolerated (see a. and b. subsequently), or more subtle, with recurrent aspiration (see c. subsequently).**
   a. Proximal esophagus blind pouch with distal TEF (87% of cases).
   b. Isolated esophageal atresia (8%).
   c. H type (4%).
   d. Diagnosis: Confirmed by barium swallow and/or inability to pass a nasogastric tube into the stomach.
   e. Treatment: Surgical repair.

H. EXTERNAL COMPRESSION.
(See section on neck masses later in this chapter.)

II. CLEFT LIP AND PALATE
A. INCIDENCE.
1. Cleft lip and palate is the second most common and significant congenital deformity, occurring in 1:1000 births (club foot is the most common).
2. The highest incidence occurs in Native Americans, followed by white infants and then African Americans.
3. Fifty percent of cases involve both cleft lip and palate; 25% cleft palate only; 20% cleft lip only; 5% cleft lip and alveolus.

B. MANIFESTATIONS.
1. Diagnosis is obvious on examination.
2. Most affected newborns have associated middle ear effusions.

10

OTOLARYNGOLOGY

3. Feeding difficulties: A longer nipple and compressible bottle are required, with more frequent burping.
4. Bifid uvula: 10% to 20% of cases are associated with a submucosal cleft palate.

C. SURGICAL REPAIR.

1. Cleft palate.
a. Early repair (10 to 12 months) is better for speech.
b. Late repair (24 to 30 months) is better for facial growth.
2. Cleft lip. Early repair (within the first year) is best.

III. EAR

A. EXTERNAL EAR. CONDITIONS THAT AFFECT THE EXTERNAL EAR INCLUDE THE FOLLOWING:

1. Congenital aural atresia.
a. Incidence is 1:10,000 to 1:20,000 births.
b. Unilateral.
   (1) Twice as common as bilateral.
   (2) Diagnosis: Auditory brainstem response (ABR) to document sensorineural hearing and contralateral hearing.
   (3) Treatment: Separate procedures for auricle and middle ear.
c. Bilateral.
   (1) Use of a bone-conducting hearing aid should begin at 6 months of age.
   (2) Surgical repair should be done at age 4 to 5 years.
2. Microtia: Varying degrees of hypoplasia of external ear with or without middle ear involvement.
3. Positional: Malformations and positional aberrations of the pinna suggest a variety of genetic defects. If it is rotated or low set, this is especially so; associated anomalies are apt to be severe (e.g., renal agenesis, CNS defects).

B. MIDDLE EAR. OTITIS MEDIA: RARE IN NEONATE.

1. Causes sepsis, fever, or both.
2. May involve gram-negative organisms in neonatal period.
3. Diagnosis: Tympanocentesis for diagnosis and culture.
4. Treatment: Intravenous antibiotics if gram-negative infection or infant <4 weeks old.

C. HEARING LOSS.

1. Incidence of severe hearing loss at birth is 1:1000.
2. Incidence of severe hearing loss in neonatal intensive care unit (NICU) is 1:60.
3. There is a high risk for hearing loss with the following conditions:
a. Family history of congenital hearing loss.
b. Birth weight <1500 g.

c. 5-minute Apgar score <5.
d. TORCH group of infections.
e. Severe hyperbilirubinemia.
   (1) >22 mg/dl in infant weighing >2000 g.
   (2) >17 mg/dl in infant weighing <2000 g.
f. Intraventricular hemorrhage.
g. Bacterial meningitis/neonatal sepsis.
h. External ear deformities.

Note: *Recent reports on the subject of universal newborn screening recommend that every infant have evoked otoacoustic emissions (EOAE) or ABR testing before 3 months of age.*

IV. FACIAL PARALYSIS
A. BIRTH TRAUMA.
1. May be related to large size, forceps delivery, or pressure through birth canal.
2. Diagnosis: Associated ecchymosis, synkinesis (contraction of unexpected facial muscles with voluntary movement).
3. Treatment: Observation; most recover spontaneously.
4. If not resolved after 14 days, serial electromyography should be performed.

B. MÖBIUS SYNDROME.
1. Usually associated with bilateral abducens nerve paralysis.
2. May also involve cranial nerves 3, 4, 7, 10, and 12.
3. May include micrognathia, club foot, and/or absence of the pectoralis muscle.
4. No treatment is available.

C. GOLDENHAR SYNDROME.
1. Oculoauriculovertebral dysplasia.
2. Hemifacial microsomia: Faulty development of first and second branchial arches.
3. Can have reconstructive surgery when older.

D. AGENESIS OF DEPRESSOR ANGULI ORIS MUSCLE.
1. Unilateral; asymmetry is prominent when baby cries.
2. Associated with cardiovascular, skeletal, and genitourinary abnormalities.

V. NECK MASSES
A. LYMPHATIC MALFORMATIONS/CYSTIC HYGROMA.
1. Soft, diffuse, painless.
2. Cystic; transilluminates; often multiloculated.
3. Often in posterior triangle of neck.
4. Can involve mucosal surfaces.

5. Does not regress.
6. Diagnosis by MRI or CT.
7. Treatment: Surgical excision.

B. HEMANGIOMA/VASCULAR MALFORMATIONS.
1. Associated skin hemangiomata in 50% of cases.
2. Usually reddish-blue, soft; often involves overlying skin.
3. Rapid growth in first 6 months.
4. Most regress by 5 years of age.
5. Treatment: Observation; surgical excision is warranted if spontaneous bleeding, airway distress, or coagulopathy occurs.

C. THYROGLOSSAL DUCT CYST.
1. Tract from tongue base to thyroid gland.
2. Painless, midline mass with normal overlying skin.
3. Most often between hyoid bone and thyroid.
4. Moves with deglutition and tongue protrusion.
5. Diagnosis by ultrasound; thyroid scan also used to discover functioning thyroid tissue other than cyst.
6. Treatment: Surgical excision (Sistrunk procedure).

D. TERATOMA.
1. All three germ layers are involved (ectoderm, mesoderm, endoderm).
2. Solid mass.
3. Plain-film x-rays reveal calcification in 50% of cases.
4. Treatment: Surgical excision.

E. STERNOCLEIDOMASTOID (SCM) TUMOR OF INFANCY.
1. Also known as fibromatosis coli.
2. Torticollis is associated with a firm, nontender nodule under the SCM muscle.
3. Occurs between 7 and 28 days of life.
4. Treatment: Massage, passive stretching, and positioning.
5. Be alert for associated congenital hip deformity.

F. BRANCHIAL CLEFT ANOMALIES.
1. Cyst: No internal or external opening; may present in adolescence or adulthood.
2. Sinus tract: External opening.
3. Fistula: Internal and external openings.
4. May involve first, second, or third branchial arches.
5. Fistulas and sinus tracts that are apparent at birth have an external opening (pit) along lower anterior border of SCM muscle.
6. Treatment is surgical excision when the child is older.

BIBLIOGRAPHY

Cotton RT: The problem of pediatric laryngotracheal stenosis. Laryngoscope 101(suppl 56):1, 1991.

Evans JNG: Management of the cleft larynx and tracheoesophageal clefts. Ann Otol Rhinol Laryngol 94:627, 1985.

Holinger LD: Etiology of stridor in the neonate, infant and child. Ann Otol Rhinol Laryngol 89:397, 1980.

Kezerian EJ, White KR, Yueh B, Sullivan SD: Cost and cost-effectiveness of universal screening for hearing loss in newborns. Otolaryngol Head Neck Surg 124:359, 2001.

Morgan DW, Baily CM: Current management of choanal atresia. Int J Pediatr Otorhinolaryngol 19:1, 1990.

National Institutes of Health: Early identification of hearing impairment in infants and young children. NIH Consensus Statement 11(1):1, 1993.

Paradise JL: Universal newborn hearing screening: Should we leap before we look? Pediatrics 103:670, 1999.

Thomsen JR, Koltai PJ: Sternomastoid tumor of infancy. Ann Otol Rhinol Laryngol 98:955, 1989.

Van Son JAM, Julsrud PR, Hagler DJ, et al: Surgical treatment of vascular rings. Mayo Clin Proc 68:1056, 1993.

10

OTOLARYNGOLOGY

Ophthalmology

Michael X. Repka

Immediate Issues in the Nursery

- Absence of or variation of the red reflex is always considered abnormal.
- Causes of neonatal cataracts include: congenital anomalies (autosomal dominant), infection (TORCH, varicella, herpes simplex virus [HSV]), chromosomal abnormalities (e.g., trisomies 18 and 21), prematurity, and metabolic disorders. Initial actions should include assessment for parental cataracts, maternal infection, maternal medication, and physical dysmorphisms. Laboratory evaluation may also be necessary.
- Corneal cloudiness is the most common sign of congenital glaucoma. Others include photophobia, corneal enlargement, and optic nerve cupping. Increased intraocular pressure is diagnostic.
- Corneal opacities can result from birth trauma (forceps delivery), glaucoma, infection, metabolic conditions, and congenital anomalies. Prompt ophthalmologic consultation is necessary to assess intraocular pressure and to initiate therapy to reduce the risk of visual impairment.

Important Reminders after Discharge

- Although esotropic (turning in) and exotropic (turning out) movements of the eyes are normal in the newborn period, these should generally cease by 4 months of age.
- Conjunctivitis in the first month of life is usually caused by infection by bacteria and *Chlamydia*. Despite the relatively low number of infections caused by *Neisseria gonorrhoeae*, consideration should be given to culturing for *N. gonorrhoeae* because of rapid spread to the cornea.
- Signs and symptoms of infantile glaucoma occur very rapidly; repeated eye examinations at well visits is an important priority.

Helpful Information for Parents

- Dacryostenosis (blocked nasolacrimal duct) often begins in the first month of life. Parents should be advised to watch for a pooling type mucoid collection in the inside corner of the eye, tears running down the cheek without crying, and crusting of the lashes/lids after sleep periods. This should be contrasted to redness of the sclera and lower lid, consistent and copious purulent discharge, and swelling of the lids that is indicative of a complicating infection.
- Subconjunctival hemorrhages are fairly common complications of vaginal delivery. They are often not noticed early on due to periorbital swelling; however, they generally resolve by 7 to 10 days of life.
- The eyes may change their color as late as 6 to 9 months of life.

I. GENERAL CONSIDERATIONS

A. **FEW INFANTS WILL HAVE ANY SIGNIFICANT ABNORMALITY DETECTABLE ON EXAMINATION.**

B. **SUBCONJUNCTIVAL HEMORRHAGE IS NOT UNUSUAL AND ORDINARILY RESOLVES SPONTANEOUSLY.**

C. **THE EXAMINATION REQUIRES A PENLIGHT TO TEST FOR A PUPILLARY LIGHT RESPONSE AND TO EXAMINE THE ANTERIOR SEGMENT, INCLUDING THE CONJUNCTIVA, SCLERA, CORNEA, ANTERIOR CHAMBER, AND IRIS.**

Direct ophthalmoscopy is necessary to examine the clarity of the media, specifically looking at the quality of the red reflex.

Note: *Disruptions in the red reflex are always abnormal and may represent a corneal opacity, cataract, vitreous hemorrhage, or retinal detachment.*

D. **THE VISUAL ACUITY OF THE FULL-TERM NEONATE IS APPROXIMATELY 20/800, ADEQUATE TO FIXATE ON A LARGE OR HIGH-CONTRAST TARGET, PARTICULARLY WHEN VIEWED UP CLOSE.**

E. **THE OCULOMOTOR SYSTEM IS WELL ESTABLISHED AT BIRTH.**

Eye movements may be tested with a doll's-head maneuver, such as by spinning the infant around the examiner, with the head held upright. The eyes will deviate in the direction opposite to the spin. Alignment need not be normal until 6 to 12 weeks after birth. During the neonatal period, intermittent esotropic (turning in) and, more frequently, exotropic (turning out) deviations of the eyes are common, but generally decrease in frequency as the child reaches 4 months of age.

F. **NEARLY ANY PROBLEM IDENTIFIED WILL REQUIRE CONSULTATION, PREFERABLY WITH AN OPHTHALMOLOGIST EXPERIENCED WITH THE OCULAR EXAMINATION OF AN INFANT.**

II. CATARACT

A. **DIAGNOSIS.**

1. The diagnosis of cataract is best made while examining the red reflex with a direct ophthalmoscope; disruption in the homogeneous red reflex is most often the result of a lens anomaly.
2. A cataract may be unilateral or bilateral.
3. A cataract may range in severity from an insignificant dotlike opacity that is not going to impair visual development through a completely white lens that completely obscures the red reflex.
4. The morphology of the cataract is rarely helpful in establishing an etiology.

B. EVALUATION.

Items to be considered in the evaluation of a cataract include the following:

1. **History.**

a. A history and eye examination of the infant's parents should be obtained for evidence of autosomal dominant cataracts, especially when bilateral.

b. Maternal drug exposure: Substances to look for include naphthalene, phenothiazines, steroids, vitamin D, and antimetabolites.

c. Maternal infection: The TORCH group of infections should be considered.

2. **Physical examination: Look for dysmorphic features that might suggest specific syndromes (e.g., trisomy 21 or Hallermann-Streiff [oculomandibulofacial dyscephaly, or "parrot nose"; bilateral cataracts, often with microphthalmia, microcornea, or glaucoma; hypotrichosis; and dwarfism are possible; all cases are sporadic]).**

3. **Laboratory evaluation.**

a. Laboratory tests should be performed when there is no history of familial infantile or juvenile cataract and the cataracts are bilateral.

b. Tests should be used selectively based on the clinical findings. Most patients will require few or no tests.

c. Blood tests should be done to determine levels of the following:
   (1) Glucose.
   (2) Calcium.
   (3) Amino acids.
   (4) TORCH titers, rapid plasma reagin (RPR).

d. Urine tests should be done to determine the presence or levels of the following:
   (1) Amino acids.
   (2) Reducing substances.
   (3) Blood and protein screens.
   (4) Lipid bodies.
   (5) Copper.

e. Specialized tests can determine the presence or levels of the following:
   (1) Red blood cell (RBC) galactose 1-phosphate uridyltransferase.
   (2) RBC glucose-6-phosphatase activity.
   (3) RBC galactokinase activity.
   (4) White blood cell (WBC) α-mannosidase activity.
   (5) Plasma phytanic acid.

C. DIFFERENTIAL DIAGNOSIS.

1. Autosomal dominant conditions are the most common cause of cataracts in otherwise healthy children.

2. Cataracts may develop after intrauterine infection with rubella, rubeola, varicella, herpes simplex virus (HSV), cytomegalovirus (CMV), or toxoplasmosis.

3. Chromosomal abnormalities: Trisomies 13, 15, 18, or 21; Turner syndrome.

4. Prematurity.
5. Cataracts can be associated with other ocular malformations or with metabolic disorders such as the following:
a. Galactosemia: Cataracts associated with galactosemia can occasionally be reversed with the prompt institution of dietary management.
b. Hypoparathyroidism and pseudohypoparathyroidism.
c. Diabetes mellitus.
d. Refsum disease.
e. Lowe oculocerebrorenal syndrome.
f. Hypoglycemia.
g. Mannosidosis.
h. Hereditary hemorrhagic nephritis (Alport syndrome).
6. Systemic syndromes.
a. Hallermann-Streiff.
b. Congenital stippled epiphysis (Conradi syndrome).
c. Smith-Lemli-Opitz (ears slanted or low set; ptosis; micrognathia; syndactyly of second and third toes; cryptorchidism; significant hypospadias).
7. Dermatologic disorders or craniofacial dysostosis.

III. CONGENITAL DEFECTS

A. ANIRIDIA.
1. Incidence is 1:75,000.
2. Autosomal dominant.
a. Chromosome 2.
b. Nystagmus, poor vision, cataracts, glaucoma.
3. Sporadic.
a. Wilms tumor develops in 25%. These patients have chromosome 11p13 deletion.
b. Associated with genitourinary anomalies and mental retardation (WAGR).

B. ALBINISM.
1. Incidence is 1:20,000.
2. Autosomal recessive, autosomal dominant, X-linked.
3. Variable visual loss especially dramatic when young, nystagmus, high refractive error.

C. MICROPHTHALMOS AND CRYPTIC EYE.
1. The reduction in the size of an eye may vary from a nearly imperceptible difference to no formed eye visible in the orbit. In the latter instance the orbit usually contains a cystic structure, which may cause the lower lid to bulge forward and the floor of the orbit to be pushed into the maxillary sinus. This structure is readily detected with imaging. Anophthalmos is extremely rare.

2. Usually unilateral.
3. 40% of affected children have other, nonocular anomalies.
4. Evaluation.
a. Ophthalmologic and pediatric examinations.
b. Orbital transillumination.
c. Consider ultrasound and neuroimaging.
5. **Management.**
a. Individualized. Includes serial aspiration or resection.
b. Lids need progressive enlargement by the use of progressively larger prostheses or orbital expanders.
6. **Prognosis: Generally poor; vision is directly related to the degree of malformation.**

D. COLOBOMA.
1. Pathogenesis: Failure of fusion of the embryonic fissure.
2. A coloboma variably affects the retina, optic nerve, iris, and choroid.
3. Types of coloboma include the following:
a. Isolated: Sporadic or autosomal dominant.
b. Part of a malformation syndrome.
  (1) CHARGE association.
    (a) Coloboma (80%).
    (b) Heart anomalies.
    (c) Choanal atresia.
    (d) Retardation.
    (e) Genital anomalies.
    (f) Ear anomalies.
  (2) Aicardi syndrome: Infantile spasms, abnormal corpus callosum, and mental retardation.
c. Associated with chromosomal abnormalities.
  (1) Trisomies 13 and 22.
  (2) Wolf-Hirschhorn (4p): Mental retardation, short stature, microcephaly, cardiac septal defects, and cleft lip or palate.
  (3) Cat's eye syndrome.
4. Vision prognosis depends on the extent of ocular involvement. Macular or optic nerve involvement causes permanently reduced visual acuity.

IV. CLOUDY CORNEA

A. A WIDE VARIETY OF ABNORMALITIES MAY BE RESPONSIBLE FOR PRODUCING A CORNEAL OPACITY AT BIRTH. CAREFUL, RAPID THERAPY IS NEEDED TO PRESERVE VISION.

B. DIFFERENTIAL DIAGNOSIS.
1. Birth trauma, often associated with a forceps delivery.
2. Infantile glaucoma (see later).
3. Infection: Rubella, HSV.

11

OPHTHALMOLOGY

4. Corneal drying (exposure keratopathy).
5. Metabolic conditions; occasionally seen at birth but more often in childhood.
a. Mucopolysaccharidosis I-H and I-S.
b. Mucolipidosis IV.
6. Corneal anomalies.
a. Replacement by dermoid tissue; most commonly a fleshy mass at the limbus.
b. Sclerocornea.
c. Corneal endothelial absence or abnormality.

C. EVALUATION.
1. Emergent determination of intraocular pressure. Such an examination may require general anesthesia or sedation.
2. Ophthalmologic examination to define diagnosis and assist in selection of therapy.
3. Echography of anterior and posterior segments.

D. MANAGEMENT.
1. Reduce elevated intraocular pressure.
2. Corneal transplant for bilateral corneal opacities, when not produced by glaucoma, within the first 12 weeks of life. The treatment of unilateral opacities must be individualized because the ultimate prognosis for vision in such a disadvantaged eye is extremely poor.

V. CONJUNCTIVITIS

A. CONJUNCTIVITIS DURING THE FIRST MONTH OF LIFE IS TERMED *OPHTHALMIA NEONATORUM*. THE INCIDENCE IS ABOUT 2% BUT RANGES FROM 0.5% TO 12%.

B. PROPHYLAXIS.
1. Erythromycin 0.5% ointment.
2. Tetracycline 1% ointment or drops.
3. Silver nitrate 1% drops.
4. All three agents are effective against *N. gonorrhoeae.*
5. None is highly effective against *Chlamydia*.
6. 2.5% povidone-iodine solution is as effective as antimicrobials and is less expensive and less toxic (not FDA approved for this indication).

C. DIFFERENTIAL DIAGNOSIS.
1. Chemical-related secondary to use of silver nitrate drops (rare).
2. Chlamydia; may represent 40% of cases in some areas.
3. Bacterial (30% to 50%)
a. *N. gonorrhoeae*(<1%): Most dangerous because of the possibility of rapid corneal perforation.
b. *Staphylococcus aureus* and *Staphylococcus epidermidis.*
c. *Streptococcus pneumoniae* and *Streptococcus viridans.*

d. *Haemophilus species.*
4. HSV (<1%).

D. EVALUATION.
1. Chemical conjunctivitis appears in the first 24 to 48 hours.
2. Always rule out *N. gonorrhoeae* and determine if the isolated strain is penicillinase producing. Make certain topical prophylaxis was given.
3. HSV usually appears later, often in the second week after delivery.
4. Microscopic evaluation and cultures are nearly always necessary.
a. Giemsa and Gram stains.
b. DNA probes for *Chlamydia.*
c. Chocolate agar in CO_2; reduced blood agar; thioglycolate broth.
d. Viral cultures as indicated.

E. THERAPY.
1. Preliminary therapy is based on clinical presentation and stains of the conjunctival scrapings.
2. *N. gonorrhoeae:* ceftriaxone 25 to 50 mg/kg per day intravenously or intramuscularly for 7 days; for hyperbilirubinemic infants, especially those who are premature, cefotaxime 50 to 100 mg/kg per day intravenously or intramuscularly in two divided doses.
3. *Chlamydia*: Erythromycin syrup, 50 mg/kg per day orally in four divided doses for 14 days. Topical therapy is ineffective. Alternative treatment: Azithromycin 20 mg/kg orally daily for 3 days.
4. HSV: Trifluridine 1%, 1 drop to affected eye every 2 hours for 7 days; should be given with ophthalmologic consultation; this treatment will control only epithelial disease. Systemic therapy with acyclovir is usually recommended.

F. PUBLIC HEALTH REFERRAL AND TREATMENT ARE NECESSARY FOR MOTHER AND ALL SEXUAL PARTNERS.

VI. INFANTILE GLAUCOMA

A. THE PRESENTATION IN INFANTS IS DIFFERENT FROM THAT IN OLDER CHILDREN AND ADULTS.
The onset may seem to be nearly instantaneous; symptoms and signs develop over just a few hours.

B. INCIDENCE IS 1:10,000.

C. SIGNS AND SYMPTOMS.
1. Cloudy cornea is the most common sign in the neonate.
2. Photophobia.
3. Corneal enlargement (buphthalmos): A horizontal diameter of 9.5 mm is normal.
4. Epiphora (increased tearing).

11

OPHTHALMOLOGY

5. Increased intraocular pressure (IOP) is needed to prove the diagnosis; it is sometimes appreciable on gentle palpation of the eye.
6. Optic nerve cupping and atrophy.
7. Poor vision is a late sign.

D. EVALUATION.

1. Intraocular pressure is measured with a tonometer in the office using topical anesthesia, or on occasion, in a facility with anesthesia. General anesthesia and sedation should be avoided because they lower the pressure. Most clinicians attempt to determine the IOP in infants in the office without medication or with ketamine sedation in the operating room.
2. Measure horizontal corneal diameter; >10.5 mm, or progressive enlargement in the infant is a reliable sign of uncontrolled pressure.

E. DIFFERENTIAL DIAGNOSIS.

1. Primary congenital open-angle glaucoma.
a. Usually occurs between 3 and 9 months but may occur in the neonate.
b. Autosomal recessive with incomplete penetrance.
2. Secondary.
a. Sturge-Weber syndrome.
b. Lowe syndrome (oculocerebrorenal).
c. Neurofibromatosis type 1.
d. Anterior segment malformation syndromes.
e. Trauma.
f. Rubella.

F. THERAPY.

1. The choice of therapy is governed by the optic nerve appearance, the IOP, and the corneal diameter.
2. Medical therapy is intended as a temporary measure.
a. Topical β-blockers may produce systemic drug levels and adverse reactions (e.g., wheezing, bradycardia) in the neonate.
b. Carbonic anhydrase inhibitors: topical agents such as dorzolamide or brinzolamide and/or oral acetazolamide at a dose of 15 mg/kg per day divided into two to four doses.
c. Alpha-adrenergic agonists work poorly and cause sedation.
3. Surgery: The objective is long-term control of the glaucoma. Multiple procedures are often needed.

VII. LEUKOCORIA

A. LEUKOCORIA (WHITE REFLEX) ALWAYS REQUIRES OPHTHALMOLOGIC EVALUATION.

B. DIFFERENTIAL DIAGNOSIS.

1. Cataract.
2. Persistent hyperplastic primary vitreous; usually unilateral, with microphthalmos.

3. Cloudy cornea.
4. Retinal detachment, including retinopathy of prematurity.
5. Vitreous hemorrhage: Think of "shaken baby" syndrome.
6. Retinal coloboma.
7. Vitreous inflammation: Toxoplasmosis.
8. Retinoblastoma, toxocariasis: Rare in the neonate but common in toddlers.

BIBLIOGRAPHY

American Academy of Pediatrics Committee on Infectious Diseases: Red Book 2003 Report of the Committee on Infectious Diseases, ed 26, Elk Grove Village, Ill, American Academy of Pediatrics, 2003.

Bell, TA, Grayston, JT, Krohn MA, Kronmal RA: The Eye Prophylaxis Study Group. Randomized trial of silver nitrate, erythromycin, and no eye prophylaxis for the prevention of conjunctivitis among newborns not at risk for gonococcal ophthalmitis. Pediatrics 92:755, 1993.

Birch EE, Stager DR: Prevalence of good visual acuity following surgery for unilateral congenital cataract, Arch Ophthalmol 106:40, 1988.

Crawford JS, Morin JD (eds): The Eye in Childhood. New York, Grune & Stratton, 1983.

Isenberg ST, Apt L, Wood M: A controlled trial of povidone-iodine as prophylaxis against ophthalmia neonatorum. N Engl J Med 332:562, 1995.

Katzman GH: Pathophysiology of neonates: Subconjunctival hemorrhage. Clin Pediatr 31:149, 1992.

Laga M, Plummer FA, Piot P, et al: Prophylaxis of gonococcal and chlamydial ophthalmia neonatorum: A comparison of silver nitrate and tetracycline. N Engl J Med 318:653, 1988.

Merin S, Crawford JS: The etiology of congenital cataracts. Can J Ophthalmol 6:178, 1971.

Nelson LB, Calhoun JH, Harley RD: Pediatric Ophthalmology. Philadelphia, WB Saunders, 1991.

Nixon RB, Helveston EM, Miller KK, et al: Incidence of strabismus in neonates. Am J Ophthalmol 100:798, 1985.

Pediatric Eye Disease Investigator Group: The clinical spectrum of congenital esotropia. Am J Ophthalmol 133:102, 2002.

Rapoza PA, Quinn TC, Kiessling LA, et al: Epidemiology of neonatal conjunctivitis. Ophthalmology 93:456, 1986.

11

OPHTHALMOLOGY

Cardiology

Joel I. Brenner

FAST FACTS

Immediate Issues in the Nursery

- An active precordium along with tachypnea, hyperpnea, muffled heart sounds, discordant blood pressures (differential blood pressures between right arm and other extremities or between upper and lower extremities), dysmorphic features, and heart murmurs are all clinical clues for congenital cardiac defects.
- A 12-lead electrocardiogram (ECG) is essential in identifying and evaluating a potential rhythm disturbance. For HR in the 220-240 range, running the ECG at double speed may help to differentiate sinus tachycardia (e.g., in sepsis) from supraventricular tachycardia (SVT).
- An echocardiogram is indicated in any newborn with: cyanosis, irregular ventricular heart beats (PVCs), cardiac arrhythmias, cardiomegaly, or when trisomy 21 is suspected.

Important Reminders After Discharge

- All infants with ongoing cardiac compromise (CHF or cyanosis) require RSV prophylaxis in the first 2 years of life.
- In the case of a large ventricular septal defect (VSD) or patent ductus arteriosus (PDA), clinical symptoms are more likely to occur after the first few weeks when the pulmonary vascular resistance falls enough to allow left-to-right shunting.
- Congestive heart failure will manifest as tachypnea, hepatomegaly, and cardiomegaly. Often a gallop is present but peripheral edema is rare. Other important clues are poor feeding, poor weight gain, and sweating during feedings.

Helpful Information for Parents

- Many parents mistake a murmur for an "extra heart beat." Take the time to explain that a murmur is a noise that blood makes as it runs through the circulatory system (the heart's chambers or valves or the blood vessels near the heart), and that the majority of murmurs heard in the newborn nursery are not associated with a heart defect. Likewise, be sure to point out that these murmurs don't "turn into" anything more serious down the road.
- If a congenital heart defect is present, explaining the medical concerns to parents can be difficult. Before direct discussion between the parents and a cardiologist, it is helpful for the family to classify the anomaly as: a problem that causes too much blood to run through the lungs; a problem that causes too little blood to run through the lungs; or a problem that causes too little blood to travel to the body.

12

I. GOAL

The goal of the primary care provider during the postpartum stay in the nursery, and through the first month of life, is to be certain that there is no abnormality of heart structure, function, or rhythm, which puts the neonate at risk. Even in an age of text messaging, high-speed data transfer, and ready availability of 2-D echocardiography, there still remains a role for a concise and organized clinical approach to accomplish this goal. The understanding and comanagement of the cardiac problems encountered in the neonate still require the ability to effectively examine the newborn and integrate laboratory data, making certain that the **clinical** findings explain the **physiologic** problem encountered.

II. FIVE TOOLS OF DIAGNOSIS

A. PHYSICAL EXAMINATION IS THE FIRST STEP BUT MAY BE DISTRESSINGLY UNIMPRESSIVE, EVEN IN INFANTS WITH CRITICAL, DUCTAL-DEPENDENT CONGENITAL HEART DISEASE (CHD).

General examination of the newborn for dysmorphic features suggestive of chromosomal or syndromic abnormalities is often very helpful in establishing the probability of a coexisting cardiac malformation (**Table 12-1**). Conversely, the recognition of certain cardiac anatomic abnormalities should alert the clinician to possible genetic associations. Auscultatory clues are often subtle in the neonate with critical heart disease, and primary care providers may not feel comfortable in affirming normal splitting of the second heart sound, or in recognizing an ejection click or a gallop rhythm in a neonate with a heart rate of 140 to 160 beats per minute. The pediatric cardiology consultant should be comfortable with these "details"

TABLE 12-1
SYNDROME-RELATED HEART DISEASE

Syndrome	Cardiac Manifestations
Trisomy 21 (Down)	Atrioventricular septal defect, tetralogy of Fallot (TOF)
Trisomy 18 (Edward)	Polyvalvular dysplasia, TOF with pulmonary atresia
Trisomy 13 (Patau)	Ventricular septal defect (VSD)
Turner (XO)	Coarctation of aorta, hyperplastic left heart (HLH)
DiGeorge (22q11)	TOF, right aortic arch, truncus arteriosus, interrupted aortic arch
VACTERL	VSD, TOF, coarctation
Noonan (12q22-qter)	Dysplastic pulmonary valve stenosis, hypertrophic cardiomyopathy
Marfan (15fbn1)	Mitral/tricuspid prolapse, aortic/pulmonary artery dilatation
Williams (microdeletion chromosome 7)	Supravalve aortic stenosis/pulmonic stenosis (AS/PS)
Heterotaxy (if X-linked, Xq26.2)	Abnormal connections—anomalous venous return, abnormal lateralization—transposed great vessels, asplenia/polysplenia

of auscultation. However, observation of the respiratory rate and pattern may provide evidence of tachypnea and suggest pulmonary venous congestion, or hyperpnea, reflecting important hypoxemia and air hunger. Recognition of an active precordium, even absent a murmur, may provide the first clue about a volume-loaded right ventricle. Abnormal perfusion with discrepant pulses in upper and lower extremities, with differential blood pressures in right arm and a leg, may be the first confirmation of an aortic arch obstruction and a ductal-dependent systemic circulation. Muffled heart sounds may reflect "insulation" of sound transmission by air or fluid: pneumopericardium (easily confirmed by chest x-ray) or pericardial effusion.

B. CHEST X-RAY IS READILY AVAILABLE AND CAN PROVIDE SPECIFIC DIAGNOSTIC INFORMATION OR SUGGEST A CATEGORY OF PROBLEM AND A TREATMENT PLAN.

Differentiation of the causes of cardiorespiratory distress requires the proper interpretation of the x-ray. In a newborn, the initial x-ray study should image from clavicles to umbilicus, permitting comment about skeletal abnormality (e.g., hemivertebrae, fused ribs), location of the stomach bubble (normally under the left hemidiaphragm) and abdominal gas pattern. Recognition of noncardiac abnormalities on the x-ray may appropriately focus attention on the increased likelihood of structural heart disease, recalling that nearly 25% of neonates and infants with structural heart disease will have associated abnormalities.

Then attention should be turned to the pulmonary vascularity and heart size. Pulmonary vascularity may be normal, decreased or, rarely in the neonate, increased. Pulmonary venous congestion is the most likely finding when a prominent pulmonary vascular pattern is noted. Increased arterial markings require a fall in pulmonary resistance. This is usually accomplished over the first 2 to 4 weeks of life, but more rapidly in preterm infants. Heart size may be normal, suggesting no volume load, or increased, confirming increased volume work. If severe cardiomegaly is noted in the first few hours or days of life, the volume load can be presumed to have been present in utero, often encountered with severe right heart enlargement due to tricuspid regurgitation. The recognition of specific cardiac contours, characteristic of malformations persisting into later infancy or childhood, such as the "coeur en sabot" or boot-shaped heart hitherto seen in tetralogy of Fallot (TOF), is no longer a dependable finding in the neonate. Neither is the "egg on a string" appearance previously seen in older infants with transposition of the great arteries (TGA) because most infants born with dextrotransposition of the great arteries (DTGA) have been surgically repaired by 2 weeks of age. As previously mentioned, an enlarged cardiac silhouette may also be observed in pericardial effusion, and a "halo" appearance around the heart, caused by air in the pericardial space, may explain distant heart sounds noted on examination.

C. PULSE OXIMETRY AND ARTERIAL BLOOD GAS INTERPRETATION IN ROOM AIR AND WITH 100% OXYGEN ARE STILL VITAL PIECES OF CLINICAL INFORMATION IN THE PHYSIOLOGIC ASSESSMENT OF THE NEONATE WITH CARDIORESPIRATORY DISTRESS.

Pre- and postductal pulse oximetry (right hand or right earlobe and either foot) will provide quick confirmation of suspected cyanosis. It may also be used to demonstrate a differential source of arterial flow in upper and lower extremities in the case of aortic arch obstruction. Lower body blood flow may derive from the pulmonary artery via a patent ductus arteriosus (PDA) to the descending aorta if there is aortic coarctation or aortic arch interruption. Severe desaturation noted with pulse oximetry should be confirmed by arterial blood gases in room air and with 100% oxygen administration to assess the adequacy of systemic circulation/degree of acidemia (pH), ventilation (pCO_2), and oxygenation. The response to varying FiO_2 should be compared with expectations for the age of the neonate (**Table 12-2**).

D. SYSTEMATIC AND COMPLETE ECHOCARDIOGRAPHIC EVALUATION OF THE NEONATE WITH SUSPECTED DUCTAL-DEPENDENT HEART DISEASE, OR OTHER NONTHREATENING CARDIAC MALFORMATION, MUST BE INTERPRETED BY A PEDIATRIC CARDIOLOGIST WITH KNOWLEDGE OF THE CLINICAL CONCERNS.

Two-dimensional echo study should demonstrate the following:
(1) the connections of the systemic and pulmonary venous pathways in to their respective atria, (2) atrial-ventricular and ventricular-great vessel

TABLE 12-2
RESPONSE TO HYPEROXIA CHALLENGE

Normal Child			Normal Neonate	
Room Air	100% O_2		Room Air	100% O_2
760 torr	760 torr	Barometric pressure— sea level (to be measured)	760 torr	760 torr
−47 torr	−47 torr	−water vapor pressure	−47 torr	−47 torr
713 torr	713 torr	BP—sea level-dry	713 torr	713 torr
× .21	× 1.0	FIO_2*	× .21	× 1.0
150 torr	713 torr	Inhaled PO_2	150 torr	713 torr
−40 torr	−40 torr	CO_2 production	−40 torr	−40 torr
110 torr	673 torr	Alveolar PaO_2	110 torr	673 torr
−11 torr	−67 torr	Physiologic atelectasis[†]	−44 torr	−268 torr
99 torr	606 torr	Pulmonary venous PaO_2 = arterial PaO_2[‡]	66 torr	405 torr

*Reader can calculate expected PaO_2 by dialing in FIO_2, barometric pressure, etc.

[†]Degree of physiologic atelectasis goes from 100%, prior to the first breath, to 10% over the course of the first few weeks of life, depending on neonatal pulmonary adaptation.

[‡]PVO_2 will equal PaO_2 absent parenchymal or structural pulmonary disease.

connections, (3) the anterior great vessel bifurcating in to the branch pulmonary arteries and the posterior great vessel branching in to the head vessels, and (4) intact flow to the descending aorta. Color flow Doppler study may allow determination of pressure relationships (e.g., bidirectional flow in the PDA predicts systemic pulmonary artery pressure), tricuspid regurgitation jet may allow quantification of RV pressure (and should be correlated with blood pressure measured at the time of the study to be maximally useful). Color flow may also facilitate recognition of obstructed outflow, valvular regurgitation, and atrial or ventricular septal defects (particularly the small muscular ventricular septal defects [VSD], which produce a loud murmur early in life and are often resolved by 1 year of age).

E. ELECTROCARDIOGRAPHY (ECG) IS SUGGESTIVE ONLY FOR STRUCTURAL ABNORMALITIES AND MYOCARDIAL DYSFUNCTION, BUT IS SPECIFIC AND PRECISE FOR DEFINITION OF HEART RHYTHM DISTURBANCE. FOR RHYTHM EVALUATION, A 12-LEAD ECG MUST BE OBTAINED. RELYING ON A RHYTHM STRIP IS UNRELIABLE AND UNWISE.

A superior frontal plane axis (e.g., marked left axis deviation or a "northwest axis") suggests abnormality of atrial-ventricular inflow, such as A-V septal defect (A-V canal, endocardial cushion defect) or tricuspid atresia. Absence of anterior and rightward electrical forces (no R wave in V_1, no S wave in V_6) suggests absence or hypoplasia of the right ventricle, which should be dominant in the neonate.

III. RECOGNITION OF THE NEONATE WITH CARDIORESPIRATORY DISTRESS DUE TO STRUCTURAL HEART DISEASE

The neonate with cardiorespiratory distress represents the greatest challenge because time lost in recognition may impact directly on morbidity and mortality. Anatomic abnormalities result in either cyanosis or congestive heart failure (CHF). Categorization of the physiologic derangement, often possible prior to and independent of the anatomic definition by echocardiography, provides the earliest information enabling the primary care provider to institute appropriate clinical managements. Using information from pulse oximetry/arterial blood gas measurements and chest x-ray, physiologic classification of the suspected cardiac abnormality can be accomplished. Most neonates with ductal-dependent heart disease can be classified in this way. In addition to the specific medical therapies discussed below, respiratory syncytial virus (RSV) prophylaxis is mandatory for all infants with ongoing cardiac compromise—either congestive heart failure or cyanosis—in the first 2 years of life. Those infants with cardiac lesions completely repaired in infancy will generally be at risk only during their first year.

A. CYANOSIS CONFIRMED TO BE DUE TO CENTRAL HYPOXEMIA AND NOT RESPONDING TO INCREASED AMBIENT OXYGEN

12

CARDIOLOGY

ADMINISTRATION AND NOT ASSOCIATED WITH X-RAY EVIDENCE OF STRUCTURAL OR PARENCHYMAL LUNG DISEASE, IS ASSUMED TO BE ON A CARDIAC BASIS.

1. Hypoxemia may result from complete or severe obstruction to pulmonary blood flow, as in tricuspid valve atresia or pulmonary valve atresia (with or without associated VSD) or severe TOF, by far the most common cause of hypoxemia associated with oligemic lung fields. TOF is seen is approximately 4% to 5% of neonates and infants with CHD, whereas tricuspid and pulmonary valve atresia are seen in less than 1%. In these malformations, systemic venous return cannot enter the pulmonary artery by traversing the right heart; therefore, right-to-left flow at the atrial level or, in the case of severe TOF, at the ventricular level, accounts for the systemic hypoxemia. The spectrum of right ventricular outflow obstruction is wide, and patients with TOF are seen in the neonatal period, but they are also identified in later infancy, in childhood, and even adulthood—if the resulting hypoxemia is minimal and the murmur does not prompt clinical evaluation.

    a. Immediate medical palliative therapy with prostaglandin E_1 ([PGE_1] Alprostadil, Prostin VR) must be instituted for the neonate with severe hypoxemia ($PaO_2 < 40$ torr) and oligemic lung fields. Immediate response to this intervention should be noted because the PDA is reopened and blood flow to the lungs is augmented. This approach can be implemented prior to anatomic confirmation by echocardiography. Conversely, if the echo were to establish the diagnosis of TOF in a 3-day-old infant with a loud murmur but no hypoxemia ($SPO_2 > 95\%$, $PaO_2 > 65$ torr), the physiologic concern would be negligible—despite a similar anatomic diagnosis—and there would be no role for urgent medical palliative therapy.

    b. If anatomic correction of the cardiac problem can be achieved, open heart surgical repair can be performed. This is rarely the case for any lesion with severe obstruction to pulmonary blood flow encountered in the neonate. Some infants with TOF may have anatomy favorable for repair in early infancy (a single VSD, acceptable pulmonary artery size and morphology, and normal coronary artery origin). Cardiac catheterization is sometimes required to resolve specific anatomic concerns, but most infants can have surgical repair with exclusively noninvasive imaging. Surgical outcome in this group is expected to be good, with >90% 1-year survival in infants without significant cardiac or noncardiac confounding factors. Palliation with systemic to pulmonary artery (Blalock-Taussig) shunt is most often required in the group with right heart atresia and no dependable source of antegrade flow into the lungs, assuring a safe source of pulmonary blood flow until a more definitive strategy can be implemented. For patients with tricuspid valve atresia, this may be a staged separation of the circulation after the initial shunt, with a bidirectional Glenn (SVC-PA) shunt and then Fontan completion—removing the IVC connection to the right atrium and incorporating it directly into the pulmonary arteries. Surgical strategies in this group result in an >80% 5-year survival rate. Those babies with pulmonary valve atresia and intact ventricular septa remain the most difficult management group in which efforts to palliate with systemic-to-pulmonary artery shunt must be combined with a strategy to decompress the RV and permit right ventricular growth. This approach is not applicable to infants with pulmonary atresia and RV-dependent coronary circulation, often resulting in no more than a 70% 5-year survival rate.

2. Hypoxemia may be encountered in venous admixture lesions in which, despite normal-appearing pulmonary vascularity on chest x-ray, profoundly low PaO_2 may be encountered. In the most common example, DTGA, hypoxemia is directly related to the degree of mixing of the venous streams. With multiple connections (ASD, VSD, PDA), the degree of cyanosis/hypoxemia is modest. With only a small atrial connection (usually a patent foramen ovale), an intact ventricular septum and closing PDA, the degree of hypoxemia may be profound, with resulting acidemia and end organ damage. DTGA is seen in approximately 4% of infants with CHD. Much less common, each less than 1%, are the other members of the admixture group. Starting at the great vessel level: common arterial trunk (truncus arteriosus); at the ventricular level: single ventricle; at the atrial level: common atrium; and at the venous level: total anomalous pulmonary venous return (TAPVR). Abnormalities of absent septation, if isolated, manifest when the fall in pulmonary vascular resistance occurs, usually long after nursery discharge. Unfortunately, most of the complete septation anomalies are associated with additional anatomic abnormality, such as obstruction to pulmonary or systemic blood flow, which will dictate the timing of presentation and the complexity of management. TAPVR is the one admixture problem that is frequently associated with obstruction to egress from the pulmonary veins into the right heart, and will manifest with hypoxemia and severe tachypnea. Unobstructed TAPVR may manifest in later infancy or even later childhood if the degree of hypoxemia and resulting cyanosis is not evident early on.

a. Medical palliation with PGE_1 in the neonate with severe hypoxemia due to DTGA is urgent, and should not await echocardiographic definition if severe hyoxemia is associated with normal pulmonary blood flow on chest x-ray and a normal PCO_2. As noted above, recognizing that the degree of hypoxemia is inversely related to the number of intracardiac connections, maintaining or reestablishing ductal patency plays an important role. Catheter palliation—balloon atrial septostomy—will optimize atrial shunting and may increase *effective pulmonary blood flow*. These two interventions may contribute to a rise in PaO_2 from 20 to 25 torr, preintervention, to 40 to 55 torr postintervention, allowing the neonate to remain "safe" prior to definitive surgical intervention (recall that the fetal PaO_2 was in the 20 to 22 torr range). In the neonate with severe hypoxemia due to TAPVR with obstruction, institution of PGE_1 therapy may be counterproductive, permitting increased access of blood flow to a pulmonary bed that cannot decompress, producing increased tachypnea due to pulmonary venous congestion and no improvement in oxygenation. *The response to PGE_1 therapy needs to be carefully monitored.*

b. Surgical repair of lesions in this category, where there are four balanced cardiac chambers, is undertaken in the neonatal period. DTGA is now corrected using the arterial switch procedure and concomitant closure of any additional septal defects. In full-term neonates with no additional confounding medical concerns, >95% survival is achieved. Surgical palliation by the atrial switch procedure (Mustard or Senning operation) is rarely done. Direct repair of TAPVR, an anastomosing of the retrocardiac common pulmonary vein directly to the left atrium, provides an anatomic solution for a hitherto difficult management problem. Pulmonary venous obstruction is most often resolved by surgery because the site of venous obstruction is encountered when (1) the anomalous pulmonary venous channel enters the right atrium, or (2) the ascending vein is compressed between the left pulmonary artery (LPA) and left bronchus or (3) the descending vein enters the portal venous system after closure of the ductus venosus. Surgical outcomes continue to improve, with >90% survival.

B. CONGESTIVE HEART FAILURE IS MANIFESTED BY TACHYPNEA (PULMONARY VENOUS CONGESTION), AND HEPATOMEGALY (SYSTEMIC VENOUS CONGESTION).

Auscultatory evidence of a gallop rhythm may be present. Rarely is peripheral edema or neck vein distention noted. And, depending on the time of presentation, there may be little historical data to support progressively poor feeding, failure to thrive, sweating with feeding, etc. A chest x-ray will almost always demonstrate cardiomegaly. The pulmonary vascularity will be increased to normal, with prominent arterial markings suggesting increased pulmonary blood flow, and venous congestion indicating left heart obstruction. Pulse oximetry will be normal in the case of a pure left-to-right shunt lesion, such as a large VSD or PDA. Some degree of arterial desaturation may be noted with progressive lung edema.

1. Congestive heart failure may result from pulmonary venous obstruction—the inability of pulmonary venous return to exit the lungs and have free access to the body. This is encountered most commonly in left heart obstructive lesions: hypoplastic left heart (HLH) syndrome, coarctation of the aorta, and aortic stenosis. Two of these lesions depend on ductal closure to become apparent; once evident, infants with HLH and coarctation of the aorta—often appearing fairly well after delivery—can present with signs of heart failure and multisystem organ failure due to inadequate systemic

blood flow. HLH and coarctation my have quite similar physical findings on initial recognition: poor pulses and systemic perfusion, a hyperactive precordium, hepatomegaly, a nonspecific systolic murmur, and gallop rhythm. Early on in neonates with coarctation, a blood pressure differential may be noted between right upper and lower extremities, but as LV function deteriorates in response to the severe aortic obstruction, this finding becomes less apparent and the two lesions have little to distinguish them. Both will show RV dominance on the ECG. Even before echocardiography, which affords a specific anatomic diagnosis and is usually all that is required for surgical intervention, PGE_1 should be administered to restore compromised systemic blood flow. The major clinical concern in delaying diagnosis in this group of neonates is sepsis. The clinical history—maternal and neonatal—needs to be reviewed for risk factors, and the physical examination, with a hyperactive precordium, gallop rhythm and hepatomegaly, may reveal the primary issue resulting in compromised perfusion and acidemia.

12

CARDIOLOGY

a. Medical palliation of coarctation of the aorta and HLH is provided with PGE_1, ventilatory support if required, and dopamine/dobutamine, if needed. Reopening the PDA permits restoration of systemic blood flow, reversing renal and GI compromise. Once stable, the neonate is able to proceed to surgical intervention. Rarely, critical aortic stenosis will compromise LV outflow to the degree that restoring ductal patency will be required. Each lesion manifests at a slightly different time in the course of neonatal care, with HLH most likely to be encountered in the first 24 to 48 hours, coarctation of the aorta at 3 to 7 days, and aortic stenosis at 1 to 2 weeks, although variability may occur. If systemic perfusion is compromised, the response should be the same, as noted earlier.

b. Surgical intervention for coarctation of the aorta, whether by the left subclavian flap procedure, resection with end-to-end repair, or patch aortoplasty, generally produces excellent short-term and long-term results. Surgical morbidity and mortality have been reduced from approximately 40% in the pre-PGE_1 era to <5% in neonates with isolated coarctation. Management of HLH is by the staged Norwood approach or cardiac transplantation. In the Norwood pathway there are three surgical procedures over a period of 4 years, resulting in the right ventricle providing systemic blood flow while systemic venous return is anastomosed directly to the pulmonary arteries. Cardiac transplantation requires maintenance of ductal patency for systemic perfusion, as well as protection of the pulmonary bed from systemic pressure, while awaiting an appropriate-sized heart. Compassionate care, previously an equally discussed and accepted form of nonintervention, is less often chosen by families because surgical survival from HLH now equals or exceeds some of the more complex forms of right heart atresias, with 5-year survival approaching

60% to 70% or better. Aortic stenosis, if compromising systemic perfusion or producing markedly elevated LV pressure with still-preserved LV function, can be successfully palliated with balloon dilatation. Adequate relief of stenosis and amelioration of symptoms, rather than complete normalization of LV pressure, are the short-term goals. LV function is generally restored following relief of the critical obstruction, hopefully avoiding the creation of severe aortic regurgitation and progressive LV volume overload. Surgical intervention may be required for severe annular hypoplasia or additional subaortic stenosis.

2. **Congestive heart failure due to left-to-right shunting is dependent on the fall in pulmonary vascular resistance (PVR) to become evident. A large VSD or PDA rarely will provide overt clues before the neonate's discharge from the nursery, more likely becoming evident by the 2-week well-baby visit. Depending on the rate of fall of the PVR, precordial hyperactivity and a soft murmur may be noted. It is the small VSD, particularly the small muscular VSD that creates a loud, long, usually blowing systolic murmur during the nursery stay, but seldom creates any true cardiac concern. When the neonate is suspected of having Down syndrome, clinical evaluation in the nursery and echocardiography are strongly suggested, given the approximately 60% prevalence of CHD in this group of babies. A-V septal defect is most common, and if this or any other form of CHD is defined, appropriate education and follow-up care can be arranged before discharge. More positively, if all is normal, cardiac issues can be safely eliminated from the problem list. Premature infants will generally have a more rapid decline in PVR and demonstrate signs of CHF earlier than term infants. If clinically ill, they offer the additional challenge of small size, requiring long-term medical management before surgical intervention.**

   a. Medical therapy of CHF in infants with large-volume left-to-right shunts has changed very little over the past 2 decades. Assuring adequate caloric intake to sustain growth in a hypermetabolic neonate is vital, with 24 to 30 kcal/oz formula and nasogastric feeding, as required. Digoxin, diuretics, and afterload reduction are still used, but earlier surgical intervention is available if the infant cannot progress with medical therapy alone.

   b. Surgical repair of membranous VSD can be accomplished with minimal risk of mortality or morbidity and with >95% survival. Large muscular defects may be difficult to approach in the young infant, and palliation with a PA band and then subsequent, combined surgical relief of the PA band with interventional catheter-device closure of the defect may offer a more favorable outcome. Surgical ligation of the large PDA associated with CHF and pulmonary artery hypertension is readily accomplished, with particular attention paid to aortic arch integrity during noninvasive preoperative imaging and postoperative physical examination. Catheter intervention plays a limited role in this group of infants.

IV. ALTERED CARDIAC MECHANICS WITHOUT STRUCTURAL HEART MALFORMATION

The neonate is at risk for noncardiac malformations that may have important impact on perinatal cardiac function. There also may be in utero exposures that adversely affect muscle performance.

A. A-V FISTULAE.

Arteriovenous fistulae, particularly intrahepatic and intracranial malformations, may provide a low-resistance circuit and cause high-output CHF in the newborn. Vein of Galen intracranial malformation will produce cardiomegaly on chest x-ray, nonspecific auscultatory findings, and possibly poor lower extremity pulses as blood is preferentially shunted to the cerebral circulation, raising false concern about coarctation of the aorta. However, there will likely be a loud continuous murmur heard over the fontanelles, enabling a high degree of clinical suspicion. When guiding the echocardiographic study to exclude intracardiac malformations, moving the transducer ever more cephalad will demonstrate a large left ventricle and aorta, along with prominent SVC return to the enlarged right heart and continuous high-velocity intracranial flow through the vein of Galen.

B. MYOCARDITIS.

Myocardial dysfunction without associated structural abnormalities, especially when associated with signs of multisystem organ inflammation, should suggest in utero infection with Coxsackie virus, enterovirus, parvovirus or the TORCH agents (**see Chapter 22**). The use of anti-inflammatory therapy and enteroviral neutralizing antibodies, along with appropriate supportive therapy, should be instituted. Inflammatory myocardial dysfunction may also be noted in the spectrum of autoimmune diseases, such as lupus and Sjögren syndrome.

C. HYPERTROPHIC CARDIOMYOPATHY.

Myocardial dysfunction producing cardiomegaly and associated with a maternal history of insulin-dependent diabetes should raise concern, not only about the increased risk of structural heart disease, but also about fetal/neonatal hypertrophic cardiomyopathy. Associated right and/or left ventricular outflow obstruction from the septal hypertrophy may be severe, but with supportive therapy and time will often regress.

D. MYOCARDIAL TUMORS.

Cardiomegaly on fetal echo evaluation or neonatal x-ray, associated with a family history of tuberous sclerosis strongly suggests myocardial rhabdomyomas. Although often large, bulky tumors—occasionally producing severe outflow obstruction or limiting ventricular inflow—they often regress, only rarely requiring surgical debulking. The neonate may be the first in the family to raise suspicion of this problem, and evaluation of first-degree family members for tuberous sclerosis should be considered.

12

CARDIOLOGY

V. CARDIAC RHYTHM DISTURBANCE

A 12-lead ECG is mandatory for adequate assessment of rhythm abnormality that was defined in utero or first recognized on neonatal examination. Even if fetal tachycardia has not been a recurrent issue postnatally, ECG evidence of ventricular preexcitation may influence follow-up care. A family history of sudden unexplained death in adolescence or early adulthood, or a history of unexplained seizures or syncope in family members should prompt an ECG to evaluate for prolonged QTc.

A. IRREGULAR HEART BEATS ARE USUALLY CAUSED BY PREMATURE ATRIAL CONTRACTIONS.

This is often noted in utero and may be found in 2% or more of healthy newborns on 24-hour Holter monitoring. They are rarely of clinical importance and rarely progress to sustained tachycardia. If the premature beats are ventricular in origin, echocardiography is indicated to assure normal cardiac function and myocardial appearance. Holter monitoring should be considered as well.

B. BRADYCARDIA WITH A SUSTAINED HEART RATE OF <100 BEATS PER MINUTE REQUIRES EVALUATION TO VERIFY THERE IS NO A-V BLOCK, EITHER SECOND OR THIRD DEGREE (COMPLETE).

The confirmation of high-degree A-V block in the neonate requires Holter monitoring to verify there are no prolonged pauses or ventricular escape beats. In addition, there should be notification of the obstetrician, so that mother can be evaluated for subclinical evidence of autoimmune disease, with measurement of anti-Ro and anti-La titers as a marker for lupus/Sjögren syndrome. Echocardiography to evaluate ventricular function and anatomy is also mandated. Profound bradycardia in the neonate due to third degree A-V block, with heart rates <50 bpm, often requires support with Isuprel or temporary transvenous/transumbilical pacing if there is evidence of low cardiac output and acidemia, followed by permanent epicardial pacemaker placement. Second-degree A-V block requires careful follow-up evaluation because of the risk of progression. If recognized early on, and associated with evidence of myocardial dysfunction, anti-inflammatory therapy may be considered—in addition to other supportive therapy.

C. TACHYCARDIA MAY BE SINUS, ATRIAL, OR VENTRICULAR.

1. Sinus tachycardia in a septic neonate *may produce heart rates in the 220 to 240 range*. Slight variability in rate will often be noted, and the ECG should be run at double speed to help define the P waves, which will be upright in leads I and aVF, confirming sinus rhythm and avoiding administration of adenosine to terminate SVT.
2. Supraventricular tachycardia (SVT) is most often a narrow QRS tachycardia at a rate of 240 to 310 in neonates. P waves are usually difficult to recognize. The majority of cases are not associated with

structural heart disease. With a structurally normal heart, typical SVT at a rate of 240 bpm can be tolerated for hours, but will eventually cause decompensation if not treated. Faster rates are progressively less well tolerated. Atrial flutter is a less common finding in the neonate, and is *often difficult to recognize if all 12 leads of the ECG are not available*. The "typical saw-tooth pattern" of the flutter waves, often at a rate of 300 to 600 in the neonate, may be recognized in only a single lead. Associated 2:1 A-V block will generally produce a ventricular rate in the 180 to 220 range, and the loss of A-V synchrony and sustained tachycardia will eventually cause CHF, depending on the ventricular rate.

a. Treatment of SVT depends on clinical presentation. If SVT is persistent and the neonate is in shock, cardioversion is essential. The initial dose of 0.5 to 1.0 watt-sec/kg is usually effective, but may be doubled if ineffective. If the infant is stable, with adequate perfusion and blood pressure, a trial of vagal maneuvers may be attempted. Gagging or rectal stimulation is easiest. A slurry of ice applied to the face for 10 seconds, taking care not to create hypothermia by repeated application, may produce the "diving reflex" and reflex bradycardia. While this is going on, adenosine should be drawn up and given if simpler maneuvers are not successful. The initial dose of 50 to 100 μg/kg intravenously—given quickly, may be doubled if no response is noted. The dose may be increased successively for two or three doses, and if no response is noted or if normal sinus rhythm is not maintained, a longer-acting medication is required. Amiodarone given intravenously is emerging as an excellent choice to obtain stable rhythm acutely, and then maintenance with beta blockers can be established. Atrial flutter, especially with clinical compromise, should be cardioverted. Recurrence is relatively rare and long-term medical therapy is not routinely required.

3. Ventricular tachycardia (VT) is a rare finding in the neonate. If a regular, wide QRS tachycardia is noted, a test dose of adenosine may help differentiate SVT with aberrancy from VT. Continuous ECG monitoring during medication administration will demonstrate the transient A-V block seen in SVT and will have little effect on VT. Heart rate in VT is usually in the 180 to 220 range in the neonate, with the loss of A-V synchrony and possible underlying ventricular dysfunction contributing to the eventual development of CHF.

a. Treatment with cardioversion, as above, or with intravenous lidocaine or amiodarone, is usually effective.

b. Echocardiography is mandatory to evaluate cardiac function, structure, and myocardial appearance.

CARDIOLOGY 12

BIBLIOGRAPHY

Ferencz C, Rubin JD, Lofredo CA, Magee CA: Epidemiology of congenital heart disease: The Baltimore-Washington Infant Study, 1981-1989. Mt. Kisco, NY, Futura, 1993.

Fost N: Bioethics of the mother, fetus and newborn. In Fanaroff AA, Martin RJ (eds): Neonatal-Perinatal Medicine, ed. 6. St Louis, Mosby, 1997.

Moller JH, Hoffman JIE: Pediatric Cardiovascular Medicine. New York, Churchill-Livingstone, 2000.

Park MK: Pediatric Cardiology for Practitioners. St. Louis, Mosby, 2002.

Pulmonary System

Siew-Jyu Wong

FAST FACTS

Immediate Issues in the Nursery

- Hypoxia can cause apnea in premature and small-for-gestational-age (SGA) infants due to delayed maturation of the autonomic nervous system.
- A hyperoxic challenge test can be used to differentiate cardiac from pulmonary causes of hypoxia. If the PaO_2 is >200 mm Hg after 10 minutes of 100% oxygen, then the cause of the hypoxia is most likely pulmonary.
- The incidence of transient tachypnea of the newborn (TTN) is increased in elective cesarean section, male infants, macrosomic infants, and in infants of mothers with asthma.
- There is increased risk for respiratory distress syndrome (RDS) with decreasing gestational age, maternal diabetes, white male infants, acute asphyxia, family history of RDS, and second deliveries in twin gestations.

Important Reminders After Discharge

- Although an infant may present after discharge with signs of respiratory distress (cyanosis, retractions, tachypnea, grunting, and nasal flaring, these signs may in fact be related to a nonrespiratory cause (e.g., cardiac, hematologic, metabolic, or infectious).
- Maternal medications and diet can have an impact on an infant's respiratory rate and overall respiratory pattern. These are usually accompanied by changes in level of alertness and in heart rate pattern.

Helpful Information for Parents

- Symptoms of meconium aspiration generally occur within the first 48 hours of life. Therefore, parents need not worry about respiratory difficulty resulting from meconium once they are discharged.
- When appropriate, be sure to fully educate parents about the usefulness of cardiorespiratory monitoring (CRM) at home. CRM has not been demonstrated to reduce the risk of sudden infant death syndrome (SIDS). CRM is indicated in documented cases of apnea, however.
- There is tremendous variation in the respiratory pattern of a newborn, in terms of rate of respirations, chest wall movement, and types of sounds emitted. Parents should be told that their baby's breathing pattern will be inconsistent and often noisy. They should follow up with their provider if the baby is having difficulty with sleeping or eating, or if their infant is persistently fussy.

Fetal breathing movements can be observed by about 11 weeks of gestation. Movements increase with gestational age but diminish sharply within 3 days of labor. These movements can be stimulated by smoking and hypercapnia and depressed by hypoxia and barbiturates. Lung liquid is reabsorbed to some extent during labor. Once the first breath is taken and the lungs inflate, there is a major stimulus to the release of lung surfactant into the alveolar spaces.

I. APNEA: CESSATION OF AIR EXCHANGE

A. TYPES.

1. Central apnea. No respiratory effort for 15 seconds; may be associated with hypoxemia and bradycardia.
2. Obstructive apnea. Resulting from airway obstruction; may be positional, functional (caused by poor tone of pharyngeal dilator [e.g., in prematurity], reflex spasms [e.g., in reaction to regurgitation of milk], or incoordination of pharyngeal muscles during feeding), or structural (see **Chapter 10**).
3. Mixed apnea. A combination of central and obstructive types.

B. CAUSES.

1. At delivery (see **Chapter 4**).
2. In the nursery, causes for central and mixed apnea include the following:
   a. Maternal drugs (e.g., sedatives, analgesics, magnesium).
   b. Metabolic imbalance (e.g., hypoglycemia, acidosis, alkalosis, hyperammonemia, electrolyte imbalance).
   c. Infection (e.g., sepsis, meningitis, necrotizing enterocolitis [NEC]).
   d. Temperature instability.
   e. Hematologic disorders (e.g., anemia or polycythemia).
   f. Seizures, especially if apnea is accompanied by tachycardia rather than bradycardia.
   g. Hypoxia. In premature and SGA infants with delayed autonomic system maturation, hypoxia triggers hypopneic response rather than hyperpneic response.
   h. Cardiovascular system (CVS) disorders (e.g., shock, patent ductus arteriosus [PDA]), with decreased blood flow to central nervous system (CNS).
   i. CNS disorders (e.g., immature CNS), congenital malformations of the CNS, chromosomal anomalies such as trisomy 13 or 18, intracranial hemorrhage, or intraventricular hemorrhage.
   j. Gastrointestinal disorders (e.g., gastroesophageal reflux and swallowing difficulties).

C. DIAGNOSIS AND MANAGEMENT.

1. History. An obstetric history should be taken to look for risk factors that could affect the pulmonary system, such as a difficult delivery, maternal fever or chorioamnionitis, drug abuse, drugs administered to the mother before and (if breast-feeding) after birth, resuscitation of the infant needed at birth, or a low Apgar score. Umbilical cord pH levels, gestational age, and events associated with apnea (e.g., drastic temperature changes, feeding, seizure activity) should also be noted.

2. Physical examination. During the physical examination, the practitioner should note the infant's temperature and the presence of either fever or hypothermia. He or she should also note the presence of dysmorphic features and malformation, skin color and perfusion, blood pressure, irritability or lethargy, tone and activity, the state of the anterior fontanel, the presence (if any) of milk in nasal and nasopharyngeal passages, the quality of respiratory effort, and the presence of any murmur, petechiae, or hepatosplenomegaly. Gestational age should also be noted. Pulse oximetry is available in most nurseries. A newborn after the first hours of life should have an SaO_2 of 94% or more in room air. A difference of >15% in the preductal (on the right upper extremity) and postductal (on the foot) SaO_2 indicates shunting through the PDA. In pulmonary hypertension and coarctation the preductal will be more than the postductal reading whereas the reverse will be true in transposition of the great arteries with coarctation. A hyperoxic challenge test could be done. If after receiving 100% O_2 for 10 minutes, arterial blood gas (ABG) measurement yields a PaO_2 of >200 mm Hg, the cause for hypoxia is most likely pulmonary. If not, an echocardiogram should be done to rule out cardiac causes or persistent pulmonary hypertension of the newborn (PPHN).

3. Laboratory evaluation (if the cause is not obvious) should be considered to assess the following: glucose and electrolyte (Ca^{++}, Mg^{++} pH, NH_3) levels, complete blood cell count (CBC) and differential, blood gases, gastric pH levels, and the possibility of sepsis. Other studies may be indicated, such as chest x-rays, a spinal tap, ultrasound of the head, electroencephalogram, or a pneumogram with an esophageal pH probe.

II. RESPIRATORY DISTRESS

Respiratory distress is indicated by the following signs, either singly or in combination: cyanosis, tachypnea, retractions, grunting, and nasal flaring. It may initially be related to nonrespiratory events.

A. CAUSES OF RESPIRATORY DISTRESS.

1. Sepsis.
2. Hematologic (polycythemia).
3. Cardiac (cyanotic and noncyanotic heart disease).
4. Shock.

13

PULMONARY SYSTEM

5. Metabolic (acidosis, hypoglycemia, hyperammonemia).
6. Respiratory.

B. RESPIRATORY-RELATED CAUSES.

1. Airway problems. At times prenatal ultrasound might detect potential airway problems such as tumors, vascular malformations, and encephaloceles in or around the nose, mouth, pharynx, or neck that cause airway obstruction. Certain congenital syndromes with craniofacial anomalies are associated with airway problems. Examples of lesions that may cause airway problems include the following:

a. Nasal obstruction. Choanal atresia/stenosis, cysts, atresia seen in CHARGE association.

b. Pharyngeal obstruction. Glossoptosis with micrognathia and central cleft palate in Pierre Robin sequence. Laryngeal mask airway (LMA) is helpful in managing this. Pharyngeal masses such as encephaloceles and polyps may also cause obstruction.

c. Vocal cord disorders. These may be functional, as seen in Arnold-Chiari malformation, or structural, as in laryngomalacia or a laryngeal web.

d. Subglottic lesions. Laryngotracheal edema may be caused by intubation related to the presence of meconium, or hemangiomas, tracheomalacia, stenosis, or atresia.

e. Paratracheal lesions (e.g., goiter, superior mediastinal masses, cystic hygromas, or vascular ring). Esophageal atresia with or without tracheoesophageal fistula (TEF) may cause aspiration into the lungs.

2. Poor respiratory muscle effort.

a. Diaphragmatic paralysis.

(1) Diaphragmatic paralysis may result from phrenic nerve injury and is usually associated with difficult delivery, shoulder dystocia, brachial plexus injury, and clavicular fracture, singly or together.

(2) Chest x-rays may show unilateral elevation of the paralyzed hemidiaphragm.

(3) Ultrasound may show absence of movement or paradoxic movement of the paralyzed leaf.

(4) Other causes include phrenic nerve compression by tumors such as neuroblastoma, and iatrogenic injury during insertion of chest tubes.

b. Myopathies, muscular dystrophies, and myasthenia.

3. Parenchymal causes.

a. Transient tachypnea of the newborn (TTN).

(1) TTN is a diagnosis of exclusion. There is an increased incidence of TTN in cesarean section deliveries (especially if they are not preceded by labor and are before 39 completed weeks of gestation), in infants who are male, in macrosomic infants, and in infants whose mothers have asthma.

(2) TTN usually involves tachypnea with minimal evidence of respiratory distress, with or without O_2 requirement.

(3) Chest x-rays show fluid in fissures (sometimes minimal), pleural effusion, and streaky parenchymal changes with hyperinflation.

(4) O_2 needs are short term; tachypnea may last longer. Follow-up chest x-rays show rapid clearing of fluid, usually within 24 hours. TTN might be complicated by pulmonary hypertension.

b. Respiratory distress syndrome (RDS).

(1) RDS occurs characteristically in preterm infants and is related to surfactant deficiency. There is an increased risk of RDS with decreasing gestational age, maternal diabetes, white male infants, acute asphyxia, second twin, and family history of RDS. PDA complicates recovery from RDS. In older gestational age infants, pulmonary hypertension might complicate management. RDS might occur in "term infants" especially if delivered by elective cesarean section at <39 completed weeks' gestation, or by precipitous delivery. If the infant is not following a typical course with response to surfactant and with improvement over time, certain cardiac lesions such as total anomalous pulmonary venous return (TAPVR) and genetic surfactant protein-B deficiency should be considered.

(2) Prevention of RDS is primary. Early prenatal care allows identification of an at-risk woman and education for all pregnant women to get them to be sensitive to the possibility of premature labor. This allows early detection of labor, improves the effectiveness of tocolysis, and permits the use of betamethasone to hasten lung maturity. Prenatal betamethasone also has been shown to decrease intraventricular hemorrhage (IVH) and periventricular leukomalacia (PVL) in very-low-birth-weight (VLBW) infants. However, multiple (i.e., more than two) courses of prenatal steroids might be deleterious. Betamethasone is the preferred prenatal steroid to dexamethasone because dexamethasone increases the risk of periventricular leukomalacia (PVL).

(3) Prompt and appropriate resuscitation at delivery decreases asphyxia-related surfactant destruction. There has been increased interest in the issue of delayed cord clamping of ≥30 seconds in preterm infants to facilitate placental transfusion—thereby decreasing the incidence of hypovolemia associated with decreased systemic flow and also increasing pulmonary capillary distention resulting in airway and alveolar stabilization.

(4) Shortly after birth, the preterm infant with RDS will start to show signs of respiratory distress, with tachypnea, retractions, grunting, and cyanosis. Chest x-rays in mild cases may show minimal underexpansion, progressing in 24 to 48 hours to the typical ground-glass reticulogranular appearance with air bronchogram. In moderate cases, RDS may start out with typical reticulogranular appearance with air bronchogram; in severe cases there is blurring of heart, diaphragm, and rib-cage borders because of marked atelectasis ("total whiteout").

13

PULMONARY SYSTEM

(5) Management includes the following:

    (a) Respiratory support in the form of early institution of nasal continuous positive airway pressure (NCPAP) might avoid the need for intubation and assisted ventilation, especially in the larger infants.

    (b) Infection and pneumonia should be ruled out; antibiotics should be used as needed; other immature organ systems should be supported.

    (c) Exogenous surfactant should be administered to infants with RDS who require endotracheal intubation for mechanical ventilatory support. Exogenous surfactant used prophylactically in very small infants at delivery has been shown to decrease the severity of RDS in the short term. The availability of exogenous surfactant is associated with decreased national neonatal and infant mortality.

    (d) Persistent pulmonary hypertension of the newborn (PPHN) is a complication of RDS, especially in infants of older gestational age.

    (e) Acute complications of barotrauma, such as pulmonary interstitial emphysema (PIE), pneumothoraces, and pneumopericardium, are constantly considered with any deterioration.

    (f) Pneumonias such as those caused by group B streptococcus (GBS) and *Ureaplasma urealyticum* should be considered when there is early appearance of PIE.

(6) Adult respiratory distress syndrome (ARDS) has been described in full-term infants and is characterized by shock, asphyxia, and aspiration.

c. Meconium aspiration syndrome (MAS).

    (1) The incidence of meconium-stained amniotic fluid depends on infant maturity; it is rare at less than 37 weeks' gestation. An associated risk of asphyxia mandates the presence of skilled personnel at delivery.

    (2) Management should be preventive. At delivery of the head, the obstetrician should clear the infant's airway, although this practice has been questioned. If the newborn is not vigorous at birth, tracheal suctioning under direct laryngoscopy should be done. Vigorous is defined by having good respiratory effort, good tone, and a heart rate of ≥100.

    (3) MAS can occur in utero. With severe stress the fetus may pass meconium and may gasp deeply causing the aspiration of meconium-mixed amniotic fluid into the lungs. At birth, this newborn will not be vigorous.

    (4) Diagnosis is by history, the presence of respiratory distress, and subsequent chest x-ray.

    (5) Management of MAS is complex, involving management for asphyxia-related multiorgan system effects especially the CNS, CVS, renal and gastrointestinal systems, in addition to the pulmonary system. Particular attention is needed to avoid further stress (e.g., hypoxia, hypercapnia, cold stress, hypoglycemia, noise, discomfort, and metabolic imbalance) to avoid or prevent worsening

of PPHN. Pneumomediastinum and pneumothorax are common; antibiotics are usually given. High-frequency ventilation without or with nitric oxide (NO), or extracorporeal membrane oxygenation (ECMO) may be life-saving.

d. Pneumonia.

(1) Risk factors for pneumonia include premature labor, premature rupture of membranes, prolonged rupture of membranes, maternal GBS colonization, maternal chorioamnionitis, maternal fever, asphyxia, difficult delivery, and tracheoesophageal fistula.

(2) Onset is usually early, with signs of respiratory distress, apnea, hypotension, shock, and secondary PPHN.

(3) Chest x-rays may show patchy or streaky infiltrates, but findings may be indistinguishable from those of RDS. Hence, in infants with RDS, pneumonia should be ruled out if antibiotics are not given.

(4) Workup includes cultures of blood, tracheal aspirate, and cerebrospinal fluid (CSF); lumbar puncture (LP) should be postponed if infant is unstable; CSF—if obtained after antibiotics were given—can be sent for rapid antigen detection in addition to the usual culture, cell count, and chemistry.

(5) Mortality remains high. Ampicillin and gentamicin remain the drugs of choice to cover GBS, *Haemophilus, Pneumococcus, Listeria, Escherichia coli,* and other gram-negative organisms. The Centers for Disease Control and Prevention (CDC) has revised guidelines for intrapartum antibiotic prophylaxis for maternal GBS colonization and chorioamnionitis (MMWR, Aug 2002). Cefotaxime instead of gentamicin is considered if there is renal compromise or strong suspicion of gram-negative meningitis. In case of maternal chorioamnionitis, anaerobic coverage might need to be considered.

(6) TORCH infections should be considered, especially in at-risk situations such as congenital syphilis and primary herpes around the time of delivery.

(7) Septic shock, PPHN, leukopenia, thrombocytopenia, and disseminated intravascular coagulation (DIC) complicate management. Aggressive volume and pressor support are used to treat septic shock. Intravenous immunoglobulin (IVIG), monoclonal antibodies, white blood cell (WBC) transfusion, and granulocyte-colony stimulating factor (G-CSF) have been used. High-frequency ventilation, without or with NO, and ECMO may be helpful when conventional ventilation fails.

e. PPHN can be primary or secondary. Secondary PPHN is defined as PPHN associated with parenchymal problems as mentioned earlier, cardiac lesions, or hypoplastic lungs. Hypoplastic lungs can occur with constraints on lung development during the critical period (<28 weeks' gestation). These include: oligohydramnios caused by prolonged, premature, or very preterm rupture of membranes, or poor renal function; intrathoracic, large, space-occupying lesions in early gestation, such as

13

PULMONARY SYSTEM

congenital diaphragmatic hernia (CDH), pleural effusions, and congenital cysts. In primary PPHN, there is no pulmonary cause. In the prenatal and intrapartum history there might be suggestions of fetal hypoxemia, distress, or conditions causing premature closure of the PDA, such as indomethacin use. An echocardiogram will provide definitive diagnosis and rule out congenital cardiac lesions as the cause of the cyanosis, although preductal and postductal O_2 saturation and PAo_2 will be of some help. PPHN can be fatal. The goal is to relax the pulmonary vasculature, keep the infant well oxygenated, avoid handling and stimulation, provide sedation and analgesia, give sodium bicarbonate to keep base deficit to zero, and provide pressure support as needed to keep systemic blood pressure higher than pulmonary pressure without causing systemic hypertension. In many cases, assisted ventilation is needed; in severe cases, high-frequency ventilation, without or with NO, is necessary. Various pharmaceutical pulmonary vasodilators, such as tolazoline, magnesium, and prostaglandins, have been tried but because of side effects they have been replaced by NO. Finally, ECMO might be needed to tide the infant over the critical period. Infants born at very high altitudes who are not genetically adapted might develop pulmonary hypertension after the first few days of life.

4. Space-occupying lesions.

a. Diaphragmatic hernia (DH).

(1) When DH is diagnosed by prenatal ultrasound, the mother should be transferred for delivery to a tertiary center with pediatric surgery capabilities. However, not all cases are anticipated prenatally.

(2) DH is one of the causes of unanticipated newborn resuscitation in a supposedly low-risk pregnancy (and hence a reason for immediate availability of trained, skilled personnel in all hospitals with delivery services).

(3) After uneventful labor and delivery, the infant may deteriorate rapidly after the first gasp; DH should be suspected when an appropriate or large-for-gestational-age newborn whose delivery is not frank breech has a scaphoid abdomen and develops acute respiratory distress.

(4) These infants should be given only endotracheal intermittent positive pressure breathing (IPPB) because ventilation by face mask will distend the herniated gastrointestinal contents and worsen the respiratory status.

(5) Pneumothoraces are common because of bilateral hypoplastic lungs. Thoracentesis may be needed in the delivery room.

(6) Ventilatory management might include permissive hypercapnia. Accompanying PPHN complicates management. High-frequency ventilation, with or without NO, or ECMO may help.

(7) DH is sometimes associated with trisomy 13 or 18 and Rubinstein-Taybi syndrome.

(8) Surgery, sometimes delayed because of pulmonary issues, is definitive treatment. Morbidity and mortality in severe DH remain high.

b. Pneumothorax and pneumomediastinum.

(1) Spontaneous pneumothorax occurs in 1% to 2% of live births. Spontaneous symptomatic pneumothorax, however, occurs in 1:1500 live births and may be associated with single umbilical artery and renal malformations. Symptomatic infants are noted to be tachypneic, with minimal retractions, grunting, and nasal flaring. They may be cyanotic in room air. On auscultation, there is diminished air entry on the affected side, muffled heart sounds, and shifting of the cardiac impulse. Transillumination may not be positive in a full-sized newborn. A chest x-ray is diagnostic. Treatment is supportive, with spontaneous resolution. Thoracentesis is indicated in cases of tension pneumothorax, which causes depression of the ipsilateral diaphragm and shift of the mediastinum to the opposite side.

(2) Most pneumothoraces are not spontaneous and are associated with iatrogenic hyperinflation during newborn resuscitation, sometimes right main stem bronchus intubation with atelectasis of the left lung and hyperinflation of the right lung, or with RDS, MAS, or hypoplastic lungs. Thoracentesis and thoracostomy are frequently needed in those with severe and persistent respiratory distress.

c. Chylothorax, pleural effusion (e.g., in fetal hydrops).

d. Other causes. Tumors, enteric or bronchial cysts, cystic adenomatoid malformation of the lungs, or congenital lobar emphysema.

III. ABNORMALITIES IN GAS EXCHANGE

Gas exchange in the alveolar-capillary unit depends on ventilation, membrane thickness and area, perfusion, ventilation-perfusion mismatch, venous gas tension, and inspired gas tension.

A. VENTILATION.

Ventilation is the movement of gas by convection, bulk flow, and molecular diffusion through the conducting airways into the alveoli, where gas exchange takes place, resulting in the elimination of CO_2 and the uptake of O_2 into the pulmonary capillary blood.

1. Hypoventilation. Inadequate gas exchange leading to increased $Paco_2$ and end-tidal Pco_2.

a. Causes.

(1) Poor respiratory effort caused by central depression, phrenic nerve injury, or respiratory muscle weakness in myopathies, myasthenia, dystrophies, or fatigue.

(2) Airway obstruction (see **Chapter 10**).

(3) Restrictive causes from within (e.g., RDS, PIE, hypoplastic lungs, or pneumonia) or from without (e.g., pneumothorax, tumors, or pleural effusion).

13

PULMONARY SYSTEM

b. Effects. Moderate increase in Pco_2 increases respiratory drive, with increase in respiratory rate and depth, heart rate, stroke volume, cardiac output, systolic blood pressure, pulse pressure with systemic vasodilation, and intrapulmonary vasoconstriction. Worsens PPHN.

c. Acute rise of Pco_2 causes CO_2 narcosis, respiratory depression, decreased myocardial contractility, hypotension, and shock.

2. **Hyperventilation. Excessive ventilation resulting in hypocapnia and decreased end-tidal Pco_2.**

a. Causes.
   (1) Compensatory for metabolic acidosis.
   (2) Response to mild-to-moderate hypoxemia.
   (3) Local limited atelectasis stimulating stretch receptors.
   (4) Iatrogenic.

b. Effects. Marked hypocapnia with alkalosis decreases ionized calcium and potassium, increases nerve and muscle excitability, decreases cerebral blood flow, and shifts the oxygen hemoglobin dissociation curve to the left with decreased O_2 release at tissue level. Systemic vasoconstriction and decreased tissue perfusion coupled with decreased O_2 release may result in tissue hypoxia. Cerebral vasoconstriction might contribute to the development of periventricular leukomalacia (PVL) in the susceptible preterm infant.

B. MEMBRANE THICKNESS AND AREA.

Increased membrane thickness and decreased area retard the rate of gas exchange. Causes include the following:

1. **Fluid in alveolar and interstitial space (seen in retained lung fluid), inflammation, or congestive heart failure.**
2. **Air, as in interstitial emphysema.**
3. **Hypoplastic lungs and atelectatic lungs with decreased area for gas exchange.**

C. PERFUSION.

Reduced pulmonary capillary blood flow is seen in PPHN (either primary or associated with various pulmonary disorders), polycythemia with its attendant hyperviscosity, and certain cyanotic congenital heart diseases (e.g., severe pulmonic stenosis, pulmonary atresia, and tetralogy of Fallot [TOF]). In both cases, the right-to-left shunt through the PDA and patent foramen into the systemic circulation decreases the O_2 saturation. After tissue extraction, the O_2 saturation in the mixed venous return is even lower. When this blood is returned to the lungs, the severe hypoxemia causes further pulmonary vasoconstriction, thereby setting off a vicious cycle of increased pulmonary vascular resistance, decreased pulmonary flow, increasing shunt, and increased systemic hypoxemia, which increases pulmonary vascular resistance.

D. VENTILATION-PERFUSION (V/Q) MISMATCH.

Wasted perfusion occurs in atelectatic alveoli, causing low V/Q. Wasted ventilation occurs in overventilated alveoli, causing high V/Q.

E. VENOUS GAS TENSION.

In cyanotic states, shock, and severe anemia, the mixed venous P_{O_2} may be extremely low. This blood is then returned to the alveolar-capillary unit. With equilibration after gas exchange, the resulting P_{O_2} may still be low. It is important to recognize the presence of these factors and rectify them if possible. Causes of poor tissue perfusion with resulting increased tissue extraction and low venous P_{O_2} include the following:

1. Hypovolemia. Hypovolemia can be caused by massive fetomaternal transfusion, twin-to-twin transfusion, fetoplacental transfusion with cord compression, placental abruption, placenta previa, vasa previa, incision into the anterior placenta at cesarean section, position of newborn at delivery and timing of cord clamping, massive internal hemorrhage (e.g., hepatic, intracranial, adrenal, subgaleal).
2. Cardiogenic shock. Causes of cardiogenic shock include myocardial depression in severe asphyxia and some congenital heart disease (e.g., hypoplastic left heart), cardiac arrhythmia, myocarditis, and myopathies.
3. Sepsis.

IV. CLINICAL APPROACH TO AN INFANT IN THE WELL-BABY NURSERY WITH RESPIRATORY SYMPTOMS:

In most hospitals, newborns <34 to 35 weeks' gestation are admitted to the special care or intensive care nursery. Therefore, most well-baby nurseries do have premature infants of gestational age 34 to 36 weeks.

In the event of being called regarding a symptomatic infant, provide resuscitation if needed. It is necessary to review the prenatal history, labor and delivery details, and the clinical presentation while doing a physical assessment and deciding the course of action. In cases of positive VDRL, HSV, GBS and intrapartum chemoprophylaxis, maternal fever and chorioamnionitis, and prolonged or premature rupture of membranes, assess for sepsis and infections. In cesarean sections and precipitous deliveries, asses for transient tachypnea. Assess for RDS in cases of preterm delivery, or elective scheduled cesarean before 39 complete weeks of gestation. Assess for hypovolemia in cases of placenta and cord related problems and in difficult deliveries, and for phrenic nerve injury in shoulder dystocia. In addition, assess for amniotic fluid, meconium, or blood aspiration, and for drug-related problems such as hypermagnesemia, maternal sedation or withdrawal from prescribed (anti-anxiety and antidepressants, methadone) or illicit drugs. Clinical presentation and timing of symptoms will provide clues such as problems with secretions since birth for esophageal atresia and tracheoesophageal fistula; association with feeding for gastroesophageal reflux; and association with lethargy and poor feeding for infections or metabolic errors. Physical examination will provide further clues. Pulse oximetry is very useful. Compare O_2 saturation of the right upper extremity and on the foot in case of doubt. Attempts should be made to pass a nasogastric tube if nasal obstruction or esophageal atresia is suspected. A chest x-ray is useful to rule out or identify lesions. The appearance of lung lesions on prenatal ultrasounds, which then seem to disappear, can be misleading and requires intensive follow-up including a chest x-ray and a CT scan. A complete sepsis workup and treatment for sepsis should be instituted promptly with clinical suspicion of sepsis.

BIBLIOGRAPHY

Centers for Disease Control and Prevention: Prevention of perinatal group B streptococcal disease: Revised guidelines from CDC. MMWR 51(RR-11):1, 2002.

Donn SM, Faix RG: Neonatal emergencies, New York, Futura, 1991.

Goldsmith JP, Karotkin EH: Assisted ventilation of the neonate, ed 4. Philadelphia, WB Saunders, 2004.

Goldsmith JP, Spitzer AR: Controversies in neonatal pulmonary care. Clin Perinatol 25:1, 1998.

Jain L, Keenan W: Resuscitation of the fetus and newborn. Clin Perinatol 26:549, 1999.

Kattwinkel J: Textbook of Neonatal Resuscitation, 4th ed. American Heart Association and American Academy of Pediatrics, 2000.

Philip AGS, Saigal S: When should we clamp the umbilical cord? Neo Rev 5:e154, 2004.

Wiswell TE, Donn SM: Update on mechanical ventilation and exogenous surfactant. Clin Perinatol 28:3, 2001.

Gastroenterology

Jose M. Saavedra

FAST FACTS

Immediate Issues in the Nursery

- Initial management of significant bloody emesis should include: assessment of cardiovascular stability; gastric lavage with warm saline; verification of vitamin K administration; inspection for petechiae; and abdominal x-rays, upper GI studies, and/or ultrasound (to evaluate for obstruction).
- In the newborn, gas is usually present in the stomach at 1 hour of life, in the cecum by 3 hours, and in the rectosigmoid by 8 to 10 hours. These times may be slightly delayed in preterm infants. Bowel gas pattern on abdominal x-ray is very important in the initial evaluation for possible bowel obstruction and should usually be the initial imaging study performed.
- Meconium ileus accounts for about one third of all neonatal small bowel obstructions, and it is almost always associated with cystic fibrosis. By contrast, meconium plug syndrome refers to colonic obstruction by meconium or mucus. This entity can be seen in infants of diabetic mothers, preterm infants, infants with cystic fibrosis, Hirschsprung disease, or with a history of maternal magnesium sulfate administration.

Important Reminders After Discharge

- If diarrhea persists for >2 weeks, causes include infection, protein allergy, malabsorption syndromes, antibiotic exposure (infant or maternal), and enterocolitis, which can even be caused by Hirschsprung disease or necrotizing enterocolitis (NEC).
- Gastroesophageal reflux (GER), persistent regurgitation alone, is caused by transient lower esophageal relaxation that is out of sync with normal swallowing and gastric contraction. Gastroesophageal reflux disease (GERD) occurs when there are symptoms of esophagitis, feeding disruption, and/or cardiorespiratory symptoms. GERD should be treated, and, when severe symptoms occur, there should be an evaluation for partial obstruction.
- Difficulty with stool passage, discomfort between stools, hard stool consistency, and an alternating stool pattern (diarrhea⇔constipation) should prompt intervention in an infant with infrequent stools.

Helpful Information for Parents

- Approximately 50% of infants will regurgitate (effortless expulsion of stomach contents that have reached the mouth) two or more times a day until about 2 months of age, and 80% of infants regurgitate formula at least once a day until about 3 months of age. Applying accurate definitions to "regurgitation," "vomiting," "spitting up," and

Continued

I. GASTROINTESTINAL (GI) DISTURBANCES

A. VOMITING/REGURGITATION.

1. General comments.

a. *Gastroesophageal reflux (GER)* is the usually passive phenomenon of passage of gastric contents into the esophagus. *Regurgitation* is the usually effortless expulsion of refluxed material which has reached the mouth (spit up). *Vomiting* is the forceful expulsion of GI contents, following an integrated reflex response involving contraction of the respiratory, abdominal, and GI muscles. The differentiation between the latter two is not always clinically obvious in newborns; but they have different pathophysiologic significance and clinical implications.

b. Regurgitation of the first few feedings in a newborn is common.

c. Approximately 50% of infants will regurgitate two or more times a day until about 2 months of age and 80% of infants regurgitate formula at least once a day until about 3 months of age.

2. **Persistent regurgitation without other signs or symptoms usually represents "uncomplicated" GER. When accompanied by pathologic signs or symptoms it is called GE reflux disease (GERD) (see GE Reflux, p. 163).**

3. **The character of vomiting is critical in suggesting potential underlying pathology.**

a. Hematemesis may represent a benign or serious condition (see GI bleeding, p. 159).

b. Bilious vomiting often indicates obstruction at or beyond the second portion of the duodenum and *represents a potential surgical emergency* (see Intestinal Obstruction, p. 162).

4. **Etiology of vomiting.**

a. Usually not bilious
  (1) Overfeeding.
  (2) Milk/formula protein allergy.
  (3) Sepsis, urinary tract infection, meningitis.
  (4) Necrotizing enterocolitis (NEC).
  (5) Central nervous system (CNS) lesion.
  (6) Pyloric stenosis.
  (7) Metabolic abnormalities (hypercalcemia, galactosemia, aminoacidopathies).
  (8) Electrolyte imbalance.
  (9) Drugs (digoxin, anticonvulsants).
  (10) Hirschsprung disease.
  (11) Lactobezoars.

b. Usually bilious.
  (1) Malrotation (with or without volvulus).
  (2) Other congenital anomalies (atresia, stenosis, web, imperforate anus).
  (3) Vascular anomalies (aberrant superior mesenteric artery [SMA], preduodenal portal vein).
  (4) Annular pancreas, persistent omphalomesenteric duct, abdominal wall defects.
  (5) Intestinal dysmotility (pseudo-obstruction, visceral myopathies and neuropathies).
  (6) Meconium ileus.

5. **Diagnosis and management.**

a. Review feeding and medication history, look for signs of infection and obtain serum electrolytes.

b. Gentle passage of gastric tube for decompression if GI obstruction is suspected.

c. Plain-film abdominal x-ray with upright or cross-table lateral view looking for specific pattern of obstruction or free air.

d. Bilious vomiting with or without hematemesis should prompt surgical consultation.

e. Upper GI series to rule out obstruction and anomalies and evaluate GI motility (usually unnecessary if complete obstruction is suspected). Abdominal ultrasound if pyloric stenosis is suspected.

f. Neurologic evaluation and central nervous system (CNS) imaging to detect CNS congenital anomalies and malformation.

g. Investigate the possibility of metabolic disorders.

B. DIARRHEA.

1. **General comments.**

a. Diarrhea indicates an increase in water content in stools, which results in decreased consistency of bowel movements, increased frequency of bowel movements, or both.

b. Stool frequency among breast-fed infants can range from once every 5 to 7 days to as many as 12 times per day. Frequency in formula-fed infants fluctuates less and is usually between one and seven stools per day.

c. Stools of breast-fed infants can normally be loose and acidic and contain reducing sugars.

d. Stool output of >10 g/kg per day suggests higher than normal stool output although this is not necessarily a practical definition.

e. Changes in daily stool volume may be more helpful to diagnosis and are usually not subtle if the etiology is infectious.

2. Etiology of diarrhea.

a. GI infections in order of frequency: viral, enteropathogenic *Escherichia coli* (EPEC), *Salmonella, Pseudomonas, Klebsiella, Enterobacter, Proteus, Staphylococcus aureus, Campylobacter fetus,* and *Shigella*. Viral infections in infants younger than 2 months of age are usually asymptomatic. After 3 months of age, rotavirus becomes the most common infectious cause of diarrhea in infants.

b. Sepsis.

c. Overfeeding.

d. Antibiotics.

e. Milk/formula protein allergy.

f. NEC.

g. Malabsorption syndromes: These can be postinfectious, or can be caused by cystic fibrosis, human immunodeficiency virus (HIV), or other congenital malabsorptive conditions (rare: Shwachman syndrome, congenital lactase deficiency, microvillus inclusion disease, glucose-galactose malabsorption, congenital sucrase-isomaltase deficiency).

h. Cholestasis (biliary atresia, Alagille syndrome).

i. Familial chloridorrhea.

j. Bowel resection (short bowel syndrome, blind loop syndrome).

k. Hirschsprung disease (enterocolitis).

l. Intestinal obstruction (diarrhea may be an initial symptom).

m. Metabolic: galactosemia, tyrosinemia, enterokinase deficiency.

n. Maternal drugs during breast-feeding (antibiotics, sulfasalazine, ergotamine).

3. Diagnosis and management.

a. Review family, feeding, and medication history. Assess and continually monitor hydration status and treat fluid and electrolyte imbalances. Obtain stool specimen for culture and assessment of leukocytes (indicative of infection) and blood; assess serum for electrolyte levels and investigate for liver or metabolic disease.

b. Obtain abdominal x-rays to assess gas distribution pattern and to seek evidence of obstruction, free air, or intestinal pneumatosis.

c. In a "sick-looking" infant, blood culture and systemic antibiotics may be necessary if infection or necrotizing enterocolitis (NEC) is suspected. Obtain surgical consult if NEC or intestinal obstruction is apparent.

d. If diarrhea persists more than 2 weeks (chronic), investigate for malabsorption of carbohydrate (stool pH <5.5, reducing sugars present) or fat (72-hour stool collection). Consider a protein hydrolysate, lactose-free or medium-chain triglyceride-containing formula if malabsorption or allergy is apparent. Pancreatic function tests, stool electrolyte levels, intestinal biopsy (for inflammatory, infectious, or malabsorptive conditions), additional imaging studies (for various etiologies) or rectal suction biopsy (for Hirschsprung disease) may be necessary for definitive diagnosis.

C. BLEEDING.
1. General comments.
a. Hematemesis usually indicates bleeding above the ligament of Treitz.
b. Grossly bloody stools usually indicate lower GI bleeding.
c. Swallowed maternal blood during delivery or breast-feeding can explain up to about 30% of neonatal "GI bleeding."
2. Etiology of bleeding.
a. Most common causes of upper GI bleeding.
  (1) Disseminated intravascular coagulation (DIC) after infection, shock, anoxia, etc.
  (2) Gastritis and gastroduodenal ulcers after severe perinatal stress or sepsis.
  (3) Pyloric stenosis.
  (4) Hemorrhagic disease of the newborn.
  (5) Coagulopathy (hemophilia rarely causes bleeding in newborns).
b. Most common causes of lower GI bleeding.
  (1) Anal fissures (most common cause of hematochezia in apparently well infants).
  (2) NEC (most frequent cause of GI bleeding in preterm infants).
  (3) Acute enterocolitis (infectious: *Salmonella, Shigella,* EPEC, *Clostridium difficile*).
  (4) Volvulus.
  (5) Intussusception.
  (6) Meckel diverticulum.
  (7) Hirschsprung disease (enterocolitis).
  (8) GI duplications.
  (9) Milk/formula protein allergy (common after first week).
 (10) Polyps, hemangiomas (rare).
 (11) Rectal injury (e.g., from thermometer).
3. Diagnosis and management.
a. Test for occult blood in vomitus or stool (hemoccult, gastroccult will confirm presence of blood).
b. The Apt test, which differentiates hemoglobin A from hemoglobin F, can differentiate maternal from infant's blood. Examine mother's nipples; pumping of breast may be helpful.

14

GASTROENTEROLOGY

c. Passage of nasogastric or orogastric tube and gastric lavage with warm saline may confirm upper GI bleeding. Never use cold saline.

d. Check to see if vitamin K was given. Check for petechiae and other bleeding sites.

e. Perform meticulous examination of the anal canal for trauma or anal fissures.

f. Obtain stool sample for culture and to examine for leukocytes and *C. difficile* toxin.

g. Obtain abdominal x-rays for evidence of obstruction, intestinal pneumatosis; upper GI series for evidence of obstruction and congenital anomalies; obtain ultrasound examination if pyloric stenosis is suspected and abdominal examination is not revealing.

h. Blood transfusion may be necessary. Supportive care and management of underlying condition are required.

i. H_2 blockers or proton pump inhibitors may be useful in suspected or confirmed gastritis, esophagitis, or ulcers.

j. Upper or lower GI endoscopy and biopsy may be indicated for definitive diagnosis.

D. DELAYED PASSAGE OF MECONIUM/CONSTIPATION.
1. General comments.
a. Approximately 70% of neonates pass meconium within 12 hours, 95% within 24 hours, and >99% within 48 hours.

b. Failure to pass meconium in the first 24 hours should raise suspicion and warrants close observation and possible workup.

c. Passage of meconium does not rule out intestinal obstruction.

d. 97% of infants have between 1 and 9 bowel movements daily in the first week.

e. 93% of infants have between 1 and 7 bowel movements daily between 2 and 20 weeks of age. The variability is greater in breast-fed infants (see earlier).

f. Consistency (hard, dry stools), difficulty with passage (excessive straining, irritability, crying during and between stools) and fluctuation in stooling pattern (alternating constipation and diarrhea) are more important in determining the need for intervention in an infant with infrequent stools.

2. Etiology.
a. Delayed passage of meconium.
　(1) Intestinal obstruction (see p. 162).
　(2) Spinal and neural tube defects (sacral agenesis, meningocele, etc).
　(3) Maternal drugs (opiates, ganglionic blocking agents, magnesium sulfate).
　(4) Meconium ileus.
　(5) Meconium plug syndrome.
　(6) Ileus (electrolyte imbalance, sepsis).
b. Infrequent passage of stools.
　(1) Hypothyroidism.

(2) Spinal and neural tube defects (sacral agenesis, meningocele, etc.).

(3) Hypotonia (Down syndrome).

(4) Drugs (antihistamines, opiates, phenothiazines).

(5) Hirschsprung disease.

(6) Idiopathic ("functional" constipation).

(7) Intestinal dysmotility (pseudo-obstruction, visceral myopathies, and neuropathies).

3. Diagnosis and management.

a. Perineal and rectal examinations are essential.

b. Investigate for causes of intestinal obstruction (see p. 162). Abdominal x-rays for evidence of obstruction; an unprepped barium enema may be used to look for a "transition zone" from normal to abnormal bowel if Hirschsprung disease is suspected. Anorectal manometry, rectal suction biopsy, or both are necessary to confirm.

c. Prolonged jaundice, lethargy, and low body temperature should prompt thyroid function and metabolic disease investigation.

d. A sweat test or screening for cystic fibrosis gene mutations is indicated in suspected or confirmed meconium ileus.

e. In the absence of a primary condition, stool softeners may help, e.g., malt soup extract (1 to 2 teaspoons three times daily) added to the infant's formula. Suppositories may also be used judiciously in the first few weeks of life.

f. Clinical or x-ray signs of intestinal obstruction and frequent or severe episodes of fecal impaction require a GI and surgical consultation.

E. ABDOMINAL DISTENTION.

1. General comments.

a. Distention may indicate the following:

(1) Increased intraluminal air (usually a result of intestinal obstruction).

(2) Pneumoperitoneum (free intra-abdominal air, usually the result of a perforation).

(3) Ascites.

b. Intraluminal air can usually be distinguished from free air on a plain-film x-ray. Cross-table lateral and upright x-rays are helpful.

2. Etiology.

a. Increased intraluminal gas (see Intestinal Obstruction, p. 162); also seen with severe aerophagia (e.g., with pain, discomfort, or stress—or after mask ventilation [bagging]).

b. Pneumoperitoneum.

(1) Spontaneous gastric perforation.

(2) Perforated Meckel diverticulum.

(3) Perforated appendix.

(4) Bowel perforation secondary to NEC, volvulus.

(5) Pulmonary air leaks can also dissect into the peritoneal cavity.

c. Ascites (may be identified prenatally by ultrasound).

(1) Urinary tract anomalies.

14

GASTROENTEROLOGY

(2) Peritonitis.

(3) Lymphatic (thoracic duct) obstruction.

(4) Hepatic or portal vein obstruction.

(5) Congenital infections.

(6) Hemolytic disease of the newborn.

(7) Cardiac or renal anomalies.

3. **Diagnosis and management: See under Intestinal Obstruction or specific conditions later in this chapter.**

Note: *When suspected, most of these conditions require GI and surgical consultations.*

F. INTESTINAL OBSTRUCTION.

1. General comments.

a. Vomiting predominates in proximal obstruction. Distention and delayed or infrequent stooling predominate in distal obstruction. Vomiting (particularly if bilious), significant abdominal distention, and constipation are the cardinal signs of intestinal obstruction, and *they constitute a potential surgical emergency.* Not all are always present.

b. Polyhydramnios is most commonly caused by congenital GI obstruction.

c. Early pooling of secretions before starting feedings and scaphoid abdomen are also indicators of possible GI obstruction (esophageal atresia without tracheoesophageal fistula).

2. Etiology.

a. Mechanical.

(1) Congenital.

(a) Malrotation, with or without volvulus.

(b) Atresia, stenosis, web, imperforate anus.

(c) Meconium ileus.

(d) Annular pancreas.

(e) Hernia (incarcerated).

(f) Hirschsprung disease.

(g) Vascular anomalies (aberrant superior mesenteric artery [SMA], preduodenal portal vein)

(h) Intestinal duplications.

(I) Persistent omphalomesenteric duct (peritoneal bands).

(2) Acquired.

(a) Pyloric stenosis.

(b) NEC.

(c) Meconium plug syndrome.

(d) Intussusception.

(e) Peritoneal adhesions (after meconium peritonitis).

(f) Mesenteric artery thrombosis.

b. Functional.

(1) Ileus (electrolyte imbalance, hypermagnesemia, NEC, sepsis, asphyxia).

(2) Maternal drugs (opiates, ganglionic blocking agents, magnesium sulfate).

(3) Hypothyroidism.

(4) Adrenal insufficiency.

3. Diagnosis and management.

a. After obtaining a history (maternal, medications, procedures), assess the infant's vital signs and hydration status. Examinations (including rectal) should be done to look for distention, masses, bleeding sites, somatic anomalies. *If obstruction is suspected, act quickly.*

b. Suspend all oral or tube feedings.

c. Decompress the stomach with a nasogastric or orogastric tube.

d. Establish intravenous access and correct fluid and electrolyte deficits.

e. Begin antibiotic therapy if sepsis is suspected.

f. Obtain emergency surgical consultation.

g. X-ray studies and findings:

(1) Plain-film abdominal x-rays are most helpful initially. In the newborn, gas is usually present in the stomach at 1 hour of life, in the cecum by 3 hours, and in the rectosigmoid by 8 to 10 hours. The progression is slower in preterm newborns.

(2) Absence of air may indicate esophageal atresia without tracheo-esophageal fistula.

(3) Mechanical causes (e.g., atresia, stenosis, Hirschsprung disease) usually result in marked distention with many air-fluid levels proximal to the obstruction and little or no gas beyond.

(4) Functional causes (e.g., electrolyte imbalance, sepsis, drugs) usually show diffuse distention with few air-fluid levels.

(5) Upper GI contrast studies are usually unnecessary in the initial evaluation and generally are contraindicated in apparent complete obstruction. Contrast enema can help in diagnosing malrotation and Hirschsprung disease; it can also be therapeutic in meconium ileus, meconium plug syndrome, and intussusception (see specific conditions discussed later in this chapter).

h. Ultrasound can help with prenatal diagnosis (e.g., polyhydramnios, echogenic bowel, ascites, duodenal atresia). It is useful if pyloric stenosis is suspected.

14

GASTROENTEROLOGY

II. SPECIFIC GASTROINTESTINAL CONDITIONS

A. GE REFLUX.

1. General comments.

a. Regurgitation secondary to GE reflux is normal in the great majority of infants. When severe or persistent, look for signs of intestinal obstruction.

b. Approximately 50% of infants will regurgitate two or more times a day until about 2 months of age and 80% of infants regurgitate formula at least once a day until about 3 months of age. Most regurgitation resolves in 80% of infants by about 6 months of age and in 90% by about 12 months.

c. Uncomplicated GER refers to persistent regurgitation without other signs or symptoms. GE reflux disease (GERD) refers to GE reflux accompanied by pathologic signs or symptoms including:

   (1) Esophagitis (pain or discomfort with regurgitation, irritability, choking, gagging, upper GI bleeding).

   (2) Cardiorespiratory symptoms (apnea, reactive airway disease, bradycardia, aspiration).

   (3) Failure to thrive (poor weight gain)—usually as a consequence of esophagitis or cardiorespiratory symptoms.

d. Transient lower esophageal sphincter relaxation (TLESR), when disassociated from normal swallowing function is the major mechanism allowing reflux and regurgitation to occur. A vagovagal reflex, composed of afferent mechanoreceptors in the proximal stomach, a brainstem pattern generator, and efferents in the LES, regulates TLESRs.

e. Potential exacerbating factors or stimuli for TLESRs and GER include:

   (1) Gastric distention (postprandially, or due to abnormal gastric emptying or air swallowing).

   (2) Straining during a TLESR—increased movement and positions that place the gastroesophageal junction below the air-fluid interface in the stomach.

   (3) Large volume or hyperosmolar feeds.

   (4) Increased respiratory effort or respiratory distress.

f. Whether GERD is caused by a higher frequency of TLESRs or by a greater incidence of reflux during TLESRs is still a matter of debate.

g. Risk factors for neonatal GER and GERD include:

   (1) Prematurity.

   (2) Neonatal stress, birth asphyxia, infection.

   (3) Neurologic compromise.

   (4) Congenital anomalies.

   (5) Drugs (xanthines, betamimetics, prostaglandins, dopamine).

   (6) Procedures (extracorporeal membrane oxygenation, chest physiotherapy).

2. Diagnosis and management of GER.

a. With significant GERD an upper GI series should be obtained to rule out a partial obstruction. Esophageal pH monitoring studies are rarely necessary if regurgitation is obvious; pH monitoring may be helpful in documenting severity of GER, subclinical reflux, and correlation with cardiorespiratory complications (e.g., apnea, bradycardia). Upper endoscopy may be necessary to rule out esophagitis when symptoms are irritability and GI blood loss. Esophageal manometry may be useful in further documenting motility abnormalities in select cases.

b. Treatment.

   (1) Supine, right lateral, and semi-seated positioning can exacerbate GER. The prone position, elevated at the head 30 degrees can improve GER. However, debate on any recommendation persists given the relationship of prone position with SIDS. Risks and benefits should be individualized.

(2) Small, frequent feeds and avoidance of hyperosmolar feedings are best.
(3) Formula can be thickened with 1 tablespoon of dry rice cereal per ounce.
(4) Pharmacologic therapy (e.g., metoclopramide, H_2 blockers and proton pump inhibitors) should be reserved for established GERD, after intestinal obstruction has been ruled out. Cisapride, although effective, is no longer available in the United States because of its potential association with cardiac rhythm abnormalities.
(5) Continuous nasogastric feedings may alleviate severe GERD, particularly when weight gain is poor.
(6) Surgery (fundoplication) may be indicated in complicated reflux refractory to other therapy.

B. PYLORIC STENOSIS.
1. General comments.
a. Pyloric stenosis is obstruction of the gastric outlet due to hypertrophy of the pyloric circular muscle. Its etiology remains unclear.
b. It usually occurs between the third and fifth weeks of life but has been observed from birth to the 12th week. It is more common in whites than in African Americans, in boys than in girls (4:1 ratio), and in infants of parents, particularly mothers, with a history of pyloric stenosis.
c. Signs and symptoms include: persistent and progressive worsening of vomiting, usually (not always) projectile, occasionally bloody, never bilious; failure to thrive and jaundice. The infant is frequently hungry after vomiting.
d. Palpation of a distinct pyloric tumor ("olive") in the epigastrium at the lateral margin of the rectus muscle, just below the liver edge, is diagnostic. A peristaltic wave seen moving from left to right in the left upper quadrant to the midline can occasionally provide additional evidence.
e. Electrolyte profile shows hypokalemic, hypochloremic metabolic alkalosis.
2. Diagnosis and management.
a. When pyloric stenosis is suspected, ultrasound can confirm the presence of a pyloric tumor (thickening of the pyloric wall) and narrowing and abnormal lengthening of the pyloric channel.
b. X-rays (usually unnecessary) show gastric distention with little or no air in the small bowel and a "string sign" (contrast in a long narrow pyloric channel) on contrast study.
c. Treatment includes hydration, correction of metabolic alkalosis, and surgical pyloromyotomy.

C. NECROTIZING ENTEROCOLITIS (NEC).
1. General comments.
a. The etiology of NEC is unclear. Several risk factors have been identified that may lead to this acute necrotizing inflammation and transmural necrosis of the large and small intestine.

14

GASTROENTEROLOGY

(1) The primary risk factor is prematurity; however, up to 20% of affected infants in some series are full term. Other risk factors include small for gestational age, maternal hemorrhage and preeclampsia, cyanotic heart disease, polycythemia, in utero cocaine exposure, umbilical catheter, exchange transfusion, and asphyxia.

(2) Precipitating factors include enteral feeding (up to 10 times more common in enteral-fed than nonenteral-fed infants), ischemia, bacteria (e.g., altered bowel flora or mucosal barrier). Drugs (glucocorticoids, indomethacin) may be contributing factors. Breast milk and low-volume early feedings ("gut priming") may be protective.

b. NEC most commonly involves the terminal ileum and proximal colon but can occur throughout. Progression can be gradual (several days) to fulminant (several hours).

c. Systemic signs and symptoms of NEC include, usually in progressive manner: lethargy, apnea, respiratory instability, temperature instability, acidosis, glucose instability, poor perfusion, sepsis, disseminated intravascular coagulation.

d. Gastrointestinal signs and symptoms, usually in a progressive manner— abdominal distention/ileus, tenderness/irritability on examination, feeding intolerance (vomiting), occult/ gross blood in stools, loose stools/diarrhea, abdominal mass, erythema of the abdominal wall, intestinal perforation.

2. Diagnosis and management.

a. Diagnosis: Usually based on the clinical picture and x-ray findings of distended intestinal loops, air fluid levels, pneumatosis intestinalis (intramural gas in the submucosa), intrahepatic air, and ascites. Free air indicates perforation.

b. Treatment is mostly supportive. The infant should receive nothing by mouth; a nasogastric tube can be used for decompression. Hypotension, anemia, and thrombocytopenia should be treated. Antibiotics should be given as needed. Serial abdominal x-rays should be taken to monitor the infant's course.

c. Surgery is indicated for perforation, peritonitis, and acidosis unresponsive to medical management.

d. Prognosis: The mortality rate for infants with NEC is 20% to 40%. Up to 10% will go on to develop a second episode. Strictures, lymphangiectasis, malabsorption, and short bowel syndrome are late complications in up to 25% of survivors.

D. MILK/FORMULA PROTEIN ALLERGY DISORDERS.

1. General comments.

a. GI manifestations of protein allergy (food allergic manifestations of the GI tract) can manifest in various forms: oral allergy (edema of the lips, tongue, palate, and throat), gastrointestinal anaphylaxis, allergic eosinophilic esophagitis, gastritis and gastroenterocolitis, allergic proctocolitis, protein-induced enterocolitis, and protein-induced enteropathy. The latter three are the more common manifestations in newborns and infants. Clinical responses to dietary changes can be diagnostically useful. Definitive diagnosis requires endoscopy and GI mucosal biopsies.

b. The GI tract also may act as a permissive and immunologic processing organ for foreign proteins in the GI tract. It may be intrinsically involved in food protein antigen processing or development of protein hypersensitivity which can lead to non-GI manifestations of protein allergy (atopic dermatitis, allergic reactive airway disease, some in later life).

2. Allergic proctocolitis: Infants may present between 1 day and 3 months of age with spots or streaks of blood and mucus in the stool and occasional mild diarrhea. Some infants may develop peripheral eosinophilia. Colonic mucosal inflammation (mild and patchy) is present. Nodular lymphoid hyperplasia is found in 25% of cases. It results most often from cow's milk protein allergy; soy sensitivity is less common. It can occur in exclusively breast-fed infants and occasionally may resolve with maternal diet allergen restriction. Non–breast-fed infants can be treated with extensively hydrolyzed protein formulas. The prognosis is excellent. It rarely causes anemia and bleeding has been reported to resolve without dietary changes.

3. Protein-induced enterocolitis: can manifest with vomiting and diarrhea between 1 week and 3 months of age. Peripheral eosinophilia is common. Stools contain occult blood, leukocytes, and eosinophils, and this persists until treated. In older infants a similar syndrome is characterized by anemia, hypoproteinemia, and failure to thrive when infants are weaned from breast milk or formula to regular cow's milk. Symptoms usually resolve within days to 1 week with use of an amino acid formula or an extensively hydrolyzed protein formula.

4. Protein-induced enteropathy: usually manifests between 1 to 3 months of age and is characterized by prolonged diarrhea, usually malabsorptive, intermittent vomiting, failure to thrive, and occasionally occult blood in the stools. Small bowel biopsy shows patchy villus atrophy with mononuclear cell inflammatory response. Reaction to food challenge as well as resolution of symptoms on removal of the offending food may take several days to weeks.

E. ESOPHAGEAL ATRESIA AND TRACHEOESOPHAGEAL (TE) FISTULA.

1. General comments.

a. Esophageal atresia with distal TE fistula is the most common form (85%); TE fistula without atresia, known as "H type" occurs in 5% of cases.

b. Esophageal atresia with a TE fistula proximal to the atretic segment is very rare.

c. About two thirds of infants with esophageal atresia and TE fistula will have associated congenital anomalies (cardiac, musculoskeletal, neurologic, renal, anorectal).

14

GASTROENTEROLOGY

2. Diagnosis and management.
   a. In esophageal atresia, polyhydramnios occurs in one third of the cases. Immediate vomiting with feedings, large amounts of secretions, and respiratory distress are present.
   b. Abdominal distention occurs if there is a distal fistula. A gasless abdomen indicates no fistula or an obliterated fistula.
   c. A soft 5F to 8F feeding tube that can't be advanced or that coils (visualized by x-ray) confirms atresia.
   d. When atresia is apparent, the infant should be placed in the upright position, with constant secretion aspiration by a catheter inserted into the esophageal pouch. Adequate hydration, nutrition, and ventilatory support should be provided until surgical correction.
   e. H-type fistulas do not often manifest with symptoms perinatally. Chronic respiratory problems or recurrent pneumonias over months or years are suggestive.

F. INTESTINAL ATRESIA (COMPLETE OBSTRUCTION OF THE LUMEN).
1. Esophageal.
a. General comments.
   (1) Polyhydramnios occurs in 30% to 60% of cases; 85% are accompanied by distal TE fistula; up to 40% are accompanied by other anomalies (e.g., imperforate anus, malrotation, cardiovascular anomalies, VACTERL syndrome [Vertebral abnormalities, Anal atresia, Cardiac abnormalities, Tracheoesophageal fistula and/or Esophageal atresia, Renal agenesis and dysplasia, and Limb defects]).
   (2) Signs and symptoms include excessive oral secretions, brisk regurgitation of feedings, abdominal distention (if TE fistula is present, see earlier), respiratory distress, and resistance on passage of a nasogastric tube.
   (3) X-ray findings include the absence of air in the bowel if there is no TE communication.
b. Diagnosis and management.
   (1) If esophageal atresia is suspected, a soft 5F to 8F feeding tube can be carefully passed until resistance is met. A plain-film x-ray after injection of a small amount of air will confirm diagnosis. The use of contrast material is usually unnecessary.
   (2) A sump tube should be passed and connected to suction. Intravenous hydration should be started promptly.
   (3) Endotracheal intubation may be necessary.
   (4) Obtain immediate surgical consultation.
2. Duodenal.
a. General comments.
   (1) Polyhydramnios is frequently associated with duodenal atresia. Obstruction is usually distal to the bile duct. Approximately 30% of infants with atresia will have Down syndrome; 50% may have

other GI anomalies (e.g., annular pancreas, malrotation, esophageal atresia, or small bowel and anorectal anomalies).
(2) Signs and symptoms include bile-stained vomitus in the first few hours, delayed passage of meconium, upper abdominal distention (may be absent), visible abdominal peristalsis, and occasionally jaundice.
b. Diagnosis and management.
(1) X-ray findings show a "double bubble" sign (dilated stomach and duodenum)with no air beyond (see Intestinal Obstruction, p. 162).
(2) Gastric decompression and surgical correction are indicated.

3. Small bowel.
a. General comments.
(1) Jejunal and ileal atresias are more common and have fewer (7%) associated anomalies than do duodenal atresias. Only 1% of cases are associated with Down syndrome. Approximately 15% of cases may manifest as meconium ileus, or occasionally as meconium peritonitis. Genders are equally represented.
(2) Signs and symptoms include delayed passage of a small amount of meconium. Vomiting, frequently bilious, and distention occur within 48 to 72 hours. Jaundice may be present.
b. Diagnosis and management.
(1) X-ray findings show dilated loops and air-fluid levels. Calcifications will be present if there was meconium peritonitis.
(2) A contrast enema should be done to rule out Hirschsprung disease and meconium ileus.
(3) Gastric decompression and surgical correction are indicated (see Intestinal Obstruction, p. 162).

G. GI DUPLICATIONS.
1. General comments.
a. GI duplications are cystic or tubular malformations lined by intestinal mucosa, with smooth muscle and sharing of a common blood supply with the adjacent gut.
b. They can occur at any level. Tubular duplications frequently communicate with the adjacent lumen. Heterotopic gastric mucosa may be present in 33% of small bowel duplications.
c. Duplications can enlarge, obstruct, bleed, or lead to volvulus or intussusception. Some may go unrecognized until adulthood.
2. Diagnosis and management.
a. Duplications should be suspected in cases involving unexplained obstruction, bleeding, mass, perforation, volvulus, or intussusception.
b. Ultrasound and computed tomography can help diagnose cystic duplications. A Meckel's scan may be positive if the duplication contains heterotopic gastric mucosa.
c. Duplications should be surgically removed (see GI bleeding and GI obstruction discussed earlier in this chapter).

14

GASTROENTEROLOGY

H. MALROTATION/VOLVULUS.

1. General comments.

a. Malrotation results from an arrest in the normal counterclockwise rotation of the bowel about the axis of the superior mesenteric artery during gestation.

b. Volvulus is the twisting of a loop of bowel about its narrow mesenteric stalk, which causes obstruction by strangulation, and ischemia. **This constitutes an extreme surgical emergency.**

c. Volvulus can occur anytime in childhood with an incidence that peaks at 1 month of age, and is more frequent in males by 2:1.

d. Signs and symptoms: Typically, the infant appears and feeds well and has normal stools. There is sudden onset of bilious vomiting, with or without distention, and passage of blood-tinged stools. Irritability and apparent pain are more constant than intermittent. Signs of cardiovascular collapse and sepsis may rapidly ensue.

2. Diagnosis and management.

a. See Diagnosis and management under Intestinal Obstruction, p. 162.

b. Plain-film x-rays show dilated proximal small bowel. The classic "double bubble" sign representing air in the stomach and duodenum in an otherwise airless abdomen frequently can be seen.

c. After stabilization, contrast enema will reveal the cecum in the right upper quadrant. Upper GI contrast study (by nasogastric tube) will show absence of the normal duodenal loop and the ligament of Treitz to the left of the midline.

d. Emergency surgery is indicated to relieve volvulus. Resection of nonviable bowel may be required and may lead to short bowel syndrome.

I. MECONIUM ILEUS.

1. General comments.

a. Meconium ileus is obstruction of distal small bowel and proximal colon caused by inspissated meconium. It is almost always (>95%) associated with cystic fibrosis and may manifest as echogenic fetal bowel on prenatal ultrasound. As many as 1 in 5 newborns with cystic fibrosis present with meconium ileus.

b. Meconium ileus accounts for about one third of neonatal small-bowel obstructions.

c. Signs and symptoms include: failure to pass meconium, even after digital examination; abdominal distention in the first 12 to 24 hours, and bilious vomiting within 48 hours after birth. Abdominal examination may indicate hard, palpable, freely movable masses.

d. Up to 30% of cases are associated with volvulus, atresia, peritonitis, or pseudocysts.

2. Diagnosis and management.

a. X-ray findings may suggest meconium peritonitis (e.g., abdominal calcifications on plain-film x-rays). If perforation has not occurred, the small bowel will appear distended, thick-walled, and granular with tiny air bubbles mixed with meconium ("ground glass" appearance). An enema with soluble contrast material will show an empty and narrow distal colon (microcolon) and may be therapeutic.

b. A sweat test (difficult in neonates) or identification of two cystic fibrosis gene mutations is confirmatory.

c. Treatment: See Intestinal Obstruction, p. 162. Once perforation and atresia are excluded, enemas with iso-osmolar contrast material or acetylcysteine may relieve the obstruction. If unsuccessful, surgical decompression, often with an enterostomy, is necessary.

J. MECONIUM PLUG SYNDROME.

1. General comments.

a. Meconium plug syndrome involves obstruction of the colon, usually distal, with meconium or mucus. Also called *small left hemicolon syndrome* or *functionally immature colon.*

b. Meconium plug syndrome is usually seen in preterm infants, infants of diabetic mothers, acutely ill neonates, or when there is a history of maternal drug abuse or magnesium sulfate therapy for preeclampsia. It may be an early manifestation of cystic fibrosis or Hirschsprung disease.

c. Signs and symptoms include failure to pass or difficulty passing stools and evidence of intestinal obstruction. Rectal examination may be enough to stimulate passage of the plug and relieve the obstruction.

2. Diagnosis and management.

a. Rectal stimulation with digital examination or glycerin suppository.

b. Soluble-contrast enema may demonstrate a narrowed distal colon and may be therapeutic, loosening inspissated material. Infants should be carefully observed for dehydration following this procedure.

c. Normal stooling pattern should resume by 48 hours after decompression. After removal of a meconium plug, the infant should be observed closely for the possible presence of Hirschsprung disease or cystic fibrosis.

K. MECKEL DIVERTICULUM.

1. General comments.

a. Meckel diverticulum is a remnant of the omphalomesenteric duct, which arises from the ileum proximal to the ileocecal valve. It is the most common congenital anomaly of the small bowel, present in approximately 2% of the general population, and becoming symptomatic approximately 2% of the time. More than 50% contain heterotopic gastric or pancreatic tissue.

b. Signs and symptoms include bleeding (usually painless), resulting from peptic ulceration. It may also manifest as intussusception.

2. Diagnosis can be made by technetium pertechnetate scan. Administration of an H_2 blocker 48 to 72 hours before the procedure will increase sensitivity of the scan.

3. Treatment is surgical excision following hemodynamic and fluid stabilization.

14

GASTROENTEROLOGY

L. ANAL FISSURE.
1. General comments.
a. An anal fissure is a slitlike tear in the anal canal, usually caused by passage of large, hard stools. Pain and irritability may be elicited with bowel movements.

b. Bright red blood can be seen on the surface of stools or occasionally isolated after defecation.

2. Diagnosis and management.
a. Examination in the knee-chest position, parting the buttocks to visualize the anal canal to the mucocutaneous junction, is all that is necessary.

b. Management includes a stool softener such as malt soup extract, 1 to 2 teaspoons three times daily, and thorough cleansing of the perianal area with water after bowel movements.

M. HIRSCHSPRUNG DISEASE.
1. General comments.
a. Hirschsprung disease is defined as congenital absence of ganglion cells of the intestinal myenteric plexus (usually distally), due to migratory arrest of vagally derived neuroblasts that usually reach the rectum by the 12th week of gestation.

b. In 80% to 90% of cases only the rectosigmoid is involved.

c. Most cases manifest in full-term infants. Only 15% of cases are diagnosed in the first month of life and 80% by 1 year. Males predominate over females by 4:1. Between 3% and 10% of infants with Down syndrome have Hirschsprung disease.

d. Signs and symptoms: 94% of infants with Hirschsprung disease do not pass meconium in the first 24 hours. Constipation, abdominal distention, and an empty rectum on digital examination (especially in long-segment disease) with rapid passage of stools after examination are suggestive.

e. Explosive stools, poor feeding, hematochezia, fever, and shock characterize associated enterocolitis, which can be fatal.

2. Diagnosis and management.
a. A "transition zone" (funnel-shaped dilatation of bowel at junction of aganglionic and normal bowel) on an unprepped contrast barium enema can be diagnostic, but is less likely to be seen in a neonate. If the clinical picture is consistent, anal manometry and rectal suction biopsy with acetylcholinesterase staining can be highly suggestive or diagnostic. Lower endoscopy can confirm ileocolitis.

b. Treatment of ileocolitis includes restoration of fluid and electrolyte balance, evacuation of the colon with a rectal tube, and administration of antibiotics.

c. Full-thickness surgical biopsy is confirmatory and helps define the length of the affected segment. Resection of the aganglionic segment can be done with a colostomy and subsequent pull-through operation, or resection and primary pull-through can be carried out in the same procedure.

N. ANORECTAL ANOMALIES.

1. General comments.

a. Anorectal anomalies are generally classified as "high"/rectal or "low"/anal depending on occurrence above or below the puborectalis levator sling.

b. More than 50% (especially high malformations) are associated with other anomalies (e.g., vertebral, genitourinary, other intestinal).

c. Low anomalies include anal stenosis, imperforate anal membrane, and anal agenesis (the most common of low anomalies). Anal agenesis usually is accompanied by a fistulous tract to the vulva or perineum.

d. High anomalies include rectal atresia (obstructing membrane above levator) and rectal agenesis (most common of all anorectal lesions, commonly accompanied by rectourethral or rectovaginal fistula).

2. Diagnosis and management.

a. Diagnosis is made by inspection and by the infant's failure to pass meconium normally.

b. Surgical correction is required, either by anoplasty or a diverting colostomy, depending on the cause.

BIBLIOGRAPHY

Godbole P, Stringer MD: Bilious vomiting in the newborn: How often is it pathologic? J Pediatr Surg 37:909, 2002.

Hussain SZ, Di Lorenzo C: Motility disorders. Diagnosis and treatment for the pediatric patient. Pediatr Clin North Am 49:27, 2002.

Jadcherla SR: Gastroesophageal reflux in the neonate. Clin Perinatol 29:135, 2002.

Kanto WP Jr, Hunter JE, Stoll BJ: Recognition and medical management of necrotizing enterocolitis. Clin Perinatol 21:335, 1994.

McCollough M, Sharieff GQ: Abdominal surgical emergencies in infants and young children. Emerg Med Clin North Am 21:909, 2003.

Okada PJ, Hicks R: Neonatal surgical emergencies. Clin Pediatr Emerg Med 3:3, 2002.

Stoll BJ, Kliegman RM: Digestive system disorders. In Behrman RE, Kliegman RM, Jenson HB (eds): Nelson Textbook of Pediatrics, 17th ed. Philadelphia, Elsevier.

14

GASTROENTEROLOGY

Genitourinary System

John P. Gearhart

FAST FACTS

Immediate Issues in the Nursery

- Information that serves as an indication for screening ultrasound:
  - Family history of polycystic kidney disease (to look for enlarged kidneys because cysts are not usually visible)
  - Prenatal ultrasound showing a renal anomaly (e.g., hydronephrosis)
  - Gross or microscopic hematuria
  - Absence of first void within 24 hours of life
  - Palpable abdominal mass
  - Single umbilical artery
- Oligohydramnios, chromosomal abnormalities, Potter facies (large, low-set, flabby ears; hypertelorism), abnormal abdominal wall musculature, cryptorchidism, cardiac anomalies, and abnormalities of the genitalia and/or anus are important clues that may suggest an underlying urologic disorder.
- Ambiguous genitalia, fluid or blood from the vagina, bladder exstrophy, patent urachus, upper tract abnormalities, persistent bleeding of circumcision are indications for immediate urologic consultation.
- Clitoromegaly may be the only sign of an ambiguous genitalia syndrome. Hypospadias combined with bilateral cryptorchidism prompt consideration of an intersex abnormality.
- Make sure to check for inguinal masses in a phenotypic female. The presence of a testis in this situation may suggest androgen insensitivity.

Things to Remember for Follow-up After Discharge from the Nursery

- Appearance of inguinal hernia with a pre-existing hydrocele or a rapidly enlarging hydrocele should prompt urologic consultation.
- It is important to ask about urinary stream if there is no witnessed voiding in the newborn nursery.
- The discovery of multiple congenital anomalies should prompt a search for renal disease via evaluation of voiding patterns, screening urinalysis, and imaging with ultrasound.
- In cases of cryptorchidism, sonography is helpful only if the testis is in the inguinal canal and MRI and CT are not usually helpful in revealing intra-abdominal testes.

Important Information for Parents

- The foreskin in an uncircumcised male should become freely mobile by 4 to 7 years of age. The foreskin should NEVER be forcibly retracted in a newborn.
- After circumcision, foreskin adhesions commonly occur. These usually break spontaneously over time.

Continued

FAST FACTS—Cont'd

- Surgical repair of hypospadias and inguinal hernias are mostly done between 6 and 12 months of life.
- Surgical repairs of undescended testis and hydrocele are generally done after 1 year of life.
- Thick mucous discharge from the vagina is common and results from stimulation by maternal hormones. It can also be tinged with blood.

I. SPECIMEN COLLECTION METHODS FOR URINALYSIS AND CULTURE

A. CLEAN CATCH.

A polyethylene bag should be attached with adhesive to the perineum and over the genitalia.

1. Cleanse area with povidone-iodine 10% (Betadine soaks) three times.
2. Rinse thoroughly with sterile water.
3. Attach bag and wait.
4. Retrieve as soon as possible after voiding, within 1 hour if findings are to be reliable.

B. SUPRAPUBIC BLADDER ASPIRATION.

A palpably distended bladder is preferable. Infant's diaper should be dry, with no indication of voiding in the previous 60 minutes.

1. Urethral diverticula, often secondary to anterior urethral valves. To prevent voiding during procedure, exert gentle anterior rectal pressure in girls, penile pressure in boys.
2. Place infant in supine, frog-leg position.
3. Cleanse area three times with povidone-iodine 10% and 70% alcohol.
4. Puncture site should be midline, 1 to 2 cm above symphysis pubis.
5. Use a syringe with a 22-gauge 1-inch needle. Insert 10 to 20 degrees to perpendicular, aimed slightly caudad.
6. Apply gentle suction as needle is introduced until urine spurts into syringe. Advance needle no more than 1 inch (2.5 cm).
7. Aspirate urine gently.

Note: Bladder aspiration is to be avoided in the event of demonstrated or possible anatomic urinary tract anomalies.

C. CATHETERIZATION.

1. Cleanse area as for clean catch.
2. Use well-lubricated, sterile no. 3 or no. 5 pediatric feeding tube.

Note: Catheterization is to be avoided unless there is concern about the reliability of previous cultures and the need for culture is great, or in the event of clinical improvement and continued bacterial growth in voided culture.

II. VOIDING PATTERNS

Oliguria, anuria, or a poor urinary stream may be an indication of a urologic emergency. Voiding will have occurred in two thirds of all neonates within 12 hours of birth and in at least 90% during the first 24 hours. Failure to void within the first 24 hours should cause concern.

A. DELAYED VOIDING WITH A PALPABLY DISTENDED BLADDER SUGGESTS POSSIBLE LOWER URINARY TRACT OBSTRUCTION (E.G., POSTERIOR URETHRAL VALVES OR OTHER STRUCTURAL ABNORMALITIES).

B. NEUROGENIC BLADDER.

Distention may be the sole, subtle clue to a neurologic defect.

C. ANURIA WITH OR WITHOUT POTTER FACIES SUGGESTS RENAL AGENESIS.

D. OLIGURIA, HEMATURIA—OR BOTH—SUGGESTS A VASCULAR CATASTROPHE, SUCH AS THE FOLLOWING:

1. Renal vein thrombosis.
2. Renal artery thrombosis.
3. Renal cortical necrosis.

E. A WEAK OR SPUTTERING URINARY STREAM IN MALES REQUIRES CAREFUL EXAMINATION OF THE PENIS DURING VOIDING. POSSIBLE CAUSES AND THEIR SIGNS INCLUDE THE FOLLOWING:

1. Posterior urethral valves: stream weak, dribbling, or absent.
2. Urethral diverticula, often secondary to anterior urethral valves (rare): stream weak, dribbling.
3. Megalourethra with inadequate corpora spongiosum: urethra dilates and fills under increased pressure of voiding.

III. CLUES TO POSSIBLE PRESENCE OF UROLOGIC DISORDER

A. HISTORY: MATERNAL, PRENATAL (PRENATAL ULTRASOUND PERFORMED, PREFERABLY AFTER 15 WEEKS), AND PERINATAL.

1. Maternal history of fetal wastage.
2. Chromosomal abnormalities (e.g., trisomies).
3. Oligohydramnios.
   a. Severe obstructive uropathy.
   b. Eagle-Barrett (prune-belly) syndrome.
   c. Renal agenesis.
4. Polyhydramnios: neonatal ovarian cysts.
5. Maternal bleeding during pregnancy, particularly first trimester.
6. Maternal illness during pregnancy (e.g., diabetes, rubella).
7. Maternal age >35 years.
8. Maternal cocaine use.

9. Toxemia of pregnancy. Therapy with magnesium sulfate during labor may cause neuromuscular blockade with generalized hypotonia and bladder distention.
10. Perinatal asphyxia.
  a. Renal cortical necrosis.
  b. Renal tubular necrosis.
  c. Renal vein thrombosis.

B. SINGLE UMBILICAL ARTERY.

Approximately 0.9% of all babies have a single umbilical artery. There is ongoing controversy regarding the urologic significance. The mortality rate is almost four times that of neonates in general; of those who die, 28% have genitourinary (GU) malformation, roughly the same percentage as those with two arteries.

Note: A sonogram is indicated in babies born with a single umbilical artery.

C. PHYSICAL EXAMINATION FINDINGS.

The following physical findings provide the most common clues to uropathy:
1. Potter facies (large, low-set, flabby ears; widely spaced eyes).
  a. Renal agenesis.
  b. Eagle-Barrett (prune-belly) syndrome.
  c. Bilateral multicystic kidneys.
2. External ear deformity.
3. Widely spaced nipples; supernumerary nipples in white babies.
4. Deficiency of abdominal musculature.
  a. Eagle-Barrett syndrome.
  b. Cryptorchidism.
5. Palpable, enlarged kidneys at first examination.
6. Abnormalities of genitalia.
7. Abnormalities of anus.
8. Sacral dermal sinus.
9. Obvious meningomyelocele; absence of sacral segments.
10. Cardiac anomalies (associated renal defects in as high as 12% of cases).
11. Imperforate anus (reported incidence of renal defect as high as 40%, particularly with high rectal atresia).
12. Tracheoesophageal fistula.
13. Polydactyly and associated anomalies of the extremities.
  a. Renal agenesis.
  b. Urethral duplication.

Note: Renal defects are associated with a number of congenital anomalies; the presence of any significant anomaly or a constellation of several minor anomalies suggests a search for renal disease, including studying voiding patterns, urinalysis, and sonography.

IV. CIRCUMCISION

The controversy surrounding newborn circumcision continues to evolve. Recent studies suggest that a decreased incidence of urinary tract infection and bacteremia is a possible benefit of circumcision; however, most of these early investigations have not been confirmed. If there is any abnormality of the penis or scrotum, circumcision should be deferred until a pediatric urologic consultation is obtained.

A. FORESKIN.
1. Without intervention, the foreskin should separate and become freely mobile by 4 to 7 years of age.

Note: The newborn's foreskin should never be forcibly retracted; additional adhesions joining foreskin to glans readily develop, with phimosis the common result.

2. Cleanliness requires attention only to what can be seen—again, there should be no forced retraction of the foreskin.

B. COMPLICATIONS OF CIRCUMCISION.
1. Bleeding.
a. Most often, local pressure will suffice to stanch bleeding; if not, sponges with 1:200,000 epinephrine should be held to the area for 10 to 15 minutes.
b. A urologic consultation should be requested if bleeding persists. (Do not cauterize without a consultation!)
2. Infection (rare).
a. Warm soaks to penis.
b. Broad-spectrum antibiotic coverage (e.g., ampicillin and gentamicin) can be given pending culture results.
c. Vaseline on the glans at diaper changes to protect glans and soften eschars.

Note: Proceed slowly. Not everything that looks infected is infected. This is a raw, healing surface. It is not necessary to delay discharge after circumcision until the infant has voided.

3. Inappropriate operative result.
a. Insufficient removal of skin. If repair is necessary, simple revision can be done when the child is older. Most often, growth solves the problem. Advise restraint and the passage of time.
b. Excessive removal of skin (common cause of litigation).
  (1) Allow healing (if excess skin removal is noted at time of circumcision immediate urologic consultation is required. Skin should be saved in sterile saline until consultant arrives).
  (2) If penis is displaced downward or otherwise distorted, mobilization of available skin and grafting may be necessary for both functional and cosmetic purposes.

15

GENITOURINARY SYSTEM

c. Injury to urethra (rare, requires immediate urologic consultation).
d. Tourniquet injury to penis from constricting gauze (rare, requires immediate urologic consultation).

V. HYPOSPADIAS

Hypospadias is common, occurring in 8:1000 live male births. It is five times more common with in vitro pregnancy. Less severe forms predominate, making up approximately 87% of the total. In 10%, the urethral meatus is on the proximal penile shaft; in 3% the meatus is in the penoscrotal or perineal region.

A. ASSOCIATED ANOMALIES.
1. Undescended testes (10%).
2. Upper urinary tract malformation. Ordinarily uncommon; potential increases to 45% in the presence of the following:
a. Imperforate anus.
b. Cardiac malformation.
c. Myelomeningocele.

Note: Renal ultrasonography and urologic consultation are essential in this event.

B. THERAPEUTIC CONSIDERATIONS.
1. Repair as early as possible between 6 and 12 months of age (current practice).
a. Extent of abnormality guides decision on exact timing.
b. Separation anxiety diminished.
c. Technical management simplified.
d. Simpler malformations may be repaired on an outpatient basis (soft silastic urethral stents are facilitative).
e. Complex malformations, such as penoscrotal or perineal hypospadias, require hospitalization and an experienced pediatric urologist.
2. In the event of association with undescended testis, consider workup for intergender anomaly.
3. Appropriate attention should be given to associated anomalies.

VI. EPISPADIAS

Epispadias may occur alone (1:112,000 births) or in combination with exstrophy (1:30,000 births). Incontinence is a common problem. Surgical correction of epispadias alone is generally deferred to about 1 year of age.

VII. THE UNDESCENDED TESTIS

Cryptorchidism is one of the most common disorders seen in the newborn. In some premature babies, birth may occur before the onset of normal testicular descent during the last trimester of gestation. Only 3% of full-term males examined at birth have a true undescended testis; nearly 30% of premature males have an undescended testis. The lower the birth weight, the greater the incidence of cryptorchidism. The cryptorchid state is usually easily determined at birth when the scrotum is relatively large, minimal subcutaneous fat exists, and the cremasteric reflex is absent. The incidence of cryptorchidism at 1 year of age is 0.8%. In 10% of patients with cryptorchidism the defect is bilateral, and in fewer than 3%, one or both of the testes are absent.

A. LOCALIZATION OF A NONPALPABLE TESTIS.
Possible locations of an undescended testis, given careful physical examination, include the following:
1. Inguinal region, obscured by abundant subcutaneous fat, small size, or both.
2. Intra-abdominal, inside a hernial sac just proximal to the internal ring (most common), and thus not palpable.
3. Intra-abdominal, not associated with a hernial sac.
4. Congenital absence.

B. MANAGEMENT.
1. In the immediate newborn period, watchful waiting and parental education are keys to management of the undescended testis.
2. With associated hypospadias, consider an intergender abnormality.
3. By 1 year of age, for the fewer than 1% that have not yet descended, consult with a pediatric urologist.
   a. Sonography is helpful only if the testis is in the inguinal canal.
   b. Magnetic resonance imaging (MRI) and computed tomography (CT) are of doubtful value for intra-abdominal study.
   c. Surgery ultimately is necessary in any event (unless the testis is definitely absent).

C. POTENTIAL THERAPEUTIC APPROACHES.
1. Hormonal stimulation (gonadotropin-releasing hormone or human chorionic gonadotropin).
   a. Use of these hormones is controversial; success in achieving full descent is relatively infrequent.
   b. Hormone stimulation is often helpful if the cryptorchidism is unilateral; it enables some descent to make the testis palpable before corrective surgery.
   c. In the event of bilateral cryptorchidism, a trial of hormonal stimulation is justified despite the low success rate.
2. Surgery for localizing the testis and placing it in the scrotum is usually done after the first birthday because descent is unlikely after 1 year.
   a. Laparoscopy is helpful to localize the testis and even to help with bringing the testis down.
   b. Histologic changes in a cryptorchid testis apparent at 24 to 30 months of age suggest the need for earlier surgery.

15

GENITOURINARY SYSTEM

c. Long-term fertility is uncertain in any event. Recent studies suggest 80% to 85% fertility in unilateral and just over 50% in bilateral cases. Further studies are necessary to validate the benefit of earlier surgery.

VIII. PRENATAL HYDRONEPHROSIS

Prenatal evaluation of the genitourinary tract with ultrasonography has become common. In some countries (e.g., England and Belgium), all pregnant women are evaluated at 16 weeks and 19 weeks of gestation in the search for malformations of the major fetal organ systems. In the U.S., routine ultrasonography was formerly limited to those with problem pregnancies or a history of an infant born with a major malformation; today, this procedure is becoming more widespread. Diagnosis and management should be guided by the following principles and steps:

A. **THE MAJORITY OF UPPER AND LOWER URINARY TRACT ANOMALIES ARE EASILY DEMONSTRATED BY 19 WEEKS OF GESTATION.**

B. **BY 22 WEEKS, THE ENTIRE TRACT IS VISIBLE AND EASILY STUDIED.**

C. **IF A MAJOR GENITOURINARY PROBLEM (E.G., HYDRONEPHROSIS) IS DISCOVERED,**
ultrasound examination should be repeated and followed during pregnancy and again just after birth, to confirm or rule out the problem. If an associated condition (e.g., oligohydramnios) is also present, weekly ultrasound examination to follow progress and to guide clinical decision making is justified.

Note: Hydronephrosis can be seen on one examination and be completely resolved on the next. Even the fetal bladder can be seen to empty and refill on ultrasonographic examination.

D. **IF A MAJOR GENITOURINARY PROBLEM PERSISTS ON POSTNATAL EXAMINATION,**
voiding cystourethrograms and appropriate upper-tract studies (e.g., diuretic renograms) can differentiate reflux from anatomic obstructive lesions of the upper or lower tract.

E. **IF AN OBSTRUCTIVE LESION IS FOUND,**
prompt surgery within a few weeks of birth is usually (but not always) indicated, with excellent expectation of normal renal growth and stable renal function.

F. **WHEN THE EXACT NATURE OF THE LESION IS NOT CLEARLY SHOWN,**
follow-up with ultrasonography or diuretic renal scans (with the guidance of the pediatric urologist) is justified until the nature of the lesion becomes apparent.

IX. ABDOMINAL MASSES COMMON TO THE URINARY TRACT

A. DIFFERENTIAL DIAGNOSIS.

The discovery of an abdominal mass on the first physical examination is a relatively common clinical finding. Many conditions must be considered in the differential diagnosis.

1. **Hydronephrosis.**
   a. Ureteropelvic junction (UPJ) obstruction. This is the most common cause of abdominal mass; 20% to 30% are bilateral, with slightly more than one half occurring in males.
   b. If bilateral, be certain that bladder outlet obstruction is not also present. This is, however, less common than the UPJ lesion.
   c. Surgical repair usually provides an excellent result.
2. **A multicystic dysplastic kidney is a common cause of abdominal mass. It is usually unilateral; cysts are usually few in number, large and varying in size, and loosely bound together.**
   a. If the condition is bilateral, it is frequently associated with Potter facies.
   b. The mass often feels lobulated.
   c. The kidney is nonfunctional on renal scanning or excretory urography.
   d. Nuclear renal scan, not ultrasonography, is used to evaluate function in the contralateral kidney.
   e. Lesions generally regress during infancy and early childhood.
   f. Surgery, usually nephrectomy, is not indicated if ultrasonography indicates regression.
3. **Renal vein thrombosis is relatively less common and is usually unilateral.**
   a. Risk factors.
      (1) Trauma.
      (2) Dehydration.
      (3) Infection.
      (4) Maternal diabetes.
      (5) Polycythemia.
   b. Clinical picture.
      (1) Firm, enlarging kidney.
      (2) Gross hematuria (caused by hemorrhagic renal infarction).
      (3) Anemia (possible, secondary to hemolysis or hematuria).
   c. Treatment.
      (1) Watchful waiting.
      (2) Nephrectomy usually is not necessary.
4. **Adrenal hemorrhage is also not uncommon.**
   a. Risk factors.
      (1) Prolonged labor.
      (2) Difficult, traumatic delivery.
      (3) Vigorous resuscitative effort.
      (4) Excessive abdominal compression for any reason.
      (5) Sepsis.
      (6) Urinary tract infection.

15

GENITOURINARY SYSTEM

b. Clinical picture.
  (1) An abdominal mass, although not always readily evident, is usually located in the flank.
  (2) Anemia, pallor.
  (3) Lethargy, even shock.
  (4) Jaundice.
  (5) Hematuria, usually microscopic.
  (6) Renal scanning indicates the kidney is displaced downward and outwardly rotated.
  (7) Demonstrable infection in urinary tract or elsewhere.
c. Differential diagnosis.
  (1) Renal vein thrombosis: usually gross hematuria.
  (2) Hydronephrosis in the upper pole of a duplicated collecting system.
  (3) Renal hemorrhage; may not be differentiated before surgery.
d. Treatment.
  (1) Fluid replacement and maintenance.
  (2) Electrolyte repair.
  (3) Steroid therapy, possible.

Note: Rarely, there is progression to bilateral involvement.

  (4) Blood transfusion should be used cautiously and only if anemia is profound.
  (5) Antibiotics are appropriate treatment for demonstrated infection.
5. **Mesoblastic nephroma. The most common renal tumor in childhood is Wilms tumor. Those discovered in neonates are most often not true Wilms tumors but mesoblastic nephromas. Clinical management is identical for either.**
a. Tumor may not, at first, be palpable on physical examination.
b. Ultrasonography or renal scans performed for other reasons may define the lesion even before a physical examination is performed.
c. Metastatic spread to lungs or bone may be demonstrated.
d. Treatment: nephrectomy.
6. **Neuroblastoma is also a common abdominal tumor of childhood. One third to one half of these tumors are found in the first year of life.**
a. Neuroblastomas are often palpable.
b. Plain-film abdominal x-rays may reveal calcification in as many as 60% of cases.
c. CT scans best define the extent of disease before surgery.
d. Radionuclide bone scans or x-ray bone survey may reveal skeletal metastases.
e. Vanillylmandelic acid (VMA) and homovanillic acid (HVA): one or both levels can be elevated in as many as 90% of cases.
f. Metastases to bone marrow, bone, and liver are most common.

g. Treatment options include surgery, chemotherapy, or radiation; requires consultation with a urologist, oncologist, or radiation therapist.

7. **Hydrometrocolpos is rare. It is the result of fluid distention of the vagina and uterus secondary to vaginal obstruction and excessive secretion of cervical glands.**

a. Associated anatomic anomalies include the following:
  (1) Vaginal atresia (the most common anomaly).
  (2) Imperforate hymen.
  (3) Imperforate anus.
  (4) Cloacal anomaly.
  (5) Ambiguous genitalia.

b. Diagnosis is based on physical examination and ultrasonography; retrograde genitography will be needed to demonstrate the level and cause of obstruction.

c. Treatment is usually surgical.

8. **Polycystic kidneys. Condition is autosomal recessive (infantile).**

a. Affects both kidneys.

b. Shows no gender preference.

c. Symptoms include palpable masses and renal failure.

d. On ultrasound, cysts are too small to see and renal size is enlarged.

e. Management includes control of hypertension, congestive heart failure, renal failure, and hepatic failure.

f. Survivors face dialysis and renal transplantation.

9. **Distended bladder. 90% of newborns void during the first 24 hours of life and essentially all void by 48 hours of life unless there is a problem such as the following:**

a. Posterior urethral valves.

b. Neurogenic bladder.

c. Pelvic/vaginal rhabdomyosarcoma (rare).

d. Ureterocele obstructing the bladder outlet.

B. DIAGNOSTIC APPROACH AFTER PHYSICAL EXAMINATION.

1. Ultrasound of abdomen and pelvis to determine if lesion is solid or cystic.

2. Voiding pattern.

3. Urinalysis to look for hematuria (gross or microscopic), proteinuria, or evidence of infection.

4. A follow-up examination, if necessary and as appropriate, should be scheduled with a pediatric urologist. Additional studies include the following:

a. Renal diuretic scan.

b. CT scan.

c. MRI.

    d. Excretory urography.

    e. Retrograde genitography.

    f. Urine culture.

    g. A variety of other studies related to associated findings.

X. AMBIGUOUS GENITALIA SHOULD BE CONSIDERED AN EMERGENCY!!!

A. CONGENITAL ADRENAL HYPERPLASIA IS A COMMON CAUSE OF AMBIGUOUS GENITALIA.

Unrecognized, the salt-losing type of adrenal hyperplasia carries a high mortality rate. Immediate evaluation and monitoring are indicated. Serum electrolytes and blood and urine steroid studies are also indicated (see p. 442).

B. GENDER IDENTIFICATION MUST BE MADE AS SOON AS POSSIBLE.

Social and emotional imperatives are on a par with anatomic and physiologic considerations.

1. Karyotyping should be performed.
2. Retrograde genitography, performed by a pediatric urologist in the radiology department, should determine the takeoff of the vagina and urethra from the urogenital sinus.

Note: Hypospadias associated with undescended testes should be thoroughly evaluated to avoid erroneous assignment of gender.

C. PARENTAL COUNSELING AND EDUCATION SHOULD BE PROVIDED.

Choose words carefully until the situation is clarified by the appropriate workup. Samples include the following:

1. Ambiguous genitalia = incomplete forming.
2. Phallus = penis, clitoris.
3. Gonads = testes, ovaries.

XI. VAGINAL DISCHARGE AND VAGINAL BLEEDING

A. MOST NEWBORN GIRLS HAVE A THICK, OFTEN PROFUSE VAGINAL DISCHARGE AS A RESULT OF PRENATAL STIMULATION BY MATERNAL HORMONES.

The discharge may be blood tinged. This is a self-limited condition requiring explanation but no intervention.

B. CAUSES OF CONCERN.

1. Discharge may be from an ectopic ureter inserting into the vagina. A clear and persistent discharge may be urine.

    a. Urinalysis is recommended.

b. Upper-tract imaging can be used to search for possible duplication of the urinary tract with ectopia.
2. Bleeding from the vagina is not common and may be caused by the following:
a. A prolapsed ectopic ureterocele descending through the bladder neck and exiting through the urethral meatus; a discolored mass may be seen.
b. Rhabdomyosarcoma of the vagina. This bleeds easily; a friable, discolored mass can be visualized.
c. Urethral prolapse.

Note: Each of these conditions mandates immediate pediatric urologic consultation.

15

XII. VULVAR ABNORMALITY
A. CLITORIS.
Hypertrophy (e.g., as the only sign of the adrenogenital syndrome.)

B. IMPERFORATE HYMEN.
May be associated with hydrocolpos or hematocolpos.

C. ABERRANT LOCATION OF URETHRAL MEATUS.
It should be just ventral to the vaginal introitus. An aberrant location indicates a possible urogenital sinus anomaly.

D. PROLAPSED URETEROCELE.
May present as a perineal mass; may be confused with hydrocolpos.

E. POORLY DEFINED URETHRAL AND VAGINAL ORIFICES.
This suggests the possibility of a urogenital sinus or cloacal outlet anomaly.
1. Careful examination of anal competence is required.
2. May be associated with an abdominal mass.

XIII. INGUINAL HERNIA AND HYDROCELE IN THE NEWBORN
A. INGUINAL HERNIA.
In clinical practice, the majority of infantile inguinal hernias appear during the first year, with the diagnosis commonly made in the first month after birth; new cases are less frequent as childhood advances. The overall incidence in the pediatric population is from 1% to 4%. In premature infants weighing <2000 g at birth, the incidence rises to >15%. The condition affects boys nine times more frequently than it does girls.
1. In recent years controversy has arisen with regard to the desirability of routine bilateral exploration in cases of apparent unilateral inguinal hernia. Clinically undiagnosed hernias on the contralateral side have been reported to occur as often as 60% of the time. However, other studies have shown that only 15% of patients developed a clinical hernia later on in childhood on the contralateral, unexplored side.

GENITOURINARY SYSTEM

Thus, it may be reasonably argued that routine operation on the second side in the younger child may be unnecessary in up to 85% of cases. When additional consideration is given to the close association of the spermatic vessels and vas deferens to the patent processus vaginalis, it will be appreciated that routine exploration is not without risk in the young infant. Indeed, there is an incidence of testicular atrophy of approximately 0.5% after infantile hernia repair.

2. Usual presentation: Many infantile inguinal hernias appear during the first month of life and a majority within the first 3 months of life; they are usually detected by the parent after discharge and manifest as a bulge in the groin after a period of crying or straining during a bowel movement. The swelling is generally absent in the morning and more noticeable in the latter part of the day. Sometimes the hernia is not clinically apparent to the clinician but the child's parent is convinced of its presence, especially during periods of infant distress.

3. Features of physical examination.

a. Roll the spermatic cord gently over the pubic tubercle; the affected side is more readily palpated and bulkier than the more delicate structure on the contralateral side.

b. Inspect the scrotum. Are both testes fully descended? Up to 6% of congenital inguinal hernias are associated with incomplete testicular descent.

c. If, in a girl, a gonad is palpable in the hernia sac at the time of surgery, one must be certain that this is an ovary and not a testis.

Note: A phenotypic female with a testis may have complete androgen insensitivity syndrome.

B. HYDROCELE.

A hydrocele is a collection of fluid between the parietal and visceral layers of the tunica vaginalis. Hydroceles usually occur during infancy but can appear even into adulthood. During infancy it is believed that a patent processus vaginalis contributes to the collection of peritoneal fluid in the tunica vaginalis. A hydrocele is common after birth, occurring in about 6% of full-term males. It causes a transilluminating, painless, oval scrotal swelling that may extend along the spermatic cord. Because a hydrocele at birth almost universally occurs secondary to a patent processus vaginalis, therapy should be delayed until after the processus closes, which may occur spontaneously within the first year of life. The patent processus vaginalis also explains why the size of an infant hydrocele may vary from time to time.

Note: Occasionally, an inguinal hernia may be suspected in a patient with a hydrocele. Careful follow-up will be needed in the first few months of life to make sure that one is dealing with a true infant hydrocele and not an inguinal hernia. There can be an association if the hydrocele persists after 1 year of life or continues to increase in size; surgical therapy will then be required.

XIV. HEMATURIA

Microscopic or gross hematuria in the neonate should be considered an emergency; gross hematuria is rare. All causes require immediate and accurate diagnosis and include the following:

A. RENAL ARTERY THROMBOSIS IS POTENTIALLY LETHAL.

There has been a recent increase in incidence.

1. It is commonly associated with umbilical artery catheterization.
2. The clinical presentation, in whole or in part, includes the following:
a. Hypertension/congestive heart failure.
b. Hematuria.
c. Proteinuria.
d. Azotemia.
e. Duskiness of lower extremities after placement of umbilical artery catheter.
f. Nonopacification of involved kidney on nuclear renal scanning.
3. Management.
a. Treatment of hypertension if present.
b. Nephrectomy should be performed only if blood pressure elevation is severe and difficult to control medically.

B. RENAL VEIN THROMBOSIS; POTENTIALLY LETHAL (SEE UNDER IX, ABDOMINAL MASSES COMMON TO THE URINARY TRACT).

C. RENAL CORTICAL NECROSIS; POTENTIALLY LETHAL.

1. Associated with the following:
a. Hypoxia/intrauterine distress.
b. Dehydration.
c. Sepsis.
d. Blood loss.
e. Birth trauma.
2. Clinical presentation not unlike bilateral renal vein thrombosis.
a. Enlarged kidneys.
b. Thrombocytopenia.
c. Anemia.
d. Azotemia.
e. Hematuria.
3. Diagnosis. Renal nuclear scanning can differentiate from renal vein thrombosis.
4. Management is supportive and includes management of renal failure.

D. OBSTRUCTIVE UROPATHY, PARTICULARLY AFTER DIFFICULT, TRAUMATIC DELIVERY (SEE UNDER IX, ABDOMINAL MASSES COMMON TO THE URINARY TRACT).

15

GENITOURINARY SYSTEM

E. RENAL TUMOR, PARTICULARLY AFTER DIFFICULT, TRAUMATIC DELIVERY (SEE UNDER IX, ABDOMINAL MASSES COMMON TO THE URINARY TRACT).

XV. URACHUS (PERSISTENT BAND OR LUMEN)

A. PRESENTATION.
1. Inversion of umbilicus, apparent pain on voiding (persistent band).
2. Draining urine at umbilicus (patent lumen). A potential of infection exists if sinuses or cysts form, involving the entire tract from umbilicus to bladder.

B. DIAGNOSIS.
1. Ultrasound of bladder and infraumbilical abdominal wall.
2. Methylene blue, instilled at umbilicus, voided in urine.
3. Carmine red dye, orally, discharged at umbilicus in the rare event of associated enteric fistula.

C. MANAGEMENT.
Surgical excision.

XVI. EXSTROPHY OF BLADDER (~1 IN 30,000 BIRTHS)

Note: Prompt referral to an experienced pediatric urologist is mandatory.

BIBLIOGRAPHY

American Academy of Pediatrics Task Force on Circumcision: Circumcision policy statement. Pediatrics 103:686, 1999.

American College of Obstetricians and Gynecologists: Ultrasound in pregnancy. Technical Bulletin 116, Washington, DC, 1988, ACOG.

Elder JS, Duckett JW: Management of the fetus and neonate with hydronephrosis detected by prenatal ultrasonography. Pediatr Ann 17:19, 1988.

Hadlock FP, Deter RL, Carpenter R, et al: Sonography of fetal urinary tract anomalies. Am J Radiol 137:261, 1981.

Lawson TL, Foley WD, Berland LL, et al: Ultrasonic evaluations of fetal kidneys. Radiology 138:153, 1988.

Mussels M, Gaudoy CL, Bason WM: Renal anomalies in the newborn found by deep palpation. Pediatrics 47:97, 1971.

Perlmutter DF, Lawrence JH, Krauss AN, Auld PAM: Voiding after neonatal circumcision. Pediatrics 96:1111, 1995.

Pinto KJ, Noe HN, Jenkins GR: Management of neonatal testicular torsion. J Urol 158:1196, 1997.

Silver RI, Rodriguez RI, Chang TS, Gearhart JP: In vitro fertilization is associated with an increased risk of hypospadias. J Urol 161:1954, 1999.

Nervous System

Rebecca N. Ichord

FAST FACTS

Immediate Issues in the Nursery

- Initial management of seizures includes correction of fluid and electrolyte imbalances; maintaining adequate oxygenation, body temperature, and blood glucose; and use of anticonvulsants in neonates with recurring seizures due to an untreatable underlying brain disorder.

- Weakness and peripheral reflexes can help to identify the cause of hypotonia. In cases of central nervous system (CNS) involvement, there is no true weakness despite decreased movements, and reflexes are normal or increased. In cases of neuromuscular disease, weakness and muscle atrophy are present along with diminished or absent reflexes.

- Early clinical signs and symptoms of hydrocephalus include: excessive head growth; suture diastasis; bulging fontanel; irritability; and poor suck/swallow. With worsening status, vomiting, VI nerve palsy, downward gaze preference, posturing, lethargy, and apnea/bradycardia occur. Cushing triad (hypertension, irregular respiration, and bradycardia) and papilledema are rare and extremely late findings.

Important Reminders After Discharge

- More than one half of all infants with congenital hydrocephalus will require a shunt. The level of residual deficits is dependent on the cause of the hydrocephalus, the presence of additional deficits, and the occurrence of shunt complications.

- With spina bifida occulta, the only clinical findings in the neonatal period may be spinal deformity, skin changes (pigmented/hairy patch, dimple), or asymmetrical lower limb movements because of tethered cord or nerve root entrapment. Be sure to question parents about stooling/voiding patterns and carefully examine for adequacy of lower extremity tone, strength, and reflexes during routine well-child examinations.

Helpful Information for Parents

- Many parents are frightened by normal twitching and spasms that occur in the neonatal period. Movements that can be stopped by a gentle touch are usually normal, as are movements that occur only during crying. Use of video recording can be extremely helpful in documenting and assessing movements that are concerning for parents.

- Parents should be encouraged to pursue genetic evaluation and counseling in most cases of severe neurologic defects. This can help to identify possible coexisting syndromes, as well as provide important information for future pregnancies.

16

I. HYDROCEPHALUS

A. FETAL VENTRICULOMEGALY.

1. Definition: enlarged ventricular diameter with enlarged head circumference (HC) for gestational age.
2. Causes: isolated in <20%; with other anomalies in >80%.
  a. Developmental anomalies: neural tube defects (NTD); aqueductal stenosis; Dandy-Walker malformation (DWM); multiple congenital anomalies; encephalocele; holoprosencephaly.
  b. Acquired in utero insults: porencephaly; infection (toxoplasmosis, cytomegalovirus [CMV]); hydranencephaly.
  c. Idiopathic communicating hydrocephalus.
3. Detection: fetal ultrasound (US) showing choroid plexus: ventricular disproportion at 12 to 22 weeks; increased ratio of lateral ventricle width: hemisphere width after 22 weeks.
4. Natural history: overall poor prognosis.
  a. Death or survival with major handicap if associated with major anomalies or congenital infection.
  b. Variable intact survival with need for postnatal shunt.
5. Evaluation: aim to define associated anomalies and/or cause prenatally.
  a. Detailed fetal MRI or ultrasound for CNS and non-CNS anomalies, or NTDs.
  b. Fetal karyotype and sex determination if pedigree shows x-linked pattern.
  c. Pedigree and indicated examination of family members.
  d. Serology for toxoplasmosis, CMV.
  e. Alpha-fetoprotein (AFP) levels.
6. Management.
  a. If prenatal diagnosis shows nonviable anomalies, major anomalies and poor prognosis, consider nonintervention or pregnancy termination with appropriate family counseling.
  b. If no major anomalies and reasonable prognosis, monitor weekly fetal US and lung maturity. If progressive or severe ventriculomegaly, deliver by cesarean section as early as feasible.
  c. In utero ventricular tap is performed only in extreme circumstances if early delivery is not feasible.
  d. In utero shunting has unproven value and high complication rate.

B. CONGENITAL HYDROCEPHALUS.

1. Definition: ventriculomegaly with macrocephaly (HC > 2 SD above mean for gestational age) or excessive head growth in first months of life.
2. Incidence: 1-3/1000 live births.
3. Causes: (same as fetal ventriculomegaly, see **A**, earlier). Also acquired disorders not apparent until postnatally, including:
  a. Posthemorrhagic: intraventricular hemorrhage; subdural/subarachnoid.

b. Postinfectious: bacterial meningitis.

c. Tumor: choroid plexus papilloma; hamartoma.

d. Vascular: vein of Galen malformation; venous sinus thrombosis.

4. Clinical signs and symptoms (in increasing order of gravity): excessive head growth; suture diastasis; bulging fontanelle; irritability; poor suck/swallow; vomiting; VI nerve palsy; downward gaze preference; posturing or hypertonia; lethargy; apnea/bradycardia. Cushing triad (hypertension, irregular respiration, and bradycardia) and papilledema are rare.

5. Natural history: high mortality if untreated; developmental handicap depends on cause and other anomalies, and occurrence of shunt complications.

a. Aqueductal stenosis and myelomeningocele: >90% with normal IQ; high risk of learning disability; majority (60% to 80%) need shunt by 6 months of age.

b. Dandy-Walker and other major CNS malformations: majority with subnormal IQ; variable motor deficits; almost all need shunt.

c. Posthemorrhagic, postinfectious: majority with major handicap; about 50% need shunt.

6. Evaluation.

a. Clinical examination for associated anomalies.

b. Neuroimaging: baseline head US if frequent ventricular monitoring anticipated; brain magnetic resonance imaging (MRI) for definitive anatomic definition for abnormalities involving hindbrain malformations, tumor, neuronal migration defect, or vascular malformation.

c. Consider lumbar puncture (LP) if communicating hydrocephalus shown on neuroimaging, and if cerebrospinal fluid (CSF) pressure and/or protein content will influence surgical decision. In normal term newborn, opening pressure is <10 cm H_2O.

d. Family pedigree and examination of indicated family members.

e. Additional studies to establish cause, as indicated by clinical examination and neuro-image: karyotype; TORCH serology; eye examination for chorioretinitis.

7. Management: aim to optimize operative risk and minimize postoperative complications; avoid shunting if possible while minimizing neurologic sequelae of elevated intracranial pressure (ICP).

a. Nonsurgical: applies if patient medically unstable, too small for surgery, or if ventriculomegaly is borderline in severity and not accompanied by symptomatic intracranial hypertension.

(1) Furosemide (1 to 2 mg/kg/day) + acetazolamide (25 mg/kg/day—divided into three daily doses), increasing up to 100 mg/kg/day if needed. Monitor and treat for electrolyte and acid/base abnormalities. Most useful in posthemorrhagic hydrocephalus.

(2) Serial LP; only in communicating hydrocephalus if diuretics are ineffective and patient is not a surgical candidate. May delay but not prevent need for shunt.

16

NERVOUS SYSTEM

(3) Ventricular drainage: via direct tap, indwelling drain or reservoir. Useful when diuretics fail and symptoms of ICP elevation dictate decompression, but hydrocephalus is noncommunicating with lumbar space. High risk of infection.

b. Surgical: applies when underlying disorder is unlikely to spontaneously resolve; ventricular enlargement is progressive or symptomatic and operative risk factors are optimal. Ventriculoperitoneal route is preferred over ventriculoatrial route.

II. NEURAL TUBE DEFECTS

A. SPINAL DEFECTS.

1. Myelomeningocele (spina bifida cystica).

a. Definition: failure of posterior neural tube closure with defects in meninges, bone, and skin, resulting in maldevelopment, injury, and dysfunction of neural elements.

b. Incidence: 0.5 to 2/1000 live births in the U.S.; 1 to 6/1000 live births in the U.K.

c. Genetics: multifactorial, unless syndromic. Preventable by maternal folate supplements. Risk is 5% if a single affected first-degree relative (sibling, parent), 10% if two affected first-degree relatives, 2% if affected second-degree relative, 1% if affected third-degree relative.

d. Clinical features.

(1) Frequency by level affected: above thoracolumbar junction 5%, thoracolumbar junction 45%, lumbar 20%, lumbosacral (L-S) junction 20%, sacral 10%.

(2) Neurologic examination: HC usually normal or small before back repair; frequent (25% to 30%) lower brainstem signs (suck-swallow dysfunction, stridor, apnea); motor and sensory deficits according to level, often asymmetrical, often sensorimotor dissociation (**Table 16-1**).

(3) Associated features: Arnold-Chiari (A-C) anomaly in all; hydrocephalus in 90% with lumbar lesions, 60% with other sites; bladder incontinence and UTI risk; foot and spine deformities.

(4) Outcome: normal IQ if nonsyndromic and no major shunt complications; mobility according to level affected (**Table 16-2**).

e. Management.

(1) Preoperative neurologic evaluation: look for associated conditions; clinically define motor and sensory levels; brain MRI to define intracranial anatomy.

(2) Urinary tract management: monitor voiding patterns, postvoid residuals; urology consultation; upper and lower tract imaging in first month.

(3) Back repair: within 48 hours of birth if possible; preoperative antibiotics if CSF leak; postoperative antibiotics at discretion of surgeon.

(4) Hydrocephalus: monitor daily for head circumference (HC), signs of increased ICP, back wound healing. Shunt when dictated by progressive symptoms.

TABLE 16-1

MOTOR AND SENSORY FINDINGS IN MYELOMENINGOCELE

Level	Motor	Sensory	Reflex
L1-2	Hip flexion	Inguinal to anterior upper thigh	
L3-4	Knee extension	Anterior lower thigh and knee to medial lower leg	Knee
L5-S1	Ankle flexion, knee extension	Lateral lower leg and medial foot to sole of foot	Ankle
S1-2	Ankle extension, hip extension	Sole of foot, posterior leg and thigh	
S3-4	Bladder and anal function	Perineum and buttocks	Anal wink

(5) Arnold-Chiari malformation: supportive care for mild brainstem symptoms; consider posterior decompressive surgery for life-threatening or progressive bulbar dysfunction.

(6) Psychosocial issues: provide a continuum of informative and supportive family counseling.

2. Occult dysraphism (spina bifida occulta).

a. Definition: incomplete bony fusion of vertebral elements with intact skin/meningeal elements, with or without neural involvement.

b. Clinical findings in neonate: overlying lumbosacral (L-S) spine, may cause CNS infection, root entrapment, tethered cord, spine deformity; rarely hydrocephalus or A-C.

(1) Skin, subcutaneous: pigmented and/or hairy patch; dimple; sinus.

(2) Vertebrae, cord: incomplete fusion; meningocele; lipomyelomeningocele; syringomyelia; diastematomyelia.

(3) Neurologic: none, or variable sphincter dysfunction; isolated L-S root syndromes; progressive paraparesis in adolescence.

c. Management: spine MRI; urinary tract and orthopedic evaluation; neurosurgical consultation; prenatal and genetic counseling. Early surgery is recommended for lipomeningocele, dermoid sinus or cyst, diastematomyelia, tethered cord.

B. CRANIAL DEFECTS:

1. Anencephaly: complete failure of anterior neural tube closure; 100% stillborn or neonatal mortality; most are detectable by fetal US or maternal AFP screening; autopsy and karyotype to rule out syndromes; family and genetic counseling needed.

TABLE 16-2

FUNCTIONAL PROGNOSIS IN MYELOMENINGOCELE WITH OPTIMAL AGGRESSIVE MANAGEMENT

Motor Level	Prognosis
Above L3	Mostly wheelchair bound
L4-S1	Partial ambulation with assistive devices
Below S1	Ambulation without assistance

2. Encephalocele: partial failure of anterior neural tube closure.
   a. Site: 75% occipital; 15% frontoethmoid; 10% other.
   b. Clinical features: microcephaly if extensive brain herniation; infection risk if skin broken; neurologic deficits depend on site (rare in frontal lesions), and extent of brain herniation; one third have spinal defects. High pre- and perinatal mortality rates for large occipital defects.
   c. Genetics: may be syndromic (e.g., Meckel syndrome); most multifactorial; recurrence risk as with myelomeningocele.
   d. Management: defer invasive management pending full evaluation of defect and family counseling.
      (1) Delivery: debatable; consider cesarean section if aggressive therapy planned.
      (2) Evaluation: HC; complete examination; karyotype if associated anomalies or syndrome is suspected; neuroimaging to define ventricular size and extent of malformation (MRI is most complete).
      (3) Treatment: aggressive surgery for frontal lesions; palliative surgery for occipital lesions; monitor and treat hydrocephalus (70% occipital lesions, 10% frontal lesions).

III. INTRACRANIAL HEMORRHAGE

A. PRETERM INFANTS.

1. A spectrum of periventricular hemorrhage (PVH) and periventricular/subcortical white matter (PVL) injuries (**Table 16-3**).
2. Incidence: increases with decreasing gestational age; varies by region and over time; 25% to 40% for <1500 g birth weight.
3. Pathogenesis: ischemia to watershed regions; hemorrhage during reperfusion into ischemic regions and histologically immature

---

TABLE 16-3

SPECTRUM OF PERIVENTRICULAR INJURIES IN PREMATURITY

Lesion	Radiologic Correlate by Ultrasound
Subependymal hemorrhage	Grade I PVH
Intraventricular hemorrhage, without ventriculomegaly	Grade II PVH
Intraventricular hemorrhage, with ventriculomegaly	Grade III PVH
Periventricular white matter hemorrhage, usually with IVH	Grade IV PVH
Periventricular or subcortical white matter ischemic changes:	
Transient edema, ischemia	Transient echodensities
Noncystic gliosis, calcification	Prolonged flare, >2 wk
Cystic necrosis	Cystic PVL
Posthemorrhage ventriculomegaly	Ventricular dilatation

IVH, intraventricular hemorrhage; PVH, periventricular or intraventricular hemorrhage; PVL, periventricular white matter injuries.

vascular bed. Risk factors include: prolonged hypotension; decreasing gestational age; ± vaginal delivery; outborn status; respiratory distress syndrome (RDS); fluctuating blood pressure (BP); coagulopathy; patent ductus arteriosus (PDA). In full-term neonates may be due to cerebral venous thrombosis.

4. Clinical features: often clinically silent. May include lethargy, bulging fontanelle, apnea/bradycardia, posturing, seizures, tone abnormalities, eye movement abnormalities, falling hematocrit. Most conditions occur in first 4 days of life.

5. Management: maternal transport; avoid hypotension, hypercarbia, wide BP fluctuations; correct coagulopathies. Serial head US for periventricular lesions; MRI for peripheral parenchymal or posterior fossa/brainstem lesions; venography if venous thrombosis is suspected. See **posthemorrhagic hydrocephalus** in part I (hydrocephalus).

6. Outcome: High mortality (30% to 50%) in grade IV PVH; grade I or II PVH—no increased risk of major handicap; grade III PVH—moderately increased risk (10% to 20%) of major handicap; grade IV PVH—majority with major handicap; PVL—variably increased risk of major handicap with increasing extent of lesions; motor handicaps predominate.

7. Promising experimental approaches to prevention: maternal phenobarbital; vitamin E; ethamsylate; muscle paralysis in first week; indomethacin.

B. FULL-TERM INFANTS

1. Types of hemorrhage: intraventricular; subarachnoid; subdural; parenchymal.

2. Causes: trauma; arteriovenous malformation; thromboembolic infarct; cerebral venous thrombosis; coagulopathy.

3. Clinical features: depends on cause, location, and severity. May include acute global encephalopathy, isolated focal seizures, signs of increased ICP, subacute focal motor deficits, craniofacial trauma. Significant intraventricular or subarachnoid blood causes chemical meningitis. At risk for acute or subacute onset hydrocephalus.

4. Evaluation: head US for initial screen and serial ventricular monitoring; brain MRI and, if venous thrombosis is suspected, do venography; cerebral angiography if AVM is suspected; rule out coagulopathy, including inherited hypercoagulable states.

5. Management: hemodynamic/respiratory support; anticonvulsants as needed; decompress symptomatic hydrocephalus; correct coagulopathy; surgery as indicated for symptomatic subdural hemorrhage and amenable AVMs. Family counseling and rehabilitation.

6. Outcome: may be very good if no diffuse hypoxic-ischemic injury and hydrocephalus is aggressively treated.

IV. SEIZURES

A. CLINICAL FEATURES: SEIZURE TYPES REFER TO INDIVIDUAL ICTAL EVENTS OF ANY CAUSE; SEIZURE SYNDROMES REFER TO RECOGNIZABLE PATTERNS OF RECURRENT SEIZURES.

1. Clinical seizure types: seizure represents paroxysmal involuntary behavior due to hypersynchronous CNS activity.
   a. Tonic: focal or generalized sustained posturing of limb(s) and/or trunk.
   b. Clonic: focal or multifocal rhythmic (1 to 3/second) jerking movements.
   c. Myoclonic: focal, multifocal, generalized fleeting, nonrhythmic spasms (predominantly flexors).
   d. Subtle, fragmentary: tonic or jerking eye movements; oral-buccal-lingual movements; limb automatisms; apneic spells; autonomic paroxysms.

2. Seizure syndromes:
   a. Benign familial neonatal convulsions: isolated clonic seizures beginning day 2 to 3; normal neurologic examination; minimally abnormal EEG; positive family history; most resolve within months.
   b. Epileptic encephalopathy: onset first week; any and all clinical seizure types; especially myoclonic seizures progressing to mixed intractable seizures and global neurologic dysfunction. A subset evolves to pattern of burst suppression EEG. May be due to inborn errors of metabolism (**Table 16-4**).

3. Differentiate from tremors, jitteriness, stimulus-provoked clonus, decerebrate posturing from ICP elevation, normal stretching, and sleep myoclonus.

TABLE 16-4
NEONATAL GENETICALLY DETERMINED METABOLIC DISEASES PRESENT AS ENCEPHALOPATHIES WITH PROMINENT SEIZURES

Acute Fulminant Metabolic Diseases, Often with Seizures	Subacute Progressive Epileptic Encephalopathy in Neonates due to Genetically Determined Inborn Errors of Metabolism
Urea cycle defects	Glycine cleavage defects
MSUD	Pyridoxine dependency, deficiency
Organic acidopathies	Sulf Ox, Mb cofactor
Electron chain defects, OxPhos defects	Folinic acid responsive defects
CPT II	Menkes disease
MTP defects	COX deficiency
	L-AAD deficiency
	MECP2
	GLUT1 DS
	AICAR/SAICAR
	Serine biosynthesis defects

AAD, L-amino acid decarboxylase; AICAR/SAICAR, 5-amino-4-imidazolecarboxamide ribosiduria and succinyl-5-amino-4-imidazolecarboxamide ribosiduria; COX, cytochrome oxidase; CPT II, carnitine palmitoyltransferase deficiency type II; GLUT1 DS, glucose transporter type 1 deficiency syndrome; MECP2, methyl-CpG-binding protein-2; MSUD, maple syrup urine disease; MTP, mitochondrial trifunctional protein deficiency; OxPhos defects, oxidative phosphorylation defects; Sulf Ox/Mb cofactor, sulfite oxidase and molybdenum cofactor deficiency.

4. EEG: Electrographic seizures without clinical events are common in NICU population. EEG more likely to correlate with focal and multifocal clonic, focal tonic, generalized myoclonic seizures.

B. CAUSES: FREQUENCY VARIES AMONG CENTERS AND POPULATIONS.

1. Hypoxic-ischemic encephalopathy (30% to 60%).
2. Vascular (20% to 30%): intracranial hemorrhage; thromboembolic arterial infarction; venous thrombosis with or without ischemic injury.
3. Infection (5% to 10%): congenital (TORCH); acquired viral encephalitis; bacterial meningitis.
4. Metabolic: transient disturbances (Ca, Na, Mg, glucose); inborn errors of metabolism (glycine, amino and organic acidopathies, peroxisomal disorders, oxidative metabolism defects (see **Table 16-4**).
5. Drugs, toxins: maternal drug withdrawal, cocaine use, xanthines.
6. Trauma: contusions, hemorrhage.
7. Genetic and malformation syndromes: phakomatoses, major CNS malformations (e.g., holoprosencephaly), migration defects (e.g., lissencephaly), chromosomal disorders (uncommon in trisomy 21).

C. EVALUATION: SEQUENTIAL, DEPENDING ON KNOWN CAUSATIVE FACTORS.

1. Carefully document nature of events and time course.
2. Screen all infants: Na, Ca, Mg, glucose, acid-base status, oxygenation.
3. Detailed examination for focal deficits, global encephalopathy, signs of intracranial hypertension, genetic/congenital syndromes.
4. Neuroimage: if no benign correctable metabolic disturbance, obtain brain MRI, consider venography.
5. Lumbar puncture (LP) if infection is suspected, or for subarachnoid hemorrhage not well documented by imaging.
6. EEG: Baseline helpful to define patterns with specific treatment (pyridoxine) or prognostic (burst suppression) meaning. Consider in paralyzed, ventilated infants at high risk for hypoxic-ischemic encephalopathy. Consider continuous video-EEG monitoring if strong clinical suspicion or if routine EEG is strongly epileptiform or has moderate to severe background abnormalities.
7. Metabolic studies: if cause not determined by other studies, consider plasma amino acids, urine organic acids, urine sulfites, blood lactate and pyruvate, plasma long-chain fatty acids, serum uric acid, CSF for glucose, lactate, neurotransmitters, amino acids.

D. MANAGEMENT

1. General: correct fluid/chemical imbalances; maintain adequate ventilation, oxygenation, perfusion; maintain normoglycemia, normothermia; avoid syndrome of inappropriate antidiuretic hormone (SIADH).

16

NERVOUS SYSTEM

TABLE 16-5

ANTICONVULSANTS IN NEWBORNS

Drug	Dosage	Comment
Phenobarbital	15-20 mg/kg IV loading	May cause respiratory, cardiac depression
	3-6 mg/kg/day maintenance IV or PO	Aim for 20-40 mg/L level
Phenytoin	15-20 mg/kg IV loading	May cause cardiac toxicity
	5-10 mg/kg/day maintenance IV	Enteric absorption erratic
	5-40 mg/kg/day maintenance PO	Aim for 15-30 mg/L level
Diazepam	0.3 mg/kg/dose IV	For status epilepticus
	0.5 mg/kg/dose rectally	For frequent runs of seizures, when other drugs are subtherapeutic
Lorazepam	0.05 mg/kg/dose IV	Alternative to diazepam. May be used as infusion
Midazolam	25-100 µg/kg bolus IV 0.25-1.00 µg/kg/min infusion	May cause hypotension, monitor infusion with continuous EEG
Clonazepam	0.25 mg loading PO 0.1 mg/day maintenance PO	For intractable or myoclonic seizures
Gabapentin	20-60 mg/kg/day	May be tried for chronic maintenance therapy in chronic epileptic encephalopathy

IV, intravenously; PO, by mouth.

2. Anticonvulsants:
   a. Who to treat: neonates with recurrent clinical seizures due to uncorrectable underlying brain disorder; recurring and especially frequent (more than one per hour) subclinical seizures.
   b. Drugs: phenobarbital (first line); phenytoin (second line); benzodiazepines (short term) for dosage (**Table 16-5**).
   c. When to stop: decrease to phenobarbital monotherapy as acute CNS injury resolves; consider discontinuation before discharge if neurologic status otherwise returns to normal; reevaluate 1 to 3 months after discharge if neurologically abnormal, and consider discontinuation if no seizures on treatment and EEG is favorable.

V. HYPOTONIA

Note: Acute cord injury manifests as hypotonia, and infants with neuromuscular disease are at risk for hypoxic-ischemic brain injury.

A. HYPOTONIA WITH PREDOMINANTLY CNS INVOLVEMENT.

1. Clinical features: diffusely low tone and diminished movement with one or more signs of CNS involvement; disturbed consciousness; cranial nerve deficits; normo- or hyperreflexia.

2. Causes: any acute encephalopathy; congenital CNS malformation; Prader-Willi syndrome; hypothyroidism; other inborn errors of metabolism or genetic syndromes.
3. Evaluation: as appropriate for acute or congenital encephalopathies, including complete examination, laboratory and metabolic screens, neuroimaging, genetic evaluation; see **B.**, subsequently if diagnosis is uncertain.

B. HYPOTONIA WITH PREDOMINANTLY NEUROMUSCULAR INVOLVEMENT.

1. Clinical features: true weakness; muscle atrophy; diminished or absent reflexes with normal level of consciousness. Signs include: ptosis; external ophthalmoplegia; bifacial weakness; dysphagia; respiratory insufficiency; limb and trunk weakness.
2. Causes: myotonic dystrophy; congenital myopathies; myasthenia gravis; spinal muscular atrophy; infantile botulism; mitochondrial encephalomyopathy; metabolic muscle diseases.
3. Evaluation.
  a. Serum creatine kinase moderately elevated in congenital dystrophy.
  b. Family history and examination (especially mother) can positively diagnose myotonic dystrophy.
  c. EMG and nerve conduction studies are useful to define neuropathic and myopathic patterns and distribution. Interpretation is difficult in neonates.
  d. Muscle US useful to guide further invasive testing.
  e. Muscle biopsy in experienced hands is useful for certain congenital myopathies but is technically limited in neonates.
  f. Look for coexisting CNS injury.
4. Management: cardiorespiratory support pending definitive evaluation; optimize nutrition; minimize orthopedic deformities; prepare family for chronic care needs.

C. ACUTE SPINAL CORD INJURY.

1. Clinical features: flaccid paralysis and hypoesthesia (sensory level) usually at cervical level, with varying respiratory insufficiency and neurogenic bladder; Horner syndrome; initially areflexic, later hyperreflexic.
2. Obstetric history is compatible with cervical trauma.
3. Evaluation: neck plain x-rays are usually nondiagnostic; spine MRI is abnormal (edema, hemorrhage); paraspinal EMG may confirm and localize diagnosis.
4. Management: avoid further neck movement acutely; maintain airway and ventilation; support BP; administer fluid conservatively; early high-dose steroid administration has been suggested but not studied in the neonate.

16

NERVOUS SYSTEM

BIBLIOGRAPHY

Allan W: The intraventricular hemorrhage complex of lesions. Neurol Clin 8(3):529, 1990.

Chervenak FA, Berkowitz RL, Tortura M, et al: The management of fetal hydrocephalus. Am J Obstet Gynecol 151:933, 1985.

Levene MI: Measurement of the growth of the lateral ventricle in preterm infant with real time ultrasound. Arch Dis Child 56:900, 1981.

Levene MI, Bennett MJ, Punt J (ed): Fetal and Neonatal Neurology and Neurosurgery. London, Churchill Livingstone, 1988.

Saudubray JM, Nassogne MC, de Lonlay P, et al: Clinical approach to inherited metabolic disorders in neonates: An overview. Semin Neonatol 7:3, 2002.

Volpe JJ (ed): Neurology of the Newborn. Philadelphia, WB Saunders, 2001.

Orthopedics

Paul D. Sponseller

FAST FACTS

Immediate Issues in the Nursery

- When an infant presents with a muscular torticollis in the nursery, x-rays of the neck should be performed to rule out a vertebral anomaly. You should also screen for an associated congenital dislocation of the hip.
- Treatment of a clavicle fracture is not necessary unless significant discomfort occurs, in which case the arm should be immobilized to the trunk with an elastic wrap or sling.
- For a floppy unstable extra digit, removal prior to discharge is recommended by tying off the digit close to the hand. Obtain surgical consultation if there is a substantial tissue bridge or if a skeletal connection exists.
- When a brachial plexus injury is suspected (large baby, difficult delivery, immobility of one of the upper extremities), obtain an x-ray of the affected limb and shoulder girdle to rule out a fracture. If both upper extremities are involved, suspect a spinal cord or a central nervous system injury. With weakness of multiple extremities and an intact Moro reflex, suspect an infectious process.

Important Reminders After Discharge

- Most (90%) of palsies resulting from brachial plexus injuries resolve spontaneously in the first 4 to 5 months of life. Watch for biceps activity (elbow flexion) as the first sign of recovery.
- Vertical talus or "rocker-bottom" sole results from plantar flexion of the hindfoot and dorsiflexion of the forefoot. Vertical talus is the most common congenital foot abnormality that will require surgical correction.
- Screening for developmental dysplasia of the hip (DDH) by physical examination (Ortolani and Barlow maneuvers) should be done at every routine health maintenance visit in the first year of life. A slide or deep "clunk" represents a positive test and should be followed up by an ultrasound and/or orthopedics referral. In accordance with the clinical practice guidelines of the American Academy of Pediatrics, an ultrasound examination at 6 weeks of age and/or an x-ray of the pelvis at 6 months of age is recommended for those infants at higher risk, e.g., a positive family history or girls born in breech position. It is important to note that any screening should be performed by an experienced pediatric ultrasonographer and that not every case can be diagnosed even when imaging is used.

Helpful Information for Parents

- Correction of syndactyly (fusion of adjacent digits) is surgical and can be done electively after 2 to 3 years of age unless there is a progressive deformity due to asymmetrical growth.

Continued

FAST FACTS—Cont'd

- Metatarsus adductus and calcaneovalgus foot deformities usually resolve spontaneously or with serial stretching/repositioning. Casting is usually done only for a clubfoot deformity. Parents are often told by older family members that deformed feet will need to be "broken and reset." The family should be reassured that this does not occur and that treatments do not involve inflicting pain or further trauma on their child.
- Be sure to inform parents that if a clavicle fracture is present, they will be able to see and/or feel a "lump" (the callus) at the fracture site within 2 to 3 weeks. Reassure them that this is a sign of proper healing and will eventually go away.
- Popping or snapping of the joints (especially knees and elbows) is very common. There is no need to worry unless the infant cries out when the joint is manipulated, suggesting that pain is present.

I. BASIC PRINCIPLES

A. GROWTH OCCURS IN RESPONSE TO FORCES APPLIED TO BONE.

Many angular and rotational abnormalities and dislocations occur in response to in utero constraints, and these deformities remodel if constraints are relieved.

B. EPIPHYSES AND GROWTH PLATES ARE LOCATED AT ENDS OF LONG BONES.

Large, unossified, cartilaginous ends of bone appear empty (radiolucent) on the x-ray of the neonate (**Fig. 17-1**). The ossification of the distal femur appears at 39 weeks of gestation, and that of the proximal tibia at 40 weeks.

C. ACUTE JOINT DISLOCATIONS NEVER OCCUR IN THE NEONATE IN RESPONSE TO TRAUMA.

More common are Salter-1 fractures. Hip and knee dislocations, which are occasionally observed at birth, are the products of prolonged, extreme malposition in utero.

D. REMODELING POTENTIAL IS GREAT IN THE NEONATE,

so exact reduction of fractures is unnecessary. Healing is fast (usually 1 to 3 weeks) until bone is clinically solid.

E. PERINATAL LIGAMENTOUS LAXITY IS GREATEST WITHIN THE FIRST 2 TO 3 DAYS.

Treatment should be started early in certain deformities (e.g., clubfoot).

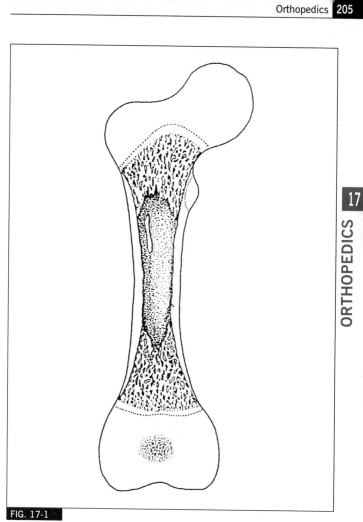

FIG. 17-1

Drawing of typical long bone (femur) in the neonate: diaphysis (shaft) is the primary ossification center, but the cortex has not developed full strength; epiphysis (secondary center) is largely cartilaginous at this stage, with small center ossification only in the distal femur.

II. REGIONAL ABNORMALITIES

A. UPPER EXTREMITIES.

1. Fractures.

a. Clavicle. Fracture occurs in 2.5% of live births; mostly with cephalic presentation (particularly with large baby or shoulder dystocia). May be either greenstick (incomplete) or complete.

    (1) Findings include localized tenderness, crepitus, hematoma; later, a firm mass of callus is noted. Pseudoparalysis is present if fracture is complete, but some hand and elbow motion is usually present.

    (2) Diagnosis. X-rays are indicated initially for diagnosis; further x-rays are not necessary as healing is uneventful.

    (3) Treatment. If discomfort is minimal, no treatment is necessary; if fracture is painful, immobilize arm to trunk with elastic bandage or sling support. Clinical healing usually takes about 10 days.

    (4) Differential diagnosis includes brachial plexus injury, congenital pseudoarthrosis of clavicle (nontender, no healing, right more often than left), infection, or humeral physeal or shaft fracture.

b. Humerus (proximal).

    (1) The etiology of proximal humerus fractures is usually hyperextension or abduction. It is usually a Salter-1 or Salter-2 fracture of the proximal humeral growth plate.

    (2) Physical findings show tenderness over the humeral neck; swelling is greater than with a clavicle fracture; it may coexist with brachial plexus injury.

    (3) X-ray findings show the metaphysis laterally or longitudinally displaced with respect to the glenoid; it often resembles shoulder dislocation because the epiphysis of the humerus is unossified.

    (4) Treatment. Using elastic bandage, wrap arm to trunk for 1 to 2 weeks.

c. Humerus (midshaft).

    (1) The etiology of midshaft fractures of the humerus is forcible traction or rotation of the arm during delivery.

    (2) Findings include decreased mobility, audible snap, and swelling; may be associated with radial nerve palsy (usually resolves in 1 to 3 months).

    (3) Treatment. Using elastic bandage, wrap arm to trunk for 2 to 3 weeks and/or apply splints made from tongue depressors.

d. Humerus (distal).

    (1) The etiology of distal humerus fractures is elbow hyperextension, usually during a breech delivery. This is a rare injury for the newborn.

    (2) Findings include decreased mobility, swelling, and crepitus.

    (3) X-ray examination often requires a comparison view because elbow ossification centers have not appeared.

    (4) Treatment. Use of a long arm splint in flexion for 2 weeks.

2. Brachial plexus injury.

a. Etiology is a stretch injury to the brachial plexus (**Fig. 17**-2), usually seen in large infants (e.g., infants of diabetic mothers) or difficult deliveries; occurs in approximately 1:1000 deliveries.

b. Types.

(1) Erb (C5-C6) palsy. Caused by downward force on the shoulder and lateral flexion of the neck; usually a cephalic delivery. Leads to loss of shoulder motion and elbow flexion (arm in "waiter's tip" position).

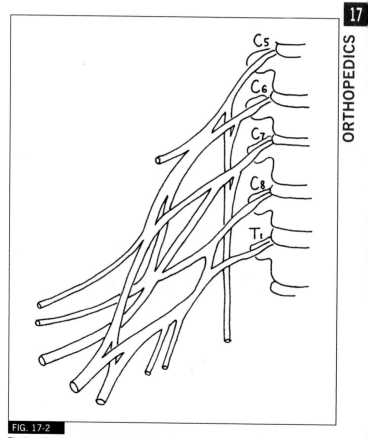

FIG. 17-2

The brachial plexus. Note that the fifth and sixth nerve roots are more vulnerable to stretch. Therefore, Erb (upper trunk) palsy is more common.

      (2) Klumpke (C8-T1) palsy. Caused by overhead traction on the arm; often in breech position. There is loss of finger and wrist flexion (absent grasp) and Horner syndrome may be present.

      (3) Combined. Entire plexus is involved.

  c. Differential diagnosis.

      (1) Fracture of clavicle/humerus. Generally there is greater swelling, pain, and crepitus, but palsy may coexist with the fracture, especially after a difficult delivery.

      (2) Central nervous system (CNS) or spinal cord injury; weakness in other extremities.

      (3) Infection. Moro reflex is usually not affected by infectious process.

  d. Evaluation.

      (1) X-rays should be obtained of the upper limb and shoulder girdle to rule out fracture.

      (2) Muscle examination.

      (3) Electromyography, magnetic resonance imaging (MRI), and myelogram are *not* useful in the neonate.

  e. Natural history.

      (1) Most palsies (90%) resolve spontaneously within the first 4 to 5 months of life. Biceps function is among the earliest to return because the muscle belly is proximal, therefore the distance for the nerve to regenerate is short. It is the easiest to monitor and is evidenced by return of elbow flexion.

      (2) Of those patients whose palsy does not recover if untreated, the most common disability is inability to rotate the arm outwardly or raise it from the shoulder (abduct). The scapula may appear to protrude ("winged"). If the palsy is very severe, some weakness of finger and wrist strength may persist.

  f. Treatment.

      (1) Passive joint exercises through range of motion should be performed by the infant's caregiver with each diaper change to compensate for specific muscle weakness. Exercises should concentrate especially on maintaining elbow extension and shoulder external rotation and abduction. Referral to a physical therapist is indicated. Unless there is motor return in first few months, orthopaedic referral is indicated.

      (2) Surgical plexus repair is an option if return of biceps function is not evident by about 5 months.

      (3) Osteotomy or shoulder muscle transfer may be used to help correct residual deformity in those who have not recovered full strength during the first few years of life.

3. Congenital malformations.

  a. Polydactyly.

      (1) Findings. Polydactyly may be preaxial (thumb side) or postaxial (little finger side) and may or may not be associated with a syndrome. The extra digit may or may not contain bone and tendons.

   (2) Treatment.
      (a) For a floppy, unstable digit, remove before discharge from the
          nursery. This may be performed surgically with a local anesthetic
          if the tissue bridge is substantial, or by tying it off if it has just a
          small skin bridge with no skeletal connection.
      (b) For a duplicated thumb or stable digit, defer resection until the
          infant is older and function may be better assessed.
 b. Syndactyly.
    (1) Findings. Fingers are joined by skin and, at times, by bone.
        Syndactyly may be associated with syndromes, such as
        acrocephalosyndactyly (Apert syndrome) or congenital constriction
        band syndrome.
    (2) Treatment. No treatment is needed in the neonatal period.
        Separation can be done early (about 6 months) if deformity
        develops as a result of asymmetrical growth; otherwise separate
        at 2 to 3 years.

B. SPINE.
1. Spinal cord injury.
a. Etiology. Caused by traction at birth; cord is less elastic than vertebral
   column, so cord damage (tear) often occurs without vertebral fracture
   or separation. Location is usually at the occiput, C2 (cephalic delivery),
   or C6-T1 (breech delivery).
b. Findings depend on location and extent of injury and may include
   diaphragmatic paralysis, initial hypotonia of extremities (spinal shock),
   absent deep tendon reflexes, and neurogenic bladder. Later, spasticity,
   contractures, and scoliosis may occur.
c. Evaluation/treatment. MRI and x-rays should be obtained of the entire
   spine; fracture and dislocation are rare. Immobilize infant if fracture/
   dislocation is confirmed. There is no role for surgery, and the role of
   steroids is unclear.
2. Congenital scoliosis.
a. Intrinsic vertebral malformation includes a wedge-shaped vertebra
   (failure of formation) or unilateral fusion of several vertebrae (failure of
   segmentation) (Fig. 17-3); may be associated with other malformations.
    (1) VACTERL association, usually partial. Components of this syndrome
        include the following: vertebral anomalies, anorectal malformations,
        cardiac defects, TE (tracheoesophageal) fistula, renal or radial
        aplasia, and limb anomalies.
    (2) Klippel-Feil (fusion of cervical vertebrae, Fig. 17-4. Sprengel
        (undescended scapula).
    (3) Hemiatrophy of extremity.
b. Findings. There is often no clinical finding in the newborn period. The
   back may appear straight; however, congenital scoliosis must be ruled
   out when the patient has one of the associated malformations. Other
   clues include the following:

17

ORTHOPEDICS

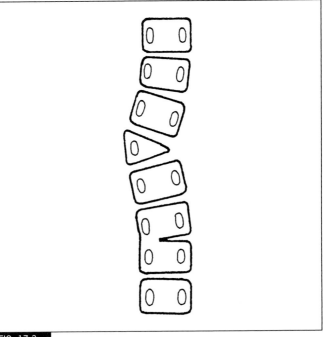

FIG. 17-3
Congenital scoliosis; should be searched for in any newborn having chest x-ray or kidney, ureter, and bladder evaluations because it is often associated with anomalies in cardiac, respiratory, or genitourinary systems. This spine drawing shows examples of both hemivertebra *(upper)* and hemifusion *(lower)*.

    (1) Abnormal hair distribution, vascular marking, or dimple over spine is occasionally seen.
    (2) X-ray findings include asymmetry of the pedicle number or spacing often noted on a chest x-ray taken for TE fistula or congenital cardiac or renal anomaly.
  c. Treatment.
    (1) Observation. Obtain an x-ray of the whole spine as a baseline for future comparison.
    (2) Serial follow-up x-rays every 6 months monitored by an orthopedist.
    (3) Approximately 50% have significant worsening of curvature. A brace does not help because this is an intrinsic problem of bone growth.

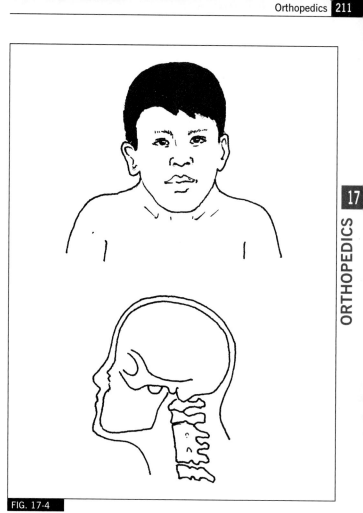

FIG. 17-4

Klippel-Feil syndrome is a triad of short neck, low hairline, and congenital cervical fusion.

(4) Ultimately, in situ fusion of the localized area of the abnormality is performed if the curve worsens more than 10 degrees from initial measurement.

3. **Myelodysplasia (spina bifida or lipomeningocele).**

a. Obtain baseline anteroposterior and lateral x-rays of the thoracolumbar spine to rule out congenital deformity and kyphosis.

b. Vertebral resection is sometimes helpful in closing a defect with severe kyphosis.

c. Perform baseline motor examination and document for further reference.

d. Serial casts/splints can be used if a clubfoot deformity is present.

e. An abduction brace can be used for subluxable hips with low lumbar myelodysplasia.

4. Muscular torticollis.

a. Definition. Sternocleidomastoid muscle contracture causing tilt of ear toward affected side and chin rotation to contralateral side.

b. Etiology is controversial; may involve a stretch injury to the muscle, usually during difficult birth, or ischemia secondary to in utero compartment syndrome.

c. Findings. Swelling of sternocleidomastoid muscle in first 3 months, then contracture, torticollis, and eventual plagiocephaly.

d. Differential diagnosis. In the newborn period, the main differential is congenital cervical vertebral anomaly.

e. Management. Take extra care to screen for associated congenital hip dislocation. X-rays of the neck should be obtained to rule out vertebral anomaly. Physical therapy and positioning of the infant to move the head to the opposite side are recommended. Surgical lengthening of the muscle may be indicated if not resolved by 1 year.

C. LOWER EXTREMITY.

1. Developmental DDH (Fig. 17-5).

a. Etiology. Gradual, acquired dislocation. There are different levels of severity as a result of malposition and ligamentous laxity. It is more frequent on the left side, in girls, those with breech position, and in those with a positive family history.

b. Physical findings. Not all physical findings are seen in any single instance. All newborns should be evaluated before discharge from the hospital. The baby should be warm and as relaxed as possible. Indications of DDH include the following:

(1) Adducted position of thigh at rest.

(2) Deep proximal thigh crease (**Fig. 17-6A**).

(3) Apparent thigh shortening in extension (see **Fig. 17-6B**) or flexion (Allis sign).

(4) Positive Barlow (dislocation) and Ortolani (relocation) tests; should feel a slide or a deep "clunk," not a "click" (see **Fig. 17-5**).

(5) Limited passive abduction (spread of legs apart); clunk with abduction or difficulty diapering in older child.

(6) Document results of examination in chart.

c. Management.

(1) Ultrasound is indicated if diagnosis is in question (e.g., equivocal Barlow, Ortolani, or Allis sign; asymmetrical abduction; consider if breech position or if family history positive); *must* be done by sonographer experienced in infant evaluation (**Fig. 17-7**).

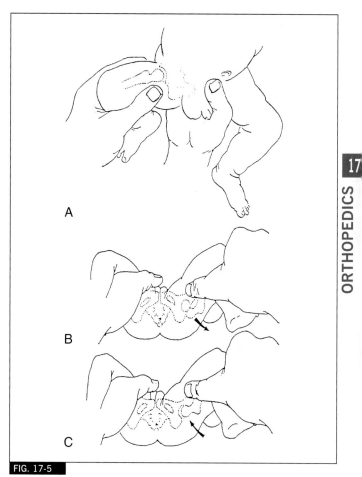

FIG. 17-5

Barlow and Ortolani tests: the definitive tests for unstable hip. **A,** Position: examine only one hip at a time; one hand around flexed thigh; feel greater trochanter with fingertips. **B,** Barlow test: causes *dislocation* by adduction, axial pressure; note sudden "clunk." **C,** Ortolani test: causes reduction by abduction, traction; note clunk with reduction.

   (2) Use Pavlik harness if hip is dislocated and child is <6 months old; reduction must be documented with ultrasound or x-ray.
   (3) Traction can be used with closed or open reduction if dislocation is diagnosed after 6 months of age or is not reduced with the Pavlik harness.

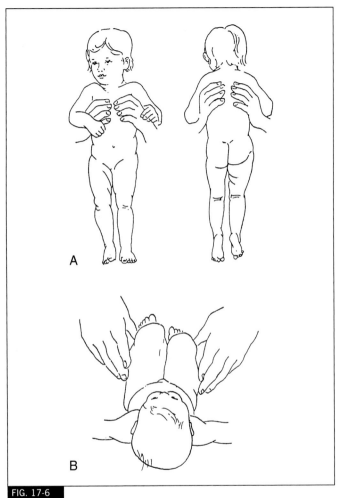

FIG. 17-6

Other signs of unstable hip in the newborn. **A,** Asymmetrical crease (extra crease in *proximal* thigh). **B,** Allis sign (apparent shortening of one thigh when pelvis is held level and both hips are flexed 90 degrees).

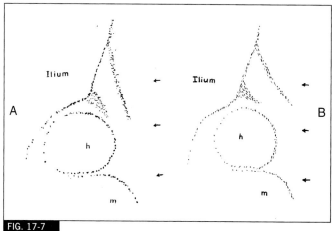

FIG. 17-7

Ultrasound of the neonatal hip in the coronal plane shows cartilaginous structures similar to the way they would appear on an x-ray later, when ossified. *Arrows* indicate ultrasound source. **A,** Normal hip, with the femoral head well covered by the acetabulum and downward-sloping labrum. The upper oblique line is the plane between the glutei. **B,** Subluxated hip. The femoral head is less than half covered by the acetabulum, and the labrum is elevated. h, femoral head; m, metaphysis.

2. **Proximal femoral focal deficiency.**
   a. Definition/etiology. Focal deficiency or absence of part or all of the upper femur. Distal anomalies may coexist; 50% are bilateral. Etiology is unknown.
   b. Diagnosis can be made by plain-film x-ray.
   c. Physical findings include shortening, anterior bowing, and external rotation of the thigh.
   d. Treatment. Obtain orthopedic consultation. Eventual bracing or reconstruction may be necessary.
3. **Congenital subluxation/dislocation of the knee.**
   a. Etiology. Caused by in utero hyperextension; may be an isolated finding, or may be associated with myelodysplasia, arthrogryposis, or Larsen syndrome (multiple joint dislocations).
   b. Findings.
      (1) Hyperextension of knee.
      (2) Limited flexion.
      (3) Posterior prominence of femoral condyles.
      (4) X-ray distinguishes subluxation from dislocation.
   c. Treatment. Serial stretching or casting. Hyperextension and subluxation usually respond to these measures; dislocation usually requires open reduction.

4. Leg/foot deformities.

a. Posteromedial bow of tibia (**Fig. 17-8**).

  (1) Definition. Angulation of distal tibia with a posterior and medial apex; foot appears in valgus, leg shortened.

  (2) Etiology. Unknown.

  (3) Diagnosis can be made by plain-film x-ray.

  (4) Treatment. Observation. There is no risk of fracture; correction usually occurs spontaneously within 5 years, but slight shortening may persist.

b. Metatarsus adductus.

  (1) Definition/etiology. Isolated medial deviation of forefoot with normal heel and ankle (**Fig. 17-9A**) secondary to in utero molding.

  (2) Treatment. In the newborn period, stretching exercises can be done by the parents; serial casts are used if there is no improvement by 8 months.

c. Clubfoot.

  (1) Definition. Contracture of posteromedial leg muscles and malrotation of foot bones, causing ankle equinus, hindfoot varus and internal rotation, and forefoot adduction (see **Fig. 17-9B**).

  (2) Etiology. Unknown; most cases are isolated, but the condition may be familial or associated with spinal cord anomaly, diastrophic dysplasia, or arthrogryposis.

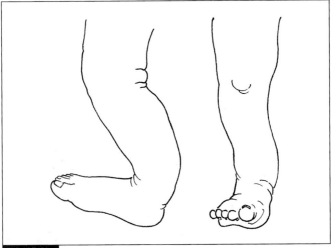

FIG. 17-8

Posteromedial bow. There is a sharp angulation in the distal tibia, with the foot in a position resembling a calcaneovalgus foot.

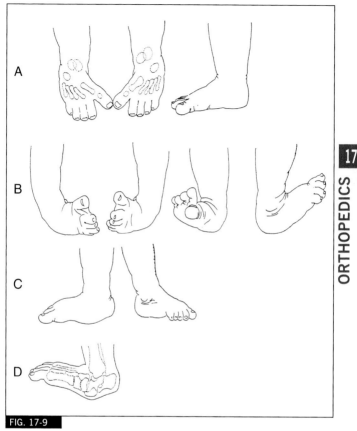

FIG. 17-9

Common foot deformities. **A,** Metatarsus adductus (forefoot medially deviated; normal hindfoot and ankle). **B,** Clubfoot (ankle equinus, hindfoot varus, and internal rotation in addition to forefoot adduction). **C,** Calcaneovalgus foot (excessive dorsiflexion valgus, but can be corrected easily past neutral). **D,** Vertical talus (rigid reversal of arch), with hindfoot plantar flexion, forefoot dorsiflexion, and dislocation of talonavicular joint.

(3) Treatment. X-rays are not needed at birth. Serial manipulations can be done from birth. Long leg casts, changed 1 or 2 times per week, can be used if there are no contraindications. Surgery can be performed at 6 to 12 months of age if condition is resistant (approximately 10% of cases).

    d. Calcaneovalgus foot.
       (1) Definition. Congenital malposition (by stretch) of foot and ankle into valgus and dorsiflexion so that the dorsum of the foot abuts the leg (see **Fig. 17-9C**).
       (2) Etiology. In utero malposition.
       (3) Findings. Foot rests in extreme calcaneus or dorsiflexion; looks serious but it is not; can be passively plantar flexed to resemble a normal foot having an arch.
       (4) Differential diagnosis. Vertical talus (calcaneus remains pulled proximally and curve is in midfoot; reverse of arch), posteromedial bow of tibia.
       (5) Treatment. Observation or serial stretching; always resolves by the time the child walks.
    e. Vertical talus.
       (1) Definition. Plantar flexion of hindfoot and dorsiflexion of forefoot producing subluxation in the middle, with reversal of the normal arch (see **Fig. 17-9D**).
       (2) Etiology. May be isolated; approximately 50% of cases are associated with a neuromuscular or chromosomal disorder.
       (3) Findings. "Rocker-bottom" sole (reversal of normal arch); head of talus is palpable where arch should be; deep crease in dorsolateral ankle and above heel; not completely correctable by passive manipulation.
       (4) Diagnosis. Lateral x-ray of foot in neutral and maximum plantar flexion.
       (5) Treatment. Serial stretching/casting to relax dorsal soft tissue; surgery virtually always needed at 6 to 12 months of age.
    f. Fibular hemimelia.
       (1) Definition. Partial or total absence of fibula, with or without other defects in the limb, primarily on the lateral side.
       (2) Findings. Valgus foot. X-rays demonstrate extent of absence. Shortening of leg. Often missing one or two lateral toes.
       (3) Treatment. Eventual reconstruction/lengthening if mild; otherwise, ankle disarticulation at age 6 to 12 months.
    g. Tibial hemimelia.
       (1) Definition. Tibia partially or completely missing; may resemble clubfoot.
       (2) Treatment. Depends on how much of the proximal tibia is available for the surgical creation of a knee and on the degree of deformity in the foot.

5. Fractures of the lower extremity.
    a. Fracture-separation of upper femoral epiphysis.
       (1) Etiology. Occurs during difficult delivery, with hyperextension and rotation; analogous to slipped capital femoral epiphysis.
       (2) Findings. Swelling, pain, minimal crepitus; leg lies in external rotation; x-ray shows displacement of entire ossified portion of the femur; resembles DDH, but acetabulum is normal.

(3) Differential diagnosis. Infection, DDH.

(4) Diagnosis is made by arthrogram.

(5) Treatment. Hip spica cast for 3 to 4 weeks.

b. Fracture of femoral shaft.

   (1) Etiology. Difficult delivery, child abuse (rare in newborn period). Also more common in children with a neuromuscular disorder, especially arthrogryposis or myelomeningocele.

   (2) Findings. Pain, swelling, crepitus, shortening of leg.

   (3) Treatment. Hip spica cast; overhead traction is associated with ischemia and is not recommended.

III. SYSTEMIC/NONREGIONAL CONDITIONS

A. INFECTION.

1. Osteomyelitis.

a. Etiology. Hematogenous spread, neonatal sepsis; often no cause is found.

b. Organisms.

   (1) Staphylococcus aureus.

   (2) Group B streptococcus.

   (3) Gram-negative organisms.

c. Findings.

   (1) Pseudoparalysis. Decreased movement of affected part.

   (2) Multiple sites may be affected, most commonly the proximal humerus, or proximal or distal femur.

   (3) Swelling, pain (appears to be less than in an older child).

   (4) Laboratory findings. Erythrocyte sedimentation rate elevated; white blood cell count variable, may be decreased; blood should be drawn for culture at same time.

   (5) X-ray findings. May be normal or show soft-tissue swelling only during early phase; osteopenia (later); periosteal reaction (last).

d. Diagnosis can be made by bone scan, ultrasound, or MRI; often confirmed by needle aspiration of bone.

e. Treatment.

   (1) If pus is obtained on aspiration, devascularization exists and area should be drained.

   (2) If no pus is present, antibiotics alone are adequate treatment.

   (3) Route. Intravenous antibiotics are given until clinical response is obtained, at which time antibiotics may be given orally if a suitable drug is available. Duration of treatment is 3 to 6 weeks, depending on the stage. Parents should be warned about risk of growth disturbance, which is greater in newborns than in older children.

2. Septic arthritis.

a. Etiology. Primary hematogenous joint seeding or spread across growth plate from adjacent osteomyelitis.

b. Organism. Same as for newborn osteomyelitis.

ORTHOPEDICS

17

c. Findings. Pseudoparalysis; swelling is less diffuse than in osteomyelitis; joint effusion; laboratory findings similar to osteomyelitis.

d. Diagnosis. Ultrasound examination can be obtained if an effusion is suspected; bone scan is not a primary procedure (this is not a *bone* problem); aspiration is key. If one infected joint is found, carefully examine all major joints (physical examination, ultrasound, or both).

e. Treatment. Surgical drainage can be performed if a major joint is involved; antibiotics should be given for 3 to 6 weeks. The parents should be counseled about possible growth disturbance, stiff joint, and arthritis.

B. CONGENITAL CONSTRICTION BANDS.

1. Amniotic bands cause creases, or partial or complete amputation. Distal (fenestrated) syndactyly is common; clubfoot and nerve compression may occur.

2. If lymphedema occurs distal to the constricting band, early Z-plasty is necessary.

3. Otherwise, band revision or syndactyly separation can be performed later in childhood.

C. ARTHROGRYPOSIS.

1. Definition. Generalized hypoplasia or aplasia of muscle, leading to stiffness of joints, including fingers.

2. Etiology. Presumed to be anterior horn cell disturbance in utero.

3. Risk of fracture is increased because limbs are so stiff.

4. Treatment. Gentle physical therapy to increase joint range of motion to the best extent possible; treatment of clubfoot or other fixed deformity.

BIBLIOGRAPHY

Carson WF, Lovell WW, Whitesides TE Jr: Congenital elevation of the scapula. J Bone Joint Surg 63A:1199, 1981.

Dobyns JH, Wood V, Bayne LG: Congenital hand deformities. In Green D (ed): Textbook of Hand Surgery, ed 3. New York, Churchill-Livingstone, 1994.

Farsetti P, Weinstein SL, Ponseti IV: Long-term follow-up of nonoperative and operative treatment of metatarsus adductus. J Bone Joint Surg 76:257, 1994.

Kling TF, Hensinger RN: Angular and torsional deformities of the lower limbs in children. Clin Orthop 176:136, 1976.

Pappas AM: Congenital posteromedial bowing of the tibia and fibula. J Pediatr Orthop 4:525, 1984.

Ponseti IV: Current concepts review: Treatment of congenital clubfoot. J Bone Joint Surg 74:448, 1992.

Rushforth GF: The natural history of hooked forefoot. J Bone Joint Surg 60B:8, 1987.

Sponseller PD: Bone joint and muscle problems. In McMillan JA(ed): Oski's Principles and Practice of Pediatrics, 4th ed. Philadelphia, Lippincott, 2005.

Staheli LT: Fundamentals of Pediatric Orthopedics, 3rd ed. Philadelphia, Lippincott, 2003.

Widhe T: Foot deformities at birth: A longitudinal prospective study over a 16-year period. J Pediatr Orthop 17:20, 1997.

Waters PM: Obstetrical palsy: A comparison of natural history, microsurgical repair. J Bone Joint Surg 81A:649, 1999.

Watson BT, Hennrikus WL: Postaxial type-B polydactyly: Prevalence and treatment. J Bone Joint Surg 79A:65, 1997.

Weinstein SL: The Pediatric Spine, 2nd ed. Philadelphia, Lippincott, 2001.

17

ORTHOPEDICS

Dermatology

Henry M. Seidel and Bernard A. Cohen

FAST FACTS

Immediate Issues in the Nursery

- Cutaneous candidiasis can manifest with generalized macules, papules, vesicles, or pustules but is generally self-limited.
- When cutaneous lesions suggestive of herpes are present, a workup including lumbar puncture (LP), chest x-ray (CXR), complete blood cell count (CBC), and liver chemistries are indicated.
- Pustular lesions of erythema toxicum can be differentiated from pustules of bacterial infection by the fact that the former appears as small pustules with a large (up to 3 cm) area of surrounding redness. Lesions of bacterial skin infection of the neonate are usually the opposite.
- Almost any lesion in the midline of the head or down the middle of the back should prompt consideration of neural tube defects.
- Plaque-like scales on the trunk, palms, and soles could be cutaneous manifestations of congenital syphilis. Lesions may also appear papular or vesicular.

Important Reminders After Discharge

- Manifestations of systemic candidiasis occur days to weeks after birth. It is more common in premature infants and does not usually cause a skin rash.
- Skin of healthy premature infants functions normally as a barrier that is comparable with a term infant by 2 weeks of age.
- Mottling that persists more than several months suggests hypothyroidism or CNS dysfunction.

Helpful Information for Parents

- In infants of color, pigmentation of genitals and paronychial skin can approximate the amount of pigmentation that is genetically determined.
- Milia, sebaceous gland hyperplasia, and erythema toxicum are all harmless and self-resolving lesions that should be pointed out to parents (and other family members) as soon as they are discovered. Reassurance for these "normal variants" will be greatly appreciated.
- Ask parents to take digital images or videos of any concerning rashes or discolorations that may occur. Many "normal" findings are often transient and may not be fully representative when the infant is seen in the office. This practice will also help prevent parents from feeling like they are overstressed, neurotic, or "imagining things."

18

I. GENERAL CONSIDERATIONS

The skin of the healthy, full-term newborn is quite mature. There is relatively more of it as compared with body weight than in the older child or adult (relatively high surface to volume ratio), making it more vulnerable to the toxic effect of topical drugs. Absorption of drugs is greater, and processing and excretion are less efficient. The premature infant, with a greater ratio of surface area to body weight, is at even greater risk. In the full-term infant, the outer barrier layer of the epidermis—the stratum corneum—is fully formed. During the last few weeks of pregnancy the skin acquires the additional protection of the vernix caseosa, which is greasy, white, and often copious. These barriers vary in efficiency and amount so that the premature infant is less well protected and, with shedding, the postmature infant is also more vulnerable. Lanugo, the delicate hair found mostly on the shoulders and back, is more prominent in the relatively premature infant (gestational age 31 to 35 weeks) and is quickly shed after birth. Given this variability, full-term infants usually develop parchment-like skin, with cracking and peeling after the first day of life. Postmature babies who develop deep cracking and peeling during the first hours after birth and premature infants with thin transparent skin have decreased skin barrier function and experience increased insensible water loss and heat loss. These babies are also susceptible to cutaneous infections and sepsis. Fortunately, regardless of the gestational age, the skin of healthy premature infants usually develops normal barrier function comparable with that of a full-term infant by 2 weeks of age.

II. OTHER OBSERVATIONS OF CONSEQUENCE

A. THE HEALTHY BABY MAY BE CYANOTIC AT BIRTH BUT TURNS TO PINK QUICKLY AS RESPIRATIONS ARE ESTABLISHED.

B. ACROCYANOSIS (CYANOSIS OF THE HANDS AND FEET, PERIPHERAL CYANOSIS) AND MOTTLING OF THE EXTREMITIES MAY APPEAR EARLY AND RECUR WITHOUT SIGNIFICANCE FOR WEEKS.

C. TEMPORARY VASCULAR INSTABILITY AND A COOL ENVIRONMENT may cause a generalized transient cyanosis or a marble-like mottling of the skin (cutis marmorata). Vascular instability may also be associated with transient erythema of the dependent half of the body (harlequin color change). Recurrent or persistent mottling beyond the first month may be a sign of hypothyroidism or central nervous system (CNS) dysfunction.

D. THE MORE FAT AND THE MORE DEVELOPED THE EPIDERMIS, the less redness of the skin; the greater the transparency (with prematurity), the greater the redness.

E. YELLOWED VERNIX AND YELLOW-TO-GREEN MECONIUM STAINING OF FINGERNAILS SUGGEST FETAL DISTRESS.

F. THE MORE PREMATURE OR POSTMATURE THE INFANT, THE MORE LIKELY ARE FISSURING AND CRACKING.

G. THE MORE TRAUMATIC THE DELIVERY, THE MORE LIKELY ARE PETECHIAE, ECCHYMOSES, LACERATIONS IN A VARIETY OF SITES, AND EDEMA AND BLEEDING IN THE SCALP.

H. THE MORE LIMITED THE AVAILABILITY OF DIRECT DAYLIGHT, THE MORE LIKELY JAUNDICE WILL BE OBSERVED.

I. MELANIN IS VARIABLE AND OFTEN SCANT AT FIRST IN BOTH BLACK AND WHITE BABIES.

Clues to normal hereditary pigmentation can be detected by examining the mid-abdominal linea nigra, genital skin, and paronychial skin.

J. POSTMATURE BABIES WITH LONGER NAILS MAY HAVE SUPERFICIAL SCRATCHES ON THE CHEEK.

No harm; these disappear quickly if ignored. Nails do not need clipping in the newborn period (or for a long time thereafter) and should not be clipped into the corners; at the most, they should be clipped straight across.

III. CARE OF NEONATAL SKIN

The goal of neonatal skin care is to achieve that smooth, soft feel so typical of a baby's buttocks. Hydration and lubrication are key and depend on ambient temperature and the dryness of the baby's skin.

A. FIRST BATH.

After delivery and when vital signs have stabilized, usually at about 2 hours of age, take the baby from the warmer for a bath with comfortably warm water; return to warmer after bath.

B. SUBSEQUENT BATHS

require water and gentle sponging; soap is not a necessity; however, any cleanser used should be fragrance-free and gentle.

C. PREMATURE BABIES

may require the humidity and warmth of the isolette (for much more than keeping their skin warm and smooth); the skin of a healthy premature infant matures in $1\frac{1}{2}$ to 2 weeks, regardless of gestational age.

D. MOISTURIZERS WILL HELP IN A DRY ENVIRONMENT,

but are not usually necessary with humidity. Petrolatum-based ointments without preservatives are best and may be safely used under a warmer They are not associated with an increased risk of infection and may actually decrease the risk by decreasing insensible water loss and improving general well being.

Note: *Beware of absorption of emulsifiers and preservatives, particularly in premature infants.*

E. AVOID FRICTION

(e.g., with tape, too much Phisoderm or similar preparations, or too-frequent monitor changes, particularly in premature infants).

F. USE SEMIPERMEABLE DRESSINGS WHEN WOUND OR OTHER PROTECTION IS NEEDED.

These dressings may also be used in some premature infants to decrease insensible water loss.

G. HAIR NEEDS GENTLE WASHING ONLY AT THE TIME OF A BATH; NO SPECIAL SHAMPOOS ARE NECESSARY.

H. POWDERS AND CORN STARCH ARE NOT NECESSARY OR APPROPRIATE.

If a mother insists on their use, suggest good dusting after application, leaving only a trace of powder; otherwise, clumping in the skin folds will facilitate irritation. Watch out for accidental talc aspiration. There is probably no reason to use talcum powder in infants. Corn starch is not associated with aspiration pneumonia, does not support the growth of yeast, and is probably as effective as talcum powder as an anti-friction agent.

IV. COMMON SKIN VARIATIONS IN THE NEWBORN (FIG. 18-1)

A. HARLEQUIN COLOR CHANGE.

Signs include erythema and pallor separated at midline when a particularly premature baby is placed on a side. The dependent side reddens, and the color change subsides readily when the baby is moved to the supine position, probably a result of immature autonomic vasomotor control.

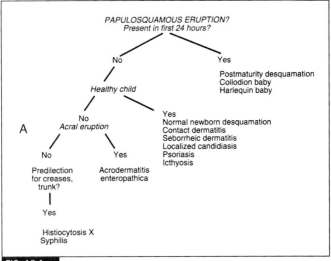

FIG. 18-1

Algorithm for evaluation of neonatal rashes. **A,** Papulosquamous eruption. (*Courtesy Dr. Bernard Cohen.*)

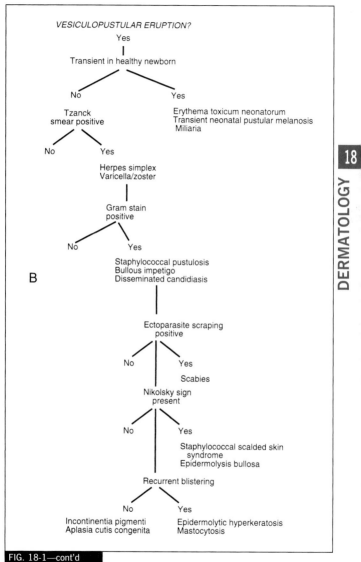

FIG. 18-1—cont'd

B, Vesiculopustular eruption.

Continued

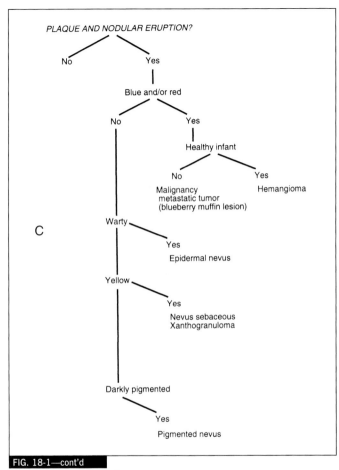

FIG. 18-1—cont'd

C, Plaque and nodular eruption.

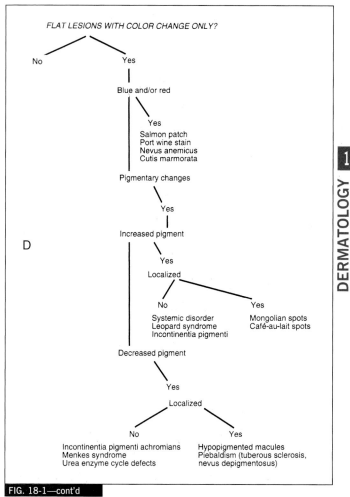

FLAT LESIONS WITH COLOR CHANGE ONLY?

No — Yes

Blue and/or red — Yes
- Salmon patch
- Port wine stain
- Nevus anemicus
- Cutis marmorata

Pigmentary changes — Yes

Increased pigment — Yes

Localized
- No
  - Systemic disorder
  - Leopard syndrome
  - Incontinentia pigmenti
- Yes
  - Mongolian spots
  - Café-au-lait spots

Decreased pigment — Yes

Localized
- No
  - Incontinentia pigmenti achromians
  - Menkes syndrome
  - Urea enzyme cycle defects
- Yes
  - Hypopigmented macules
  - Piebaldism (tuberous sclerosis, nevus depigmentosus)

D

FIG. 18-1—cont'd

D, Flat lesions with color change only.

Do not confuse with harlequin fetus, a life-threatening autosomal recessive ichthyotic disorder characterized by scaling, ectropion, and fissures and tightening of the skin which restricts breathing.

B. MOTTLING (CUTIS MARMORATA).

Splotchiness with pale red patches forming a sometimes continuous, sometimes discontinuous fishnet-like pattern; macular; more common with cooling, tends to disappear with warming. Persistence for more than a few months suggests hypothyroidism or CNS dysfunction. Lability of appearance and disappearance with warmth are characteristic; poorly developed autonomic vasomotor control is the probable cause.

C. MILIA (PLATE 1).

Multiple, scattered, white, keratin-filled cysts (miniature epidermal inclusion cysts), about 1 mm in diameter, raised, most often on the face; no therapy other than routine cleanliness. They rupture and disappear within days to a few weeks without visible trace. May be confused with sebaceous gland hyperplasia.

D. SEBACEOUS GLAND HYPERPLASIA (PLATE 2).

Multiple scattered, yellowish macules or papules, occurring principally on the nose and cheeks at the site of pilosebaceous follicles. No "therapy" other than routine cleanliness. They tend to disappear within a few days to as many as several months without visible trace. May be confused with milia.

E. ERYTHEMA TOXICUM (PLATE 3).

1. Splotchy, reddish macules, scattered on the face, upper body, and upper extremities; may be as much as 3 cm in diameter, many with a tiny central papule or pustule, giving a "flea-bitten" appearance. Wright stain of contents reveals eosinophils.
2. Lesions appear within about 48 hours of birth and begin to disappear within 4 to 5 days. New lesions may appear for up to 10 days. Common, particularly in the full-term infant.
3. Peripheral blood examination, not a routine need, often reveals eosinophilia.
4. No therapy needed. Pathophysiologic significance is unclear.

F. TRANSIENT NEONATAL PUSTULAR MELANOSIS (PLATE 4).

1. Multiple vesicles and pustules, frequently ruptured, are characterized by a collarette of scale and are scattered over the body, particularly the scalp, face, sacrum, and even the palms and soles. They are more frequent in black males.
2. Lesions may be present at birth and may last about 5 days. Subsequent pigmented macules may last many more weeks before disappearing. Sometimes macules are the only lesions present at birth.
3. Wright stain of a pustule reveals neutrophils; pathophysiologic significance is unknown.
4. No treatment necessary.
5. May occasionally be confused with herpes or bacterial infection.

G. SUBCUTANEOUS FAT NECROSIS.

1. Relatively hard and well-demarcated subcutaneous plaques and nodules of necrotic fat, appearing within the first few days of life

and up to about 2 weeks; trauma and cold are likely contributing factors (e.g., forceps delivery).

2. Cheeks, arms, legs, and buttocks are common sites.
3. No treatment necessary. Resolution is usually within a few weeks, and the babies are usually otherwise healthy and seemingly unconcerned.
4. Might be confused with cellulitis, which is usually accompanied by the appearance of illness.
5. Hypercalcemia is an occasional finding and may be more common than believed. It may not develop until several months of age and may be associated with poor weight gain.

H. SUCKING BLISTERS ON FINGERS, WRISTS, AND FOREARMS

are sometimes seen in the first hours of life and are presumably the result of vigorous in utero or neonatal sucking. No treatment is necessary, but these blisters should not be confused with herpes or impetigo. In bullous disorders, blistering tends to be more widespread.

18

DERMATOLOGY

V. COMMON, USUALLY TRANSIENT SKIN DISEASES OF THE NEWBORN

A. NEONATAL ACNE (PLATE 5).

1. Rarely seen in the newborn, occurs usually at about 2 to 4 weeks of age. Multiple discrete papules and, occasionally, blackheads are scattered on the face, chest, back, and groin; may evolve into pustules.
2. Will most often subside without treatment. Topical 2.5% benzoyl peroxide gel may help in the severe circumstance.

B. CUTANEOUS CANDIDIASIS.

1. Contracted from an ascending intrauterine infection; evident at birth or within a few hours.
2. Generalized distribution (including palms and soles) of red macules, papules, vesicles, and pustules; may be confused with staphylococcal scalded skin syndrome. Generally self-limited in full-term infants and involves subsequent peeling of skin. May become disseminated in premature infants.
3. Pseudohyphae and budding yeast can be seen on direct microscopy of scales or smear of pustule.

Note: *Systemic candidiasis, which is much more dangerous, does not usually cause skin rash. It is contracted at birth in the vagina but may not become manifest for many days to a week. A rare condition, the risks are greatest in premature infants, those with low Apgar scores, and sick babies during a long hospital stay and after much manipulation, e.g., intubation.*

C. NEONATAL HERPES SIMPLEX VIRUS (CUTANEOUS) (PLATE 6).

Grouped vesicles with a red base, anywhere on the body (particularly presenting body parts), often found on the scalp or buttocks; sometimes seen at birth, but onset after several days is more common. Type 2 (herpes genitalis, common to the genital region) predominates by far over type 1 (herpes labialis, common to the facial area, particularly the mouth and nose); more than one half of those infected have skin lesions. Maternal birth canal infection is the usual source.

Note: *Early diagnosis and expeditious therapy are essential. With cutaneous herpes alone, a complete workup is essential: LP, CXR, CBC, and liver chemistries.*

1. Varicella or impetigo, particularly with bullae, may confuse, but they lack the uniform clustered vesicles of herpes.
2. Systemic herpetic infection, particularly involving the CNS, may dominate the clinical picture.
3. On a Tzanck test, or stained cells smeared from the base of a vesicle with Wright or Giemsa stains, multinucleated giant cells and balloon cells are characteristic; however, only 60% to 70% are sensitive even under the best circumstances.
4. Confirmation is with fluorescein-tagged anti-herpes simplex virus-specific antibody on vesicle smears or snap-frozen biopsy sections of skin. Polymerase chain reaction is even more sensitive and can be performed with a sample of fluid swabbed from a vesicle and placed in viral transport medium.
5. Culture is usually positive at 12 to 24 after birth hours but may take as long as 5 days and should not delay treatment.
6. Treatment of choice is acyclovir, 10 mg/kg intravenously every 8 hours for 10 to 14 days.

D. IMPETIGO.
Bullae, flaccid, often ruptured, involving any part of the body, particularly the head, periumbilical, and diaper areas. Shallow, erythematous base involving only the outer epidermis. When *Staphylococcus aureus* is present, the erythema may be fringed with remnants of ruptured bullae.

1. Commonly caused by *S. aureus;* at times, group A streptococci or enterococci may be the culprit.
2. Culture of bullous contents can confirm etiology; Gram stain may give an early indication.
3. Therapy should be immediate with systemic antibiotics appropriate to the organism to forestall spread, sepsis, and staphylococcal scalded skin syndrome.

E. PETECHIAE AND PURPURA.
1. Petechiae and purpura are frequent harbingers of congenital infection with thrombocytopenia, particularly the TORCH group ("blueberry muffin" rash) (**PLATE 7**).

2. Occasionally there may be a few scattered petechiae on the upper body (after vertex delivery) or lower body (after breech delivery) that are transient and unaccompanied by other evidence of illness.

3. Larger, isolated ecchymotic areas unaccompanied by other evidence of illness suggest trauma (e.g., with forceps). The shape of the bruise may give a clue to the cause.

F. PUSTULES.

1. Discrete yellow papules or vesicles usually ringed with erythema, up to 1 cm in diameter, that appear in a scattered distribution after delivery, often within a few hours. In erythema toxicum, the pustule is small and the surrounding erythema is large. With bacterial pustules, the pustule is relatively large and the ring of erythema is small.

2. Infection and sepsis (e.g., with prolonged rupture of the membranes) must be a first consideration.

3. Culture of pustule contents is indicated, in addition to other investigations for sepsis guided by history and a full physical examination. Wright stain of the contents usually reveals neutrophils and, occasionally, bacteria. Although eosinophils are found in the pustules of erythema toxicum, do not be fooled by the presence of eosinophils in bacterial infections.

4. Other common conditions in the differential diagnosis include the following:

a. Benign pustular eruptions.
   (1) Erythema toxicum (see **PLATE 3**).
   (2) Pustular melanosis (see **PLATE 4**).
b. Herpes simplex (usually clustered vesicles, not pustules) (see **PLATE 6**).
c. Candidiasis (usually, but not always limited to diaper and intertriginous areas; sometimes pustular).
d. Listeriosis, early and late forms; the former is associated with "blueberry muffin" lesions and the latter with disseminated papulopustules, particularly on the back and lumbar area.

G. SCLEREMA.

1. Diffuse, nonpitting hardening of the skin, more common in the premature infant, characterized by tight immobility and a glistening quality.

2. A very ill infant with severe underlying disease is more susceptible; mortality is apt to be high.

3. Diagnosis tends to be easy.

4. Treatment is guided by the underlying disorder, and maintenance of temperature and nutrition are apt to be difficult.

18

DERMATOLOGY

5. Cold and immature autonomic vasomotor control resulting in cutaneous ischemia and increased fibroblast activity appear to contribute to causation.

H. STAPHYLOCOCCAL SCALDED SKIN SYNDROME (RITTER DISEASE).

1. Generalized erythema appearing as early as 24 to 48 hours of age, followed by scattered superficial bullae, rupture, and widespread exfoliation, particularly involving the head, neck, diaper area, skin folds, and periumbilical area.
2. Caused by exotoxins from phage group II staphylococci.
3. Not to be confused with toxic epidermal necrolysis, an immunologic, drug-related form of erythema multiforme, which occurs only rarely in a newborn.
4. Culture of the primary skin lesion (e.g., from the umbilicus or circumcision site) is most often apt to give a positive result but most areas of skin do not harbor the organism.
5. Therapy includes immediate administration of systemic antibiotic appropriate to the organism; infant should be isolated. Widespread "scalding" requires meticulous attention to fluid and electrolyte balance. However, the blistering is superficial and reepithelialization occurs quickly in most cases.

I. VARICELLA (CONGENITAL).

1. Rare; may be confused with herpes simplex.
2. There should be a maternal history of infection 14 to 21 days before delivery. Appears in infants as it does in older children and adults, with red macules appearing first and progressing to red papules, delicate vesiculation, rupture, umbilication, and crusting. Lesions may occur anywhere on skin and mucous membranes, beginning usually by 10 days of age.
3. The course may be severe and is occasionally fatal.
4. Herpes simplex or impetigo, particularly with bullae, may confuse. In herpes, vesicles are usually clustered and uniform. Except in areas of trauma, varicella vesicles are in various stages of development and scattered over the entire skin surface.
5. Stained cells from a vesicle show multinucleated giant and balloon cells which are suggestive but not pathognomonic; Tzanck test will not distinguish between herpes and varicella.
6. Confirmation is with fluorescein-tagged anti-herpes zoster virus-specific antibody on vesicle smears or snap-frozen biopsy sections of skin. Polymerase chain reaction is sensitive and specific and, as with herpes simplex infection, a swab of blister fluid can be sent in viral transport medium.
7. Culture takes 7 to 14 days and should not delay treatment.
8. Therapy. Acyclovir, 10 mg/kg intravenously every 8 hours for 10 to 14 days if the infant is severely ill; varicella-zoster immune globulin

may limit the number of vesicles, particularly if maternal infection is within 14 to 21 days of delivery.

Note: *Varicella-zoster immune globulin should be given to the newborn of any mother who develops varicella within 3 weeks of delivery. It will also have to be given to any accidentally exposed roommates in the nursery.*

VI. BIRTHMARKS

Birthmarks are benign hamartomas that may be formed from any component of the skin. They may offer clues to a variety of more generalized diseases (e.g., the café au lait spots of neurofibromatosis or the connective tissue nevi [shagreen patches] of tuberous sclerosis).

A. VASCULAR BIRTHMARKS.
1. Cutis marmorata telangiectatica congenita (congenital phlebectasia). Rare; a reddish-purple vascular malformation, reticulated, spotted with blanching, usually affecting one extremity but occasionally more widespread. Lesions are persistent but may become more subtle in later childhood; may be associated with other congenital defects but is usually isolated. Pathogenesis is not understood; careful attention should be paid to social and emotional impacts.
2. Blue rubber bleb nevus syndrome.
a. Rare; multiple diffuse cutaneous and visceral vascular malformations that are blue, several millimeters to centimeters in diameter, appear in skin and in virtually any other organ.
b. Gastrointestinal hemorrhage may occur. Accessible lesions can be pressed free of blood, refilling slowly.
c. Number and location of lesions may influence management and prognosis (e.g., significant intestinal bleeds, compromised cardiovascular efficiency).
d. Management includes periodic CBC, stool hemoccult examinations. Surgical excision of isolated, delicately situated lesions may be indicated; laser therapy should be considered.
3. Hemangiomas (**PLATE 8**) are not usually apparent in the neonate; a few telangiectases amid blanched skin may be a herald. There is a superficial and/or deep component. Superficial types are bright red. Both types are composed of proliferated, mostly unchanneled endothelial cells. Deep lesions are darker, tend to be deep purple or blue, and feel spongy. All become raised, but not necessarily in the neonate. These lesions tend to grow faster than the baby for 2 to 3 months, although growth up to about 1 year is possible. Most lesions begin to involute by 12 to 15 months of age; more than 75% disappear by first grade and 90% by 10 years of age.
a. Few hemangiomas require treatment in the newborn; bleeding is rarely a problem. A subglottic or intraoral cavernous hemangioma may

DERMATOLOGY

18

obstruct the airway, and a large hemangioma external to the trachea may compress it; these require immediate attention. Similarly, hemangiomas in or near vital structures (e.g., eye, ear canal, alae nasi, urethra, or anus) that might obstruct the associated passage require intervention. Rarely, hemangiomas may be associated with Kasabach-Merritt syndrome (disseminated intravascular coagulation [DIC]). Surgery or laser excision may then be the first-line treatment. Given less urgency, prednisone, 2 to 5 mg/kg daily or every other day, is effective. Tracheostomy may, on occasion, be necessary. Interferon is an effective alternative but may be associated with neurologic complications.

b. Females are usually more cosmetically compromised by problem hemangiomas than are males. Hemangiomas occur more often in girls than in boys, generally 3 or 4:1.

c. Usually, anticipatory guidance is all that is indicated; schooling the parents in the natural history, informing them of available therapy, warning against deleterious radiation or cryotherapy treatments, and planning follow-up examinations in which measurements and photographs will be taken beginning at age 2 weeks is recommended. On consultation with parents, a small hemangioma in a potentially disfiguring location and with uncertainty about its course may be treated.

d. Although hemangiomas are not usually associated with extracutaneous features, large segmental lesions may be. These include lesions in the genital area where an ultrasound (before 6 months of age) and MRI (after 6 months of age) are required to exclude anomalies of the lumbosacral spine. Lesions in the beard area are associated with airway hemangiomas, and massive hemangiomas of the face and neck are associated with PHACE syndrome (posterior fossa brain malformations, hemangioma, arterial anomalies, coarctation of the aorta, cardiac anomalies, and eye defects).

4. Port-wine stain (nevus flammeus) (PLATE 9).

a. Port-wine stains are flat, intensely red or purple stains that are usually large. They are often seen on the face, and sometimes on the arms and legs. They are usually unilateral and do not cross the midline. They are cosmetically difficult.

b. A stain on the face involving the forehead, temple, extending onto the frontal and parietal scalp (distribution of ophthalmic branch of the trigeminal nerve), may be associated with Sturge-Weber syndrome, which includes seizures, cognitive impairment, and glaucoma. A hemangiomatous area of brain may become calcified; computed tomography (CT) or magnetic resonance imaging (MRI) studies are indicated, although most stains are not associated with Sturge-Weber syndrome.

c. A stain on an extremity, with associated soft tissue or bony hypertrophy, suggests Klippel-Trénaunay-Weber syndrome; malformations of the deep venous system occur in 25% of those affected.

d. Eradication can be successfully achieved with pulsed-dye laser. This will also minimize the risk of late complications, such as soft tissue hypertrophy and superficial papules, which tend to develop in adolescence or later. Excellent results are probable and therapy is indicated—the earlier the better. Parents need support and counseling; social and emotional impacts may be heavy.

5. Salmon patch (nevus simplex) (**PLATE 10**). Often called *stork bites.* Light red, blanching patch, most commonly on glabella, upper eyelids, sacrum, or nape of neck; common in whites; perhaps as many as one half gradually disappear, often in a year, sometimes longer. Adult remnants, particularly at the nape of the neck, are not ordinarily cosmetic problems. Lesions on the forehead in individuals with light complexion may become more prominent with fever and intense physical activity. No treatment is indicated unless the patch is prominent and persistent in a psychosocially important area.

B. LYMPHATIC BIRTHMARKS (LYMPHANGIOMAS).

1. There are a variety of forms of lymphangiomas, from well-demarcated, superficial papular investments of the skin, often in a cluster of thick-walled, skin-colored lesions, ("frog-spawn" appearance; lymphangioma circumscriptum) to deeper, more cavernous, irregular hamartomatous growths of great size (cystic hygromas).
2. Size and location (e.g., the neck) may require immediate surgical intervention (decompression of trachea) or more deliberately considered intervention for cosmetic reasons.
3. There may be hemangiomatous involvement, usually of a cavernous type, which adds a degree of bluish-red color. Recurrent lymphangitis and lymphedema may complicate large lesions.
4. Superficial lesions may be confused with herpes, but they have a more gelatinous substance and do not show multinucleated giant cells on Wright stain; deep lesions may be confused with nodes, lipomas, or neurofibromas. Sonography is helpful in differentiation.
5. Surgery may be complicated depending on the extent of neural and vascular proximities and is generally unsatisfactory; avoid radiation or steroid therapy. There may be a role for embolization in select lesions.

C. PIGMENTED BIRTHMARKS.

1. Blue nevus. Uncommon; bluish or blue-black, well demarcated. Papular, occurring on face, buttocks, dorsum of hands and feet; usually no more than 1 cm in diameter. Although the risk of melanoma is low and no greater than with other pigmented nevi, unusual changing lesions may require excision.
2. (Café-au-lait spots (**PLATE 11**). Well-demarcated, irregularly shaped, light-brown macules, occurring anywhere on the body, usually solitary; much more common in blacks than in whites; six or more with

18

DERMATOLOGY

diameters of 0.5 cm or more suggest type I neurofibromatosis. This may be confusing in that numbers can increase with age and the correlation with neurofibromatosis is not absolute. Usually not cosmetically difficult. No treatment. Spots do not generally disappear during childhood.

3. Congenital melanocytic nevi.

a. Small lesions occur in 1% of newborns; rarely there is large, often grotesque involvement of the skin in a "garment" or "bathing trunk" distribution; may be macular or raised, involving the dermal-epidermal junction (junctional nevocellular nevi) and dermis (compound nevi), or deeper dermis alone (intradermal nevi). Lesions vary in color from light tan to intense black.

b. Midline lesions on the back may be associated with spina bifida or meningomyelocele; lesions on the head and large lesions on the trunk may be associated with meningeal melanocytosis and seizures or other CNS findings.

c. Malignant melanoma may occur in 5% to 6% of giant nevi, particularly midline lesions on the back of the scalp extending onto the scalp, often in the first 5 years; there is uncertain frequency but low risk in smaller nevi, and then usually after puberty.

d. Management is dictated by prevention of malignancy and by the cosmetic requirements. Intervention is not usually indicated in the newborn. Small and medium nevi can be observed and removed with local anesthetic during adolescence, if necessary.

4. Mongolian spots (**PLATE 12**).

a. Mongolian spots are almost as common as salmon patches, and are more prevalent in blacks (90%), Asians (75%), and Native Americans (10%).

b. Large, irregular, blue-green macules can be found almost anywhere on the body, most often on the back and buttocks.

c. Spots will disappear or fade significantly by 2 years of age, particularly as an infant's skin darkens, although there may occasionally be a trace in the adult. Provide parental counseling only; no treatment is required. *Special variants:* Nevus of Ota on the face and nevus of Ito on the shoulder are persistent and respond well to laser treatment designed for pigmented lesions.

5. Urticaria pigmentosa (mastocytosis).

a. Solitary lesions that occur in about one half of affected infants are usually present at birth.

b. Multiple lesions tend to develop from a few weeks to about 2 years of age.

c. Mastocytomas are brown or red-brown papules, usually under 2 cm in diameter; the trunk and extremities are most commonly involved, but lesions on the face and scalp are not infrequent.

d. Should be considered in the differential diagnosis of pigmented neonatal lesions.

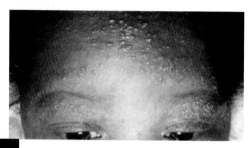

PLATE 1

Milia. (From Cohen BA: *Atlas of pediatric dermatology,* London, 1993, Wolfe Publishing, Mosby.)

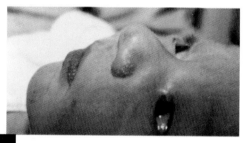

PLATE 2

Sebaceous gland hyperplasia. (From Zitelli BJ, Davis HW: *Atlas of pediatric physical diagnosis,* ed 2, St. Louis, 1991, Mosby.)

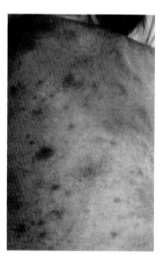

PLATE 3

Erythemia toxicum. Blotchy, erythematous macules and plaques with multiple papules and pustules. (From Weston WW, Lane AT: *Color textbook of pediatric dermatology,* St. Louis, 1996, Mosby, p 225.)

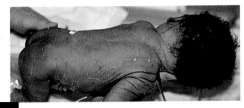

PLATE 4
Transient neonatal pustular melanosis.

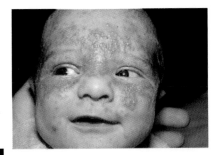

PLATE 5
Neonatal acne. Red papules, closed comedones, and pustules on face of a 1-month-old.
(Courtesy Bernard A. Cohen, MD.)

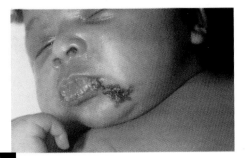

PLATE 6
Neonatal herpes. (From Cohen BA: *Atlas of pediatric dermatology,* London, 1993,
Wolfe Publishing, Mosby.)

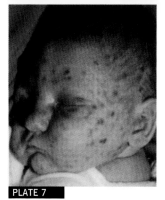

PLATE 7
"Blueberry muffin" rash.

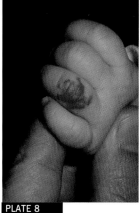

PLATE 8
Hemangioma. Courtesy, Kasia Miller.

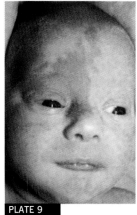

PLATE 9
Nevus flammeus.

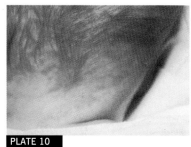

PLATE 10
Salmon patch.

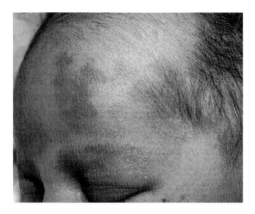

PLATE 11
Café-au-lait spots.

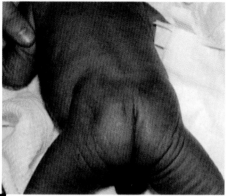

PLATE 12
Mongolian spots.

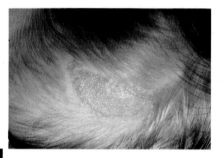

PLATE 13
Nevus sebaceous. Yellow cobblestone-like, hairless plaque on scalp. (Courtesy Bernard A. Cohen, MD.)

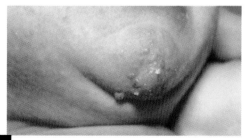

PLATE 14
Juvenile xanthogranuloma. (From Cohen BA: *Atlas of pediatric dematology,* London, 1993, Wolfe Publishing, Mosby.)

e. Darier sign (rubbing produces an urticarial wheal as histamine is released) is a helpful, usually diagnostic test; biopsy is definitive.

f. No treatment is indicated unless there is significant histamine release; cutaneous lesions most often resolve by adolescence, sometimes leaving brown spots. Ordinarily, activity decreases with increasing age.

g. Rarely, with diffuse lesions at birth, there may be blistering, flushing, and dermographism with Darier sign.

h. Parents should be counseled to avoid giving the child aspirin, polymyxin, codeine, or medication with opiates (anything stimulating histamine release).

D. HYPOPIGMENTATION.

All hypopigmented lesions occur infrequently; none lends itself to therapeutic intervention.

1. Oculocutaneous albinism. Hair is white and fine, eyes are gray, skin is uniformly white or pink. Nystagmus may be readily detected, along with a suggestion of photophobia. Of several pathogenetic mechanisms, absence or decreased activity of tyrosinase, essential to production of melanin, is most common. There is autosomal recessive inheritance, and the phenotype may be only partially expressed. Discovery of the related genes has allowed for specific diagnosis of variants.

2. Ash-leaf spots. Hypopigmented macules; classic lesions are leaf-shaped, but may be any shape, and range in size from pinpoint to 4 to 5 cm. Ash-leaf spots are the only neonatal manifestation of tuberous sclerosis. If there is a family history, a Wood lamp may highlight otherwise hard-to-see macules in light-pigmented infants. In a child with a solitary spot and no other signs of tuberous sclerosis, the term *nevus depigmentosus* should probably be used. Nevus depigmentosus may follow a dermatome distribution and may be present in up to 0.5% of newborns.

3. Chédiak-Higashi syndrome. Involves general pigment dilution, with blond hair, blue eyes, and lighter skin than other relatives. Abnormal melanosomes and lysosomes result in defective pigmentation, neurologic deterioration, and increased skin infections.

4. Hypomelanosis of Ito (incontinentia pigmenti achromians). Lesions most often manifest at birth and may intensify with age. Causes irregular, whorled, widespread areas of hypopigmented skin, often unilateral, involving the whole of one side, or it may be generalized; it is frequently associated with abnormalities of teeth, hair, nails, bone, and CNS. This is a marker of genetic mosaicism that may be demonstrated by chromosomal studies of peripheral lymphocytes and/or involved and normal skin. Stable hyperpigmented lesions (hypermelanosis of Ito) in the same pattern have similar implications. It is probably reasonable to avoid eponyms and think of all of these lesions as markers of genetic mosaicism. Late embryologic

nonhereditary mutations, resulting in segmental or Blaschko lines (pigmentary changes), are relatively common and require a thorough physical examination, review of systems, and careful neurodevelopmental monitoring. In healthy infants these pigmentary anomalies are usually isolated findings and not associated with extracutaneous findings.

5. Nevus anemicus. Congenital, pale macule, appearing anywhere on the body; pseudodepigmented. Pallor is result of vasoconstriction of blood vessels, not hypopigmentation. It is a permanent defect that may be transiently highlighted by rubbing; the surrounding area reddens, the macule does not. It does not enhance with a Wood light.

6. Phenylketonuria. Hair blond, eyes blue, skin pallid. Mandatory screening for phenylalanine should easily differentiate from albinism or Chédiak-Higashi syndrome.

7. Piebaldism, a variant of partial albinism. An autosomal-dominant condition characterized at birth by scattered depigmented patches of skin interspersed with bits of normal pigmentation or hyperpigmentation. Severe CNS disorder may become evident with age. Waardenburg syndrome, also autosomal dominant, is a variant characterized by a flip of white frontal hair (white forelock), congenital deafness, hypertelorism, and heterochromia irides, among other features.

E. ORGANOID NEVI.
Hamartomatous proliferations of any of the constituents of the epidermis and/or dermis. Usually present at birth but may not become apparent for several months.

1. Epidermal nevi.
a. Usually linear, oval, streaky; benign papular lesions, usually along Blaschko embryonic cleavage lines. May be hard to see or feel in the neonate, but will progress from smooth to rough and warty, and from waxy to red or much more intensely pigmented as hyperplasia of skin occurs.

b. There is no indicated treatment in the neonate. Surgical excision, laser ablation, or keratolytic agents (e.g., 0.05% retinoic acid cream, alpha-glycolic acid cream) may ultimately be necessary, depending on cosmetic compromise.

c. All patients with epidermal nevi, particularly large lesions on the head and neck, need careful neurodevelopmental follow-up.

2. Nevus comedonicus.
a. Present at birth; a proliferation of gaping pilosebaceous follicles stuffed with keratin, generally on the face and scalp but can involve any site; may become pustular.

b. May require retinoic acid cream, 0.05% twice daily, or possibly meticulous surgical excision.

3. Sebaceous nevi (**PLATES 13 and 14**).
a. Present at birth; characteristic yellow-orange color; usually linear, sometimes oval; well defined, raised, hairless; commonly found on the scalp.

b. Immediate treatment unnecessary; parental counseling should anticipate growth and intensity with puberty.

c. Hyperplasia of nevus usually occurs at puberty. Occasional malignant changes in later life may justify removal when preadolescent or teen will cooperate with local anesthesia or assure long-term careful observation.

4. **Connective tissue nevi. Rare proliferations of collagen, elastin, or both; scattered skin-colored papules and plaques with thickened skin; those primarily of collagen (collagenomas) may be multiple and follow a dermatomal distribution; those primarily of elastin (elastinomas) are, when multiple, sometimes part of Buschke-Ollendorf syndrome, appearing particularly on the lower trunk and extremities; may be a marker for tuberous sclerosis. No treatment indicated.**

VII. APLASIA CUTIS CONGENITA

Rare cutaneous defect of varying depth, not truly a birthmark; hairless, 1 to 2 cm in diameter; primarily in midline of posterior scalp, sometimes on face or trunk; sometimes associated with other readily discernible congenital defects. May appear as healing crust, atrophic scar, or large full-thickness ulcer, and, rarely, extend through skull. Do not confuse with possible trauma during delivery.

VIII. NEURAL TUBE DEFECTS

Tufts of hair, hemangiomas, nevi, or café-au-lait spots (almost anything) in the midline of the head and down the back suggest defects; hair is usually associated with dimples and is usually long and black; defects may not be immediately obvious. In infants younger than 6 months of age, an ultrasound of the lumbosacral spine is an adequate screening tool. Older children will require MRI (with sedation for most infants and toddlers).

IX. ICHTHYOSES

A. SEVERE VARIANTS INCLUDE LAMELLAR ICHTHYOSIS AND ICHTHYOSIFORM ERYTHRODERMA (DIFFUSE ERYTHEMA AND SCALE).

Ichthyosis vulgaris, described later in this chapter, is an exception. Genetically determined, ichthyosis may be heralded in the neonate by a "collodion membrane," an encasement of the baby with a tight, reddish, shiny membrane that restricts movement and may cause ectropion (eversion of the eyelids) and eclabium (eversion of the lips). After the membrane is shed; normal skin is rarely the result and lamellar ichthyosis generally ensues.

B. X-LINKED ICHTHYOSIS

begins with upper-body scaling that is yellowish-brownish and increases in intensity and distribution with age, giving a dirty-scale appearance; palms and soles are not involved. There is a defect in aryl sulfatase A. Mother may have corneal opacities.

C. LAMELLAR ICHTHYOSIS.

Autosomal recessive; frequently heralded by a collodion membrane; scales are present of varying degrees of coarseness (do not try to differentiate types by how fine the scales are); palms and soles are thickened. Ectropion and eclabium are common.

D. EPIDERMOLYTIC HYPERKERATOSIS (BULLOUS ICHTHYOSIS).

Autosomal dominant; significant scaliness at birth, reddened skin, progressing to widespread bullous formations; susceptible to secondary infection in the neonate. Do not confuse with epidermolysis bullosa.

E. NONBULLOUS ICHTHYOSIFORM ERYTHRODERMA.

Rare; autosomal recessive; 100% of body surface red and scaly starting at birth, may evolve to more specific clinical variants.

F. HARLEQUIN FETUS.

Autosomal recessive; most severe of all the ichthyoses; at birth, extensive thick scales invest the entire body; yellow skin with red fissures; there is significant malformation of soft tissues and skeleton; survival is unlikely; condition is probably a result of defects in fat and protein metabolism.

G. ICHTHYOSIS VULGARIS.

Autosomal dominant; affects 3% to 5% of population; does not appear in the neonate, but may appear by 3 to 5 months of age, generally as dry, scaly skin; not life-threatening.

H. THE ICHTHYOSES ARE NOT READILY TREATED.

Occlusive emollients should be used with care. There may be a role for topical organic, acid-containing products (e.g., lactic acid, glycolic acid). Severe variants may respond to oral retinoids. The relatively large surface area of a neonate mandates caution before widespread application of anything to the skin. Consultation with a pediatric dermatologist is essential. Parents should be counseled about the long-term follow-up that will be required. These conditions do not modify with age in any meaningful way.

X. NEONATAL SKIN MANIFESTATIONS OF CHRONIC DISEASE

A. ACRODERMATITIS ENTEROPATHICA.

Autosomal recessive defect of zinc metabolism; indistinguishable from rash of zinc, biotin, or essential fatty acids deficiency; the skin is moist and red, and peeling involves hands and feet, perioral and perianal areas, and creases of the diaper area, arms, and legs. Associated signs are diarrhea, listlessness, hair loss, and failure to thrive. Rare in the newborn; usually becomes manifest at 2 to 3 weeks of age or at a point when a breast-fed baby is weaned. Breast milk contains a protein that helps with zinc absorption even in babies with acrodermatitis enteropathica. This disorder may be an early manifestation of cystic fibrosis—in which zinc deficiency occurs with calorie and protein malnutrition.

B. CONGENITAL SYPHILIS.
Usually manifests as plaquelike scales on the trunk and extremities; occasionally papular or vesicular, particularly on the palms and soles; occurs at birth or shortly thereafter (**see Chapter 22**).

C. EPIDERMOLYSIS BULLOSA.
Inherited mechanobullous disorders defined by split in skin, inheritance pattern, biochemical markers, and specific gene defect where known; may be manifest at birth. Any easily traumatized area is vulnerable to the development of bullae. Specific diagnosis is based on electron microscopic studies, immunomapping, and identification of the gene in child and parents. Prenatal diagnosis is available for severe variants.

D. LANGERHANS CELL HISTIOCYTOSIS.
Generalized scaly, crusted rash associated with petechiae and purpura, particularly of the head and neck and body creases; frequently seen as a persistent diaper rash. Skin biopsy, even in the newborn, will reveal typical histiocytic cells; hepatosplenomegaly and lymphadenopathy may be present. A "benign" regressing newborn variant with 5 to 10 scattered, crusted 4- to 6-mm papules may be associated with the development of visceral disease years later.

E. INCONTINENTIA PIGMENTI.
X-linked dominant, usually lethal in utero to males. At birth, clusters of vesicles are present in a linear, bandlike arrangement, particularly on the extremities and trunk, progressing in 2 to 3 weeks to hyperkeratotic, wartlike lesions, which after several months become hyperpigmented. In time the reticulated hyperpigmented plaques resolve leaving subtle atrophic lesions. Mothers may have scattered or localized scarring as the only residual marker. May be confused with herpes or impetigo in the newborn, but Tzank smear for herpes and cultures can differentiate. Skin biopsy may be helpful. There is no available treatment, but most affected children do well. Associated with eye, dental, and bony anomalies, and rarely with seizure disorder. Genetic counseling is indicated.

Acknowledgment
The outline for this section was originally guided by Neonatal Dermatology. In Weston WW, Lane AT: Color Textbook of Pediatric Dermatology, St. Louis, Mosby, 1991.

The algorithms for Primary Care of the Newborn were adapted from Cohen BA: Pediatric Dermatology, 2nd ed. London, Mosby, 1999.

18

DERMATOLOGY

BIBLIOGRAPHY

Cohen BA: Pediatric Dermatology, 2nd ed. London, Mosby, 1999.

Cohen BA, Lehmann C: dermatlas.org

Vasiloudes P, Morell JG, Weston WL: A guide to rashes in newborns. Contemp Pediatr 14:156, 1997.

Weinberg S, Prose NS: Color Atlas of Pediatric Dermatology, 2nd ed. New York, McGraw-Hill, 1990.

Weston WL, Lane AT: Color Textbook of Pediatric Dermatology. St. Louis, Mosby, 1991.

Zitelli BJ, Davis HW: Atlas of Pediatric Physical Diagnosis, 4th ed. St. Louis, Mosby, 2002.

Hematology[*]

Gregory J. Kato, James F. Casella, and Henry M. Seidel

FAST FACTS

Immediate Issues in the Nursery

- Maternal noninfectious entities that can affect the newborn via transplacental transfer of antibodies include systemic lupus erythematosus (SLE)—causing thrombocytopenia, leukopenia, malar rash, congenital heart block, anemia, hepatosplenomegaly; hyperthyroidism—causing thrombocytopenia, jaundice, hepatosplenomegaly, hyperviscosity; and alloimmune disease—causing antibody-mediated destruction of red blood cells (RBCs, ABO or Rh), platelets, or white blood cells (WBCs). Also, antiphospholipid antibodies can increase the risk of thrombosis in newborns.

- Almost one half of all infants of mothers with diabetes mellitus will have a hematocrit ≥65. Although, this doesn't usually require treatment, it can lead to hyperviscosity, hyperbilirubinemia, and increased risk of thrombosis. Attention to feeding and hydration status is very important.

- In autoimmune hemolytic disease of the newborn, manifestations (anemia and jaundice) generally occur in the first 24 hours of life. Rh sensitization is more severe than ABO sensitization. About 15% of whites are Rh negative, compared with 5% of blacks and 0% of Asians. Boys are more likely to be severely affected than girls. Prematurity increases the risk of kernicterus. Obstetric risk factors that increase the possibility of maternal fetal blood mixing include: toxemia, trauma, amniocentesis, cesarean section, breech delivery, and prior abortion or childbirth.

- A positive Coombs test can occur when there is no ABO or Rh blood group mismatch. This occurs when there is an incompatibility of minor blood group antigens (Kell, C, E, Duffy [Fya], and Kidd [JKa]).

- Neutropenia is commonly caused by infection, so an appropriate clinical workup for infection and sepsis should be done whenever the absolute neutrophil count (ANC) is <1500 cells/mm^3. The ratio of immature cells (bands) to total neutrophils (I/T ratio) should be elevated (>0.2) when infection is present and can be as high as 0.4 to 0.8. Maternal diabetes, hypoglycemia, meconium aspiration, and Apgar score <6 at 5 minutes can all result in an increased I/T ratio but generally will not be associated with neutropenia.

Continued

[*]Portions of this chapter are from Oski FA, Naiman JL: Hematologic Problems in the Newborn, ed 3. Philadelphia, WB Saunders, 1982.

FAST FACTS—Cont'd

Important Reminders After Discharge

- The timing of anemia in the neonate can suggest the cause. For onset at birth, generally hemorrhage or alloimmunization is the cause. Within the first 2 days, hemorrhage, external or internal, is the cause. For cases manifesting after the first 2 days of life, the cause is hemolytic; usually associated with jaundice.

- Symptoms of hyperviscosity usually occur in 48 to 72 hours after birth. By definition, hyperviscosity occurs with a venous hematocrit level above 65%, but levels between 60% and 64% may also result in hyperviscosity. Measurement by capillary samples should be confirmed by venous levels. Although most cases are idiopathic, other factors that increase the risk for polycythemia can result in increased blood viscosity. These include intrauterine growth retardation (IUGR), small for gestational age (SGA), postmaturity, maternal diabetes, trisomy 21, and delayed cord clamping.

- Hemoglobin C is a relatively common type of abnormal hemoglobin that is present in persons of African, Mediterranean, Middle Eastern, and Native American descents. It is likely to be detected via the neonatal phenylketonuria (PKU) metabolic screening panel. Heterozygous hemoglobin AC is not associated with clinically significant disease, whereas homozygous hemoglobin CC causes a moderate hemolytic anemia that is generally easy to manage. Hemoglobin sickle cell (SC) disease is generally milder than homozygous sickle cell (SS) disease, but can result in a complex medical course.

Helpful Information for Parents

- When an infant is large for gestational age (LGA) or there is a precipitous delivery, parents should be alerted to the risk and or presence of "appropriate complications" (e.g., bruising, cephalohematoma, and petechiae). Being pre-emptive and describing these complications can often prevent anxiety and allow parents to focus on normal bonding that is necessary for effective feeding and healthy parent-infant interactions.

- Injection of the mother with RhoGAM (Rh immunoglobulin), 300 μg, within 72 hours of delivery after the first Rh-incompatible pregnancy is highly effective (protection rate of at least 90%) at preventing hemolysis from Rh incompatibility with subsequent pregnancies. Although some mothers have been reported to be sensitized during a first pregnancy, this is not common.

- When a history of maternal immune-mediated thrombocytopenia is present, consultation with a pediatric hematologist is helpful for evaluation of the infant after birth and assessment of risk for subsequent pregnancies.

I. MATERNAL-FETAL RELATIONSHIP: HEMATOLOGIC CONCERNS

A. IRON ENTERS THE PLACENTA BOUND TO MATERNAL TRANSFERRIN AND, IN THE PLACENTA, TO TRANSFERRIN RECEPTORS.

1. In full-term neonates, serum iron is initially higher than in the mother, then it drops rapidly, and rises in 2 weeks.
2. The fetus effectively extracts iron from the mother; if she is severely iron deficient, the infant may suffer.
3. Prematurity intensifies the problem; there is not enough time to extract iron from the mother.
4. On average, a newborn has a total of 0.3 to 0.5 g of iron, an adult about 5 g.
5. Iron gain and stability derive from the infant's diet.

B. TRANSPLACENTAL TRANSMISSION OF MATERNAL DISEASE

with neonatal hematologic manifestations (**Tables 19-1** and **19-2**). is possible with the following diseases:

1. Congenital syphilis (see p. 383).
2. Toxoplasmosis (generalized) (see p. 380).
3. Cytomegalovirus (CMV) infection (see p. 374).
4. Rubella (see p. 376).
5. Malaria. In endemic areas, as many as 9% of neonates may have a form of congenital malaria, which causes fever, failure to thrive, a sometimes profound anemia, relentless jaundice, and reticulocytosis; occasionally it may cause stillbirth.
6. Coxsackie B virus. 10% to 15% of cases may develop disseminated intravascular coagulation (DIC).
7. Echovirus II. Potentially severe, leading to DIC.
8. Epstein-Barr virus. Probably more common than suspected; transient jaundice and mild to moderate anemia are most likely; severe in utero infection may cause multiple congenital and hematologic anomalies (e.g., thrombocytopenia, persistent atypical lymphocytosis).

19

HEMATOLOGY

TABLE 19-1

HEMATOLOGIC FEATURES OF CONGENITAL INFECTIONS

Infection	Common Abnormality	Associated Disorders
Rubella	Thrombocytopenia	Hemolytic anemia
Cytomegalovirus	Thrombocytopenia	Hemolytic anemia
Toxoplasmosis	Hemolytic anemia	Thrombocytopenia Eosinophilia
Syphilis	Hemolytic anemia	Thrombocytopenia Leukemoid reaction
Malaria	Hemolytic anemia	
Herpes	Disseminated intravascular coagulation	Hemolytic anemia

From Lukens JN: Clin Haematol 7:155, 1978.

TABLE 19-2
MATERNAL EVENTS ASSOCIATED WITH HEMATOLOGIC ABNORMALITIES IN THE NEWBORN INFANT

	Maternal Events	Hematologic Abnormalities in the Infant
Infection	Cytomegalic inclusion disease	Jaundice, hemolytic anemia, and thrombocytopenia
	Toxoplasmosis	
	Syphilis	
	Rubella	
	Coxsackie B virus	
	Herpes simplex	
	Malaria	
Illness	Lupus erythematosus	Thrombocytopenia, leukopenia, and anemia
	Malignant melanoma	Melanoma, hemolytic anemia, and thrombocytopenia
	Hodgkin disease	Hodgkin disease in infancy (rare)
	Leukemia	Leukemia in late infancy (rare)
	Diabetes	Polycythemia, jaundice, increase in hemoglobin A_{1c} + F, thrombosis
	Hypertension	Neutropenia
	Hyperthyroidism	Thrombocytopenia, plethora
	Idiopathic thrombocytopenic purpura	Thrombocytopenia
	Autoimmune hemolytic anemia	Hemolytic anemia, thrombocytopenia
	Eclampsia	Thrombocytopenia, disseminated intravascular coagulation
Sensitization	Erythrocytes	Hemolytic anemia
	Leukocytes	Leukopenia
	Platelets	Thrombocytopenia

Drug investigation	Thiazides	Thrombocytopenia (?), leukopenia, hemolytic anemia (?)
	Hydralazine	Thrombocytopenia, leukopenia
	Quinine	Thrombocytopenia
	Mothballs, antimalarials, sulfonamides, fava beans, nitrofurantoins	Hemolytic anemia if infant has G6PD deficiency
	Methylene blue (intra-amniotic-insertion)	Hemolytic anemia
	Dicumarol	Hemorrhage
	Hydantoins/barbiturates	Hemorrhage
	Acetylsalicylic acid	Hemorrhage, prolonged bleeding time
	Penicillin	Coombs-positive hemolytic anemia
	Epidural analgesics prilocaine bupivicaine	Methemoglobinemia
	Oxytocins in excess	Jaundice, decreased red cell deformability
		Jaundice, increased red cell osmotic fragility
	Methadone	Thrombocytosis

From Oski FA, Naiman JL: Hematologic Problems in the Newborn, ed 3. Philadelphia, WB Saunders 1982.

HEMATOLOGY

19

9. Systemic lupus erythematosus. Intrauterine transfer of autoantibodies can result in thrombocytopenia, sometimes severe anemia, and leukopenia; a rough, red scale involving the face primarily and other parts of the body may leave scars; congenital heart block and hepatosplenomegaly are typical of severe neonatal disease. Transplacentally acquired Ro/SS-A antibody disappears within the first year and the disease subsides. Confirmation is by detection of antinuclear antibodies (ANA) and Ro/SS-A. Protect infant from sunlight. Prednisone administration may be necessary.

10. Malignancy. Maternal disease does not usually spread to the infant; exceptions include malignant melanoma and hematologic malignancy.

11. Maternal hyperthyroidism. Placentally passed thyroid antibodies may result in neonatal thyrotoxicosis with thrombocytopenia, jaundice, hepatosplenomegaly, plethora (sometimes with hyperviscosity), and possibly congestive heart failure.

12. Alloimmune hematologic disease. Red cell hemolysis (e.g., ABO incompatibility [see **p. 263**], Rh incompatibility [see **p. 260**], thrombocytopenia [see **p. 284**]), neutropenia (see **p. 279**).

13. Diabetes mellitus. Hyperviscosity, hyperbilirubinemia, hyperaggregation of platelets, and increased incidence of thrombosis are all possible. Nearly one half of infants of diabetic mothers will have hematocrit levels ≥ 65. These findings are usually transient and seldom require treatment.

14. Maternal drug use.

15. Human immunodeficiency virus (HIV) (see **p. 377**).

16. Herpes virus (see **p. 371**).

17. Treatment of the mother with steroids may result in significant leukocytosis in the newborn.

C. MATERNAL HEMATOLOGIC FACTORS CAN AFFECT THE FETUS IN OTHER WAYS.

Maternal factors such as factor V Leiden, antiphospholipid antibodies, and other inherited and acquired prothrombotic factors can have a profound effect on the placenta and the fetus—resulting in such diverse problems as spontaneous abortions, stillbirths, placental insufficiency, IUGR (small-for-gestational-age [SGA] babies), and overt thrombosis in the infant. Postnatal problems, such as cerebral palsy may also be related to thrombotic risk.

II. APPROACH TO ANEMIA IN THE NEWBORN

Possible causes of anemia in the newborn include blood loss, hemolysis, or impaired production of RBCs. If, in the first 24 hours, hypovolemia is present, a severe degree (Hgb ≤ 5 g/dl) of anemia may be life-threatening; hemorrhage or hemolysis related to alloimmunization is then more likely, and immediate transfusion may be necessary. However, diagnosis unobscured by transfusion is preferable. Once past the first day, other causes become more likely.

A. HEMORRHAGE.

1. Clinical findings. If bleeding is significant, pallor is often obvious at birth, particularly in the mucous membranes; respiration may be irregular and gasping, but without retractions; pulses are weak and rapid; blood pressure is often unobtainable; notably, there is no edema or organomegaly. This contrasts with asphyxia, in which case the associated pallor improves with oxygen, the pulse is slow, and respiration may be labored or absent. Severe alloimmunization or other causes of severe, chronic anemia may result in pallor associated with hepatosplenomegaly and edema (Box 19-1).

2. Diagnosis.

a. Obstetric history may include vaginal spotting during the last trimester, placenta previa, abruptio placentae, nonelective cesarean section, and compromise of the umbilical vessels.

b. Additional considerations.

   (1) Degree of prematurity. Small infants do more poorly with blood loss and the associated hypovolemia and anemia.

   (2) Hemoglobin level. Best determined using venous blood, not a heel stick. An initially high hemoglobin level may be illusory; it may drop quickly as the body compensates for hypovolemia.

   (3) Occult blood loss: fetal hemorrhage into maternal circulation.

   (a) Blood loss may be acute or chronic; for differentiation, see **Table 19-3**.

   (b) Direct Coombs test result is negative; jaundice is generally absent.

   (c) Diagnosis can be confirmed only by demonstrating fetal red cells in maternal circulation (Kleihauer-Betke elution test) and after ruling out alloimmunization (Coombs test) and evidence of other hemorrhage.

   (4) Occult blood loss: twin-to-twin.

   (a) Most common with monochorionic placenta.

   (b) Donor twin is pale at birth, perhaps in shock, and when the process is chronic, is smaller than the usually plethoric recipient.

   (c) Suggested when the hemoglobin difference is >5 g/dl and the donor shows evidence of reticulocytosis, increased numbers of nucleated RBCs, and at times thrombocytopenia.

   (d) Prenatal sonogram might reveal oligohydramnios in the donor amniotic sac, or polyhydramnios in the recipient.

   (5) Occult blood loss: internal hemorrhage.

   (a) Anemia occurring at 24 to 72 hours without jaundice may be the result of internal hemorrhage after traumatic delivery.

   (i) Cephalohematoma may be large, leading to significant loss. Subaponeurotic blood loss may also be great—covering, at times, the whole of the calvaria—particularly after vacuum extraction or neglect in giving vitamin K. Estimated blood loss in this event equals 38 ml times the number of centimeter increase over expected head circumference. As red cells disintegrate, jaundice results.

BOX 19-1
TYPES OF HEMORRHAGE IN THE NEWBORN
OBSTETRIC ACCIDENTS, MALFORMATIONS OF THE PLACENTA AND CORD
Rupture of a normal umbilical cord
Precipitous delivery
Entanglement
Hematoma of the cord or placenta
Rupture of an abnormal umbilical cord
Varices
Aneurysm
Rupture of anomalous vessels
Aberrant vessel
Velamentous insertion
Communicating vessels in multilobed placenta
Incision of placenta during cesarean section
Placenta previa
Abruptio placentae
OCCULT HEMORRHAGE BEFORE BIRTH
Fetoplacental
Tight nuchal cord
Cesarean section
Placental hematoma
Fetomaternal
Traumatic amniocentesis
After external cephalic version, manual removal of placenta, use of oxytocin
Spontaneous
Chorioangioma of the placenta
Choriocarcinoma
Twin-to-twin
Chronic
Acute
INTERNAL HEMORRHAGE
Intracranial
Giant cephalohematoma, subgaleal, caput succedaneum
Adrenal
Retroperitoneal
Ruptured liver, ruptured spleen
Pulmonary
IATROGENIC BLOOD LOSS

From Oski FA, Naiman JL: Hematologic Problems in the Newborn, ed 3. Philadelphia, WB Saunders, 1982.

TABLE 19-3

CHARACTERISTICS OF ACUTE AND CHRONIC BLOOD LOSS IN THE NEWBORN

Characteristic	Acute Blood Loss	Chronic Blood Loss
Clinical	Acute distress; pallor; shallow, rapid, and often irregular respiration; tachycardia; weak or absent peripheral pulses; low or absent blood pressure; no hepatosplenomegaly	Marked pallor disproportionate to evidence of distress; on occasion, signs of congestive heart failure may be present, including hepatomegaly
Venous pressure	Low	Normal or elevated
Laboratory		
Hemoglobin concentration	May be normal initially; then drops quickly during first 24 hours of life	Low at birth
Red cell morphology	Normochromic and macrocytic	Hypochromic and microcytic; anisocytosis and poikilocytosis
Serum iron	Normal at birth	Low at birth
Course	Prompt treatment of anemia and shock necessary to prevent death	Generally uneventful
Treatment	Intravenous fluids and whole blood; iron therapy later	Iron therapy; packed red cells may be necessary on occasion

From Oski FA, Naiman JL: Hematologic Problems in the Newborn, ed 3. Philadelphia, WB Saunders 1982.

19

HEMATOLOGY

     (ii) Intracranial hemorrhage (as much as 10% to 15% of blood volume) is more common in the infant who weighs <1500 g.

     (iii) Breech delivery may traumatize the perineum and abdominal contents, most commonly the adrenals, kidneys, and spleen.

  (b) Hemorrhage into the adrenals may result in precipitous collapse; sonography is helpful.

  (c) Rupture of the liver may remain subcapsular or cause free blood in the peritoneal cavity; undetected, shock is common after 24 to 48 hours; a mass contiguous with the liver may be palpated. Flat x-rays of the abdomen—taken in both erect and supine positions—or paracentesis can confirm blood in the abdomen. Prognosis is guarded.

  (d) Rupture of the spleen is more likely when it is enlarged for any reason (e.g., erythroblastosis fetalis). Pallor, abdominal distention, scrotal swelling, and, noted on x-rays, peritoneal effusion without free air suggest this diagnosis. Rupture may occur during exchange transfusion, leading to a drop in venous pressure rather than the expected rise.

Note: *Internal hemorrhage should prompt (at minimum) a detailed family bleeding history and assessment of platelet count, PT, and aPTT; occasionally, neonatal hemorrhage is an initial sign of a hemorrhagic diathesis, such as hemophilia A or B.*

      (6) Placental/cord blood loss.

         (a) Placental hematoma. Inspection of the placenta may reveal a hematoma or avulsion of the cord large enough to cause significant anemia.

         (b) Umbilical cord hematoma. Significant hemorrhage into the cord should be readily apparent at birth.

3. Treatment depends on the degree of anemia, hypovolemia, and chronicity of blood loss. Shock may result if there is an acute loss of 20% to 25% of blood volume. Otherwise, hypotension is a relatively late manifestation of blood loss.

a. If an infant is severely anemic (<8 g/dl) and in distress at birth, get help from a second physician.

    (1) Clear airway, give oxygen, perform artificial ventilation if necessary.

    (2) Obtain blood from umbilical vein for crossmatch and hemoglobin level. Insert catheter into vein and leave in place to measure venous pressure and to provide access for fluids.

    (3) After asphyxia has been eliminated as a diagnosis, transfuse with first-available isotonic fluid (e.g., O-negative blood, plasma, Ringer's lactate, D_5 normal saline, or Dextran). Give a 20-ml/kg bolus of available fluid. Repeat with 10 to 20 ml/kg of whole blood within 1 hour, particularly if whole blood was not used at first. If whole blood is unavailable, use packed RBCs plus plasma.

    (4) Recheck placenta and umbilical cord for abnormalities; if a bleeding site is not discovered, draw maternal blood to test for fetal hemoglobin.

    (5) Follow transfusion with iron therapy to ensure adequate replacement of iron stores.

b. If the infant is in congestive heart failure, give furosemide, 1 mg/kg intravenously before transfusion. Alternatively, partial exchange transfusion can be effective.

c. If the infant is mildly anemic (not unusual in the event of chronic blood loss), transfusion is usually not necessary. Treat with ferrous sulfate, 2 mg/kg elemental iron, three times daily for about 3 months. Check progress with periodic determinations of hemoglobin level. Continue iron 1 to 2 months after normalization of the hemoglobin.

d. If the problem is twin-to-twin transfusion

    (1) Do not forget the plethoric twin and the possible need for partial exchange transfusion if the infant is symptomatic and polycythemic (**p. 276**).

    (2) Check hematocrits shortly after birth for clinically inapparent anemia or polycythemia on all isosexual twins.

B. HEMOLYTIC ANEMIA IS A COMMON PROBLEM IN THE FIRST WEEK OF LIFE AND HAS MULTIPLE ETIOLOGIES (BOX 19-2).

The lifespan of the RBC is shortened, and hyperbilirubinemia is almost always present. It does not take much breakdown of hemoglobin to raise

BOX 19-2
CAUSES OF A HEMOLYTIC PROCESS IN THE NEONATAL PERIOD
IMMUNE
Rh incompatibility
ABO incompatibility
Minor blood group incompatibility
Maternal autoimmune hemolytic anemia
Drug-induced hemolytic anemia
INFECTION
Bacterial sepsis
Congenital infections
Syphilis
Malaria
Cytomegalovirus
Rubella
Toxoplasmosis
Disseminated herpes
DISSEMINATED INTRAVASCULAR COAGULATION
MACROANGIOPATHIC AND MICROANGIOPATHIC HEMOLYTIC ANEMIAS
Cavernous hemangioma
Large-vessel thrombi
Renal artery stenosis
Severe coarctation of the aorta
GALACTOSEMIA
PROLONGED OR RECURRENT ACIDOSIS OF A METABOLIC OR RESPIRATORY NATURE
HEREDITARY DISORDERS OF THE RED CELL MEMBRANE
Hereditary spherocytosis
Hereditary elliptocytosis
Hereditary stomatocytosis
Other rare membrane disorders
PYKNOCYTOSIS
RED CELL ENZYME DEFICIENCIES
Most common are glucose-6-phosphate dehydrogenase deficiency, pyruvate kinase deficiency, 5′-nucleotidase deficiency, and glucose phosphate isomerase deficiency
α-THALASSEMIA SYNDROME
ALPHA CHAIN STRUCTURAL ABNORMALITIES
GAMMA THALASSEMIA SYNDROMES
GAMMA CHAIN STRUCTURAL ABNORMALITIES

From Oski FA, Naiman JL: *Hematologic problems in the newborn,* ed 3, Philadelphia, 1982, WB Saunders.

the bilirubin significantly; anemia may not be noted at first. The three etiologic categories are as follows:

1. **Alloimmunization. Maternal-fetal incompatibility in Rh, ABO, or other blood-group systems.**
2. **Congenital defect of the erythrocyte.**
a. Enzymopathy (e.g., glucose-6-phosphate dehydrogenase [G6PD] or pyruvate kinase deficiency).
b. Membranopathy (or membrane abnormalities) (e.g., hereditary spherocytosis).
c. Abnormal hemoglobins (or hemoglobinopathy) (e.g., hemoglobin H disease [β-chain defects such as sickle cell disease rarely cause anemia before several months of age]).
3. **Acquired defect of the erythrocyte (most frequent cause).**
a. Drugs (e.g., penicillin).
b. Toxins.
c. Congenital infections, particularly viral.
d. Profound acidosis, shock, asphyxia; secondary at times to DIC.

C. IMPAIRED RBC PRODUCTION.

Rare in the newborn; *always* requires consultation with a pediatric hematologist. Disorders include Diamond-Blackfan syndrome (congenital hypoplastic anemia, congenital pure red-cell aplasia, erythrogenesis imperfecta), parvovirus B19-induced anemia and hydrops fetalis, transcobalamin II deficiency, and congenital sideroblastic anemia.

D. DIFFERENTIAL DIAGNOSIS OF ANEMIA IN THE NEONATE.

Note: *Profound anemia in the neonate requires rapid action (**Fig. 19-1, Box 19-3**).*

1. **Family history should be checked for anemia, jaundice, cholelithiasis, or splenectomy. Hereditary factors to consider include spherocytosis or other cytoskeletal defect, enzymatic red-cell defect, or hemoglobinopathy.**
2. **Maternal history.**
a. Drug ingestion near term.
    (1) G6PD deficiency (e.g., sulfonamides).
    (2) Recent exposure to naphthalene mothballs.
b. Obstetric history.
    (1) Vaginal bleeding during pregnancy.
    (2) Placenta previa, abruptio placentae, vasa previa, cesarean section.
    (3) Traumatic delivery.
    (4) Cord rupture.
    (5) Multiple birth.
c. Age of onset.
    (1) At birth: generally hemorrhage or alloimmunization.
    (2) First 2 days: hemorrhage, external or internal.
    (3) After first 2 days: hemolytic, usually associated with jaundice.

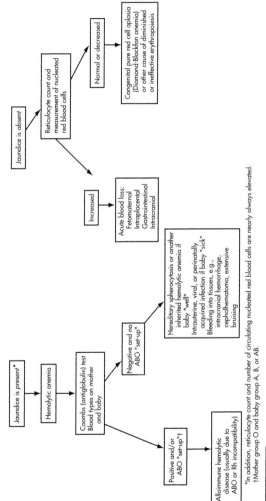

FIG. 19-1

Diagnostic approach to anemia in the newborn infant (hemoglobin ≤14 g/dl, with or without symptoms). The most likely diagnoses are provided in the boxes. *(Modified from Oski FA, Naiman JL: Hematologic Problems in the Newborn, ed 3. Philadelphia, WB Saunders, 1982.)*

*In addition, reticulocyte count and number of circulating nucleated red blood cells are nearly always elevated.

†Mother group O and baby group A, B, or AB.

HEMATOLOGY 19

```
BOX 19-3
DIFFERENTIAL DIAGNOSIS OF PALLOR IN THE NEWBORN
ASPHYXIA
Respiratory findings: retractions, response to oxygen, cyanosis
Moribund appearance
Bradycardia
Stable hemoglobin
ACUTE SEVERE BLOOD LOSS
Decrease in venous and arterial pressures
Rapid, shallow respirations
Acyanosis
Tachycardia
Drop in hemoglobin
HEMOLYTIC DISEASE
Hepatosplenomegaly, jaundice
Positive Coombs test
Anemia
```

Modified from Kirkman HN, Riley HD Jr: Pediatrics 24:97, 1959.

3. Laboratory studies.
a. Hemoglobin level, WBC and platelet counts (included now in most complete blood counts [CBCs]).
b. RBC indices; if hypochromic or microcytic, consider iron deficiency.
   (1) Fetomaternal or twin-to-twin chronic transfusion.
   (2) α-Thalassemia trait.
c. Reticulocyte count.
   (1) If elevated, consider hemorrhage or hemolysis.
   (2) If depressed, consider Diamond-Blackfan syndrome or parvovirus infection.
d. Peripheral blood smear.
e. Direct Coombs test on infant's blood; if positive, alloimmunization is likely.
f. Maternal blood smear for fetal erythrocytes (Kleihauer-Betke test).
g. Blood typing of infant and mother if result of direct Coombs test on infant is positive. Search for maternal antibodies.
h. Blood and urine cultures, viral serologies, if infection is suspected.
i. Bone marrow aspirate, particularly in the presence of reticulocytopenia.
4. Other useful findings include the following:
a. Spherocytes or elliptocytes, indicating hereditary disorders of RBC cytoskeleton.
b. "Drug reactor cells" (blister cells or parachute cells) or pyknocytes, suggesting pyknocytosis or G6PD deficiency.
c. Normocytic, normochromic RBCs, suggesting possible acute blood loss or congenital enzymatic defect of RBCs.
d. Excessive red cell fragmentation, suggesting DIC or other microangiopathic process.

Note: *Jaundice or hepatosplenomegaly does not usually accompany acute blood loss; pallor or shock may. Fetal cells in maternal circulation can confirm a traumatic delivery with internal hemorrhage.*

e. In the presence of hemolytic anemia and jaundice without evidence of alloimmunization, enzymatic defect of RBCs is likely.
   (1) G6PD deficiency, particularly in Mediterranean and Asian male infants.
   (2) Pyruvate kinase deficiency.
   (3) Hexokinase deficiency.

Note: *Infection (e.g., from TORCH complex) can disrupt RBC morphology and cause anemia and jaundice. Cultures and serologic studies are necessary. Neutropenia and thrombocytopenia should be a red flag. DIC is a strong possibility with sepsis, acidosis, or hypoxia.*

E. PHYSIOLOGIC ANEMIA OF INFANCY.

The hemoglobin concentration of full-term infants decreases over the first 8 to 12 weeks of life—the so-called *physiologic anemia of infancy*—then rises slowly to expected levels after that age. It is not associated with discoverable abnormalities; there is a greater decrease in premature infants, corresponding to the degree of prematurity; hemoglobin generally returns to expected levels by 5 months of age.

1. Iron. Supplementation for prevention of iron deficiency anemia is indicated, certainly by 2 months of age; dosage of elemental iron is 2 to 3 mg/kg per day.
2. Vitamin E (α-tocopherol). The newborn is in a state of relative vitamin E deficiency; the smaller the infant, the greater the deficiency. Hemolytic anemia is a possibility, particularly in infants <1500 g. Correction of anemia is possible with 50 to 200 units of vitamin E per day for 14 days. Prevention is possible with 10 to 15 mg per day for 6 to 8 weeks. Currently available commercial formulas are generally adequate in this regard.
3. Folic acid (pteroylglutamic acid). Deficiency results in megaloblastic anemia. Diarrhea and prematurity contribute. Prevention is possible with 20 to 50 µg per day, which is available in commercial formulas. Parenteral supplementation may be necessary in infants with diarrhea or infection.

III. HEMOLYTIC DISEASE OF THE NEWBORN: ERYTHROBLASTOSIS FETALIS

Blood-group incompatibilities are the most common and, if undetected and untreated, are potentially the most severe of the hemolytic anemias. Most common is ABO incompatibility; however, the potential for harm from Rh incompatibility (usually D epitope) is by far the greatest if not prevented. Minor blood-group incompatibilities (e.g., C, Kell, Duffy, Kidd, E) are infrequent, but can be severe.

A. GENERAL CONSIDERATIONS.

1. Boys are more likely to be severely affected than girls.
2. Racial differences are clear: 15% of whites are Rh negative, compared with 5.5% of blacks in the United States and 0% of Asians.
3. The potential of a clinical problem is increased by an increase in maternal-fetal sharing of blood resulting from obstetric determinants (e.g., toxemia, trauma, amniocentesis, cesarean section, breech delivery, prior abortion or childbirth).
4. The size and configuration of maternally produced antibody molecules are also a determinant (e.g., anti-A and anti-B in IgG will cross over; naturally occurring anti-A and anti-B in IgM will not).
5. Antibody destruction of red cells results in anemia and hyperbilirubinemia; the degree of anemia depends on the infant's ability to keep pace with the hemolytic process.
6. The principal risk with hyperbilirubinemia is to the central nervous system (CNS); the amount of unconjugated bilirubin deposited in nerve tissue determines the extent of brain damage (kernicterus).
7. The liver of the normal newborn, particularly that of the premature infant, is unable to deal effectively with an increased bilirubin load; thus, even minimal degrees of hemolysis may result in pronounced hyperbilirubinemia. Age, individual variation, prematurity, and concurrent illness can all contribute. Improved bilirubin binding capacity does not begin until the third to fifth day of life and may not be fully achieved until 5 to 6 months of age.

B. RH INCOMPATIBILITY.

1. Clinical findings.

a. Jaundice. Generally absent at birth, may be evident at 4 to 5 hours, reaching a peak by 3 to 4 days. Daylight is best for detection, a white fluorescent lamp is second best. Finger pressure to blanch skin is helpful. If jaundice first appears after 24 hours of age, causes other than hemolytic anemia must be considered (see **Chapter 19**).

b. Kernicterus. Risk increases as serum indirect bilirubin level approaches or exceeds 20 mg/dl. Lower levels are hazardous in premature infants with acidosis, hypoglycemia, sepsis, or hypothermia. Lethargy, hypotonia, and loss of sucking reflex are early signs. Opisthotonos and generalized spasticity come later. Even mild onset can be followed by severe neurologic problems in time, such as deafness, mental retardation, and choreoathetoid cerebral palsy. Kernicterus as the result of hyperbilirubinemia must be prevented. Once present, it is *not* reversible.

Note: *Do not be misled by the myth that risk decreases after 4 days of life; fully mature bilirubin binding capacity may take months or longer to achieve.*

c. Anemia. Compensatory erythropoiesis can moderate degree; severe anemia can compromise cardiac function, leading to generalized edema, failure, weak heart sounds—the picture of hydrops fetalis.

Note: *Hydrops may occur from nonimmune causes (**Box 19-4**).*

BOX 19-4

NONIMMUNE HYDROPS FETALIS: CAUSES AND ASSOCIATIONS

FETAL

Hematologic
  Homozygous α-thalassemia (four-gene deletion)
  Chronic fetomaternal transfusion
  Twin-to-twin transfusion (recipient or donor)
  Multiple gestation with "parasitic" fetus
Cardiovascular
  Severe congenital heart disease (atrial septal defect, ventricular septal defect,
    hypoplastic left heart, pulmonary valve insufficiency, Ebstein anomaly, subaortic
    stenosis)
  Premature closure of foramen ovale
  Myocarditis
  Large arteriovenous malformation
  Tachyarrhythmias: paroxysmal supraventricular tachycardia, atrial flutter
  Bradyarrhythmias: heart block
  Fibroelastosis
Pulmonary
  Cystic adenomatoid malformation of lung
  Pulmonary lymphangiectasia
  Pulmonary hypoplasia (diaphragmatic hernia)
Renal
  Congenital nephrosis
  Renal vein thrombosis
Intrauterine infections
  Syphilis
  Toxoplasmosis
  Cytomegalovirus
  Leptospirosis
  Chagas disease
  Congenital hepatitis
  Parvovirus
Congenital anomalies
  Achondroplasia
  E trisomy
  Multiple anomalies
  Turner syndrome
Miscellaneous
  Meconium peritonitis
  Fetal neuroblastomatosis
  Dysmaturity
  Tuberous sclerosis
  Storage disease
  Small bowel volvulus

Continued

BOX 19-4—Cont'd

NONIMMUNE HYDROPS FETALIS: CAUSES AND ASSOCIATIONS

PLACENTAL

Umbilical vein thrombosis

Chorionic vein thrombosis

Chorioangioma

MATERNAL

Diabetes mellitus

Toxemia

IDIOPATHIC

From Etches PC, Lemons JA: Pediatrics 64:326, 1979.

d. Hepatosplenomegaly. Varies with severity of disease, from none to the huge enlargement noted with hydrops.
e. Hemorrhage. Petechiae and purpura are bad prognostic signs, suggesting onset of a condition simulating DIC.
f. Maternal polyhydramnios and preeclamptic toxemia are frequent precursors.
g. Degree of severity increases with subsequent sensitized pregnancies.
2. Laboratory findings.
a. Hemoglobin concentration. Values <14 g/dl are worrisome. Determinations are best done using venous blood (e.g., from the cord). Capillary blood may give inappropriately high result.
b. Reticulocyte count. May be as high as 30%.
c. Nucleated RBCs. Concentrations of >10:100 WBCs are common.
d. Spherocytes. Usually seen only with ABO incompatibility.
e. Platelets. Number may be decreased if anemia is severe.
f. Hypoglycemia. Hyperinsulinism is common in severely affected babies; mechanism remains unclear. Blood glucose level should be closely followed.
g. Coombs test. Direct test with infant's washed RBCs is usually clearly positive with Rh incompatibility, but not at all or only weakly so with ABO incompatibility. An indirect test searches for free anti-A or anti-B antibodies in infant serum and is usually positive with clinically significant ABO incompatibility.
h. Serum bilirubin levels. Cord blood value at birth >4 mg/dl suggests severe disease. The concern is with indirect bilirubin. It is helpful to know the level of direct bilirubin before initiating any type of therapy. The figure of 20 mg/dl as the "risk point" for kernicterus refers to indirect bilirubin in Rh hemolytic disease. That risk point drops with increasing prematurity.
i. Bilirubin binding capacity of serum albumin. Indirect (unconjugated) bilirubin bound to albumin in the serum is harmless; only the amount unbound or "free" is toxic to the CNS. There is no clinically useful test for this binding capacity.

Note: *Diagnosis can be facilitated with an approach suggested in **Fig. 19-1**.*

3. Treatment. Prevention of RH incompatibility is the primary goal.

a. Injection of the mother with RhoGAM (Rh immunoglobulin), 300 µg, within 72 hours of delivery after the first Rh-incompatible pregnancy; highly effective, with a protection rate of at least 90%; although some mothers have been reported to be sensitized during a first pregnancy, this is not common. A larger RhoGAM dose is required for fetomaternal hemorrhage.

b. Exchange transfusion. Not an innocuous procedure, with an estimated mortality rate of 1%; hyperkalemia, hypocalcemia, hypomagnesemia, introduction of citrated blood, acidosis, and hypoglycemia are potential complications; hemodynamic changes may result in myocardial dysfunction; serum IgG levels in the first year of life tend to be lower. Still, a bilirubin level >4 mg/dl at birth and a hemoglobin concentration <14 g/dl suggest the need for urgent exchange transfusion. Portal vein thrombosis and necrotizing enterocolitis (NEC) are possible complications; moderate anemia is not uncommon after exchange.

Note: *Effective use of RhoGAM prophylaxis has rendered Rh hemolytic disease so rare today that many primary care pediatricians have never performed exchange transfusion in the neonate, or have not done so for many years. Because of the significant mortality rate of the procedure, its use should be determined and undertaken only by highly trained and experienced personnel.*

c. Intrauterine intraperitoneal (or intravascular) transfusion. Should be used only in fetuses with early evidence of severe incompatibility and who are seriously ill; an experienced operator is essential.

d. Intrauterine plasmapheresis. Should be used only with fetuses otherwise certain to die and in the hands of an experienced operator. A good indication is a previous pregnancy ending in stillbirth before 24 to 26 weeks of gestation.

e. Phototherapy (see **p. 345**).

f. Persistent reticulocytopenia after birth can result in late anemia for months after birth. Erythropoietin therapy may shorten the period of postnatal transfusion requirement.

g. Recently, the use of intravenous immune globulin G (IVIgG) to reduce hemolysis in infants with Rh disease has been suggested. This issue is discussed in **Chapter 21**.

C. ABO INCOMPATIBILITY.

Currently, ABO incompatibility is the most common cause of alloimmune hemolytic disease of the newborn. It is the result of interaction between maternal anti-A and anti-B antibodies and the corresponding A and B erythrocytes in the baby. A potential for it exists in about 15% of white and black births in the United States; Asian babies are at less risk. The clinical manifestations are generally relatively mild. Only one infant in five develops clinically significant jaundice, which is generally more severe in blacks.

1. Clinical findings. (For comparison with Rh incompatibility, see **Table 19-4**.)

19

HEMATOLOGY

TABLE 19-4

COMPARISON OF Rh AND ABO INCOMPATIBILITY

	Rh	ABO
Blood group setup		
Mother	Negative	O
Infant	Positive	A or B
Type of antibody	Incomplete (IgG)	Immune(IgG)
Clinical aspects		
Occurrence in firstborn	5%	40%-50%
Predictable severity in subsequent pregnancies	Usually	No
Stillbirth or hydrops	Frequent	Rare
Severe anemia	Frequent	Rare
Degree of jaundice	+++	+
Hepatosplenomegaly	+++	+
Laboratory findings		
Direct Coombs test (infant)	+	+ or −
Maternal antibodies	Always present	Not clear-cut
Spherocytes	0	+
Treatment		
Need for antenatal measures	Yes	No
Value of phototherapy	Limited	Great
Exchange transfusion		
Frequency	Approximately two thirds	Approximately 1%
Donor blood type	Rh-negative; group specific when possible	Rh same as infant group O only possible
Incidence of late anemia	Common	Rare

From Oski FA, Naiman JL Hematologic Problems in the Newborn, ed 3. Philadelphia, WB Saunders 1982.

a. Jaundice. Usually appears within the first 24 hours; usually mild, rarely sufficiently intense to cause kernicterus.
b. Pallor. Uncommon.
c. Anemia. Mild or absent.
d. Hydrops fetalis/stillbirth. Extremely rare.
e. Hepatosplenomegaly. Minimal, if at all.
f. One half of affected infants are firstborn; there is no predictor for subsequent infants.
g. Degree of severity is not directly related to the number of pregnancies; there is no predictable progression of severity with succeeding pregnancies.

2. Laboratory findings.
a. Hemoglobin concentration. Usually normal, rarely as low as 8 g/dl; may be accompanied by an increase in nucleated RBCs.
b. Microspherocytosis. Common, accompanied by increased osmotic fragility; can help to distinguish from Rh alloimmunization, in which spherocytes are uncommon.

c. Bilirubin levels. The earlier the rise, the more likely there is to be a high ultimate bilirubinemia.

d. Serologic findings. Incompatibility is almost always O with A or B—rarely A with B or B with A. Direct Coombs test result is usually weakly positive, and may even be negative. Indirect Coombs test may be helpful in such cases.

Note: *A positive direct Coombs test suggests greater need for therapeutic intervention. The indirect Coombs test is more frequently positive, but the positive direct Coombs test suggests greater severity.*

3. **Treatment. Directed toward control of hyperbilirubinemia. Routine blood typing and direct Coombs test should be performed on all infants born of type-O mothers; follow-up with serial bilirubin levels can readily identify the baby at risk. The first appropriate intervention is phototherapy. Exposure to blue light (overhead lamp or fiberoptic vest) will reduce serum bilirubin concentration promptly and safely in many infants. Phototherapy is more effective with the milder hyperbilirubinemia of ABO incompatibility than with that of Rh; it drastically reduces the need for exchange in the former condition and limits the number of exchanges in the latter.**

a. Cautions.
   (1) Bronze baby syndrome is an infrequent complication in babies with impaired biliary secretion and a greater level of direct bilirubin.
   (2) Side effects (e.g., rash, diarrhea, lethargy, mild hypocalcemia, and mild drop in platelets) are transient and usually not significant.
   (3) Eyes must be protected when overhead lamp is in use.
   (4) Phototherapy must *not* be used as a substitute for accurate diagnosis.

b. Indications.
   (1) For phototherapy guidelines for ABO incompatibility, see **Chapter 21.**
   (2) Phenobarbital enhances bilirubin conjugation and excretion; however, the slow rise in blood level over several days limits its value. Phenobarbital cannot be substituted for phototherapy.
   (3) Exchange transfusion should be considered in ABO hemolytic disease when the rate of bilirubin increase exceeds 1 mg/dl/hour, hemoglobin concentration is 10 g/dl or less, or if bilirubin level exceeds 15 mg/dl in the first 24 hours of life; all are possible but infrequent occurrences.
   (4) Recently, the use of IVIgG to reduce hemolysis in ABO disease has been proposed. The potential use of this therapy is addressed in **Chapter 21**.

D. MINOR BLOOD GROUP INCOMPATIBILITIES.

Since the introduction of Rh immunoglobulin (RhoGAM), the proportion of cases of hemolytic disease caused by "minor group" antibodies

19

HEMATOLOGY

(e.g., Kell, C, E, Duffy [Fya], and Kidd [JK^a]) has increased. Most infants affected by these antibodies show only mild evidence of hemolysis. Diagnosis depends on the clinical picture of jaundice, some evidence of hemolysis, and a positive direct Coombs test that cannot be explained by an Rh or ABO incompatibility. Consult a hematologist to pursue exact identification of the antibody.

1. Prenatal management. Screening of all pregnant women for atypical antibodies early in pregnancy and, if negative, at 28 and 34 weeks of gestation. If serial titers indicate a significant rise, intrauterine transfusion or plasmapheresis may rarely be indicated.
2. Postnatal management is similar to that of infants with ABO incompatibility.

Note: *In the unusual event of a need for exchange transfusion, donor blood lacking the antigen to which antibodies have developed must be used.*

IV. DISORDERS OF RBC METABOLISM

A. INHERITED, TRANSIENT, OR ACQUIRED RBC DEFECTS MAY CAUSE HEMOLYTIC DISEASE OF THE NEWBORN.

These defects are characterized by shortened RBC lifespan and varying clinical manifestations depending on the infant's ability to compensate with increased erythropoiesis and bilirubin clearance.

B. GENERALLY, THE DESTRUCTION OF 1 G OF HEMOGLOBIN WILL RESULT IN THE PRODUCTION OF 35 MG OF BILIRUBIN.

C. BECAUSE OF THE NEONATE'S LIMITED ABILITY TO COMPENSATE, SIGNIFICANT HYPERBILIRUBINEMIA CAN OCCUR WITH EVEN MINIMAL HEMOLYSIS.

Kernicterus is generally a risk only with Rh hemolytic disease, but it can occur with other causes of hyperbilirubinemia; profound anemia is always a possibility; hepatosplenomegaly is a variable finding.

D. FETAL ERYTHROCYTES DIFFER FROM THOSE OF OLDER INFANTS AND CHILDREN IN THEIR MEMBRANE PROPERTIES, HEMOGLOBINS, UNIQUE METABOLIC PROFILE, AND MUCH SHORTER LIFESPAN.

Genetic factors, acquired disease, and maternal and gestationally derived factors may contribute; the clinical picture can vary from that of the older child or adult.

E. THE NEWBORN'S RED CELLS ARE OSMOTICALLY AND MECHANICALLY MORE FRAGILE

and more prone to hemolysis in the presence of drugs, acidosis, oxidant stress, and genetic and congenital metabolic defects (**Box 19-5**).

BOX 19-5
CAUSES OF HEMOLYTIC DISEASE IN THE NEWBORN
ISOIMMUNIZATION (ERYTHROBLASTOSIS FETALIS)
ENZYMATIC DEFICIENCIES OF THE RED CELL
Glycolytic enzymes
Hexokinase
Glucose phosphate isomerase
Phosphofructokinase
Aldolase
Triose phosphate isomerase
2,3-DPG mutase
Phosphoglycerate kinase
Pyruvate kinase
Glucose-6-phosphate dehydrogenase
Galactose 1-phosphate uridyltransferase deficiency-galactosemia
Nonglycolytic enzymes
Glutathione peroxidase (?)
Glutathione synthetase
γ-GLUTAMYL-CYSTEINE SYNTHETASE
ATPase
Adenylate kinase
Adenosine deaminase
Pyrimidine-5′-nucleotidase
DRUGS AND TOXINS
Heinz body anemia
DEFECTS CHARACTERIZED BY ABNORMALITIES OF RED CELL MORPHOLOGY
Hereditary spherocytosis
Hereditary elliptocytosis
Hereditary stomatocytosis
Infantile pyknocytosis
Pyropoikilocytosis
INFECTIONS
Bacterial
Viral (cytomegalic inclusion disease, hepatitis)
Toxoplasmosis
Syphilis
DEFECTS IN HEMOGLOBIN SYNTHESIS
Hemoglobin Barts (α-thalassemia)
Unstable hemoglobins (congenital Heinz body anemias)
MISCELLANEOUS
Erythropoietic porphyria
Disseminated intravascular coagulation

From Oski FA, Naiman JL: Hematologic Problems in the Newborn, ed 3. Philadelphia, WB Saunders, 1982.

19

HEMATOLOGY

F. ENZYMATIC DEFICIENCIES IN THE NEONATAL RED CELL.

Enzymatic deficiencies are a heterogeneous group, each of which is capable of causing congenital nonspherocytic hemolytic anemia. They demonstrate normal osmotic fragility, few or no spherocytes, and normal hemoglobin; many do not respond to splenectomy. They can all cause jaundice and anemia, usually mild and possibly escaping detection until later in life. Except for G6PD deficiency, which affects as many as 100 million or more persons in the world, these disorders are rare. Consultation with a pediatric hematologist is needed.

1. **Defects of the Embden-Meyerhof pathway. More than 90% of red cell glucose is metabolized by this pathway; hyperbilirubinemia, anemia, and reticulocytosis may occur, possibly with bilirubin levels >20 mg/dl and hemoglobin concentrations <10 g/dl; blood smear reveals a few spherocytes, a random poikilocyte, and a variety of morphologic disorders typical of hemolysis. Pyruvate kinase deficiency is the most common of these defects. Therapy requires control of hyperbilirubinemia and correction of anemia. The use of transfusion, phototherapy, and exchange transfusion is guided by principles similar to those outlined in the treatment of blood-group incompatibilities (see pp. 259-266).**

2. **Defects of the pentose phosphate pathway and disorders of glutathione metabolism.**

a. Hemolysis is the result of oxidative injury to the red cell—usually mild unless triggered by a drug, infection, or acidosis; G6PD deficiency is by far the most common among several otherwise rare conditions and is discovered primarily in the Mediterranean region and among blacks, Sardinians, Greeks, Iranians, and Sephardic Jews.

b. Fewer than 10% of affected neonates have clinically significant jaundice or anemia. If present, the jaundice usually becomes apparent after the first 24 hours and sometimes not for several days. Bilirubin levels may exceed 20 mg/dl by 3 to 5 days, sometimes into the second week. If there is early-onset jaundice, note the mother's drug history.

Note: *The risk of kernicterus does not necessarily diminish with time.*

c. Hemoglobin levels may drop.

d. Reticulocytes will increase.

e. Blood smear will show nucleated red cells, blister cells, spherocytes, poikilocytosis, and other morphologic disruptions.

f. Screening tests will reveal sharply diminished G6PD activity. In patients with unstable enzymes, activity levels may be falsely normal if reticulocytosis is present, a result of the higher enzymatic activity of young cells.

g. Screening is indicated in any baby with clinical evidence of hemolysis who is a member of a high-incidence ethnic group (African or Mediterranean descent).

h. Treatment may involve phenobarbital, phototherapy, and exchange transfusion. There is some evidence that phototherapy may be less helpful and phenobarbital more so in avoiding or reducing the number of exchange transfusions. In any event, avoidance of "trigger" drugs and careful tracking of hyperbilirubinemia are essential (see **Chapter 21**).

3. **Additional uncommon RBC metabolic abnormalities.**

a. Adenosine triphosphate deficiency.

b. Adenylate kinase deficiency; probably autosomal recessive.

c. Adenosine deaminase deficiency.

d. Pyrimidine-5′-nucleotidase deficiency. Basophilic stippling of red cells is a striking characteristic; autosomal recessive.

e. Galactose-1-phosphate uridyltransferase deficiency (galactosemia). Not generally considered a primary red-cell disorder but may cause hemolytic anemia; the mechanism is unclear. When hyperbilirubinemia is unexplained, urine should be examined for a non–glucose-reducing substance.

Note: *The clinical manifestations and treatment approaches for these disorders parallel those for the other hemolytic anemias.*

V. DEFECTS ASSOCIATED WITH ABNORMALITIES IN RBC MORPHOLOGY

These disorders may all occur in the neonate, although often they manifest after the neonatal period.

A. HEREDITARY SPHEROCYTOSIS. RBCs ARE SPHEROCYTIC AND ABNORMALLY FRAGILE.

Inheritance is usually autosomal dominant and is probably more common in northern Europeans. Autosomal recessive mutations with no parental anemia cause a minority of cases.

1. **Clinical findings.**

a. Neonatal jaundice is common, usually occurring by 48 hours, but as late as 7 days, after birth.

b. Hyperbilirubinemia may exceed 20 mg/dl and be sufficient to cause kernicterus.

c. Splenomegaly is usually minimal.

d. Anemia is generally mild; hemoglobin level is rarely <10 g/dl.

e. Reticulocytes are increased.

f. Peripheral blood smear reveals characteristic spherocyte, but some neonates may not have many at first. The spherocyte is smaller in diameter and the central pallor is absent, indicating a dense cell.

g. The red-cell osmotic fragility test is usually strongly positive. Neonatal controls are required.

h. Haptoglobin levels are not helpful. The haptoglobin level is low in most normal newborns, rendering such test results difficult to interpret in the newborn with anemia, although it is a useful test after 1 year of age.

i. The most helpful diagnostic findings are spherocytes, reticulocytosis, and low haptoglobin in a parent; this may be confirmed by osmotic fragility test.

2. Treatment:

a. If the diagnosis is secure, red cell transfusions should be reserved for very severe anemia (hemoglobin < 6 gm/dl) or symptomatic anemia (poor feeding due to tachypnea, congestive failure).

b. Splenectomy is very helpful in moderate to severe cases, but because of risk of overwhelming sepsis, surgery before 4 to 6 years of age should be avoided, if possible.

Note: *ABO incompatibility in the presence of spherocytes does not necessarily establish the incompatibility as the cause of hemolytic anemia. A negative Coombs test can be helpful. Chronicity may be the ultimate determinant; hereditary spherocytosis is lifelong.*

B. HEREDITARY ELLIPTOCYTOSIS.

A group of rare disorders characterized by varying numbers of oval and elliptical red blood cells in the peripheral blood; often autosomal dominant, but genetically heterogeneous.

1. Neonatal anemia and jaundice are uncommon.
2. Demonstration of elliptical cells in the infant and at least one of the parents may be diagnostic—although the blood smear may be confusing, requiring hematologic consultation. An unusual number of pyknocytes may obscure the diagnosis.

C. HEREDITARY PYROPOIKILOCYTOSIS.

Rare membranopathy; occurs in early infancy as severe, transfusion-dependent hemolytic anemia with significant disruption of RBC morphology. RBCs are heat labile. Call for hematologic consultation.

D. HEREDITARY STOMATOCYTOSIS (HYDROCYTOSIS).

Rare; an area of pallor in the RBC resembles a mouth and disrupts cell morphology; probably variable inheritance. Call for hematologic consultation.

E. INFANTILE PYKNOCYTOSIS.

Transient abnormality of the first few months of life. Pyknocytic RBCs are smaller than the normal red cell, misshapen, irregular in outline, densely stained, and contain spiny projections. A few are seen in all infants, more so in premature infants, and disappear after about 3 months. The disorder is caused by an increased number of pyknocytes and is characterized by jaundice, anemia, reticulocytosis, and frequently splenomegaly. It may be clinically evident in the first week, and rarely may require exchange transfusion.

F. HEINZ BODY ANEMIA.

Neonates, particularly premature infants, are susceptible to the development of a hemolytic anemia characterized by Heinz bodies within the RBCs. These inclusions, when stained with a supravital dye, appear as minute, refractile, irregularly shaped bodies, usually near the periphery of the cell. They are not seen in routinely stained smears. They represent hemoglobin precipitation caused by oxidative damage. Heinz bodies can be seen in G6PD deficiency, disorders of the pentose phosphate pathway, and some unstable hemoglobin disorders.

1. Triggers in the neonate (swallowed by the neonate or mother, or applied to the neonate's skin) include the following:
a. Naphthalene.
b. Phenylhydrazine.
c. Primaquine.
d. Menadione (vitamin K_3).
e. Synthetic water-soluble analogs of K_3, Synkayvite, and menadione.
f. Henna (commonly used in Middle Eastern neonatal skin dyes).
g. Aniline dyes.
h. Nitrobenzene derivatives (formerly used for making diapers).
i. Skin lotions with resorcin.
j. Sulfonamides.

2. Clinical findings.
a. Jaundice usually appears after 24 hours and may be prolonged.
b. Severe anemia takes 2 to 3 weeks to develop.

3. Diagnosis.
a. Identification of the Heinz bodies with supravital stains.
b. Usually, red-cell fragmentation, blister cells, and some spherocytosis; G6PD deficiency and the presence of an unstable hemoglobin should be evaluated.

4. Treatment.
a. Removal of the offending trigger agent.
b. Exchange transfusion for hyperbilirubinemia.
c. Simple transfusion for progressive and severe anemia.

VI. DISORDERS OF HEMOGLOBIN SYNTHESIS AND METABOLISM

A. NORMAL HEMOGLOBIN PHYSIOLOGY.

1. Hemoglobin enables the RBC to transport oxygen from lungs to tissues. Oxygenation results from the combination of oxygen with the ferrous iron (Fe^{++}) of heme, a totally reversible, non–energy-dependent reaction essential for oxygen transport. Should ferrous iron be oxidized to a ferric (Fe^{+++}) state, methemoglobin incapable of oxygen transport is the result. Normal adult hemoglobins (A, A_2) may vary somewhat in the constitution of their polypeptide chains without loss of oxygenation capacity. Some abnormal hemoglobins can interfere with this function in a manner dependent on their individual characteristics. Hemoglobin F, unlike adult hemoglobins, resists denaturation by strong acid or alkali solutions.

2. The cord blood of the normal neonate contains Hb F, Hb A, and Hb A_2 in varying fractions, with F predominating by far. Hb A is present in small amounts in the first trimester and begins to rise in the third trimester.

3. As the fetus approaches term, Hb A begins to replace Hb F. The process is slower in small-for-gestational-age (SGA) babies. Normally, Hb F declines to levels of 10% to 15% in the first few months, then more slowly after that to levels of <1% at 6 months of age.

4. The γ polypeptide chains of intrauterine life are replaced by the β polypeptide chains of adult life, the γ-β switch. This relatively delicate process can be confounded in a number of ways. Embryonic hemoglobins typical of the first trimester of pregnancy (e.g., Hb Gower 1, Hb Gower 2, Hb Portland) may persist in trisomy 13 or other D-group translocations.

B. DISORDERS OF HEME SYNTHESIS.

Congenital erythropoietic porphyria is rare and is characterized by skin vesicles, red urine, and hemolytic anemia. Red urine is possible in normal neonates of mothers with porphyria; "passive porphyria" disappears within 48 hours.

C. DISORDERS OF GLOBIN SYNTHESIS.

Many disorders of globin synthesis may be detected in the neonate.

1. Hemoglobinopathies are qualitative disorders in which an amino acid substitution in one of the polypeptide chains results in a variant hemoglobin; more than 400 have been described; only a few cause disease and have significant prevalence.

a. Sickle hemoglobin (Hb S) is the most important and prevalent.

b. Hb C is also common. Sickle cell syndromes are inherited, predominantly in blacks but also in Arabs, Asians, Native Americans, and persons of Mediterranean descent. The heterozygous form (Hb S with Hb A) occurs in 8% of blacks in the United States; the homozygous form (Hb SS) occurs in 1:500. The homozygous disease tends to be severe; Hb SC is less severe but still has the potential for handicap; Hb AC is not clinically significant; Hb CC causes mild hemolytic anemia that is generally easily managed.

2. Thalassemia syndromes. Characterized by a decreased rate of synthesis of one of the normal polypeptide chains.

a. α-Thalassemia syndromes. Reduced rate of synthesis of α chains; inherited; varying clinical manifestations; common in Southeast Asia and in black populations; most cases require no therapy, although occasional transfusion may be necessary. The severity varies with the number of deleted/abnormal genes.

(1) Homozygous (four alpha gene deletion) infants generally die in utero with profound hydrops, which is sometimes detectable with sonography. Infants with increased, although not predominant, levels of Hb Bart's (tetramers of γ chains) at birth may have a lifelong hypochromic, microcytic anemia requiring no diagnostic or therapeutic intervention. Five syndromes have been defined (**Table 19-5**).

(2) Silent carrier.

(3) α-Thalassemia trait. Newborns may show mild anemia, microcytosis.

(4) Hb H disease. Newborns may show anemia and hemolysis, striking microcytosis, hypochromia, and target cells; there is a significant percentage of unstable Hb Bart's, which switches to Hb H after the newborn period.

TABLE 19-5
FEATURE OF α-THALASSEMIA SYNDROMES

Syndrome	CLINICAL FEATURES		HEMOGLOBIN PATTERN			Number of Genes Affected by Thal Mutation
	Birth	Later life	Birth	Later life	β/α ratio	
Silent carrier	No anemia or microcytosis	No anemia or microcytosis	1%-2% Hb Bart's	Normal	Sl > 1	1
Thalassemia trait	Mild anemia and microcytosis	Mild anemia and microcytosis	3%-10% Hb Bart's	Normal	1.2/1	2
Hb H disease	Moderate microcytic hypochromic hemolytic anemia	Same	20%-40% Hb Bart's	5%-30% Hb H	2.5/1	3
Fetal hydrops syndrome	Moderate to severe hypochromic microcytic anemia	Lethal	≈80%Hb Bart's 0%-20% Hb H Small amount of Hb Portland	—	∞	4

From Oski FA, Naiman JL: Hematologic Problems in the Newborn, ed 3. Philadelphia, WB Saunders 1982.

HEMATOLOGY 19

(5) Fetal hydrops. Most severe of the α-thalassemias; total absence of α-chain synthesis; fetuses born prematurely, stillborn, or die soon after birth; particularly noted in Southeast Asia; universal edema, profound anemia, massive hepatosplenomegaly, microcytosis, hypochromia, negative Coombs test. Hb Bart's predominates. Intrauterine transfusion can be life-saving.

(6) Hb Constant spring. A minor Hb variant associated with α-thalassemia. Newborns, usually Asians, may have mild anemia and microcytosis. The clinical abnormalities are more severe in the presence of multiple α-thalassemias, and can be associated with Hb H disease.

b. β-Thalassemia syndromes. Reduced synthesis of β-hemoglobin chains; autosomal inheritance.

(1) Thalassemia major (Cooley anemia). Homozygous, severe, requiring frequent blood transfusions to sustain life; marked hepatosplenomegaly; failure to thrive; significant compensatory elevations in Hb F in neonate delay clinical manifestation beyond newborn period for as long as 6 months.

(2) Thalassemia minor. Heterozygous, mild microcytic, hypochromic anemia, not usually clinically significant; can be nonanemic with erythrocytosis; notably in individuals of Greek and Italian descents. Usually becomes apparent after several months of age as β-chain synthesis increases.

(3) $\gamma\delta\beta$ Thalassemia. Rare; occurs in the neonate with a clinical picture resembling erythroblastosis fetalis; milder presentations are possible.

3. Diagnosis. These disorders manifest only rarely in the neonate. Nevertheless, intrauterine diagnosis and early confirmation or detection in the neonate are important to the medical care of the affected individual; some important diagnostic signs (e.g., elevated hemoglobin Bart's in α-thalassemia minor) may be detected only in the neonatal period.

a. Chorionic villus biopsy at 10 to 12 weeks of gestation is the method of choice for detection of possible serious thalassemic disorders, provided the parental mutations are known and detectable by genetic testing.

Note: *Chorionic villus biopsy is not recommended before 10 weeks of gestation because of potential for congenital abnormalities of the digits.*

b. Fetal blood sampling by fetoscopy or placental aspiration offers another method of detection; in the second trimester, β-chain synthesis can be detected by 12 weeks of gestation. Sensitivity and specificity are high.

c. Amniocentesis for fetal fibroblasts may be used as for chorionic villus sampling mentioned earlier.

d. Hemoglobin electrophoresis or isoelectric focusing is reliable in the neonate: ordinary screening tests with metabisulfate or dithionate are insensitive to the scant amount of Hb S in neonatal red cells; Hb C and α- and β-thalassemias can be readily detected with cord-blood electrophoresis. Many states have sophisticated newborn hemoglobin screening programs to detect hemoglobinopathies at birth.

Note: *Fatal intravascular sickling is rare but is more likely in a premature infant transfused with blood from a donor with sickle trait. A prior sickle test on donor blood is preventive.*

D. METHEMOGLOBINEMIA.

Excessive red-cell methemoglobin is unable to transport oxygen, resulting in slate-gray, diffuse cyanosis in the neonate; it should always be included in the differential diagnosis of neonatal cyanosis.

1. Causes.

a. Hereditary deficiency of enzymes needed for reduction of methemoglobin.

b. Presence of abnormal Hb M.

c. Triggers. Drugs or toxic agents that oxidize hemoglobin directly (e.g., nitrates [contaminated well water; conversion to nitrites required], benzocaine, aniline dyes) (**Table 19-6**).

2. Clinical features.

a. Generalized cyanosis, including mucous membranes, nose, fingers, and toes.

b. No respiratory distress unless methemoglobin level is extraordinarily high.

c. Onset of cyanosis in a previously pink infant (suggests a toxic agent).

3. Confirmation.

a. At bedside. Expose a drop of infant's capillary blood on filter paper to air for 30 seconds. Use a drop of normal adult blood as a control. The infant's blood appears chocolate brown as compared with the red color of the control; methemoglobin level may be high enough to warrant treatment.

b. Association of normal arterial Po_2 with low oxygen saturation by pulse oximeter or co-oximeter.

c. Spectroscopic analysis of venous or arterial blood, performed on most arterial blood gas machines. Levels of methemoglobin sufficient to cause cyanosis may range from 10% to as high as 60% to 70% in the severely affected infant.

19

HEMATOLOGY

TABLE 19-6

AGENTS THAT MAY CAUSE METHEMOGLOBINEMIA IN THE NEWBORN

Agents	Source
Nitrate (→nitrites)	Well water (contaminated)
	Bismuth subnitrate (antidiarrheal)
Nitrites (ethyl)	Sweet spirit of nitre
Aniline derivatives	Diaper-making dyes
	Disinfectants (e.g.,TCC, or tricholorocarbanilide)
	Benzocaine (skin application)
Resorcin	Skin applications
Acetophenetidin	Analgesic compounds
Prilocaine	Local obstetric analgesic
Sulfonamides (older)	Sulfanilamide, sulfathiazole, sulfapyridine

From Oski FA, Naiman JL: Hematologic Problems in the Newborn, ed 3. Philadelphia, WB Saunders 1982.

4. Treatment.
   a. Start with a single intravenous dose of methylene blue, an effective reducing agent, 1 to 2 mg/kg in a 1% solution in normal saline. Cyanosis will generally disappear within 60 minutes, confirmed by a sharp drop in methemoglobin level.

Note: *Larger or more concentrated doses may damage red cells. Lack of response may be seen with G6PD deficiency.*

   b. Search for and remove potential toxic agent; after its elimination, there should be no recurrence and no further need for treatment.
   c. With hereditary methemoglobinemia, continued therapy is indicated with oral methylene blue (anticipate stained diapers) or ascorbic acid, 300 to 400 mg per day orally.
5. Hemoglobin M disease. Rare; autosomal dominant inheritance, may be familial in occurrence. Clinically obvious cyanosis does not respond to treatment with methylene blue; confirm with hemoglobin electrophoresis. This eliminates the need for more extensive pulmonary or cardiac workup.

Note: *Methylene blue may be used in the differential diagnosis of normoxemic neonatal cyanosis when an obvious source is unclear.*

VII. POLYCYTHEMIA AND HYPERVISCOSITY (NEONATAL THICK BLOOD SYNDROME)

Hyperviscosity and polycythemia are not synonymous. Viscosity relates to hematocrit, deformability of red blood cells, and plasma viscosity; the hematocrit is the most important variable. Viscosity increases exponentially at higher hematocrit levels, leading to poor peripheral flow and perfusion and occasional persistent pulmonary hypertension.

A. DEFINITION.

Venous hematocrit level ≥65 (hemoglobin ≥22); occasionally, hematocrit level of 60 to 64 may result in hyperviscosity.

Note: *Measurements of venous hematocrit are more reliable than capillary hematocrits and should always serve as a check on the capillary values, particularly at the extremes of the normal range.*

B. INCIDENCE.

Occurs in 1% to 2% of newborns; one half of these may be symptomatic; there is a higher incidence (4% to 5%) at higher elevations.

C. PREDISPOSITIONS TO POLYCYTHEMIA

(* indicates particular risks).
1. Active (increased intrauterine erythropoiesis).

   a. Intrauterine hypoxia.
     (1) Intrauterine growth retardation (IUGR).*
     (2) SGA (rarely in the very premature).*
     (3) Postmaturity.*
     (4) Placental insufficiency.
     (5) Toxemia of pregnancy.
     (6) Drugs (propranolol).
     (7) Severe maternal heart disease.
     (8) Maternal smoking.
     (9) Cyanotic congenital heart disease.
   b. Maternal diabetes.*
   c. Neonatal thyrotoxicosis.
   d. Congenital adrenal hyperplasia.
   e. Chromosome abnormalities.
     (1) Trisomy 13.
     (2) Trisomy 18.
     (3) Trisomy 21 (Down syndrome).*
     (4) Hyperplastic visceromegaly (Beckwith syndrome).
   f. Decreased fetal erythrocyte deformability.
   g. Pregnancy at high altitude.
  2. Passive (secondary to erythrocyte transfusion).
   a. Delayed cord clamping.*
     (1) Intentional.
     (2) Unassisted delivery.
   b. Maternal-fetal transfusion.
   c. Twin-twin transfusion.

Note: *Infants actively responding to prolonged intrauterine hypoxia are often born with increased numbers of reticulocytes and nucleated red blood cells in peripheral circulation.*

Note: *Idiopathic is probably the most common diagnosis.*

D. CLINICAL FINDINGS.

There is considerable variability in the clinical picture; symptoms and signs usually appear in 48 to 72 hours and may include the following:
  1. Plethora (most common).
  2. Lethargy; hypotonia; weak suck; poor feeding.
  3. Difficult to arouse; irritable when aroused.
  4. Cyanosis while active.
  5. Vomiting.
  6. Tremulousness; easily startled; myoclonic jerks.
  7. Hepatomegaly.
  8. Jaundice (more RBCs to break down).
  9. Poor response to light.
 10. Increased respiratory rate.
 11. Oliguria.

E. LABORATORY FINDINGS, WHICH CAN HAVE CONSIDERABLE VARIABILITY, INCLUDE THE FOLLOWING:

1. Venous hematocrit ≥65%.
2. Hyperviscosity.
3. Thrombocytopenia.
4. Reticulocytosis.
5. Normoblastemia.
6. Hypoglycemia (one third of affected infants).
7. Hypocalcemia (less common).
8. Hyperbilirubinemia.
9. Abnormal electroencephalogram (EEG) (not generally indicated).
10. Abnormal electrocardiogram (ECG) (only on indication).
11. Urinalysis may reveal hematuria, proteinuria, hemoglobinuria.
12. Evidence of increased vascularity, pleural fluid, hyperaeration, alveolar infiltrates, and cardiomegaly on chest x-ray.

F. POSSIBLE COMPLICATIONS, WHICH CAN HAVE GREAT VARIABILITY, INCLUDE THE FOLLOWING:

1. Respiratory distress.
2. Congestive heart failure.
3. Convulsions and a variety of neurologic sequelae (e.g., spastic diplegia, hypotonia, tremor).
4. Peripheral gangrene.
5. Priapism.
6. NEC (especially in SGA babies).
7. Ileus.
8. Acute renal failure (hemoglobinuria, hematuria, proteinuria, oliguria, rarely azotemia).
9. Thromboses (CNS, renal).

G. MANAGEMENT.

1. Obtain careful prenatal and perinatal history for risk factors (see list of causative or related factors).
2. Obtain capillary hematocrit on all infants at 4 to 6 hours of life.
3. Measure venous hematocrit level if capillary hematocrit level is ≥65.
4. Perform careful repeat examination of every infant with a venous hematocrit level ≥60.
5. Obtain blood glucose and calcium levels on all infants with a venous hematocrit level ≥65.

H. TREATMENT.

1. The symptomatic baby should be treated; however, the decision to treat an asymptomatic baby is controversial. Some evidence suggests at least subtle difficulty, particularly neurologic, in later childhood for the presumably asymptomatic newborn. In the face of controversy, the higher the hematocrit level, the more likely treatment becomes.

2. Partial exchange transfusion is the recommended procedure. The goal is to reduce the venous hematocrit level to about 50% to 55%, using 5% albumin, normal saline, or lactated Ringer's solution. Avoid fresh frozen plasma; *never* use simple phlebotomy without volume replacement.

Volume of exchange (ml) (approximate) =
(Weight in kg × 80 ml/kg) × (Current Hct − Desired Hct) ÷ Current Hct

3. Perform exchange in 10- to 20-ml aliquots; *do not* exceed 5% of the blood volume (approximately 4 ml/kg).
4. Repeat measurement of hematocrit level before exchange is ended and catheter is removed.
5. Repeat exchange if there is recurrence or persistence of symptoms.

VIII. DISORDERS OF LEUKOCYTES

A. NEUTROPENIA.

1. Definition. Absolute neutrophil count <1500/mm^3; a count <500/mm^3 is extraordinarily worrisome.
2. Neutrophil function. At best, the neutrophil in the newborn does not function up to par, thus putting the neonate at considerable risk for infection. Deficiencies may be quantitative, qualitative, or an interplay of both. Qualitative defects may involve the phagocytic process, including the following:
   a. Motility. Random motility may be reduced (delayed detachment of cord suggests this defect) or chemotaxis limited.
   b. Defective opsonization (deficiencies in IgM antibodies and various complement components, including alternative pathway).
   c. Defective phagocytosis and pseudopod formation under stress.
   d. Defective intracellular bactericidal capability, particularly during stress (e.g., sepsis, meconium aspiration, hemolytic jaundice).
3. Reaction to infection. Ordinarily, the total neutrophil count during the first day of life peaks at 12 to 14 hours with a range of 7800 to 14,500 cells/mm^3. By 72 hours, the count can be as low as 1750, with a gradual return to as many as 5500 by 5 days of age. Bands may range from 0 to 1400, averaging 500 by 5 days of age. The ratio of immature cells to total neutrophils in the first few hours is 0.16, dropping gradually to 0.13 by 5 days, and after that averaging about 0.12.
   a. Infection alters these numbers; the incidence of infection varies inversely with neutrophil count; neutropenia is more common than leukocytosis; band count increases; an elevated ratio, as much as 0.4 is common, and may even be 0.8 with sepsis.
   b. Infection also (but not always) alters WBC morphology (e.g., increased toxic granulation, vacuolization, Döhle bodies).
4. Conditions with neutropenia. Disorders may involve immune or metabolic disturbance, genetic predetermination, decreased neutrophil survival, myelodysplastic processes; no unifying pathogenic classification.

a. Infection, viral or bacterial; bacterial sepsis is the most common cause, but consider herpes simplex virus (HSV).

b. Maternal drug-induced neutropenia (e.g., thiazides, sulfonamides, propylthiouracil, methimazole, gold salts [common]).

c. Maternal hypertension (common, usually not severe).

d. Transplacental transfer of maternal IgG against antigens on infant's neutrophils.

   (1) Alloimmune. Maternal sensitization to fetal neutrophil antigen, analogous to Rh or ABO red cell alloimmunization or platelet alloimmunization.

   (2) Maternal autoimmune. Mother with autoimmune neutropenia, often subclinical.

   (3) Infection (e.g., omphalitis) may occur but is not frequent.

e. Cyclic neutropenia (autosomal dominant when familial; not usually diagnosed in the neonate).

f. Benign congenital neutropenia (a variety of heritable or random conditions, rarely a clinical problem in the newborn).

g. Kostmann syndrome (severe congenital neutropenia, can be autosomal dominant or recessive; may be clinically obvious on the first day of life).

h. Concurrent immune deficiencies (IgG, IgA); occasionally eczema/polyarthralgia/infection, neutropenia, eosinophilia (similar to Wiskott-Aldrich syndrome).

i. Exocrine pancreatic insufficiency/dwarfism/malabsorption (Shwachman-Diamond syndrome); autosomal recessive; normal sweat test result. (Treatment of malabsorption does not relieve the neutropenia.)

j. Cartilage hair hypoplasia syndrome.

k. Reticular dysgenesis (rare, severe, *all* leukocytes deficient).

l. Severe asphyxia.

m. Periventricular hemorrhage.

n. Repeated exchange transfusion (transient; not a worrisome circumstance).

o. Maternal lupus erythematosus (rare).

5. **Conditions that may be associated with increased band/neutrophil ratio (all of these ratios generally return to normal quickly).**

a. Maternal diabetes.

b. Hypoglycemia.

c. Meconium aspiration.

d. Apgar score <6 at 5 minutes.

6. **Diagnosis and management.**

a. Consideration of infection a first priority; sepsis is the most common cause in the neonate—therefore, one should presume infection until it is ruled out.

b. Neutrophil count and band-to-neutrophil ratio should be followed carefully.

c. Obtain erythrocyte sedimentation rate (ESR), C-reactive protein (optional).

d. Obtain appropriate cultures, bacterial and viral (e.g., blood, urine, spinal fluid, and others as suggested by history and physical examination).

e. Initiate antibiotic therapy based on findings, history, clinical judgment.

f. If infection is not found and neutropenia persists, check for maternal hypertension, familial history of antineutrophil antibody formation, or maternal drug history.

g. If these factors are absent and neutropenia persists, examine the following:
(1) Maternal neutrophil counts.
(2) Does mother have disease or history of drug use?
(3) Family member neutrophil counts.
(4) Antineutrophil antibody determinations on infant and mother.
(5) Consider immune-mediated disease.
(6) Bone marrow aspirate.
(7) Consider leukemia, neoplasm, aplastic anemia.
(8) In vitro granulocyte colony cultures to classify mechanism of neutropenia.
(9) Follow neutrophil counts twice weekly for 2 months.
(10) Consider cyclic neutropenia.

7. **Specific therapy.**
a. Geared to the particular diagnosis.
b. Meticulous attention to good hygiene (e.g., hand washing, gloves).
c. Granulocyte-colony stimulating factor (G-CSF) often can stimulate transient neutrophil production in many neutropenic disorders.
d. Granulocyte transfusions (only during life-threatening sepsis).
e. Prophylactic antibiotic schedules when infection is not discovered (to be considered individually, based on severity).

B. DISORDERS OF NEUTROPHIL FUNCTION

generally express themselves clinically beyond the newborn period and are generally uncommon (e.g., leukocyte adhesion disorder, lazy leukocyte syndrome, impairment of phagocytosis, degranulation [Chédiak-Higashi syndrome], neutrophil killing [chronic granulomatous disease]).

C. LYMPHOCYTES IN THE NEWBORN.

1. Infants generally have more lymphocytes than older children and adults; the range is 3000 to 5000/mm^3 at birth, with a transitory decline and a rise to about 6000 around the 10th day. There is a predominance of large and medium cells as compared with those of an adult; the proportion of B cells in cord blood is greater than in adults and relatively mature in function; T cells are relatively inefficient at birth but can release interferon.

2. **Lymphopenia.**
a. Definition. Absolute count <1500/mm^3.
b. Causes.
(1) Infection. There are many viral processes (e.g., CMV, rubella).
(2) Maternal collagen vascular disease (e.g., the hematologic and serologic findings observed in women with SLE) may be seen in the infant.
(3) Immunodeficiency syndromes.
(4) Reticular dysgenesis.
(5) Agammaglobulinemia of the Swiss type.

(6) Agammaglobulinemia associated with short-limb dwarfism.
(7) X-linked recessive agammaglobulinemia (thymic alymphoplasia).
(8) Lymphopenia with dysgammaglobulinemia (Nezelof syndrome).
(9) Wiskott-Aldrich syndrome (sometimes lymphopenic).
(10) Adrenocorticoid excesses.
(11) Iatrogenic, from steroid treatment (in mother, infant, or both).
(12) Some instances of congenital adrenal hyperplasia.
(13) Excessive lymphocyte losses.
   (a) Intestinal lymphangiectasia.
   (b) Thoracic duct drainage (including congenital and acquired chylothorax).
c. Diagnosis and management.
   (1) Perform immunologic studies for defects of cellular and humoral immune function, including serum immunoglobulin determination and B-cell evaluation.
   (2) Withhold live virus vaccines until clinical picture is clarified.
   (3) Use only irradiated blood products for transfusion (prevent graft-host disease after engraftment with donor lymphocytes).

D. EOSINOPHILIA IN THE NEWBORN.
1. Definition. Normal infants have <1200 cells/mm^3 during first few days of life. At birth, a peak number of 1000/mm^3 is common, with 1200/mm^3 by 1 week and a drop to 600/mm^3 by 4 weeks. Anything in excess should be considered abnormal.
2. Incidence. Common, particularly in premature infants.
3. Significance. Uncertain. The usual causes in older children and infants are not usually detectable or considered in the neonate. The day of peak eosinophilia is consistently related to the day birth weight is regained. May be related to endotracheal intubation or parenteral nutrition, but there is no consistency in any finding. It may be a response, presumably immature, to foreign antigens.
4. Management. Watchful waiting; keep immune deficiency in mind but do nothing further during the newborn period without complementary clinical findings.

E. LEUKEMIA IN THE VERY YOUNG INFANT.
1. Definition. Congenital leukemia, indistinguishable from that in older children and adults, may occur in the first few days of life; neonatal leukemia, a semantic hair-splitting, occurs in the first 4 to 6 weeks and is equally undifferentiated.
a. Acute myeloid leukemia (AML) is far more frequent than other types. The etiology is unknown; a relationship exists with heritable disorders, including Down syndrome, Bloom syndrome, trisomy 13, Turner syndrome, Ellis-van Creveld syndrome.
b. AML in patients with Down syndrome is often of the megakaryocytic subtype.

2. **Clinical findings.**
a. Skin. Large, blue-gray nodules with fibroma-like feel, petechiae, ecchymoses; nodules are an early manifestation.
b. Hepatosplenomegaly.
c. Lymphadenopathy (infrequent).
d. Failure to thrive.
e. Fever.
f. Diarrhea; after several days to a few weeks of age.
g. Pallor; after several days.
h. Clinical presentation does not distinguish type.

3. **Laboratory findings.**
a. Sharply increased WBC count (as high as several hundred thousand/mm^3; may also be in normal range).
b. Predominance of immature forms.
c. Distorted RBC morphology.
d. Thrombocytopenia at times.
e. Confirmatory bone marrow study is hypercellular, with immature forms, decreased megakaryocytes, and erythrocyte and granulocyte precursors; cytochemical staining, chromosomal analysis or flow cytometry may be necessary to distinguish type.

4. **Differential diagnosis.**
a. Frequent confusion with bacterial infection, erythroblastosis fetalis, congenital syphilis, CMV infection, toxoplasmosis, histiocytosis X, metastatic neuroblastoma, and overwhelming viral disease.
b. Down syndrome patients can have a transient myeloproliferative disease resembling acute myeloid leukemia, but they also are predisposed to bona fide acute myeloid leukemia, often of megakaryocytic lineage.

Note: *Accurate diagnosis is needed to guide therapy; bone marrow aspiration must be undertaken in parallel with steps to exclude other possibilities.*

5. **Treatment.** The prognosis for neonates with congenital leukemia is generally poor, and optimal outcome is dependent on the most current treatment protocols.

IX. DISORDERS OF PLATELETS

Deficiency of platelet numbers, qualitative impairment of platelet function, or a generalized systemic illness may lead to bleeding. This is often signaled by generalized petechiae and purpuric spots that recur in crops over the first few days of life and is usually much more dramatic than the few, nonrecurring petechiae limited to the head and chest of normal newborns after vertex delivery and to the lower limbs after breech presentation. Newborn platelets are highly susceptible to maternal influences, particularly in premature infants. Associated bleeding is common from mucous membranes and at needle puncture sites.

19

HEMATOLOGY

A. THROMBOCYTOPENIA.

1. Definition.

a. Platelet counts in healthy, full-term newborns. Most infants have counts >150,000/mm^3; a small number are in the 100,000 to 150,000/mm^3 range. Recheck of a somewhat lower count is mandatory in a potentially ill infant. Counts <100,000/mm^3 are always abnormal; however, severe bleeding is unlikely with counts >30,000/mm^3.

b. Platelet counts in otherwise healthy preterm newborns. Unrelated to the degree of prematurity; there is a somewhat greater tendency to lower counts than in the full-term baby, but at rates insufficient to change approach; recheck counts <150,000/mm^3; define significant thrombocytopenia as a count <100,000/mm^3.

c. Severe thrombocytopenia at birth (platelet count <30,000/mm^3) is rare and usually the result of alloimmune disease.

2. Pathogenesis. The numbers of platelets related to rates of production and destruction. Ordinarily, platelets survive about 8 to 10 days; larger platelets may be seen in cases of rapid platelet turnover; defects may be heritable or acquired, and the acquired ones may be subject to a great variety of perinatal influences (Boxes 19-6 and 19-7)

BOX 19-6

PERINATAL INFLUENCES ON NEONATAL THROMBOCYTOPENIA

MATERNAL

Drugs

Antibodies

Infections

Procoagulants (DIC)

Severe hypertension (HELLP–hypertension, elevated liver chemistries, low platelets)

PLACENTA

Chorangioma

Vascular thrombi

Abruptio placentae

INFANT SUSCEPTIBILITY

Illness Associated with Thrombocytopenia

    Hypoxic (with or without DIC)

    Sepsis (with or without DIC)

    Localized thrombonecrotizing enterocolitis, renal vein thrombosis, etc.

    Giant hemangioma

    Polycythemia

Therapeutic Measures Causing Thrombocytopenia

EXCHANGE TRANSFUSION

PHOTOTHERAPY

INDWELLING VASCULAR CATHETERS (THROMBI)

From Oski FA, Naiman JL: Hematologic Problems in the Newborn, ed 3. Philadelphia, WB Saunders, 1982.

BOX 19-7
ETIOLOGIC CLASSIFICATION OF NEONATAL THROMBOCYTOPENIA

Immune Disorders
  Passive (acquired from mother)-ITP, drug-induced thrombocytopenia, systemic
    lupus erythematosus
Active
  Isoimmune-platelet group incompatibility
  Associated with erythroblastosis fetalis-caused by the disease or exchange transfusion
Infections
  Bacterial
  Nonbacterial
    TORCH group
    Congenital syphilis
    Echovirus II
Drugs (administered to mother) (e.g., Thiazides [?], Tolbutamide, Hydralazine)
Congenital Megakaryocytic Hypoplasia: Associations
  Congenital anomalies (chromosomes normal)
    Absent radii (TAR syndrome)
    Microcephaly
    Rubella syndrome
Pancytopenia
  With congenital anomalies (Fanconi anemia)
  Without congenital anomalies
  Trisomy syndromes 13, 18
Bone marrow disease
  Congenital leukemia
Disseminated intravascular coagulation (DIC)
  Obstetric complication—abruptio placentae, toxemia, amniotic fluid embolism,
    dead twin fetus
  Hypoxia
  Sepsis
  Giant hemangioma (including placental chorioangioma)
Inherited thrombocytopenias
Miscellaneous
  Extensive localized thrombosis/stasis—intracardiac thrombosis, vascular catheters,
    renal vein thrombosis, placental vascular thrombi, necrotizing enterocolitis,
    polycythemia, thrombotic thrombocytopenic purpura
  Inherited metabolic disorders
  The high-risk infant—respiratory distress syndrome, perinatal aspiration, sepsis
Phototherapy
Congenital thyrotoxicosis

From Oski FA, Naiman JL: Hematologic problems in the newborn, ed 3, Philadelphia, 1982, WB Saunders.

19

HEMATOLOGY

3. Immune thrombocytopenia. May be autoimmune (passive transfer of maternal antiplatelet autoantibody) or alloimmune (passive transfer of maternal antibody formed against antigen on neonate's platelets).

a. Autoimmune.

(1) Maternal idiopathic thrombocytopenic purpura (ITP). There is a risk to the newborn if there is a maternal history of ITP before pregnancy, ITP treated with splenectomy, or circulating antibodies detectable in the mother; it is usually transient over a period of weeks to 4 months; may be fatal; the presence of a circulating antibody in a mother with a normal platelet count still places an infant at risk.

(a) The greatest risk is during and immediately after birth; risk of intracranial hemorrhage may be reduced by delivering at-risk babies by cesarean section if the mother's hemorrhagic tendency allows it; objective evidence for this approach is lacking.

(b) Test the mother for platelet count and circulating antiplatelet antibody when there is a history of ITP. Consultation with a pediatric hematologist is advisable.

(c) Platelet count can be obtained on fetal scalp blood, but reliability is limited; umbilical vein sampling to determine infant's platelet counts may be considered in select cases but involves significant risk to fetus.

Note: *Scalp blood sampling may result in falsely low counts because of platelet clumping or clotting. It should be relied on only when performed by experienced personnel; a low count may justify cesarean section.*

(d) Consider prenatal IVIgG for mother, or steroid therapy; the effect is uncertain and insufficient by itself to avoid cesarean section unless the infant's platelet count is determined to be normal.

(e) Platelet counts in infants may be as low as $5000/mm^3$ or, in asymptomatic infants, close to normal; there is poor correlation with maternal platelet counts.

(f) Platelet transfusion, IVIgG, and possibly steroids should form the basis of treatment (in consultation with a hematologist).

(g) Repeat counts should be obtained in an infant with near-normal counts at birth because there may be a significant drop after several hours to days.

(h) Anemia is not ordinarily a factor unless blood loss is great.

(i) Hepatosplenomegaly is not ordinarily seen.

(j) Most infants are mildly affected and recover without specific therapy; risk diminishes after the first few days of life.

(2) Drug-induced thrombocytopenia in the mother is the result of a postulated immune reaction with antibody formation and passive transfer to baby (e.g., quinidine, sulfonamides, thiazide diuretics, phenytoin, methyldopa, ampicillin, cephalexin, meprobamate).

(3) Maternal SLE. Placental transmission of LE factor is well documented; relatively few babies become thrombocytopenic; those that do attain normal counts in 3 to 4 weeks and may not demonstrate clinical signs; those that do not may require therapy, usually with steroids.

b. Alloimmune.

(1) Neonatal alloimmune thrombocytopenic (NAIT) purpura. Not as rare as originally believed, NAIT is the most common cause of severe thrombocytopenia in the first day of life. The mother forms antibodies to infant platelets and then transfers antibodies passively. There is a wide variation in clinical presentation, with greater severity than in autoimmune disease. The firstborn child is often affected. Platelet antigens are genetically determined (e.g., mother is Pl^{A1}-negative, baby and father are positive [as in Rh incompatibility]).

(2) Petechiae may appear almost immediately after birth or in a few hours; purpura, ecchymoses, and cephalohematoma are not uncommon. Thrombocytopenia can occur during the second trimester. Intrauterine intracranial hemorrhage is common with Pl^{A1} antibody and can occur with other antigens.

(3) In subsequent pregnancies, the infant of a sensitized mother may be delivered by cesarean section to avoid birth trauma; this is not always successful. Severity of thrombocytopenia tends to increase with subsequent pregnancies.

(4) Hepatosplenomegaly is not ordinarily a factor.

(5) Platelet count may be as low as 1000/mm^3.

(6) Anemia is ordinarily not a factor unless blood loss is great.

(7) Jaundice is common and may require therapy.

(8) Platelet transfusion with Pl^{A1} or other specific antigen-negative platelets (i.e., from the mother) and intravenous immunoglobulin are the therapeutic options (in consultation with a hematologist). Both can be used prenatally as well as postnatally.

c. Thrombocytopenia with erythroblastosis or exchange transfusion may occur as a result of bilirubin toxicity, DIC, or possibly on an alloimmune basis. Occasionally independent of the severity of the hemolytic disease, platelet counts may drop well below 50,000/mm^3. Most often, thrombocytopenia with erythroblastosis is corrected by exchange transfusion. The hazard of the transfusion can be minimized by the use of fresh whole blood collected within 12 hours of the transfusion. Freezing blood destroys platelets.

d. With infection (common in newborns).

(1) Bacterial infection. Platelet counts can fall rapidly with the onset of infection; serial counts can be helpful in diagnosing sepsis; the peak drop usually occurs by 4 days and is the result of increased platelet destruction, possibly with DIC, or bacterial exotoxins. Bleeding tends not to be severe and is generally limited to infants with counts <20,000/mm^3. Petechiae are the most common manifestation. Need for treatment is rare; at most, 1 U of platelet concentrate is needed to raise the platelet count above 40,000/mm^3.

(2) Nonbacterial infection. Most commonly occurs with TORCH group of infections, syphilis, and echoviruses. These infants are generally otherwise ill, depending on the specific organism. Hemolytic anemia is common, with reticulocytosis and increased nucleated RBCs on smear. With greater severity, DIC is a risk. Treatment with platelet concentrate is suggested for counts <20,000/mm^3, with goal of ≥40,000. One unit usually suffices.

e. Thrombocytopenia with DIC is possible in a variety of circumstances; platelets and other coagulation factors are depleted during the clotting process.

(1) Obstetric complications, including abruptio placentae, toxemia, amniotic fluid embolism, or dead twin fetus.

(2) Hypoxia.

(3) Sepsis.

(4) Giant hemangioma, obvious at birth, usually huge and solitary, but may be disseminated; thrombocytopenia and associated bleeding correlate with sudden increases in size and firmness of hemangioma. Bleeding is rare. Platelet count is commonly <50,000/mm^3; sequestered and destroyed in tumor. Extreme variability in response to therapy. Treatment options to consider include surgical or laser excision, steroids, fibrinolytic inhibitors, anticoagulants, antiplatelet agents, perhaps fresh frozen plasma or cryoprecipitate for coagulation factors, RBC transfusion for anemia, and α-interferon. Interferon use has been limited by a high incidence of spastic diplegia. Platelet transfusions are controversial and may increase the size of the lesion by providing growth factors. Vincristine therapy shows promise in the treatment of these lesions.

Note: *Consultations with a hematologist and surgeon are necessary. Fatalities can occur secondary to airway compression, hemorrhage, or infection.*

f. Thrombocytopenia with use of antepartum drugs is not common; maternal platelet count is normal, and platelet antibodies are absent (nonimmune). Thiazides can be a cause when given over many weeks during preeclampsia, as can tolbutamide and hydralazine. Purpura is seen at or soon after birth; platelet counts are often well under 30,000/mm^3; leukopenia is associated. Steroids are not usually helpful.

g. With megakaryocytic hypoplasia, platelets are not produced; bone marrow is deficient in megakaryocytes or megakaryocyte release is inhibited. Purpura is usually an early manifestation; platelet counts are in the range of 10,000 to 30,000/mm^3. There is occasional leukocytosis; anemia is possible if blood loss is severe. Steroids and splenectomy are not helpful. Transfusion with platelet concentrates is recommended for severe bleeding and with RBCs for anemia. It is most commonly associated with obvious anomalies; the causative factor is often obscure.

(1) Thrombocytopenia, absent radius (TAR). May be associated with other skeletal, renal, cardiac abnormalities.

(2) Microcephaly.

(3) Trisomies 13 and 18.

(4) Chromosome 11 q deletions (Paris-Trousseau/Jacobsen syndrome).

(5) Fanconi anemia (pancytopenia, short stature, microcephaly, thumb, skin, and renal defects).

(6) Congenital rubella syndrome.

(7) Noonan syndrome, often associated with splenomegaly.

(8) Possibly other congenital anomalies.

(9) Pancytopenia.

h. Inherited thrombocytopenia. Bleeding in the newborn is uncommon. Inheritance is usually autosomal dominant or gender-linked recessive. The degree of thrombocytopenia generally is not severe, with counts ranging from 20,000 to 100,000/mm^3; diagnosis is difficult in newborns unless there is a positive family history or associated findings to provide the clue; definitive diagnosis is usually made in the older infant who has unexplained thrombocytopenia.

(1) Gender-linked recessive.

   (a) Wiskott-Aldrich syndrome (eczema, immune deficiency). The patient is ill from infancy; melena in the neonatal period often is a first clue. Platelet life is shortened by intrinsic defect; platelets are smaller than in other conditions; this is the most common laboratory abnormality. Splenectomy should be considered but delayed until later in life, if possible, because of concurrent immune deficiency.

   (b) Without associated findings (milder form of Wiskott-Aldrich).

(2) X-linked or autosomal dominant.

   (a) May-Hegglin anomaly (giant platelets; Döhle bodies in neutrophils).

   (b) Alport syndrome (nephritis and nerve deafness, along with May-Hegglin anomaly); similar to Fechtner, Sebastian, and Epstein syndromes.

(3) Autosomal recessive.

   (a) Hermansky-Pudlak syndrome (giant platelets, ceroid accumulation in marrow, albinism).

   (b) Bernard-Soulier syndrome (deficiency of von Willebrand factor receptor on platelets).

   (c) Alport syndrome (same as above, but some cases recessive).

i. Thrombocytopenia with associated findings. Causal relationships are not necessarily clear.

(1) Localized thrombi with respiratory distress syndrome and severe hypoxia.

(2) Large thrombosis of umbilical vessels and chorion (usual range is 15,000 to 20,000/mm^3).

(3) NEC (usual range is 50,000 to 60,000/mm^3).

(4) Hyperviscosity, polycythemia; platelets return with resolution of hyperviscosity.

(5) Inborn errors of metabolism, probably related to severe acidosis and other metabolic factors: methylmalonic acidemia, ketotic glycinemia, isovaleric acidemia, holocarboxylase synthetase deficiency.

(6) Phototherapy. Thrombocytopenia may occur in infants with meager marrow reserves as platelets are destroyed by phototherapy.

(7) Hemolytic-uremic syndrome.

(8) Cyanotic congenital heart disease.

(9) Hypersplenism.

(10) Hypertension.

(11) Down syndrome.

(12) Intravascular catheter (often associated with thrombi).

(13) High-risk infant. Increasing survivability of the very premature and very ill infant has enabled more frequent finding of thrombocytopenia than in the past. These infants are more apt to be thrombocytopenic and, if so, are more likely to die. A mother with a high-risk pregnancy (e.g., preeclampsia, eclampsia, placenta previa, abruptio placentae, hypertension) is at greater risk for thrombocytopenia; the infant's platelet counts may correlate with hers.

4. Diagnosis and management of neonatal thrombocytopenia (Tables 19-7 and 19-8, Fig. 19-2).

a. Maternal history and laboratory evaluation.

(1) Previous bleeding (idiopathic thrombocytopenic purpura) (e.g., easy bruising, frequent nosebleeds).

(2) Illness, previous infants with purpura, rubella in first trimester, SLE, drugs (e.g., quinidine, quinine, hydralazine, tolbutamide, thiazides).

(3) Placenta. Possibility of chorangioma.

(4) Serologic test for syphilis.

(5) Low platelet count.

(a) Maternal ITP, SLE.

(b) Drug-induced purpura.

(c) Inherited thrombocytopenia.

b. Physical examination of the infant; findings may be varied—including among others—pallor, petechiae, hepato- and splenomegaly, lethargy:

(1) Absence of unusual findings, however, does not necessarily exclude many of the following:

(a) Alloimmune purpura.

(b) Drugs.

(c) Inherited thrombocytopenia.

(d) Early congenital aplastic anemia.

(e) Metabolic disorders.

(f) Hepatosplenomegaly (with or without jaundice).

(g) Bacterial infections.

(h) Nonbacterial infections.

(i) TORCH group.

(ii) Echovirus II.

(iii) Human immunodeficiency virus (HIV).

(i) Congenital syphilis.

(j) Congenital leukemia.

TABLE 19-7
DIAGNOSTIC FEATURES OF VARIOUS TYPES OF NEONATAL THROMBOCYTOPENIC PURPURA

	HISTORY				PHYSICAL FINDINGS		
	Previous Infants Affected	Maternal Illness	Maternal Drugs	Jaundice*	Hepatosplenomegaly	Congenial Anomalies	
Immune disorders							
Maternal ITP	+/0	Purpura	0	0	0	0	
Drug purpura	+/0	Purpura	Quinine, quinidine Sedormid	0	0	0	
Maternal SLE renal	+/0	Rash, arthritis,	0	0	0	Congenital heart block	
Isoimmune	+/0	0	0	+/0	0	0	
Infections							
Bacterial							
Viral	0	+/0	0	+	+	0	
Protozoal	+/0	0	+	0	0	0	
Drugs (nonimmune type)							
Congenital							
Megakaryocytic Hypoplasia							
Associated anomalies							
Absent radii	0	0	0	0	+/0	Cardiac, skeletal, etc.	
Rubella syndrome	0	Rash in T_1	0	+/0	+/0	Eye, cardiac	
With pancytopenia (no anomalies)	0	0	0	0	0	0	

Continued

TABLE 19-7
DIAGNOSTIC FEATURES OF VARIOUS TYPES OF NEONATAL THROMBOCYTOPENIC PURPURA—cont'd

| | HISTORY | | | PHYSICAL FINDINGS | | |
	Previous Infants Affected	Maternal Illness	Maternal Drugs	Jaundice*	Hepatosplenomegaly	Congenital Anomalies
Bone marrow disease						
Congenital leukemia	O	O	O	+/O	+	O
Giant hemangioma (including chorioangioma)	O	O	O	O	O	Hemangioma
Inherited						
Thrombocytopenia	+/O	Purpura only if carrier	O	O	O	O

*May occur in any types from enclosed hemorrhage.
ITP, Idiopathic thrombocytopenic purpura; SLE, systemic lupus erythematosus
From Oski FA, Naiman JL: Hematologic Problems in the Newborn, ed 3. Philadelphia, 1982, WB Saunders.

TABLE 19-8

LABORATORY STUDY RESULTS TYPICAL OF NEONATAL THROMBOCYTOPENIC PURPURA

	Associated Hematologic Abnormalities*	LABORATORY STUDIES			Duration of Thrombocytopenia
		Bone Marrow Megakaryocytes	Platelet Antibodies (mother)	Maternal Thrombocytopenia	
Immune disorders					
Maternal ITP	0	$\uparrow$ (or $\downarrow$)	+	+	Up to 3-4 mo
Drug purpura	0	$\uparrow$ (or $\downarrow$)	+	+	Up to 1 wk
Maternal SLE	± Anemia, neutropenia	?	+	+	Up to 1 wk
Isoimmune	0	$\uparrow$ (or $\downarrow$)	+	0	Above 60,000 mm² by 2-3 wk
Infections					
Bacterial	± Coagulation defects				Parallels activity of infection; often months
Viral	Anemia (hemolytic)	?	0	0	
Protozoal					
Drugs (nonimmune type)					
Congenital	± Leukopenia	$\downarrow$	0	0	2-12 wk
Megakaryocytic Hypoplasia					
Associated anomalies					
Associated anomalies					
Absent radii	Leukemoid reaction	$\downarrow\downarrow$ or 0	0	0	Life-long
Rubella syndrome	± Leukopenia	$\downarrow$	0	0	Up to 2 mo
With pancytopenia (no anomalies)	Late pancytopenia	$\downarrow\downarrow$ or 0	0	0	Life-long

Continued

19

HEMATOLOGY

TABLE 19-8
LABORATORY STUDY RESULTS TYPICAL OF NEONATAL THROMBOCYTOPENIC PURPURA—cont'd

| | Associated Hematologic Abnormalities* | LABORATORY STUDIES | | | Duration of Thrombocytopenia |
		Bone Marrow Megakaryocytes	Platelet Antibodies (mother)	Maternal Thrombocytopenia	
Bone marrow disease					
Congenital leukemia	Anemia, leukocytosis	(↓ Blasts ++)	0	0	Fatal
Giant hemangioma (including chorioangioma)	Coagulation defects	↑	0	0	Disappear with hemangioma
Inherited					
Thrombocytopenia	0	Normal or decreased	0	+/0	Life-long, may remit with splenectomy

*Anemia in any type if bleeding is severe.
ITP, Idiopathic thrombocytopenic purpura; SLE systemic lupus erythematosus.
From Oski FA, Naiman JL: Hematologic Problems in the Newborn, ed 3. Philadelphia, WB Saunders, 1982.

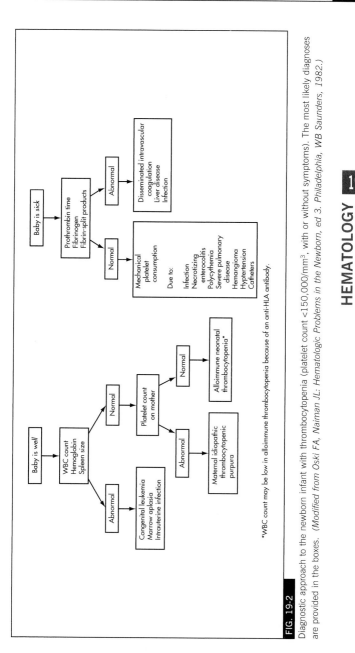

FIG. 19-2

Diagnostic approach to the newborn infant with thrombocytopenia (platelet count <150,000/mm³, with or without symptoms). The most likely diagnoses are provided in the boxes. (Modified from Oski FA, Naiman JL: Hematologic Problems in the Newborn, ed 3. Philadelphia, WB Saunders, 1982.)

HEMATOLOGY

19

Text within the figure:

Baby is sick
- Prohrombin time / Fibrinogen / Fibrin-split products
  - Abnormal → Disseminated intravascular coagulation / Liver disease / Infection
  - Normal → Mechanical platelet consumption

    Due to:
    - Infection
    - Necrotizing enterocolitis
    - Polycythemia
    - Severe pulmonary disease
    - Hemangioma
    - Hypertension
    - Catheters

Baby is well
- WBC count / Hemoglobin / Spleen size
  - Abnormal → Congenital leukemia / Marrow aplasia / Intrauterine infection
  - Normal → Platelet count on mother
    - Normal → Alloimmune neonatal thrombocytopenia*
    - Abnormal → Maternal idiopathic thrombocytopenic purpura

*WBC count may be low in alloimmune thrombocytopenia because of an anti-HLA antibody.

    (k) Congenital anomalies.
    (l) Giant hemangioma.
    (m) Rubella syndrome.
    (n) Absent radii.
    (o) Trisomy syndromes.
    (p) Noonan syndrome.
    (q) Constitutional aplasia (e.g., Fanconi anemia).

c. The general approach should emphasize the following:
  (1) Careful consideration of the mother's history and her platelet status.
  (2) Determination of risk in the pregnancy.
  (3) Those ill with respiratory disorders, NEC, and other serious, even life-threatening conditions.
  (4) Consideration of particular diagnostic features (see **Tables 19-7** and **19-8**).
  (5) Consultation with pediatric hematologist.

d. Laboratory studies should include some or all of the following:
  (1) CBC.
    (a) Platelet count.
    (b) Hemoglobin level. Associated anemia may be caused by blood loss, concurrent hemolysis, marrow infiltration (e.g., congenital leukemia).
    (c) WBC count. Leukocytosis or neutropenia suggests infection; may be associated with hemolysis or blood loss.
    (d) Smear.
  (2) Bone marrow test. Increased megakaryocyte count suggests consumptive coagulopathy, immune thrombocytopenia (bone marrow may not be necessary if latter diagnosis seems clear and infant is otherwise well).
  (3) Serologic tests can indicate immune disorders. These are complex and require consultation with a hematologist.

e. Treatment.
  (1) When intervention is necessary.
    (a) Platelet transfusion (stored at room temperature); should be undertaken with hematology consultation; usually, 1 U is sufficient to attain a rise to at least 40,000 to 50,000/mm^3, more often as high as 75,000 to 100,000/mm^3; after transfusion, count will drop by about 10% per day; follow-up counts are necessary to judge the need for repeat transfusion; washed maternal platelets may be helpful in the event of alloimmunization from maternal/fetal platelet incompatibility.
    (b) Infusion in any event should be warm and slow.
  (2) Specific therapy is indicated by the underlying disease, as discussed previously.

B. PLATELET DYSFUNCTION.

1. **Drug-induced.**

a. Aspirin and other salicylates may cause platelet dysfunction as a result of irreversible inhibition of platelet cyclooxygenase, which is essential for normal platelet function; they can prolong the bleeding time for days.

b. Other nonsteroidal anti-inflammatory drugs (NSAIDs), including indomethacin, cause reversible inhibition of platelet cyclooxygenase; effects wane 12 to 24 hours after the drug is discontinued.

c. β-Lactams. Ticarcillin, carbenicillin, and rarely, some cephalosporins have been implicated.

2. Uremia. This has been clearly known for many years, but the precise mechanism is unknown.

3. Liver disease. Unclear defects in platelet function have been reported and these complicate the coagulopathy and thrombocytopenia that often accompany liver failure.

4. Congenital. These are quite rare. Temporary hemostasis may usually be obtained by platelet transfusion, but sometimes this runs the risk of inducing immunization to a congenitally absent platelet protein.

a. Glanzmann thrombasthenia. A deficiency of the fibrinogen receptor on platelets; there is a relatively high prevalence in Middle Eastern countries.

b. Bernard-Soulier syndrome. Large platelets; deficiency of the receptor on platelets that binds von Willebrand factor.

c. Wiskott-Aldrich syndrome. Small platelets, thrombocytopenia, defective adhesion.

d. Gray platelet syndrome. Absence of alpha granules.

e. Storage pool syndrome. Deficiency of dense granule contents; includes Hermansky-Pudlak and Chédiak-Higashi syndromes.

f. Cyclooxygenase deficiency. Clinically resembles drug-induced platelet dysfunction.

g. Scott syndrome. Unknown defect in platelet procoagulant activity.

19

HEMATOLOGY

C. THROMBOCYTOSIS.

1. Definition is difficult because the upper limits of normal are not well defined.

2. Provocative conditions include the following:

a. Low birth weight. Generally apparent after 2 weeks of age and up to several months of age in a range up to about 700,000/mm^3. Etiology is unknown; there is an apparently physiologic change, generally not complicated by thrombosis.

b. Acute inflammation.

c. Acute blood loss.

d. Hemolysis.

e. Nutritional deficiency (e.g., iron, vitamin E, hyperalimentation with lipid emulsions).

f. Asplenia.

g. Leukemia-like syndromes (e.g., as with Down syndrome).

h. Neuroblastoma.

i. Maternal abuse of many drugs.

3. Management.

a. Watchful waiting and therapy directed to the underlying condition are generally appropriate.

b. No direct intervention is ordinarily necessary.

c. Thrombosis is an extremely rare event.

d. Preventive drug therapy (e.g., aspirin, dipyridamole) is not well tested in neonates and not proved efficacious in older children.

X. DISORDERS OF BLOOD COAGULATION

As many as 1 neonate in 100 will have a problem with bleeding or thrombosis; the numbers are probably higher in intensive care nurseries (**Table 19-9**).

TABLE 19-9

AGE-SPECIFIC COAGULATION VALUES

Coagulation Tests	Preterm infant 30-36 wk, Day of Life #1	Term Infant, Day of Life #1
PT (sec)	15.4 (14.6-16.9)	13.0 (10.1-15.9)
INR	—	—A
aPTT (sec)	108 (80-168)	42.9 (31.3-54.3)
Fibrinogen (g/l)	2.43 (1.50-3.73)	2.83 (1.67-3.09)
Bleeding time (min)	—	—
Thrombin time (sec)	14 (11-17)	12 (10-16)
II (U/ml)	0.45 (0.20-0.77)	0.48 (0.26-0.70)
V (U/ml)	0.88 (0.41-1.44)	0.72 (0.43-1.08)
VII (U/ml)	0.67 (0.21-1.13)	0.66 (0.28-1.04)
VIII (U/ml)	1.11 (0.50-2.13)	1.00 (0.50-1.78)
vWF (U/ml)	1.36 (0.78-2.10)	1.53 (0.50-2.87)
IX (U/ml)	0.35 (0.19-0.65)	0.53 (0.15-0.91)
X (U/ml)	0.41 (0.11-0.71)	0.40 (0.12-0.68)
XI (U/ml)	0.30 (0.08-0.52)	0.38 (0.10-0.66)
XII (U/ml)	0.38 (0.10-0.66)	0.53 (0.13-0.93)
PK (U/ml)	0.33 (0.09-0.57)	0.37 (0.18-0.69)
HMWK (U/ml)	0.49 (0.09-0.89)	0.54 (0.06-1.02)
XIIIa (U/ml)	0.70 (0.32-1.08)	0.79 (0.27-1.31)
XIIIs (U/ml)	0.81 (0.35-1.27)	0.76 (0.30-1.22)
d-Dimer	—	—
FDPs	—	—
COAGULATION INHIBITORS		
ATIII (U/ml)	0.38 (0.14-0.62)	0.63 (0.39-0.97)
α_2-M (U/ml)	1.10 (0.56-1.82)	1.39 (0.95-1.83)
C_1-Inh (U/ml)	0.65 (0.31-0.99)	0.72 (0.36-1.08)
α_2-AT (U/ml)	0.90 (0.36-1.44)	0.93 (0.49-1.37)
Protein C (U/ml)	0.28 (0.12-0.44)	0.35 (0.17-0.53)
Protein S (U/ml)	0.26 (0.14-0.38)	0.36 (0.12-0.60)
FIBRINOLYTIC SYSTEM		
Plasminogen (U/ml)	1.70 (1.12-2.48)	1.95 (1.60-2.30)
TPA (ng/ml)	—	—
α_2-AP (U/ml)	0.78 (0.48-1.16)	0.85 (0.70-1.00)
PAI (U/ml)	—	—

α_2-AP, α_2-Antiplasmin; α_2-AT, α_2-antitrypsin; α_2-M, α_2-macroglobulin; ATIII, antithrombin III; HMWK, high-molecular-weight kininogen; PAI, plasminogen activitor inhibitor; PK, prekallikrein; TPA, tissue plasminogen activator; VIII, factor VIII procoagulant.

Data from Andrew M, et al: Blood 1987; 70;165; Andrew M, et al: Blood 1988; 72:1651; and Andrew M, et al: Blood 1992; 8:1998.

A. BLEEDING RESULTS FROM THE FOLLOWING:

1. Transient "immaturity" of coagulation mechanism in the newborn period (**Table 19-10**).
2. Transient insult to coagulation mechanism (e.g., DIC).
3. Inherited, permanent coagulation disorders.
4. Abnormal or insufficient platelets.
5. Vascular abnormalities.
6. Trauma with or without associated abnormality.

B. LABORATORY TESTING FOR COAGULATION DEFECTS.

Because the infant can be bleeding at birth or shortly thereafter, be sure the blood is the infant's and not the mother's.

1. If there is any question, the Apt test (**Box 19-8**) can be used to settle the issue with any bloody body discharge (e.g., vomitus, stool).
2. Additionally, great care must be taken with collection of blood:
a. Too much squeezing may contaminate the sample with tissue factor, which activates clotting, causing artifactual consumption of factors.
b. Samples may be contaminated by heparinized catheters.
c. When anticoagulant is added, the proper amount is determined relative to the hematocrit level (discuss with laboratory).
d. Collect minimal amounts of blood; microtechniques allow many studies on as little as 1 ml or less.
e. Collect blood to test for fibrin degradation products in tubes containing a fibrinolytic inhibitor.

19

HEMATOLOGY

TABLE 19-10
BLOOD CLOTTING FACTORS

Procoagulants	Synonyms
Factor I	Fibrinogen
Factor II	Prothrombin (vitamin K-dependent protein)
Factor III	Tissue factor, thromboplastin
Factor IV	Calcium
Factor V	Proaccelerin, labile factor
Factor VI	Number no longer employed, previously recognized as active form of factors V
Factor VII	Proconvertin, stable factor (vitamin K-dependent protein)
Factor VIII	Antihemophilic factor (AHF), antihemophilic globulin (AHG)
Factor IX	Plasma thromboplastin component (PTC), Christmas factor (vitamin K-dependent protein)
Factor X	Stuart-Prower factor (vitamin K-dependent protein)
Factor XI	Plasma thromboplastin antecedent (PTA)
Factor XII	Hageman factor
Factor XIII	Fibrin-stabilizing factor
Prekallikrein	Fletcher factor
High-molecular-weight kininogen	Fitzgerald, Flaujac, Williams factor

From Oski FA, Naiman JL: Hematologic Problems in the Newborn, ed 3. Philadelphia, WB Saunders, 1982.

BOX 19-8

APT TEST FOR DIFFERENTIATION OF FETAL AND ADULT (MATERNAL) HEMOGLOBIN IN STOOL OR VOMITUS

- Mix 1 part discharge with 5 parts water.
- Centrifuge 3-4 minutes at 2000 rev/min.
- Decant pink supernate (contains hemoglobin).
- Add 1 ml 1% NaOH to 4 ml supernate.
  Adult blood: supernate becomes yellow-brown (hemoglobin A).
  Infant blood: pink supernate remains (hemoglobin F).
- Run control tube with infant's peripheral blood.

Modified from Apt KL, Downey WS: J Pediatr 47:6, 1955.

---

f. Cord-blood collection requires double clamping as soon as possible after delivery (be sure clamps are not too close together), with blood drawn quickly from the intervening segment using a tube with anticoagulant.

3. Screening tests.

a. Cover slip smear of peripheral blood. Clumped platelets or many platelets in one oil immersion field suggests *no* significant thrombocytopenia (clumping will not be seen if anticoagulant has been added); examine both cover slip preparations from a single drop of blood because platelets may adhere to only one cover slip.

b. Whole-blood coagulation time. Generally not a useful test; requires a large volume of blood and the test is not highly specific.

c. Bleeding time.
  (1) Basically, the time needed for a standardized wound to stop bleeding; prolonged in thrombocytopenia, von Willebrand disease, functional platelet disorders, and DIC; usually normal in hemophilia and other congenital factor deficiencies.
  (2) Not recommended when thrombocytopenia is already documented or highly probable.
  (3) Not thoroughly standardized for neonates.

d. Activated partial thromboplastin time (aPTT).
  (1) Sensitive for most plasma procoagulant factors, except VII and XIII.
  (2) Prolonged with factor XII, Fletcher factor, kininogen deficiencies, and other deficiencies not associated with bleeding; also with heparin and other circulating anticoagulants.

e. Prothrombin time (PT) (Quick test). Measures activities of factors II, V, VII, X, and fibrinogen; less disturbed by heparin than aPTT.

f. Thrombin clotting time. Measures plasma clotting time after addition of thrombin; prolonged with fibrinogen deficiency, heparin, or fibrin split products.

g. Fibrin degradation products (FDP).
  (1) Formed by the lysis of fibrin or fibrinogen by plasmin. FDP accumulate in DIC and thrombotic states. D-dimers are a subset of FDP, seen only in fibrinolysis (not in fibrinogenolysis).

(2) Can also accumulate without DIC with functional impairment of the liver or kidney, sites where fibrin degradation products are normally cleared.

C. PRINCIPLES OF NEONATAL BLOOD COAGULATION.

1. Coagulation status represents a balance between procoagulant and anticoagulant systems. On the whole, neonates appear to be in a relatively prothrombotic state.
2. Almost immediately at birth, there is a decrease in vitamin K-dependent factors, which, if profound after the first few days of life, may result in hemorrhage.
3. The clotting activity of all factors involved in initial activation of intrinsic clotting system is decreased in varying degrees. Interpretation requires consulting neonatal norms.
4. Illness may further depress naturally low levels of some factors.
5. Fibrinogen levels, on the other hand, approximate those of the adult, except in the rare case of congenital afibrinogenemia.
6. Regardless, thrombin time is generally abnormal, for obscure reasons.
7. Overall, fibrinolytic activity is increased at birth and decreases to adult levels within about 6 hours of age. It is somewhat less in premature babies, particularly those with respiratory distress.
8. Whole-blood clotting time is shortened in healthy newborns.

D. VITAMIN K IS REQUIRED FOR CONVERSION OF PRECURSOR PROTEINS

into proteins with procoagulant and anticoagulant activity; it is additionally involved in protein conversion in bone, kidney, spleen, pancreas, lung, and placenta.

1. Coumarin and coumarin analogs block its action; heparin does not cross the placenta and is preferable if the mother requires anticoagulation therapy; coumarin can be resumed after delivery because it does not appear in breast milk in significant amounts.
2. If precursor protein is diminished, sufficient vitamin K cannot prevent hemorrhage; however, administration of vitamin K to a healthy full-term infant prevents decrease in prothrombin activity and the prolonged PT generally found in the first hours and days of life.
3. The premature infant, especially when very small, responds to vitamin K less predictably and often minimally. An immature liver unable to synthesize precursor proteins is the probable reason.
4. Large doses of synthetic, water-soluble, vitamin K analogs may provoke hyperbilirubinemia, or even kernicterus. Small doses of natural vitamin K do not. In any event, giving large (not recommended) doses does not increase activity or response.
5. Vitamin K administration to the mother during pregnancy may be helpful to the infant, but timing relevant to delivery is hard to judge. It must be given at least 12 hours before delivery to be sure transplacental

19

HEMATOLOGY

passage is affected; this is difficult to ensure and is the reason it is given to the baby.

6. The recommended approach to safe and easy prevention of hemorrhage resulting from neonatal vitamin K deficiency is immediate administration of vitamin K (K_1, phytonadione) to the newborn immediately after birth, 0.5 to 1 mg intramuscularly.

7. Repeat doses may be necessary for offspring of mothers treated with anticoagulants or anticonvulsants; these infants are particularly susceptible; clotting studies may be normal in the mother but abnormal in the infant.

Note: *Oral vitamin K administration, in use in several countries, is not recommended in the United States.*

E. HEMORRHAGIC DISEASE OF THE NEWBORN

is a form of self-limited, generalized hemorrhagic disease usually clinically evident on the second or third day of life, but possible on the first day or many days later; rarely, it can occur weeks or months later. The gastrointestinal tract is the most common site of bleeding; other sites (e.g., adrenal, CNS, nose, skin, umbilical cord; indeed, any body area) may also be involved.

1. **Cause. Vitamin K deficiency and consequent deficiencies of factor II, VII, IX, and X activities. The activities of protein C and S are also diminished.**

a. Diet has an impact on the coagulation process; the earlier the feeding the better; cow's milk has four times the vitamin K of breast milk; hemorrhagic disease is more common in breast-fed babies not provided preventive vitamin K (phytonadione, 0.5 to 1 mg intramuscularly).

b. Vitamin K is not well carried across the placenta.

c. Response to treatment is rapid, within a few hours.

2. **Diagnosis.**

a. Bleeding anywhere in the neonate.

b. Prolonged PT and aPTT.

c. CBC otherwise noncontributory.

3. **Treatment. Intravenous or intramuscular administration of 1 mg of vitamin K (K_1, Konakion), preferably intravenously; expectation is of rapid response, certainly within 6 to 12 hours. If hemorrhage is serious, fresh frozen plasma should be administered while waiting for vitamin K effect.**

F. DIC IS AN ACQUIRED DYSFUNCTION

distinguished by intravascular consumption of platelets and of plasma clotting factors; fibrinogen; factors II, V, VIII, and XIII; protein C; protein S; and antithrombin. Intravascular coagulation leads to widespread deposition of fibrin, thrombi, and hemorrhage as platelets and clotting factors are exhausted. Intravascular fibrinolysis and fibrinogenolysis lead to accumulation of fibrin degradation products. Red cells are fragmented and decreased in number, leading to anemia. DIC is common in sick newborns, much more so than other causes of bleeding; it is characterized particularly by hemorrhage in the lungs and brain.

1. Cause. DIC occurs only in response to an associated disorder. Obstetric, respiratory, and septic processes predominate.

2. Clinical findings are varying and depend on the associated disease process. Oozing may be noted at puncture sites; petechiae and bleeding anywhere and everywhere—umbilicus to CNS—may be present, with symptoms and signs dependent on site and extent of bleeding.

3. Diagnosis.

a. Prolonged PT and aPTT.

b. Thrombocytopenia.

c. Abnormalities of several coagulation factors, particularly reduced factor V and VIII activities, low fibrinogen and antithrombin; elevated fibrin degradation products, including D-dimer.

d. Hemolytic anemia. RBC fragmentation on peripheral smear (microangiopathy).

e. Toxic granulation in leukocytes.

f. Probable elevated WBC with many immature forms.

g. Additionally, findings related to associated disease factors (e.g., liver disease) can confuse the picture and make diagnosis more difficult.

4. Treatment consists of attention to the underlying disease process and the repair of coagulation deficiencies. In general, success with the first will correct the second: antibiotics, appropriate fluid and electrolyte maintenance, adequate oxygen, and maintenance of blood pressure may be required. Among therapeutic possibilities for coagulation repair, consider exchange transfusion, fresh frozen plasma/platelets, and cryoprecipitate (limits volume expansion, increases factor VIII and fibrinogen). Fresh frozen plasma helps to maintain appropriate levels of antithrombin needed for heparin effectiveness. None of these is uniformly successful if the associated disease process does not respond; hemostatic support provides time to give primary therapy a chance. Appropriate schedules include the following:

a. Fresh frozen plasma, 10 to 15 ml/kg every 12 hours.

b. 1 U of platelets every 12 hours when count is ≤50,000/mm^3.

c. Exchange transfusion with anticoagulated fresh blood, repeated every 12 hours if coagulation deficiency persists; exchange helps avoid fluid overload in very sick premature infants.

d. Heparin should be used in the event of thrombosis of an artery or deep vein or purpura fulminans, 75 U/kg in initial intravenous bolus and 28 U/kg every hour in a constant intravenous drip; adjust to keep aPTT 1.5 to 2 times normal control; premature babies may need a larger initial bolus and faster drip; maintain platelets at a minimum of 50,000/mm^3.

Note: *Consultation with a hematologist or neonatologist is mandatory. The process may play havoc with a variety of the coagulation factors in unanticipated ways.*

19

HEMATOLOGY

G. LIVER DISEASE AND NEONATAL BLEEDING.

The liver is the site of manufacture of most clotting proteins; severe compromise of liver function by any underlying process may lead to bleeding; ascites is a complicating factor because the coagulation proteins may "drain" into the ascitic fluid.

1. **If there is associated bleeding, the following factors must be considered:**
   a. PT and aPTT are prolonged; sometimes the PT is disproportionately prolonged relative to the aPTT.
   b. Factors V, VII, and fibrinogen are reduced, in addition to other liver-derived coagulation factors.
   c. Factor VIII is usually increased or normal—a point that distinguishes this from DIC.
   d. Platelets are normal or decreased; associated DIC or splenic sequestration may be seen.
2. **Treatment parallels that of DIC; ensure vitamin K administration. Consultation with a hematologist may be important.**

H. THROMBOSIS.

Sick infants are particularly susceptible, often after vascular catheterization. Catheters require careful attention.

1. **Other predisposing pathophysiologic events include the following:**
   a. Protein C, protein S, AT III (antithrombin) deficiencies, factor V Leiden, plasminogen or plasminogen activator abnormalities, prothrombin 20210 mutation.
   b. Maternal diabetes, toxemia, hypertension, antiphospholipid antibody syndrome.
   c. Polycythemia.
   d. Sepsis.
   e. Dehydration.
   f. Congenital nephrosis.
   g. Vascular injury or stasis.
   h. Placental vascular anomalies or thrombosis.
   i. Hyperhomocystinemia or homocystinuria.
2. **The clinical picture depends on the extent and site of thrombosis; gangrene is a possibility.**
3. **Treatment considerations include the following:**
   a. Remove catheters or other potential inciting factors; specific attention should be paid to the particular area compromised by the thrombosis.
   b. Provide heparin in a 75-U/kg bolus followed by 28 U/kg/hour in a constant intravenous drip; adjust the infusion to keep the aPTT 1.5 to 2 times control. Low-molecular-weight heparin can be used, reduces but does not eliminate the need for monitoring. Average of 1 mg/kg/dose needed in children older than 2 months of age to achieve therapeutic anti-Xa levels, average of 1.7 mg/kg/dose in infants younger than 2 months (range 0.96 to 2.36 mg/kg/dose) to achieve therapeutic anti-Xa levels.

Note: *Preterm infants may require a slightly larger loading dose and infusion rate. Consider urokinase or tissue plasminogen activator (tPA) therapy, depending on the site of thrombosis and risk of intracranial hemorrhage. Risks of hemorrhagic complications of thrombolysis in preterm infants and infants in the first week of life are higher.*

c. Fresh frozen plasma. Some inherited disorders (e.g., severe protein C deficiency) do not respond to heparin; consider replacement therapy if specific deficiency is known.

d. Ensure that platelet count is maintained at about 50,000/mm^3; platelet transfusion may be necessary.

e. Consultation with a hematologist. Heparinization can be extraordinarily difficult in the newborn.

19

HEMATOLOGY

I. CONGENITAL DEFICIENCIES OF PROCOAGULANT FACTORS

may manifest in the newborn; often, clinical presentation is delayed several weeks, even into toddler time. Circumcision is a common precipitating event; intracranial and umbilical cord bleeding are relatively uncommon. Massive cephalohematoma, intracranial hemorrhage, or protracted bleeding from scalp puncture, circumcision, or other laceration, no matter the size, should suggest the possibility of a deficiency. The reason for relatively fewer occurrences during the neonatal period is not clear.

1. Hemophilias. Hemophilia A (factor VIII deficiency) and hemophilia B (Christmas disease, factor IX deficiency) are X-linked recessive traits; females are heterozygous carriers and are often free of symptoms; however, bleeding can be seen. Prenatal diagnosis is possible in most cases, requiring chorionic villus sampling, amniocentesis, or fetoscopy. Hemophilia C (factor XI deficiency) is autosomal recessive, occurring most often in Ashkenazi Jews; it should be considered if an infant bleeds excessively after ritual circumcision. Hemophilias A and B are most common, but other deficiencies among the factors must be considered, particularly von Willebrand disease, fibrinogen, and factors II, V, VII, X, and XIII deficiencies. Factor XIII deficiency may cause delayed bleeding after cord separation or circumcision (with normal PT and aPTT).

2. Diagnosis. A neonate's aPTT is generally somewhat prolonged. Therefore, prolongation of aPTT with normal PT cannot be used to confirm hemophilia in the newborn. Confirmation comes from a positive family history and from specific factor assays performed on the infant's and mother's blood, starting with factors VIII and IX.

3. Treatment. Replacement of deficient factors is essential and should be guided by a pediatric hematologist.

a. Hemophilia A. Concentrates that have undergone viral inactivation have replaced cryoprecipitate; recombinant factor VIII is now considered the treatment of choice by most hematologists for newborns diagnosed with hemophilia A. The dose should be 10 to 50 U/kg, depending on the severity of bleeding. One unit of factor VIII activity equals the activity in

1 ml of average normal human plasma. In general, 1 U/kg body weight will yield a 2% rise in circulating factor VIII level; half-life after infusion may be as long as 14 hours, but initial half-life is usually shorter (6 to 8 hours). Administration of 10 to 20 U/kg should achieve the usual goal, a minimum level of 20% to 40%. Concentrates allow this with smaller volumes. In the event of more serious bleeding (e.g., large cephalohematoma or constant umbilical or gastrointestinal loss), continuous infusion may facilitate maintenance of a level of at least 40% for at least 48 hours.

b. Hemophilia B. Recombinant factor IX concentrate should be used at a dose of 20 to 100 U/kg, depending on the severity of bleeding. Factor IX deficiency requires the same approach as factor VIII deficiency; however, 1 U factor IX/kg body weight will generally yield a 0.8% rise in level with recombinant factor IX; initial half-life may be 6 hours or less, but subsequent half-life is approximately 24 hours.

c. von Willebrand disease. Viral inactivated concentrates containing von Willebrand factor are preferred to cryoprecipitate for safety reasons.

d. Cryoprecipitate may, with hematologic consultation, be considered for afibrinogenemia.

e. Fresh frozen plasma (FFP) (10 ml/kg) may be necessary with significant hemorrhage in an unidentified coagulopathy.

f. Precautions are necessary to avoid the transmission of hepatitis B and HIV infection.

g. Mandates immediate hepatitis B immunization (administer subcutaneously unless factor replacement has been given).

h. Suspected or known hemophiliacs should receive vitamin K prophylaxis subcutaneously or by mouth instead of intramuscularly because of the risk of muscle hematoma. Avoid or defer circumcision until the infant can receive appropriate factor dosing for the procedure.

XI. DIAGNOSTIC AND THERAPEUTIC APPROACHES TO THE BLEEDING INFANT

A. DIAGNOSIS.

Bleeding infants may, aside from the hemorrhage, give the impression of either "wellness" or "illness."

1. If a bleeding infant looks "well," the differential diagnosis includes the following:

a. Hemorrhagic disease of the newborn.

b. Inherited coagulation disorders.

c. Immune-induced thrombocytopenia.

d. Drug-induced thrombocytopenia.

e. Trauma (e.g., local vascular lesion, superficial or deep [gastrointestinal tract, abdominal cavity, retroperitoneal space]).

f. Collagen disorders such as Ehlers-Danlos syndrome.

2. If the bleeding infant seems "ill," consider the following:

a. DIC.

b. Liver disease.

c. Platelet consumption (e.g., infection, NEC, renal vein or other thrombosis).

d. The impact of associated prematurity, acidosis, hypoxia, hyperosmolarity.

e. Mechanical or immune-complex mediated thrombocytopenia.

f. Local vascular lesions (e.g., periventricular hemorrhage).

3. The diagnostic workup includes the following (Fig. 19-3):

a. Family history; often the most helpful factor. More than 50% of patients with factors VIII, IX, and XIII deficiencies have a positive family history.

b. Maternal history.

  (1) History of hemorrhagic symptoms or disorder, especially autosomal dominant (e.g., von Willebrand disease).

  (2) Drug ingestion (e.g., coumarin, anticonvulsants, barbiturates, or aspirin).

  (3) Recent or past history of thrombocytopenia, rubella, or syphilis.

  (4) Preeclampsia.

  (5) Repeated abortion (factor XIII deficiency).

  (6) Splenectomy for ITP.

c. Neonate's history.

  (1) Vitamin K_1 administered.

  (2) Trauma.

  (3) Prolonged anoxia.

  (4) Degree of prematurity.

  (5) Sites of bleeding.

d. Physical examination.

  (1) Types and sites of bleeding.

    (a) In hemophilia, skin lesions seem to be ecchymoses; they are often palpable and not petechiae; muscle and joints may be involved rarely; symptoms are not typical of hemophilia in older individuals.

    (b) Oozing from circumcision, umbilical cord, puncture sites, or lacerations suggests DIC or deficiency of vitamin K or factor VIII, IX, or XIII.

    (c) Hemorrhage in more than one area makes a hemostatic disorder more likely.

    (d) Vomiting of blood with no other site involved may suggest swallowed maternal blood. The Apt test helps differentiate maternal from fetal blood (see **Box 19-8**).

  (2) Indicators of sepsis.

  (3) Jaundice (may be the result of cephalohematoma or other large, enclosed hematoma).

  (4) Hepatosplenomegaly. Sepsis indicators, jaundice, and hepatosplenomegaly may together or singly suggest infection (e.g., toxoplasmosis, herpes simplex, syphilis, or cytomegalic inclusion disease).

  (5) Syndactylism (factor V deficiency).

  (6) Cephalohematoma (e.g., vitamin K deficiency, congenital disturbances of coagulation, trauma).

  (7) Hemangiomas; may trap platelets, leading to consumptive coagulopathy; sonogram may reveal retroperitoneal site.

  (8) General clinical status.

19

HEMATOLOGY

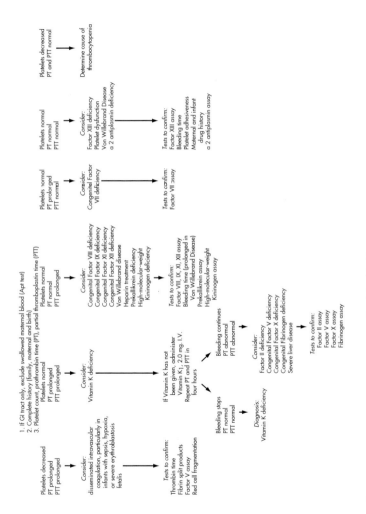

1. If GI tract only, exclude swallowed maternal blood (Apt test)
2. Complete history (family, maternal and birth)
3. Platelet count, prothrombin time (PT), partial thromboplastin time (PTT)

Platelets decreased
PT prolonged
PTT prolonged

Consider:
disseminated intravascular coagulation, particularly in infants with sepsis, hypoxia, or severe erythroblastosis fetalis

Tests to confirm:
Thrombin time
Fibrin split products
Factor V assay
Red cell fragmentation

Platelets normal
PT prolonged
PTT prolonged

Consider:
Vitamin K deficiency

If Vitamin K has not been given, administer Vitamin K₁, 2.0 mg. I.V. Repeat PT and PTT in four hours

Bleeding stops
PT normal
PTT normal

Diagnosis:
Vitamin K deficiency

Bleeding continues
PT abnormal
PTT abnormal

Consider:
Factor II deficiency
Congenital Factor V deficiency
Congenital Factor X deficiency
Congenital Fibrinogen deficiency
Severe liver disease

Tests to confirm:
Factor II assay
Factor V assay
Factor X assay
Fibrinogen assay

Platelets normal
PT normal
PTT prolonged

Consider:
Congenital Factor VIII deficiency
Congenital Factor IX deficiency
Congenital Factor XI deficiency
Congenital Factor XII deficiency
Von Willebrand disease
Heparin treatment
Prekallikrein deficiency
High-molecular-weight Kininogen deficiency

Tests to confirm:
Factor VIII, IX, XI, XII assay
Bleeding time (prolonged in Von Willebrand Disease)
Prekallikrein assay
High-molecular-weight Kininogen assay

Platelets normal
PT prolonged
PTT normal

Consider:
Congenital Factor VII deficiency

Tests to confirm:
Factor VII assay

Platelets normal
PT normal
PTT normal

Consider:
Factor XIII deficiency
Platelet dysfunction
Von Willebrand Disease
α 2 antiplasmin deficiency

Tests to confirm:
Factor XIII assay
Bleeding time
Platelet adhesiveness
Maternal and infant drug history
α 2 antiplasmin assay

Platelets decreased
PT and PTT normal

Determine cause of thrombocytopenia

TABLE 19-11

LABORATORY EVALUATION OF THE BLEEDING INFANT

	Platelet Count	PT	APTT	Fibrinogen	Factor VIII
Well infant					
Thrombocytopenia	↓	N	N	N	N
Vitamin K deficiency	N	↑	↑	N	N
Classic hemophilia	N	N	↑	N	↓↓
Sick infant					
DIC	↓	↑	↑	↓↓	↓↓
Liver disease	N-↓	↑	↑	SI ↓	N-↑
Infection	N-↓	N	N-↑	↑	↑

*N, normal; SI, slightly

From Fanaroff AA, Martin RJ: Neonatal-Perinatal Medicine: Diseases of the Fetus and Infant, ed 4. St. Louis, Mosby 1987

e. Laboratory studies (**Table 19-11**).

(1) To determine platelet adequacy, use a well-prepared cover slip smear of peripheral blood, or determine direct platelet count; determine PT and aPTT.

Note *Give vitamin K, 1 to 2 mg subcutaneously or orally, while waiting for results.*

(2) If platelet count is abnormal, consider causes of isolated thrombocytopenia.

(3) If platelet count is decreased and PT and aPTT are prolonged, consider DIC, particularly in a very sick infant with sepsis, hypoxia, or acidosis. Confirmation of this diagnosis requires a decrease in factor V, VIII, antithrombin or fibrinogen, the presence of fibrin degradation products in plasma, and RBC fragmentation.

(4) If the platelet count is normal and PT and aPTT are prolonged, consider vitamin K deficiency. Prothrombin time should be significantly prolonged, more than 25 seconds. Repeat tests 4 hours after vitamin K is given; cessation of bleeding and drops in PT and aPTT times are confirmatory. Liver dysfunction may contribute to a sluggish response to vitamin K therapy.

(5) If the platelet count is normal and PT and aPTT remain prolonged after vitamin K is given, consider congenital deficiencies of factor II, V, or X or fibrinogen. If all vitamin K-dependent factors are normal but one, there is probably a congenital deficiency in that one.

(6) If a prolonged PT is the sole abnormal test result, and it does not normalize after vitamin K treatment, consider congenital deficiency of factor II or VII.

←

FIG. 19-3

A diagnostic approach to the bleeding newborn. *(Modified from Oski FA, Naiman JL: Hematologic Problems in the Newborn, ed 3. Philadelphia, WB Saunders, 1982.)*

(7) If a prolonged aPTT is the sole abnormal test result, consider von Willebrand disease and, among others, congenital deficiencies of factors VIII, IX, XI, and XII. Also, heparin administration or contamination should be ruled out. Specific factor assays can help determine a particular coagulation defect.

(8) If a congenital defect is a strong possibility or confirmed, study the family. A genetic pattern can provide a clue.

(9) If there are no abnormal platelet, PT, or aPTT results, consider congenital deficiency of factor XIII or antiplasmin, or a defect in platelet function. Disorders of connective tissue (such as Ehlers-Danlos syndrome) and vascular anomalies (such as Osler-Weber-Rendu syndrome) can cause hemorrhage without disorders in the platelets or coagulation factors. Transient platelet dysfunction may be associated with maternal aspirin ingestion.

B. MANAGEMENT.

The immediate approach depends on the site and extent of the bleeding.

1. Red cell transfusion if bleeding is extensive.
2. Vitamin K_1 administration if it has not been given; give anyway if there is uncertainty.
3. In the event of DIC, consider administration of plasma, platelets, heparin, or exchange transfusion (**see pp. 302-303**).
4. In the event of congenital disturbance of coagulation, provide fresh frozen plasma (10 to 15 ml/kg every 12 hours) or fresh whole blood in similar amounts until specific abnormality is detected; if anemia is profound, supplement plasma (administered more rapidly) with packed RBCs.
5. At the time of identification of specific coagulation abnormality, substitute specific replacement (when it is available) for fresh frozen plasma. Determine frequency of administration by the severity of the bleeding. In this regard, pediatric hematology consultation is essential.
6. Topical therapy may include thrombin or an absorbable gauze (e.g., Gelfoam or Oxycel).
a. Do not use nonabsorbable materials. They stick and cause further bleeding on removal.
b. Do not suture or cauterize, if possible; avoid further trauma.
c. Anticipation and prevention. In the event of a contemplated circumcision, careful maternal and family histories are helpful; bleeding times and other, more sophisticated studies, generally are not and should not be done routinely.

BIBLIOGRAPHY

American Academy of Pediatrics: Controversies concerning vitamin K and the newborn. Pediatrics 91:1001, 1993.

Committee on Nutrition, American Academy of Pediatrics: Vitamin K compounds and the water-soluble analogs: Use in therapy and prophylaxis in pediatrics. Pediatrics 28:501, 1961.

Casella JF, Bowers DC, Pelidis MA: Disorders of coagulation. In McMillan JA, DeAngelis JA, Feigin RD, Warshaw JB (eds): Oski's Pediatrics, ed 3. Philadelphia, Lippincott, Williams & Wilkins, 1999.

Fanaroff AA, Martin RJ: Neonatal-Perinatal Medicine: Diseases of the Fetus and Infant, ed 5. St. Louis, Mosby, 1992.

Ho SH, Wu JK, Hamilton DP, et al: An assessment of published pediatric dosage guidelines for enoxaparin: A retrospective review. J Pediatr Hematol Oncol 26(9):561, 2004.

Miqdad AM, Abdelbasit OB, Shaheed MM, et al: Intravenous immunoglobulin G (IVIG) therapy for significant hyperbilirubinemia in ABO hemolytic disease of the newborn. J Matern Fetal Neonatal Med 16(3):163, 2004.

Nathan DG, Orkin SH: Hematology of infancy and childhood, ed 6. Philadelphia, WB Saunders, 2003.

Nathan DG, Oski FA: Hematology of Infancy and Childhood, ed 4. Philadelphia, WB Saunders, 1993.

Osborne LM, Lenarsky C, Oakes RC, et al: Phototherapy in full term infants with hemolytic disease secondary to ABO incompatibility. Pediatrics 74:371, 1984.

Oski FA, Naiman JL: Hematologic Problems in the Newborn, ed 3. Philadelphia, WB Saunders, 1982.

Samuels P, Bussell JB, Braitman LE, et al: Estimation of the risk of thrombocytopenia in the offspring of pregnant women with presumed immune thrombocytopenia purpura. N Engl J Med 323:229, 1990.

19

HEMATOLOGY

Birth Injuries

Beryl J. Rosenstein

FAST FACTS

Immediate Issues in the Nursery

- Erb palsy (injury to C5-C6 nerve roots) accounts for 90% to 95% of all brachial plexus injuries. When present, x-rays of the clavicle, humerus, and shoulder should be done to rule out associated injuries.

- Fractures of the long bones can occur in association with a difficult fetal extraction. These occur mostly during breech delivery, but fractures may also occur during cesarean section. They mostly involve the metaphysis or diaphysis of the humerus and femur and usually produce immediate signs on examination.

- Subgaleal bleeding occurs when blood extravasates beneath the aponeuroses of the scalp. An enlarging collection of blood appears under the scalp, crosses suture lines, and produces significant fluctuance and tension in the scalp. It is associated with prolonged use of a vacuum. In the absence of a history of vacuum extraction, a bleeding diathesis should be suspected. Serial head circumference measurements are useful in gauging severity, and cardiovascular status should be carefully monitored.

Important Reminders After Discharge

- Linear skull fractures can be caused by pressure against the maternal symphysis or ischial spines, although they are usually from forceps pressure. They are seen in up to 5% of patients with a cephalhematoma. When discovered, it is recommended to obtain a skull x-ray at 2 to 3 months of age to ensure that the fracture has healed.

- Because 80% of clavicular fractures have no symptoms and only minimal displacement, the diagnosis is often missed on the initial newborn examination. A knot on the clavicle at 2 to 4 weeks of age is a common presentation (usually lateral segment; 2:1 right:left).

- Traumatic extracranial bleeding (caput, cephalhematoma, and often subgaleal) usually resolves spontaneously over a period of days to weeks. However, there can be calcification of the blood collection or true exostoses seen on physical examination after several months. Also, large closed-space bleeds can result in significant hyperbilirubinemia.

Helpful Information for Parents

- Ninety percent of infants with acquired facial nerve palsy secondary to birth trauma will regain full function by 5 weeks of age.

- Because fractures associated with birth trauma may not be clinically evident in the first few days, when significant risk factors

Continued

for birth trauma are present (e.g., macrosomia, shoulder dystocia, precipitous delivery, prolonged second stage of labor, breech delivery, use of forceps/vacuum), parents should be alerted to watch for fussiness during dressing/diapering, decreased movement of an extremity, or the presence of a "knot" over the collarbone. This information should be balanced with the statement that most fractures requiring treatment are diagnosed before discharge from the nursery.

- Care and consideration should be taken when discussing the etiology and outcome of a birth-related injury with parents. Acknowledging that many factors exist which cannot be controlled and that consequences can result from medically necessary interventions is important. Similarly, the obstetrician can be included in the discussion so that parents receive appropriate and accurate information regarding the circumstances of the injury.

I. RISK FACTORS FOR NEONATAL BIRTH INJURIES

A. MATERNAL FACTORS.
1. Diabetes.
2. Obesity.
3. Undersized pelvis.
4. Postmaturity.
5. Primiparity.

B. FETAL FACTORS.
1. Macrosomia (associated with multiparity, advanced maternal age, obesity, gestational diabetes, previous macrosomic infant).
2. Increased ratio of chest circumference to head circumference.
3. Breech position.

C. OBSTETRIC FACTORS.
1. Shoulder dystocia (major factor in pathogenesis of birth injuries).
2. Forceps (especially midforceps) delivery.
3. Vacuum extraction.
4. Prolonged second stage of labor.
5. Precipitous delivery.

Note: *Infants who are large for gestational age (>4500 g) and who are delivered vaginally (especially with forceps or vacuum extraction) are at increased risk for fractured clavicle, fractured humerus, brachial plexus injury, asphyxia, hypoglycemia, and cephalhematoma. Newborns >5000 g are at increased risk for perinatal mortality.*

D. VACUUM EXTRACTION.

1. May be safer than forceps, but complications include the following:

a. Cephalhematoma (10%).

b. Scalp abrasions and lacerations (1% to 2%).

c. Necrosis and avulsion of the scalp.

d. Subgaleal (subaponeurotic) hemorrhage (0.5% to 1%).

e. Skull fractures.

f. Intracranial bleeding (0.2%).

g. Supratentorial hemorrhage; subdural hematoma.

h. Brachial plexus injury.

2. No evidence of increased incidence of neurologic sequelae after use of vacuum extraction exists; however, whenever there are clinical signs of neurologic compromise after vacuum extraction, evaluation by computed tomography (CT), magnetic resonance imaging (MRI), or ultrasonography is indicated.

E. FORCEPS.

1. Complications include the following:

a. Facial nerve injury.

b. Intraventricular hemorrhage.

c. Brachial plexus injury.

2. Sequential use of vacuum and forceps significantly increases the rates of traumatic complications.

II. HEAD TRAUMA

A. CAPUT SUCCEDANEUM.

1. Caput succedaneum is a collection of edema fluid in the subcutaneous tissues of the scalp involving the portion of the head that presents in a vertex delivery.

2. Swelling is not limited by suture lines; discoloration of the scalp may occur secondary to ecchymosis.

3. There is spontaneous resolution, without sequelae, over a period of several days.

4. Rarely, there may be massive hemorrhage in the scalp secondary to bleeding within the subaponeurotic layer (sometimes classified as a *hemorrhagic caput succedaneum*).

B. CEPHALHEMATOMA. TRAUMATIC SUBPERIOSTEAL HEMORRHAGE USUALLY INVOLVING A PARIETAL BONE; SEEN IN 0.5% TO 1.5% OF BIRTHS; RARE IN <36-WEEK GESTATION.

1. Predisposing factors: large size, primiparity, prolonged labor, male gender, vacuum extraction, forceps delivery (most important).

2. Clinical features.

a. More than 95% involve parietal bone; 90% to 95% are unilateral, right more than left (2:1).

20

BIRTH INJURIES

b. Firm swelling is fixed at the suture lines; the overlying skin is not discolored.

c. May not become apparent until several hours to several days after birth.

d. Any neurologic signs and symptoms are probably related to underlying central nervous system (CNS) trauma.

e. An underlying skull fracture occurs in 1% to 5% of cases, almost always in association with use of forceps; the fracture is usually linear, nondepressed, and clinically insignificant; routine skull x-rays are not indicated.

3. Course and prognosis.

a. Spontaneous resolution occurs over a period of several weeks; 1% to 2% will calcify.

b. Complications include hyperbilirubinemia and anemia (rare), exostoses, and infection.

4. Treatment.

a. None required, except for associated complications.

b. If neurologic signs and symptoms are present, workup for underlying CNS trauma is indicated.

c. Primary infection is rare; infection is usually seen in association with sepsis or meningitis. The most frequently isolated pathogen is *Escherichia coli.* Aspiration of the cephalhematoma is indicated if there is evidence of local infection (e.g., increasing size, local erythema, fluctuance, osteomyelitis of the underlying calvarium), relapse of systemic infection, or a delay in the resolution of clinical symptoms of systemic infection.

C. SUBGALEAL (SUBAPONEUROTIC) HEMORRHAGE.

1. Collection of blood beneath the galea; may cross suture lines and dissect over entire calvarial vault.

2. Most cases are associated with difficult and often prolonged (>10 minutes) vacuum extraction.

3. Presentation.

a. Onset from 1 hour to as late as 4 days after birth.

b. Diffuse swelling of scalp, which may pit on pressure: expanding head circumference: over time fluctuance gives way to tension and fontanel may become obscured; ecchymoses around orbits and behind ears.

c. Lethargy, hypotonia, weak suck, pallor, jaundice, tachypnea, seizures.

d. Hypovolemic shock.

e. Silent presentations resulting in neonatal death with unremarkable clinical findings have been described.

4. Ultrasound, CT, and MRI can be used to confirm the diagnosis.

5. Treatment.

a. Hemodynamic stabilization.

b. Inotropic and ventilatory support.

c. Surgical evacuation of the hematoma (for infants with evidence of cerebral compression).

d. Pressure wrapping of the head is controversial and not generally recommended.

6. Mortality may be as high as 25%.

D. SKULL FRACTURES.

1. Linear.

a. Linear fractures are seen in 1% to 5% of patients with a cephalhematoma; they are secondary to forceps pressure or pressure against the maternal symphysis or ischial spines and usually involve the parietal bone.

b. These fractures are rarely clinically significant, but a follow-up x-ray is recommended at several months of age to ensure that healing has occurred and that the fracture has not increased in width.

2. Depressed.

a. Depressed fractures are the result of excessive molding and compression of the fetal skull by the maternal symphysis or ischial spines or occur secondary to forceps pressure; they are usually "ping-pong ball"–type fractures and are secondary to inward buckling of the resilient bone.

b. The need for treatment remains controversial.

   (1) Fractures almost always elevate spontaneously over a period of months.

   (2) If the patient is neurologically and behaviorally asymptomatic, treatment is probably not necessary.

   (3) Surgical elevation may be indicated if the depression is >5 mm.

E. INTRACRANIAL HEMORRHAGE; RARE IN THE FULL-TERM NEWBORN; MAY BE SECONDARY TO BIRTH TRAUMA, SEVERE ASPHYXIA, OR A COAGULATION DEFECT.

1. Subarachnoid hemorrhage is the most frequent form of traumatic intracranial bleeding in the term neonate. It is usually of limited degree and rarely of clinical significance. It is probably secondary to birth trauma.

a. Clinical features.

   (1) May be asymptomatic.

   (2) Intermittent seizures beginning on second or third day.

   (3) Lethargy, irritability, retinal hemorrhages.

b. Diagnosis.

   (1) Red blood cells (RBCs) in cerebrospinal fluid (CSF) may be difficult to interpret because of the frequency of traumatic taps; look for xanthochromia in centrifuged supernatant and count the RBCs in the first and third tubes of CSF.

   (2) CT is the neuroradiologic study of choice; ultrasound is not useful.

c. Prognosis.

   (1) There are usually no long-term sequelae, but hydrocephalus may be a late complication.

   (2) With evidence of other bleeding or cerebral contusion, prognosis is poor.

20

BIRTH INJURIES

2. Subdural hemorrhage, now a rare occurrence, is caused by severe molding of the cranium with dural venous lacerations or rupture of the bridging veins over the convexities.
   a. Predisposing factors.
      (1) Large infant delivered to a primipara mother.
      (2) Infant born in breech position or with difficult forceps delivery.
      (3) Precipitous delivery in a multipara mother.
      (4) Macrosomia.
   b. Clinical features.
      (1) Posterior fossa.
         (a) Lethargy, irritability, vomiting, irregular respirations, tense anterior fontanel, split sutures, increasing head circumference, anemia, blood in CSF, hypertonia or hypotonia, nystagmus, cranial nerve palsies, seizures.
         (b) With a slowly expanding hematoma, symptoms may be delayed up to 96 hours.
      (2) Over cerebral hemispheres.
         (a) May be clinically silent.
         (b) Signs of increased intracranial pressure with anemia and jaundice.
         (c) Increased head circumference, poor feeding, vomiting, altered mental status, seizures.
   c. Diagnosis.
      (1) Ultrasound may be diagnostic; can be done as initial screen.
      (2) CT is the definitive diagnostic study.
      (3) Lumbar puncture (LP) should be avoided because of risk of herniation.
   d. Treatment depends on symptoms, from supportive treatment to craniotomy with removal of subdural collections of blood; one third of cases require a subsequent shunt procedure because of hydrocephalus.
3. **Intraventricular hemorrhage.**
   a. Rare in full-term neonates—*not* related to trauma. May be associated with intrapartum asphyxia or bleeding diatheses.
   b. Usual site of bleeding is the choroid plexus in full-term infants and the subependymal germinal matrix in preterm infants.
   c. Hemorrhage is often clinically silent but may cause hypotonia, hyperreflexia, decreased activity, irritability, poor feeding, seizures, and hyperpyrexia.
   d. May be associated with pulmonary hemorrhage and cardiac defects.
   e. CT is the best diagnostic procedure.
   f. Treatment is supportive including seizure control.
4. **Epidural hemorrhage.** Rare in the full-term neonate, epidural hemorrhage is secondary to bleeding from a laceration of the middle meningeal artery after fracture of the temporal bone.
   a. Predisposing factor: difficult forceps delivery.

b. Clinical features.

   (1) Signs of increased intracranial pressure.

   (2) Anemia.

   (3) Asymmetrical or focal neurologic signs.

c. Diagnosis is by CT.

d. Treatment includes evacuation of blood and ligation of the bleeding vessel.

5. Intracerebral hemorrhage.

a. Intracerebral hemorrhage is a rare type of bleeding in the full-term neonate.

b. Clinical features include convulsions, hemiparesis, signs of increased intracranial pressure, lethargy, and irritability.

c. Diagnosis is by CT.

III. EYE INJURIES

Birth injuries to the eye and its adnexa are common. These include the following:

A. RETINAL HEMORRHAGE IS SEEN IN UP TO 50% OF VAGINAL DELIVERIES.

It resolves over several days to 2 weeks and requires no specific intervention.

B. SUBCONJUNCTIVAL HEMORRHAGE.

C. CORNEAL EDEMA.

D. EYELID ECCHYMOSIS.

E. RUPTURE OF DESCEMET MEMBRANE.

F. ORBITAL HEMORRHAGE WITH PROPTOSIS.

G. FRACTURE OF THE ORBIT.

H. INJURIES TO THE EXTRAOCULAR MUSCLES.

I. DISLOCATION OF THE GLOBE OUTSIDE THE EYELIDS.

J. EVERSION OF THE EYELIDS.

K. BLEPHAROPTOSIS.

L. MARGINAL EYELID LACERATIONS.

M. LACERATION OF THE LACRIMAL CANALICULUS.

N. HYPHEMA.

Note: *In cases of suspected eye injury, other than retinal hemorrhage, lid ecchymosis, and subconjunctival hemorrhage, immediate ophthalmologic consultation is mandatory.*

IV. NERVE INJURIES

A. BRACHIAL PLEXUS INJURY IS A MECHANICAL DISRUPTION OF THE BRACHIAL PLEXUS NERVE ROOTS SECONDARY TO TRACTION AND LATERAL FLEXION DURING A DIFFICULT VAGINAL DELIVERY; AVULSION OF THE ROOTS IS RARE.

1. Incidence. 0.5 to 2 per 1000 live births; may occur in up to 10% of cases of shoulder dystocia.

2. Predisposing factors. The major risk factor is shoulder dystocia. Associated factors include fetal macrosomia, breech delivery, multiparity, prolonged or precipitous second-stage labor, and instrument delivery.

Note: *Neonatal injuries are most frequent when shoulder dystocia is unanticipated or unrecognized, which is often the case.*

3. Clinical features.
a. Erb palsy. Secondary to injury of C5-C6 nerve roots; accounts for 90% to 95% of brachial plexus injuries.
 (1) Absence or decreased spontaneous movement of involved extremity; asymmetrical Moro reflex.
 (2) Shoulder is internally rotated, forearm prone, elbow extended, and wrist and fingers flexed (waiter's tip position); winging of the scapula; diminished to absent deep tendon reflexes (DTRs); hypesthesia.
 (3) Right side predominates 2:1; usually unilateral, but in breech delivery may be bilateral.
 (4) Associated findings include fetal asphyxia, facial palsy, fractured clavicle, fractured humerus, cephalhematoma, cervical cord injury, and diaphragmatic paralysis (5% of cases).
b. Klumpke paralysis. Secondary to injury to C7, C8-T1 nerve roots.
 (1) Hand is flaccid; loss of wrist movement and grasp.
 (2) Associated findings are those outlined for Erb, plus ipsilateral Horner syndrome (ptosis, miosis, anhidrosis).
c. Combination paresis.

4. Diagnosis.
a. Physical examination.
b. Electromyography (EMG) and nerve conduction studies can be helpful in delineating the location and extent of the injury and in assessing the degree of recovery.
c. X-rays of the clavicle, shoulder, and humerus may help in the diagnosis of associated injuries.

5. Treatment.
a. For the first 7 to 10 days the arm should be wrapped against the body to prevent further injury.
b. After 10 days, passive range-of-motion exercises should be carried out.
c. Hand/wrist splints may help prevent contractures in Klumpke paralysis.
d. The role of early microsurgical nerve repair is controversial and is not indicated in the first 3 months.
e. Infants who do not show good recovery by 6 to 9 months may benefit from neurosurgical intervention.

6. Prognosis.
a. Generally good; 75% to 90% of injuries resolve spontaneously without sequelae; recovery is better for Erb than for Klumpke or mixed pareses (the presence of Horner syndrome is a bad prognostic sign).

b. In most cases recovery takes place within weeks to 3 months, but there may be gradual improvement up to 1 year of age. All cases that show complete recovery show some improvement by 2 weeks.

Note: *Serial neurologic examinations can be useful in predicting recovery. Return to antigravity strength in the biceps, triceps, and deltoid by 6 months of age is predictive of good recovery. There is evidence that if perceptible muscle contractions have not returned to the deltoid and the biceps by the end of the third month, the ultimate functional recovery of the shoulder and arm will be unsatisfactory.*

B. FACIAL NERVE PALSY MAY BE DEVELOPMENTAL OR ACQUIRED; IT IS SEEN IN APPROXIMATELY 1 TO 2:1000 BIRTHS.

20

BIRTH INJURIES

1. Clinical features.
a. Developmental (rare); seen in association with the following:
   (1) Möbius syndrome including bilateral facial palsy, failure to abduct eyes, multiple cranial nerve abnormalities (III, IV, VI, VII, X, XII), micrognathia, club feet, and absence of pectoralis muscles.
   (2) Hemifacial microsomia.
   (3) Agenesis of the depressor anguli oris muscle. Unilateral facial palsy; prominent asymmetry when baby cries (asymmetrical crying facies syndrome); thinning of lateral portion of lower lip; forehead wrinkling, eye closure, and nasolabial folds are symmetrical; may be associated with cardiovascular, skeletal, or genitourinary anomalies.
b. Acquired (common).
   (1) Unilateral; all divisions of the facial nerve are involved.
   (2) Secondary to birth trauma; compression of the facial nerve within the mastoid segment or just outside the sternomastoid foramen.
   (3) Predisposing factors including large size, primiparity, prolonged second-stage labor, and use of forceps (most important).
   (4) Clinical features include decreased forehead wrinkling, increased eye opening, decreased nasolabial fold, and flattening of the corner of the mouth.
   (5) Often associated with facial bruises or lacerations, hematotympanum, temporal bone fracture, or other birth injuries.
   (6) Ninety percent show full recovery, most often within days to weeks, but some may take up to 2 years; 10% show only partial or no return of function.

2. Diagnosis.
a. Based on birth history, physical examination, x-ray studies, and associated findings.
b. Facial nerve conduction studies can be helpful and are indicated starting on day 1 or 2 in any newborn in whom the etiology of the palsy is uncertain.

3. Management.
a. Developmental. Patient should have complete neurodiagnostic evaluation to guide treatment decisions.

b. Acquired. Ninety percent show complete resolution within 1 month without treatment, but surgical intervention may be helpful in highly select cases. Criteria for surgical exploration of the facial canal and nerve decompression include the following:

    (1) Unilateral complete paralysis.

    (2) Hematotympanum and depressed fracture of the petrous bone.

    (3) Absence of voluntary and evoked motor unit responses in all muscles innervated by the facial nerve by 3 to 5 days of life.

    (4) No return of facial nerve function clinically or electrophysiologically at 5 weeks of age.

Note: *Observing every patient is prudent for at least 5 weeks for evidence of spontaneous recovery before considering surgical exploration (some experts would wait even longer).*

C. MISCELLANEOUS NERVE INJURIES.

1. The hypoglossal nerve may be injured during a difficult delivery. Clinical features include weak or hoarse cry (vocal cord paralysis), difficulty feeding, difficulty with secretions, and fasciculations and deviations of the tongue. The injury is usually self-limited.

2. Phrenic nerve.

a. Stretch injury of anterior cervical nerve roots 3, 4, and 5 may occur after a traumatic delivery (breech delivery or shoulder dystocia), leading to paralysis of the diaphragm. Symptoms may begin on the first day of life or may be delayed for as long as a month.

b. Most cases occur in association with an ipsilateral Erb palsy, but isolated phrenic nerve injury has been reported.

c. Clinical features include respiratory distress, cyanosis, and flaring of the chest on the involved side during inspiration. Most cases involve the right side.

d. Fluoroscopy (elevated diaphragm with paradoxical movement) is diagnostic.

e. On EMG there is failure of diaphragmatic response to phrenic nerve stimulation.

f. Initially, the patient may require oxygen, chest physical therapy (PT), continuous positive airway pressure (CPAP), or ventilatory support, but in most cases there is complete recovery over a period of several months. If early recovery of diaphragmatic function is going to occur, it will usually be evident within 2 weeks. In the rare case in which recovery does not occur, surgical plication or partial excision of the involved diaphragm may be helpful.

3. Peripheral nerve injuries. The radial, median, sciatic, and peroneal nerves may rarely be injured, either prenatally (constriction by umbilical cord or amniotic bands) or perinatally (pressure on the nerve during the delivery by bony compression, forceps trauma, or fracture).

D. SPINAL CORD INJURY.

Spinal cord injury in newborns results from the general laxity of the infantile spine in relation to the more inelastic and fragile cord. Excessive longitudinal stretch and torsional and flexion-extension forces can result in disruption of the dura, vascular supply, and neuronal structures. The lower cervical and upper thoracic areas are usually involved. Up to 10% of all neonatal deaths may have an associated spinal cord injury.

1. Predisposing factors.

a. Difficult vaginal delivery of a breech or transverse presentation.

b. Mid-to-high forceps delivery.

c. Prematurity, shoulder dystocia, precipitous delivery.

2. Clinical features.

a. A "snap" or "pop" may be heard at the time of delivery.

b. Profound hypotonia, absent deep-tendon reflexes, obvious sensory level, flaccid extremities, Horner syndrome.

c. Temperature instability.

d. Diaphragmatic paralysis (absent respiratory effort, paradoxical breathing, bell-shaped thorax).

e. Neurogenic bladder (urinary retention).

f. Two thirds have hypoxic-ischemic encephalopathy (i.e., neonatal seizures, cranial CT abnormalities, and subsequent developmental delay).

Note: *Fracture or dislocation of the spinal column is seen in <1% of cases of spinal cord injury.*

3. Differential diagnosis.

a. Hypotonia secondary to birth asphyxia.

b. Neuromuscular disease.

c. Congenital spinal cord tumor; syringomyelia.

4. Diagnosis.

a. Plain-film x-ray of the spine is rarely helpful.

b. Myelography with CT, ultrasound, nerve conduction studies, EMG, and somatosensory evoked potentials may be helpful but often fail to localize or define the lesion.

c. MRI is the best diagnostic test available. It is the only modality that produces a direct image of the spinal cord. Advantages of MRI include the following:

(1) MRI provides excellent soft-tissue definition.

(2) It can differentiate an extramedullary from intramedullary lesion.

(3) It can be performed even in ventilator-dependent patients.

5. Treatment.

a. If there is a possibility of spinal instability, immobilization of the head and neck is mandatory.

b. Management is best carried out in a tertiary-care facility.

c. Treatment is usually conservative (reduction obtained with light traction); laminectomy and surgical exploration are rarely of any benefit.

d. Patient may eventually require a posterior stabilization procedure.

6. Prognosis depends on the extent of neurologic injury. Presence of intra-cord hemorrhage is a bad prognostic sign.

V. FRACTURES AND DISLOCATIONS

A. FRACTURED CLAVICLE.

This is the most frequently fractured bone in the neonate and is present in 1% to 3% of vaginal deliveries.

1. Clinical features.

a. Predisposing factors include large size and shoulder dystocia; most fractures occur after traumatic vaginal deliveries.

b. Usually involves the lateral segment of the clavicle.

c. There is a higher frequency on the right (2:1).

d. The most common finding is minimal swelling or fullness over the fracture site; there may also be crepitus, decreased arm movement, irritability during movement of the arm, and asymmetrical Moro reflex. However, 80% have no symptoms and only minimal physical findings; displacement is rare.

e. The diagnosis is often missed on the initial newborn examination and becomes obvious only when a calcified swelling (callus) is noted at the 2- to 4-week examination.

f. An associated Erb palsy is present in 2% to 5% of cases.

2. Diagnosis.

a. Based on careful physical examination.

b. X-rays or ultrasound studies are not usually indicated, but ultrasound may be helpful to rule out brachial plexus injury.

3. Differential diagnosis.

a. Brachial plexus injury.

b. Traumatic separation of the proximal humeral epiphysis.

c. Humeral shaft fracture.

d. Shoulder dislocation.

4. Treatment.

a. Specific intervention not indicated (if both ends of the bone are in the same room, good healing will occur!).

b. Advise parents to avoid tension on the affected arm.

c. Prognosis is excellent; sequelae are rare.

B. LONG BONE FRACTURES MAY INVOLVE DIAPHYSEAL OR METAPHYSEAL FRACTURES OF THE HUMERUS AND FEMUR, ALTHOUGH OTHER BONES MAY BE AFFECTED.

1. Predisposing factors.

a. Usually seen after difficult extraction of infant in breech position.

b. Most occur during vaginal deliveries but can occur secondary to difficult extraction at cesarean section.

2. **Clinical features.**
a. Swelling and tenderness of the extremity.
b. Decreased mobility.
c. Audible or palpable click; crepitus.

3. **Diagnosis.**
a. Physical examination.
b. X-rays.

4. **Treatment.**
a. Splinting, soft cast, or hard cast, depending on location and severity of fracture.
b. Prognosis is excellent.

C. NASAL SEPTAL DEFORMITIES ARE SEEN IN 0.1% TO 1% OF BIRTHS; THEY ARE SECONDARY TO SLIPPING OF THE TRIANGULAR CARTILAGE OF THE NASAL SEPTUM FROM ITS PROPER POSITION IN THE VOMERINE GROOVE.

1. **Etiology.** The nasal septum is mainly cartilaginous in the newborn. The tip of the nose is particularly vulnerable to trauma during rotation of the head during delivery. Deformities may also occur secondary to intrauterine forces.

2. **Clinical features.**
a. Outward deformity of the nose to one side accompanied by leaning of the columella to the side opposite the dislocation.
b. Loss of nasal tip stability.
c. Flattening of the nasal aperture on the side of dislocation.
d. Diminished movement of ala during inspiration.

3. **Diagnosis.**
a. Physical examination. Pass a probe or cotton-tipped applicator along the floor of the nose and feel the subluxated septum.
b. Compression on the tip of the nose will accentuate asymmetry of the nares.

Note: *Septal deviation must be differentiated from the more common transient flattening or twisting of the nose that resolves spontaneously over several days.*

4. **Treatment.** The septal cartilage should be replaced in the vomerine groove by the third day of life. This manual reduction can be done in the nursery by an otolaryngologist using a special elevator instrument.

5. **Prognosis.** If untreated, there is no spontaneous resolution. Although the nose may appear to straighten, there is an increased incidence of septal and cosmetic deformities.

D. MANDIBULAR FRACTURE

1. Usually secondary to traumatic forceps delivery.
2. Clinical features include facial asymmetry, swelling and ecchymosis over the fracture site, poor feeding, and palpable bony deformity.

20

BIRTH INJURIES

3. Diagnosis is by physical examination and x-rays.
4. Treatment consists of immediate reduction followed by maxillomandibular fixation.

VI. MISCELLANEOUS INJURIES

A. MYOGLOBINURIC RENAL FAILURE.

Rarely, rhabdomyolysis and subsequent myoglobinuric renal failure have been reported in newborns secondary to asphyxia and birth trauma.

B. HEMOPERITONEUM.

1. Intra-abdominal bleeding is rare. Risk factors include large size, hepatomegaly, breech extraction, and forceful manipulation during delivery.
2. Bleeding can occur from the liver, adrenals, spleen, mesentery, umbilical vein, or kidney, but the liver is the most common site. There is usually a slowly expanding subcapsular hematoma that ruptures into the free peritoneal cavity. Rupture of a subcapsular cavernous angioma has also been reported.
3. Hemoperitoneum should be suspected in the newborn with pallor, abdominal distention, anemia, and shock without an obvious source of bleeding. A bluish discoloration of the overlying abdominal skin and scrotal ecchymosis and enlargement may be present. Diagnosis is confirmed by paracentesis and laparotomy.
4. Subcapsular hematoma is the most common form of liver injury; rupture may occur up to 1 week of age.
   a. If the hematoma is large there may be nonspecific prerupture symptoms of poor feeding, lethargy, jaundice, and slowly progressive anemia; a right-upper-quadrant mass may be palpable.
   b. Differentiation from a solid tumor can be made by ultrasonography or CT.
   c. Treatment includes prompt resuscitation, correction of any coagulation defect, evacuation of the hematoma, and repair and drainage of the lacerated liver.
   d. In cases in which the laceration or hematoma is small, careful observation with serial ultrasonography may be appropriate.
5. Adrenal injuries may occur in large babies and those born by breech or otherwise difficult delivery; 90% are unilateral, with 75% occurring on the right side.
   a. Symptoms, which usually appear in the first week, relate to the degree of hemorrhage; when small in amount there may be poor feeding, lethargy, irritability, inguinoscrotal bruising, hematuria and jaundice; when large, there may be an abdominal mass and signs of shock.
   b. When both glands are involved there may be signs and symptoms of adrenal insufficiency.
   c. Abdominal ultrasonography may show a suprarenal mass with downward displacement of the kidney and compression of its

upper pole. Calcification may occur as early as 12 days and is usually rimlike in distribution.

d. Treatment depends on the degree of bleeding; it may vary from expectant (blood loss is mild and within the capsule) to evacuation of the hematoma or adrenalectomy.

C. PNEUMOPERITONEUM.

1. Pneumoperitoneum occurs rarely as a direct result of birth injury, but it may also be the indirect result of birth asphyxia and mucosal ischemia.
2. Symptoms include abdominal distention and vomiting.
3. Diagnosis is by abdominal x-ray, especially the left lateral decubitus view.
4. Treatment includes resuscitation and immediate surgical exploration and repair.

D. PHARYNGEAL INJURY.

1. Pharyngeal perforation may be restricted to the mucosa and submucosa or may extend into the mediastinum or pleural cavity; it occurs secondary to postpartum suctioning, digital injury during a breech delivery, or attempts to pass a nasogastric or endotracheal tube.
2. Symptoms include excessive oropharyngeal secretions and regurgitation of feedings.
3. Diagnosis is established by water-contrast x-ray.
4. Treatment of superficial injuries consists of antibiotics and placement of a soft nasogastric tube. More extensive injuries may require drainage, tube thoracostomy, closure of the perforation, and parenteral nutrition.

E. LIMB ISCHEMIA AND GANGRENE.

1. Limb ischemia and gangrene may be due to a variety of prenatal or perinatal events that result in occlusive vascular disruption. The etiology is usually not evident but may be secondary to compression by an encircling umbilical cord, compound presentation of the arm and head, acute asphyxia, or thromboembolic events (possibly related to poorly controlled maternal diabetes).
2. When gangrene is established at birth, surgical amputation, autoamputation, or some loss of function is the usual outcome.
3. In cases in which ischemia develops within hours of birth secondary to a thromboembolic event, surgical thrombectomy may be successful.

F. TESTICULAR INJURY.

1. Among newborns who are delivered vaginally in the breech position, approximately 10% show injury to the genital area, half of whom have testicular damage. In many of these cases the injured testis will remain abnormal. No specific treatment exists.

20

BIRTH INJURIES

2. Common causes of progressive scrotal findings in the newborn include hydrocele, hernia with incarceration, testicular torsion, and trauma. Scrotal discoloration can result from retroperitoneal and intraperitoneal bleeding.

BIBLIOGRAPHY

Amar AP, Aryan HE, Meltzer HS, Levy ML: Neonatal subgaleal hematoma causing brain compression: Report of two cases and review of the literature. Neurosurgery 52:1470, 2003.

Boulet SL, Alexander GR, Salihu HM, Pass M: Macrosomic births in the United States: Determinant, outcomes and proposed grades of risk. Am J Obstet Gynecol 188:1372, 2003.

Falco NA, Eriksson E: Facial nerve palsy in the newborn: Incidence and outcome. Plast Reconstr Surg 85:1, 1990.

Gonik B, Hollyer VL, Allen R: Shoulder dystocia recognition: Differences in neonatal risks for injury. Am J Perinatol 8:31, 1991.

Hazbi B: Subluxation of the nasal septum in the newborn: Etiology, diagnosis, and treatment. Otolaryngol Clin North Am 10:125, 1977.

Hernandez C, Wendel GD: Shoulder dystocia. Clin Obstet Gynecol 33:526, 1990.

Joseph PR, Rosenfeld W: Clavicular fractures in neonates. Am J Dis Child 144:165, 1990.

LeBranc CMA, Allen UD, Ventpureyra E: Cephalhematomas revisited: When should a diagnostic tap be performed? Clin Pediatr 34:86, 1995.

Mills JF, Dargaville PA, Coleman LT, et al: Upper cervical spinal cord injury in neonates: The use of magnetic resonance imaging. J Pediatr 138:105, 2001.

Painter MJ, Bergman I: Obstetrical trauma to the neonatal central and peripheral nervous system. Semin Perinatol 6:89, 1982.

Poggi SH, Stallings SP, Ghidini A, et al: Intrapartum risk factors for permanent brachial plexus injury. Am J Obstet Gynecol 189:725, 2003.

Schullinger JN: Birth trauma. Pediatr Clin North Am 40:1351, 1993.

Serfontein GL, Rom S, Stein S: Posterior fossa subdural hemorrhage in the newborn. Pediatrics 65:40, 1980.

Siegel MJ, Gado MH, Shackelford G, et al: Cranial computed tomography and real-time sonography in full-term neonates and infants. Pediatr Radiol 149:111, 1983.

Tiwary CM: Testicular injury in breech delivery: Possible implications. Pediatr Urol 34:210, 1989.

Turpenny PD, Stahl S, Bowers D, Bingham P: Peripheral ischemia and gangrene presenting at birth. Eur J Pediatr 151:550, 1992.

Wen SW, Shiliang L, Kramer MS, et al: Comparison of maternal and infant outcomes between vacuum extraction and forceps deliveries. Am J Epidemiol 153:103, 2001.

Yasunaga S, Rivera R: Cephalhematoma in the newborn. Clin Pediatr 13:256, 1974.

Jaundice

Ambadas Pathak

FAST FACTS

Immediate Issues in the Nursery

- Recent studies indicate that in a mixed race population where 60% to 70% of infants are breast-fed, the 95th percentile for bilirubin level at various ages is as follows: 8 mg/dl at 24 hours; 10 mg/dl at 36 hours; 12 mg/dl at 48 hours; 16 mg/dl at 72 hours; and 17 to 18 mg/dl at 120 hours.

- Per the recommended clinical guidelines of the American Academy of Pediatrics, nursing staff should be allowed to evaluate an infant for hyperbilirubinemia by obtaining blood for total serum bilirubin. Likewise, all jaundiced infants < 24 hours old should have blood drawn for bilirubin level. The initial measurement should include a fractionated bilirubin (indirect and direct) level.

- If the total serum bilirubin (TSB) is < 5 mg/dl, a direct or conjugated bilirubin of > 1 mg/dl is generally considered abnormal. For a TSB value of > 5 mg/dl, a direct bilirubin value of > 20% of TSB is considered abnormal. Neonatal hepatitis, biliary atresia, and α_1-antitrypsin deficiency are the three most common causes, with an approximate incidence of 1:5000, 1:10,000, and 1:20,000, respectively.

- In an infant of Asian, Middle Eastern, or African descent with a significantly elevated bilirubin level, consideration should be given to the possibility of hemolysis secondary to G6PD deficiency.

Important Reminders After Discharge

- Infants with cholestatic jaundice may pass colored stools at first. By 3 to 5 weeks, conjugated hyperbilirubinemia can develop along with enlarged liver and lighter stools.

- Babies with umbilical hernia and hyperbilirubinemia (prolonged unconjugated or later-onset conjugated) should be considered at risk of having hypothyroidism. Appropriate follow-up with the results of the newborn screening and attention to the physical examination (macroglossia, large anterior fontanel, cool mottled skin) are therefore warranted.

- Extensive laboratory testing and intensive therapies are NOT warranted for infants who have the following features: jaundice after day 1 of life; serum bilirubin rate of rise < 5 mg/dl per day; peak bilirubin level of < 13 mg/dl (term), < 15 mg/dl (preterm); direct bilirubin level < 2 mg/dl; and a healthy clinical appearance.

Continued

21

FAST FACTS—Cont'd

Helpful Information for Parents

- An infant with a sibling who experienced clinically significant jaundice is at greater risk of also having jaundice. Other factors that increase the risk of clinically significant jaundice include cephalhematoma, excessive bruising, gestational age < 37 weeks, and a blood group mismatch.
- Parents and family members are often comforted when they receive a thorough description of the issues around hyperbilirubinemia. This is especially true if repeated blood sampling is necessary. Likewise, parents often feel empowered by the fact that their attention to feeding and elimination can help to improve the situation.
- In 20% to 30% of all breast-fed infants, indirect hyperbilirubinemia persists beyond 2 to 3 weeks and in some up to 3 months.

I. INDIRECT HYPERBILIRUBINEMIA

A. GENERAL CONSIDERATIONS.

1. Jaundice is a common occurrence in the newborn period. Two of three full-term newborns develop clinical jaundice; most of them have unconjugated hyperbilirubinemia. Male infants tend to have higher levels of bilirubin than female infants, Asians, whites, and African Americans develop hyperbilirubinemia with decreasing frequency.
2. The newborn's susceptibility to jaundice is the result of shortened red cell lifespan and immaturity of liver function. If one newborn has significant jaundice, subsequent siblings are at significantly increased risk.
3. Breakdown of 1 g of hemoglobin results in production of 35 mg of bilirubin.
4. A normal full-term infant produces 8 to 10 mg/kg per day of bilirubin.
5. There is a considerable variation in TSB levels in normal full-term and near-term infants, as shown in **Fig. 21-1**. Factors contributing to this are ethnic background and feeding practices.
6. There is considerable variation in measured bilirubin from laboratory to laboratory. Accuracy of this measurement is ±5%.
7. Serial measurements to determine rate of rise are necessary.
8. The degree of jaundice may be assessed initially by the number of dermal zones involved (**Table 21-1**). As jaundice begins, it advances from head to toe; it fades uniformly throughout without significant progression.

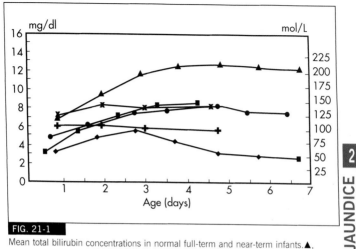

FIG. 21-1

Mean total bilirubin concentrations in normal full-term and near-term infants. ▲, Fifty healthy Japanese newborn infants, 37 to 42 weeks of gestation, all breast-fed. Excludes Rh and ABO incompatibility. *(Data from Yamauchi Y, Yamanouchi I: Acta Paediatr Jpn 31:65, 1989.)* ×, One hundred seventy-six term breast-fed Canadian infants. Excludes Rh hemolytic disease, but includes nine ABO incompatible infants with positive Coombs tests. Seventeen infants received phototherapy. +, One hundred sixty-four Canadian term formula-fed infants, seven ABO incompatible with positive Coombs tests, and three received phototherapy. *(Data from Maisels MJ, 1999.)* ■, One thousand eighty-seven term Israeli infants, 78% fully or partially breast-fed. *(Data from D. Seidman, personal communication, 1988.)* ●, Fifty-six Nigerian term appropriate-for-gestational-age (AGA) infants. Excludes ABO or Rh incompatibility and G6PD deficiency. Infants were "largely breast-fed." *(Data from Maisels MJ, 1999.)* ◆, Twenty-nine full-term American infants, all formula-fed, about 50% African American and 50% white. *(Data from Maisels MJ: Neonatal jaundice. In Avery BG, Fletcher MA, MacDonald MG (eds): Neonatology, Pathophysiology, and Management of the Newborn, 5th ed. Philadelphia, Lippincott Williams & Wilkins, 1999.)*

TABLE 21-1

DERMAL ZONES AND SERUM BILIRUBIN LEVELS

Dermal Zone	Mean Serum Bilirubin (mg/dl)
1. Head and neck	6
2. Trunk to umbilicus	9
3. Groin including upper thighs	12
4. Knees and elbows to ankles and wrists	15
5. Feet and hands including palms and soles	>15

Modified from Kramer LI: Am J Dis Child 118:454, 1969.

21

JAUNDICE

The reliability of visual assessment has recently been questioned, particularly in darkly pigmented infants.

B. CAUSES OF INDIRECT HYPERBILIRUBINEMIA ARE SUMMARIZED IN BOX 21-1.

1. Hemolytic disease of the newborn. Erythroblastosis fetalis is discussed fully in **Chapter 19**.

BOX 21-1

CAUSES OF A PATHOLOGIC INDIRECT HYPERBILIRUBINEMIA IN NEWBORN INFANTS

Increased production or bilirubin load on the liver

Hemolytic disease

Immune

   Rh, ABO, and other blood group incompatibilities

   Heritable

   Red cell membrane defects (hereditary spherocytosis, elliptocytosis, stomatocytosis, and pyknocytosis)

   Red cell deficiencies (glucose-6-phosphate dehydrogenase [G6PD] deficiency,* pyruvate kinase deficiency, and other erythrocyte enzyme deficiencies)

   Hemoglobinopathies (α-Thalassemia, β-γ-thalassemia)

Other causes of increased production

Sepsis*†

Extravasation of blood; hematoma; pulmonary, cerebral, or occult hemorrhage

Polycythemia

Macrosomic infants of diabetic mothers

Increased enteropathic circulation of bilirubin

Breast-milk jaundice

Pyloric stenosis*

Small or large bowel obstruction or ileus

Decreased clearance

Prematurity

G6PD deficiency

Inborn errors of metabolism

Crigler-Najjar syndrome, types I and II, and Gilbert syndrome

Galactosemia†

Tyrosinemia†

Hypermethioninemia†

Metabolic

Hypothyroidism

Hypopituitarism†

Modified from Maisels MJ: Neonatal jaundice. In Avery BG, Fletcher MA, MacDonald MG (eds): Neonatology, Pathophysiology, and Management of the Newborn, 5th ed. Philadelphia, Lippincott Williams & Wilkins, 1999.

*Decreased clearance also part of pathogenesis.

†Elevation of direct-reading bilirubin also occurs.

2. Extravascular blood. Cephalhematomas, cerebral and pulmonary hemorrhage, and severe bruising secondary to breech presentation contribute to prolonged hyperbilirubinemia.

3. Polycythemia. Result of twin-twin transfusion, maternal-fetal transfusion, or delayed clamping of cord; the additional bilirubin load for the liver causes hyperbilirubinemia.

4. Pyloric stenosis. The absolute decrease in glucuronyl transferase activity and increased enterohepatic circulation in this condition leads to prolonged jaundice.

5. Congenital nonhemolytic unconjugated hyperbilirubinemia. Crigler-Najjar syndrome and Gilbert syndrome are examples; bilirubin uridine diphosphate glucuronyl transferase (UDPGT) activity is undetectable (in vitro) in the former and is 20% to 30% of normal in the latter.

6. Congenital hypothyroidism. Characteristic prolonged unconjugated hyperbilirubinemia without hemolysis; now easily detectable with neonatal thyroid screening.

7. Sepsis. May occur, though rarely, with jaundice alone; after the first week, elevation of direct fraction is common, but before that nearly all bilirubin is indirect reacting. Congenital syphilis; toxoplasmosis, other (congenital syphilis and viruses), rubella, cytomegalovirus, and herpes simplex virus (TORCH) infections; and coxsackievirus B infection deserve consideration.

8. Galactosemia. Jaundice has a hemolytic and hepatic component secondary to ingestion of galactose.

9. Breast milk jaundice. There is an association between breast-feeding and neonatal hyperbilirubinemia. Studies have shown that breast-fed infants are three times more likely to develop TSB levels of 12 mg/dl or higher and 6 times more likely to develop levels of 15 mg/dl or higher when compared with formula-fed infants. There is a considerable overlap between "breast-feeding jaundice syndrome" and "breast-milk jaundice syndrome." The former appears in the first 2 to 4 days, and the latter at 4 to 7 days. In 20% to 30% of all breast-fed infants, indirect hyperbilirubinemia persists beyond 2 to 3 weeks and in some up to 3 months. A decreased caloric intake and an increase in enterohepatic circulation of bilirubin are main contributors. **Box 21**-2 lists measures to prevent and treat jaundice associated with breast-feeding.

10. Glucose-6 phosphate dehydrogenase (G6PD) deficiency. Seen in infants of African American, East Asian, and Mediterranean descents, G6PD is accompanied by moderate indirect hyperbilirubinemia and, rarely, kernicterus. These infants have increased bilirubin production caused by hemolysis and abnormal bilirubin elimination.

BOX 21-2

APPROACHES TO THE PREVENTION AND TREATMENT OF JAUNDICE
ASSOCIATED WITH BREAST-FEEDING

PREVENTION

1. Encourage frequent nursing (i.e., at least 8 times per day)
2. Do not supplement with water or dextrose water.

TREATMENT OPTIONS

1. Observe.
2. Discontinue nursing, substitute formula.
3. Alternate feedings of breast milk and formula.
4. Discontinue nursing, administer phototherapy.
5. Continue nursing, administer phototherapy.

From Maisels MJ: Neonatal jaundice. In Avery BG, Fletcher MA, MacDonald MG (eds):
Neonatology, Pathophysiology, and Management of the Newborn, 5th ed. Philadelphia, Lippincott
Williams & Wilkins, 1999.

C. EVALUATION OF A JAUNDICED FULL-TERM NEONATE (TABLE 21-2).

1. History should include details of the pregnancy including the mother's
   general health, blood type, diabetes, hemolytic anemia, gallstones,
   splenectomy, medications, familial disorders, or jaundice in previous
   children.
2. Physical examination should include assessments of cry, color, and
   activity; check for the presence of petechiae, ecchymoses, or
   hepatosplenomegaly, and review neurologic status as indicated by
   tone and reflexes.
3. Laboratory studies should include a complete blood count (CBC)
   including reticulocyte count, peripheral smear, blood group of mother
   and infant, Coombs' test, and urinalysis.

Note: *A diagnostic approach proposed by Maisels is recommended (**Fig. 21-2**).*

D. MANAGEMENT.

The American Academy of Pediatrics Subcommittee on Hyperbilirubinemia
has published an updated guideline providing a framework for the
prevention and management of hyperbilirubinemia in newborn infants of
35 or more weeks' gestation. The clinical algorithm proposed is presented
in **Fig. 21-3**. The salient features of the guideline follow:

1. The nursery policies should promote breast-feeding.
2. A protocol for identification and evaluation of hyperbilirubinemia
   should be available.
3. Jaundice should be assessed whenever the infant's vital signs are
   measured but no less than every 8 to 12 hours.
4. The nursing staff should be able to obtain a TSB value (or a
   transcutaneous bilirubin [TcB] value, when available) as clinically
   indicated.

TABLE 21-2

DATA COLLECTION IN THE DIAGNOSIS OF NEONATAL JAUNDICE

Information	Significance
FAMILY HISTORY	
Parent or sibling with history of jaundice or anemia	Suggests hereditary hemolytic anemia such as hereditary spherocytosis
Previous sibling with neonatal jaundice	Suggests hemolytic disease caused by ABO or Rh isoimmunization
History of liver disease in siblings or disorders such as cystic fibrosis, galactosemia, tyrosinemia, hypermethioninemia, Crigler-Najjar syndrome, or α_1-antitrypsin deficiency	All associated with neonatal hyperbilirubinemia
MATERNAL HISTORY	
Unexplained illness during pregnancy	Consider congenital infections such as rubella, cytomegalovirus, toxoplasmosis, herpes, syphilis, hepatitis A or B, Epstein-Barr virus
Diabetes mellitus	Increased incidence of jaundice among infants of diabetic mothers
Drug ingestion during pregnancy	Ingestion of sulfonamides, nitrofurantoins, antimalarials may initiate hemolysis in G6PD-deficient infant
HISTORY OF LABOR AND DELIVERY	
Vacuum extraction	Increased incidence of cephalhematoma and jaundice
Oxytocin-induced labor	Increased incidence of hyperbilirubinemia
Delayed cord clamping	Increased incidence of hyperbilirubinemia among polycythemic infants
Apgar score	Increased incidence of jaundice in asphyxiated infants
INFANT'S HISTORY	
Delayed passage of meconium or infrequent stools	Increased enterohepatic circulation of bilirubin; consider intestinal atresia, annular pancreas, Hirschsprung disease, meconium plug, drug-induced ileus (hexamethonium)
Caloric intake	Inadequate caloric intake results in delay in bilirubin conjugation
Vomiting	Suspect sepsis, galactosemia, or pyloric stenosis; all associated with hyperbilirubinemia
INFANT'S PHYSICAL EXAMINATION	
Small for gestational age	Infants frequently polycythemic and jaundiced
Head size	Microcephaly seen with intrauterine infections associated with jaundice

From Madan A, MacMahon JR, Stevenson DK: Management of neonatal hyperbilirubinemia. In Taeusch H, Ballard RA, Gleason CA (eds): Avery's Diseases of the Newborn, 8th ed. Philadelphia, Elsevier Saunders, 2004.

21

JAUNDICE

Continued

TABLE 21-2

DATA COLLECTION IN THE DIAGNOSIS OF NEONATAL JAUNDICE—cont'd

Information	Significance
INFANT'S PHYSICAL EXAMINATION—cont'd	
Cephalhematoma	Entrapped hemorrhage associated with hyperbilirubinemia
Plethora	Polycythemia
Pallor	Suspect hemolytic anemia
Petechiae	Suspect congenital infection, overwhelming sepsis, or severe hemolytic disease as cause of jaundice
Appearance of umbilical stump	Omphalitis and sepsis may produce jaundice
Hepatosplenomegaly	Suspect hemolytic anemia or congenital infection
Optic fundi	Chorioretinitis suggests congenital infection as cause of jaundice
Umbilical hernia	Consider hypothyroidism
Congenital anomalies	Jaundice occurs with increased frequency among infants with trisomic conditions
LABORATORY DATA	
Maternal	
Blood group and indirect Coombs test	Necessary for evaluation of possible ABO or Rh incompatibility
Serology	Rule out congenital syphilis
Infant	
Hemoglobin	Anemia suggests hemolytic disease or large entrapped hemorrhage; hemoglobin above 22 gm/dl associated with increased incidence of jaundice
Reticulocyte count	Elevation suggests hemolytic disease
Red cell morphology	Spherocytes suggest ABO incompatibility or hereditary spherocytosis; red cell fragmentation is seen in disseminated intravascular coagulation
Platelet count	Thrombocytopenia suggests infection
White cell count	Total white cell count $< 5000/mm^3$ or band/neutrophil ratio > 0.2 suggests infection
Sedimentation rate	Values in excess of 5 during the first 48 hours indicate infection or ABO incompatibility
Direct bilirubin	Elevation suggests infection or severe Rh incompatibility
Immunoglobulin M	Elevation indicates infection
Blood group and direct and indirect Coombs tests	Required to rule out hemolytic disease as a result of isoimmunization
Carboxyhemoglobin level	Elevated in infants with hemolytic disease or entrapped hemorrhage
Urinalysis	Presence of reducing substance suggests diagnosis of galactosemia

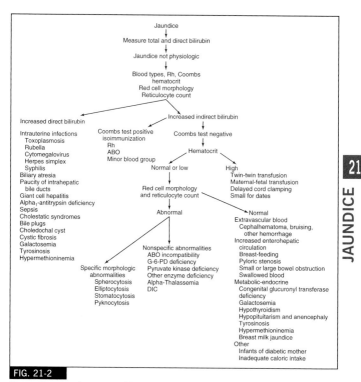

FIG. 21-2

Diagnostic approach to neonatal jaundice. *(From Maisels MJ: Neonatal jaundice. In Avery GB, Fletcher MA, MacDonald MG (eds): Neonatology, Pathophysiology, and Management of the Newborn, 5th ed. Philadelphia, Lippincott Williams & Wilkins, 1999.)*

5. Any infant who is jaundiced in the first 24 hours of life should have a serum bilirubin measurement. The need for subsequent determination of TSB will depend on the zone in which the value falls (**Fig. 21-4**), age of the infant, and evolution of jaundice.

Note: *Fig. 21-4 does not represent the natural history of neonatal hyperbilirubinemia, particularly after 48 and 72 hours of age, as the lower zones are spuriously elevated due to sampling bias.*

6. All TSB levels should be interpreted according to the infant's age in hours.
7. Infant's level of risk is determined according to the risk factors present (**Fig. 21-5**).
8. Guidelines for phototherapy are presented in **Fig. 21-6**. These are based on limited evidence, and the levels shown are approximations.

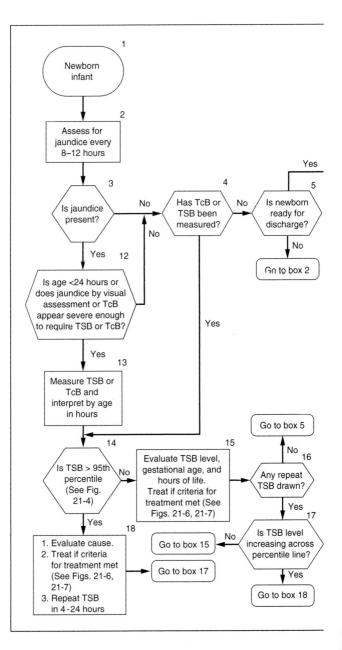

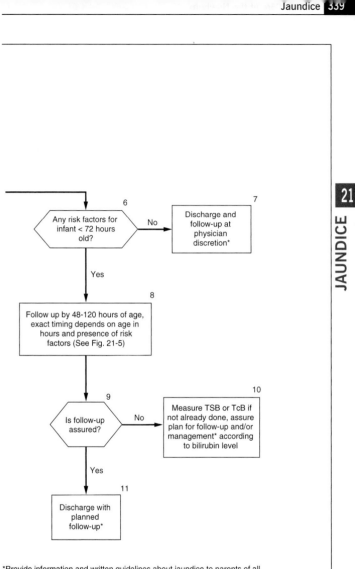

*Provide information and written guidelines about jaundice to parents of all newborns at discharge.

FIG. 21-3

Algorithm for the management of jaundice in the newborn nursery. *(Modified from American Academy of Pediatrics Subcommittee on Hyperbilirubinemia: Management of hyperbilirubinemia in the newborn infant 35 or more weeks of gestation. Pediatrics 114:297, 2004.)*

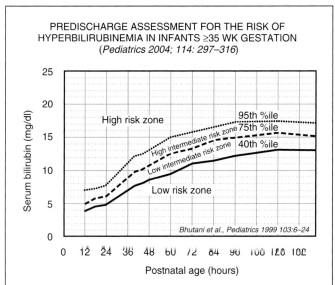

PREDISCHARGE ASSESSMENT FOR THE RISK OF
HYPERBILIRUBINEMIA IN INFANTS ≥35 WK GESTATION
(*Pediatrics 2004; 114: 297–316*)

Date	Time	Age (hrs)	TcB	TSB	Initials

TcB–Transcutaneous bilirubin
TSB–Total serum bilirubin/direct

9. Only intensive phototherapy should be used.

10. If the TSB level approaches or exceeds the exchange transfusion line (**Fig. 21-7**), the sides of the bassinet, incubator, or warmer should be lined with aluminum foil to increase the surface area exposed to the light.

11. If TSB fails to decline or continues to rise despite intensive phototherapy, suspect hemolysis.

12. The levels suggested for exchange transfusion represent a consensus of most of the committee but are based on limited evidence, and the levels shown are approximations.

13. If an infant shows signs of acute bilirubin encephalopathy or if TSB is ≥ 5 mg/dl above the line (see **Fig. 21-7**), perform immediate exchange transfusion even if the TSB levels are falling.

14. Exchange transfusion should be performed only by trained personnel and in a neonatal intensive care unit with full monitoring and resuscitation capabilities.

15. Intravenous administration of gamma globulin (0.5 to 1 g/kg over 2 hours) is recommended for infants with isoimmune hemolytic disease if the TSB continues to increase despite aggressive phototherapy, or it is within 2 to 3 mg/dl of the exchange level. This can be repeated in 12 hours, if necessary.

16. Discharge planning should include providing parents with written and verbal information about newborn jaundice. Parent information handout in English and Spanish is available on the American Academy of Pediatrics website *(www.aap.org/family/jaundicefaq.htm)*.

17. Based on the age at discharge and the risk assessment, provide appropriate follow-up. During follow-up, infant's weight and percent change from birth weight, adequacy of intake, pattern of voiding and stooling, and the presence or absence of jaundice should be assessed. If there is any doubt about the degree of jaundice, TSB should be measured.

Note: *Attention to fluid and caloric intake, frequency of stools, and general health of the infant is important. Breast-feeding at frequent intervals should be encouraged.*

18. Tin-mesoporphyrin, a drug that inhibits the production of heme oxygenase, is effective in preventing or treating hyperbilirubinemia. However, it is not approved by the U.S. Food and Drug Administration.

19. **Table 21-3** provides a clinical pathway for the management of a newborn readmitted for phototherapy or exchange transfusion.

21

JAUNDICE

FIG. 21-4

Predischarge assessment for the risk of hyperbilirubinemia in infants 35 or more weeks of gestation. *(Modified by Maisels MJ from the American Academy of Pediatrics Subcommittee on Hyperbilirubinemia: Management of hyperbilirubinemia in the newborn infant 35 or more weeks of gestation. Pediatrics 114:297, 2004.)*

RISK FACTORS FOR DEVELOPMENT OF SEVERE HYPERBILIRUBINEMIA*

Risk Factors	Major Risk	✓	Minor Risk	✓	Decreased Risk
Predischarge TSB or TcB (see nomogram in Fig. 21-4)	In high risk zone (>95%)		In high intermediate risk zone (>75%)		Low risk zone (<40%)
Visible jaundice	First 24 hrs		Before discharge		
Gestational age	35-36 wk		37-38 wk		≥41 wk
Previous sibling	Received phototherapy		Jaundiced, no phototherapy		
Blood groups Hemolytic disease	Blood grp. incompatibility with +DAT. Other known hemolytic disease (e.g., G6PD deficiency)				
Feeding	Exclusive breast (↑risk if poor feeder or ↑wt. loss)		Breast-fed, nursing well		Exclusive formula feeding
Race	East Asian		Hispanic (Mexican)?		African American *unless G6PD deficient –12% are G6PD deficient
Other factors	Cephalhematoma or significant bruising		Macrosomic infant of IDM, male gender, maternal age ≥25 yr		Discharged from hospital after 72 hr.

*The more risk factors present, the greater the risk of developing severe hyperbilirubinemia.

Follow-up should be provided as follows:
Any infant discharged before age 72 hours should be seen within 2 days of discharge.

*If an infant is discharged before age 72 hours AND if you plan to follow up in more than 2 days, please document your reasons in the chart.

FIG. 21-5

Risk factors for development of severe hyperbilirubinemia. *(Modified by Maisels MJ from the American Academy of Pediatrics Subcommittee on Hyperbilirubinemia: Management of hyperbilirubinemia in the newborn infant 35 or more weeks of gestation. Pediatrics 114:297, 2004.)*

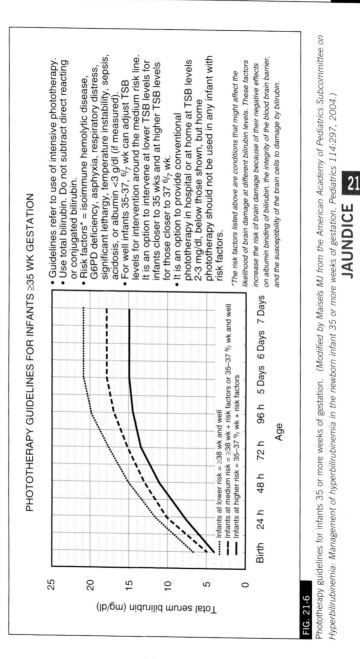

PHOTOTHERAPY GUIDELINES FOR INFANTS ≥35 WK GESTATION

- Guidelines refer to use of intensive phototherapy.
- Use total bilirubin. Do not subtract direct reacting or conjugated bilirubin.
- Risk factors* = isoimmune hemolytic disease, G6PD deficiency, asphyxia, respiratory distress, significant lethargy, temperature instability, sepsis, acidosis, or albumin <3 g/dl (if measured).
- For well infants 35-37, $6/7$ wk can adjust TSB levels for intervention around the medium risk line. It is an option to intervene at lower TSB levels for infants closer to 35 wks and at higher TSB levels for those closer to 37 $6/7$ wk.
- It is an option to provide conventional phototherapy in hospital or at home at TSB levels 2-3 mg/dl, below those shown, but home phototherapy should not be used in any infant with risk factors.

*The risk factors listed above are conditions that might affect the likelihood of brain damage at different bilirubin levels. These factors increase the risk of brain damage because of their negative effects on albumin binding of bilirubin, the integrity of the blood brain barrier, and the susceptibility of the brain cells to damage by bilirubin.

Total serum bilirubin (mg/dl)

Age: Birth, 24 h, 48 h, 72 h, 96 h, 5 Days, 6 Days, 7 Days

······ Infants at lower risk = ≥38 wk and well

─ ─ ─ Infants at medium risk = ≥38 wk + risk factors or 35-37 $6/7$ wk and well

──── Infants at higher risk = 35-37 $6/7$ wk + risk factors

FIG. 21-6

Phototherapy guidelines for infants 35 or more weeks of gestation. (Modified by Maisels MJ from the American Academy of Pediatrics Subcommittee on Hyperbilirubinemia: Management of hyperbilirubinemia in the newborn infant 35 or more weeks of gestation. Pediatrics 114:297, 2004.)

21

JAUNDICE

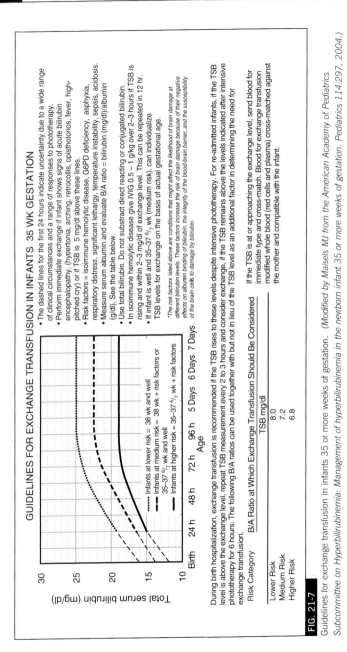

GUIDELINES FOR EXCHANGE TRANSFUSION IN INFANTS 35 WK GESTATION

- The dashed lines for the first 24 hours indicate uncertainty due to a wide range of clinical circumstances and a range of responses to phototherapy.
- Perform immediate exchange if infant shows signs of acute bilirubin encephalopathy, (hypertonia, arching, retrocollis, opisthotonos, fever, high-pitched cry) or if TSB is 5 mg/dl above these lines.
- Risk factors = isoimmune hemolytic disease, G6PD deficiency, asphyxia, respiratory distress, significant lethargy, temperature instability, sepsis, acidosis.
- Measure serum albumin and evaluate B/A ratio = bilirubin (mg/dl)/albumin (g/dl). See the table below.
- Use total bilirubin. Do not subtract direct reacting or conjugated bilirubin.
- In isoimmune hemolytic disease give IVIG 0.5 – 1 g/kg over 2–3 hours if TSB is rising and within 2–3 mg/dl of exchange level. This can be repeated in 12 hr.
- If infant is well and 35–37 $^{6}/_{7}$ wk (medium risk), can individualize TSB levels for exchange on the basis of actual gestational age.

The risk factors listed above are conditions that might affect the likelihood of brain damage at different bilirubin levels. These factors increase the risk of brain damage because of their negative effects on albumin binding of bilirubin, the integrity of the blood-brain barrier, and the susceptibility of the brain cells to damage by bilirubin.

If the TSB is at or approaching the exchange level, send blood for immediate type and cross-match. Blood for exchange transfusion modified whole blood (red cells and plasma) cross-matched against the mother and compatible with the infant.

······ Infants at lower risk = 38 wk and well

━ ━ Infants at medium risk = 38 wk with risk factors or 35–37 $^{6}/_{7}$ wk and well

━━ Infants at higher risk = 35–37 $^{6}/_{7}$ wk + risk factors

During birth hospitalization, exchange transfusion is recommended if the TSB rises to these levels despite intensive phototherapy. For re-admitted infants, if the TSB level is above the exchange level, repeat TSB measurement every 2 to 3 hours and consider exchange, if the TSB remains above the levels indicated after intensive phototherapy for 6 hours. The following B/A ratios can be used together with but not in lieu of the TSB level as an additional factor in determining the need for exchange transfusion.

Risk Category	B/A Ratio at Which Exchange Transfusion Should Be Considered
	TSB mg/dl
Lower Risk	8.0
Medium Risk	7.2
Higher Risk	6.8

FIG. 21-7

Guidelines for exchange transfusion in infants 35 or more weeks of gestation. *(Modified by Maisels MJ from the American Academy of Pediatrics Subcommittee on Hyperbilirubinemia: Management of hyperbilirubinemia in the newborn infant 35 or more weeks of gestation. Pediatrics 114:297, 2004.)*

TABLE 21-3

MANAGEMENT OF THE NEWBORN INFANT RE-ADMITTED FOR PHOTOTHERAPY OR EXCHANGE TRANSFUSION

TREATMENT

Use intensive phototherapy and/or exchange transfusion as indicated in **Figs. 21-6** and **21-7**

LABORATORY TESTS

TSB and direct bilirubin levels

Blood type (ABO, Rh)

Direct antibody test (Coombs)

Serum albumin

Complete blood cell count with differential and smear for red cell morphology

Reticulocyte count

$ETCO_c$ (if available)

G6PD if suggested by ethnic or geographic origin or if poor response to phototherapy

Urine for reducing substances

If history and/or presentation suggest sepsis, perform blood culture, urine culture, and celebrospinal fluid for protein, glucose, cell count, and culture

INTERVENTIONS

If TSB ≥ 25 mg/dl (428 μmol/L) or ≥ 20 mg/dl (342 μmol/L) in a sick infant or infant < 38 wks' gestation, obtain a type and crossmatch, and request blood in case an exchange transfusion is necessary

In infants with isoimmune hemolytic disease and TSB level rising in spite of intensive phototherapy or within 2-3 mg/dl (34-51 μmol /L) of exchange level (**Fig. 21-7**), adminster intravenous immunoglobulin 0.5-1 g/kg over 2 h and repeat in 12 h if necessary

If infant's weight loss from birth is > 12% or there is clinical or biochemical evidence of dehydration, recommend formula or expressed breast milk. If oral intake is in question, give intravenous fluids.

FOR INFANTS RECEIVING INTENSIVE PHOTOTHERAPY

Breast-feed or bottle-feed (formula or expressed breast milk) every 2-3 h

If TSB ≥ 25 mg/dl (428 μmol/L), repeat TSB within 2-3 h

If TSB 20-25 mg/dl (342-428 μmol /L), repeat within 3-4 h. If TSB < 20 mg/dl (342 μmol /L), repeat in 4-6 h. If TSB continues to fall, repeat in 8-12 h

If TSB is not decreasing or is moving closer to level for exchange transfusion or the TSB/albumin ratio exceeds levels shown in **Fig. 21-7**, consider exchange transfusion (see **Fig. 21-7** for exchange transfusion recommendations)

When TSB is < 13-14 mg/dl (239 μmol/L), discontinue phototherapy

Depending on the cause of the hyperbilirubinemia, it is an option to measure TSB 24 h after discharge to check for rebound

TSB, total serum bilirubin.

From the American Academy of Pediatrics Subcommittee on Hyperbilirubinemia: Management of hyperbilirubinemia in the newborn infant 35 or more weeks of gestation. Pediatrics 114:297, 2004.

E. PHOTOTHERAPY.

1. Phototherapy converts bilirubin to its photo products, which are less lipophilic and can bypass hepatic conjugation and be excreted without further metabolism.

2. A standard phototherapy unit has a bank of eight fluorescent lights: four special blue and four daylight bulbs.

3. For effective phototherapy, a minimum irradiance of 4 $\mu W/cm^2/nm$ in the blue spectrum is necessary. Response is dose related; a saturation point is reached at 23 $\mu W/cm^2/nm$. Irradiance should be monitored by using a photometer.

4. With the naked infant in a bassinet, lights may be kept at a distance of 10 cm without overheating the infant. When halogen phototherapy lamps are used, manufacturer's recommendations should be followed to avoid the risk of a burn.

5. A wraparound fiberoptic unit that has been shown to be effective for standard phototherapy is available; it has the advantage of promoting mother–infant bonding and avoiding the complications associated with fluorescent light phototherapy. However, these units have a low spectral power.

6. Bilirubin measurements every 12 hours are necessary; evaluation of skin color is unreliable.

7. Usually 2 to 3 days of continuous therapy are necessary; serum bilirubin decreases by 2.5 to 3 mg per day in the absence of excessive production. The use of standard phototherapy systems leads to a decrease of 6% to 20% of initial bilirubin level In 24 hours, whereas intensive phototherapy results in a decrease of 30% to 40% of initial bilirubin level in 24 hours. Performing periodic checks of phototherapy units is important to assure delivery of adequate irradiance.

8. Intensive phototherapy implies the use of high levels of irradiance in the 430 to 490 nm band (usually 30 $\mu W/cm^2/nm$ or higher) delivered to as much of the infant's surface area as possible.

9. On discontinuation of phototherapy, primarily in babies with hemolytic jaundice, the serum bilirubin level should be measured after 12 hours to detect rebound phenomenon; rarely this requires restarting of phototherapy.

10. Complications of phototherapy include increased water loss, elevation of temperature, skin rash, hypocalcemia, abdominal distention, displaced eye patches causing respiratory distress, and bronze baby syndrome.

11. Home phototherapy should not be used in any infant with risk factors.

12. Neither visual assessment of jaundice nor TcB measurements are reliable in infants undergoing phototherapy, as phototherapy "bleaches" the skin.

13. An absolute contraindication for phototherapy is congenital porphyria or a family history of porphyria, as is the concomitant use of photosensitizers.

F. PHYSIOLOGIC JAUNDICE.

1. Physiologic jaundice is by far the most common type of jaundice, and it accounts for 50% of cases.

2. Proposed criteria.

a. Jaundice appearing after day 1.

b. Rate of increase in serum bilirubin <5 mg/dl per day.
c. Serum bilirubin level does not exceed 13 mg/dl in full-term and 15 mg/dl in preterm infants.
d. Direct bilirubin fraction is <2 mg/dl.
e. Jaundice does not last beyond 1 week in full-term and beyond 2 weeks in preterm infants.
3. Infant does not present with any signs of illness (e.g., lethargy, poor feeding, temperature instability).
4. Elaborate laboratory evaluation and aggressive therapeutic intervention are *not* indicated.

G. KERNICTERUS.

An apparent resurgence of kernicterus has occurred in the past decade. The reported cases were in infants with G6PD deficiency, sick newborns with low bilirubin levels, and in apparently healthy term and near-term newborns with high (usually ≥30 mg/dl) bilirubin levels.

II. CHOLESTASIS (REDUCTION IN BILE FLOW)

A. GENERAL CONSIDERATIONS.

1. Cholestasis, defined as jaundice caused by elevated conjugated bilirubin, is an uncommon but potentially serious problem resulting from hepatobiliary dysfunction.
2. If the TSB is < 5 mg/dl, a direct or conjugated bilirubin > 1 mg/dl is generally considered abnormal. For a TSB value of greater than 5 mg/dl, a direct bilirubin value greater than 20% of total serum bilirubin is considered abnormal.
3. Compared with unconjugated hyperbilirubinemia, cholestatic jaundice is much more likely to have a serious etiology.
4. For its successful treatment and a favorable prognosis, early detection of cholestatic jaundice by the primary care physician and an accurate diagnosis by the pediatric gastroenterologist are essential.
5. Cholestasis results from extrahepatic obstruction or hepatocellular injury, either primary or secondary to many infectious, metabolic, and toxic causes.
6. The newborn is particularly susceptible because of immature hepatobiliary function, with decreases in bile acid pool size, rate of synthesis, intraluminal concentration, and ileal uptake. Consequently, intraluminal fat digestion is impaired, and cholestatic effects of various endogenous and exogenous substances are enhanced.
7. In a study reported from Spain, biliary sludge was found in 1 of 300 fetuses studied ultrasonographically. On follow-up, these infants remained asymptomatic and had normal sonograms.

B. CLINICAL SYNDROMES (BOX 21-3).

Neonatal cholestasis occurs in 1:2500 births, with extrahepatic obstruction accounting for half of the cases. Neonatal hepatitis, biliary atresia, and

21

JAUNDICE

BOX 21-3

DIFFERENTIAL DIAGNOSIS OF NEONATAL CHOLESTASIS

EXTRAHEPATIC BILIARY DISEASE

Extrahepatic biliary atresia

Choledochal cyst

Bile-duct stenosis

Spontaneous perforation of the bile duct

Neoplasm

Cholelithiasis

INTRAHEPATIC BILIARY DISEASE

Intrahepatic bile-duct paucity

    Syndromic form (Alagille syndrome)

    Nonsyndromic forms

Inspissated bile

Caroli disease (cystic dilation of the intrahepatic bile ducts)

Congenital hepatic fibrosis and infantile polycystic disease

HEPATOCELLULAR DISEASE

Metabolic and genetic diseases

    Disorders of amino acid metabolism (tyrosinemia)

    Disorders of lipid metabolism

        Wolman disease

        Niemann-Pick disease

        Gaucher disease

    Disorders of carbohydrate metabolism

        Galactosemia

        Hereditary fructose intolerance

        Glycogenosis type IV

    Peroxisomal disorders

        Zellweger syndrome (cerebrohepatorenal syndrome)

        Adrenoleukodystrophy

        Glutaric aciduria type II

        Olivocerebellar atrophy

    Endocrine disorders

        Idiopathic hypopituitarism

        Hypothyroidism

    Familial with uncharacterized excretory defect

        Dubin-Johnson syndrome

        Rotor syndrome

        Byler syndrome

        Aagenaes syndrome (hereditary cholestasis with lymphedema)

        Familial benign recurrent intrahepatic cholestasis

    Defective bile acid synthesis (trihydroxycoprostanic acidemia)

    Defective protein synthesis

        α_1-Antitrypsin deficiency

        Cystic fibrosis

Continued

BOX 21-3—Cont'd
DIFFERENTIAL DIAGNOSIS OF NEONATAL CHOLESTASIS
Chromosomal disorders
Trisomy 21
Trisomy 17-18
Donahue leprechaunism
Infectious
Viral
Cytomegalovirus
Rubella
Herpes
Toxoplasmosis
Syphilis
Hepatitis B
Hepatitis C
Varicella
Coxsackievirus
Enteric cytopathogenic human orphan (ECHO) virus
Bacterial-sepsis, urinary tract infection, gastroenteritis, listeriosis
Iatrogenic
Total parenteral nutrition
Drug or toxin
Idiopathic (neonatal hepatitis)
Miscellaneous (shock or hypoperfusion)

From Haber BA, Lake AM: Clin Perinatol 17:483, 1990.

α_1-antitrypsin deficiency are the three most common causes, with an approximate incidence of 1:5000, 1:10,000, and 1:20,000, respectively.

1. **Extrahepatic biliary disease.**
a. Extrahepatic biliary atresia. Infants with biliary atresia are usually well nourished and more likely to be female. At first, infants pass "normal-colored" stools. In established cases, stools are acholic or faintly pigmented. By 3 to 5 weeks, conjugated hyperbilirubinemia develops. In addition to clinical icterus, these infants may have an enlarged liver and, occasionally, an enlarged spleen. Associated anomalies include polysplenia, preduodenal portal vein, malrotation, and congenital heart disease. Obstruction to bile flow is at the porta hepatis in the majority of infants. Establishing the patency of the extrahepatic biliary tree early to allow prompt surgical intervention is important. Magnetic resonance cholangiography may be useful in excluding biliary atresia. Hepatic portoenterostomy (Kasai procedure) is used on the basis of the results of the operative cholangiogram and histopathology of the liver. If operated on before 60 days of age, postoperative bile flow is restored in 70% to 80% of cases, but if operated on after 120 days of age, bile flow is restored in only 10% to 20% of cases. Therefore it is absolutely essential to make an early diagnosis.

b. Choledochal cyst. A choledochal cyst is a dilation of the extrahepatic biliary tree that produces signs and symptoms of obstruction that mimic extrahepatic biliary atresia. It is 5 times more common in girls than in boys. Complete surgical excision is the treatment of choice and prevents cirrhosis, portal hypertension, and cholangiocarcinoma.

2. Intrahepatic biliary disease.
a. Paucity of interlobular bile ducts.
   (1) Syndromic. Alagille syndrome (arteriohepatic dysplasia) consists of hypoplastic intrahepatic bile ducts; chronic cholestasis; and extra-hepatic anomalies including characteristic facies (small, pointed chin; broad forehead; hypertelorism), vertebral defects (butterfly and hemivertebrae), cardiovascular abnormalities (peripheral pulmonary stenosis, coarctation of the aorta), growth retardation, and anomalies of the anterior chamber angle of the eye. Autosomal dominant inheritance with low penetrance is probable. Prognosis is variable but more favorable than the nonsyndromic form.
   (2) Nonsyndromic. A progressive cholangiolitic insult leads to paucity of intrahepatic bile ducts; it is also seen as a late complication in infants with biliary atresia and as a feature of liver involvement in graft-versus-host disease. Congenital rubella, cytomegalovirus (CMV), hepatitis B, trisomies 18 and 21, and α_1-antitrypsin deficiency have been associated.
b. Inspissated bile. Results from bilirubin overload in 10% of newborns with hemolytic anemia resulting from Rh or ABO incompatibility, spherocytosis, and G6PD deficiency. Conjugated bilirubin is elevated in cord blood because of intrauterine hemolysis. Hepatosplenomegaly is marked; transaminase levels are normal or mildly elevated, and cholestasis lasts for 4 weeks or longer.

3. Hepatocellular disease.
a. Metabolic and genetic defects.
   (1) α_1-Antitrypsin deficiency accounts for 5% to 15% of infants with cholestasis; jaundice appears at about 8 weeks of age and in 15% of cases is resolved by 7 months. Infants may have conjugated hyperbilirubinemia, jaundice, acholic stools, dark urine, and liver enlargement. After a prolonged period of apparently normal health, cirrhosis and its complications may lead to death in late childhood or early adulthood. Diagnosis is confirmed by serum α_1-antitrypsin determination and by protease inhibitor phenotyping. Liver transplantation is the only treatment.
   (2) Dubin-Johnson syndrome and Rotor syndrome are autosomal recessive conditions that cause nonhemolytic conjugated hyperbilirubinemia. Transaminase and bile acid levels are normal; prognosis is excellent.
   (3) With benign recurrent intrahepatic cholestasis, infants develop intermittent jaundice, pruritus, dark urine, pale stools, and elevated alkaline phosphatase without progressive liver disease.

(4) Peroxisomal disorders. Zellweger cerebrohepatorenal syndrome is an autosomal recessive disorder. Clinical features include cholestatic jaundice, hepatomegaly, mental retardation, hypotonia, renal cortical cysts, and abnormal facies with epicanthal folds, hypertelorism, and prominent forehead. The defect consists of absence of peroxisomes and derangement of mitochondria. Diagnosis is confirmed by the presence of abnormal levels of very long chain fatty acids in the serum. Most infants die within 1 year, and survivors have severe mental retardation and seizures. Other cholestatic disorders in this category include adrenoleukodystrophy, glutaric aciduria type II, and olivocerebellar atrophy.

(5) Cystic fibrosis rarely causes conjugated hyperbilirubinemia. Meconium ileus may be seen in half of the cases. Jaundice resolves gradually, with increased risk of liver disease later in life.

(6) Galactosemia is an autosomal recessive disorder of carbohydrate metabolism resulting from deficiency of galactose-1-phosphate uridyltransferase, with an incidence of 1:100,000. Clinical features include lethargy, emesis, anorexia, growth failure, cholestasis, and lenticular cataract formation. Elimination of lactose- and galactose-containing products from the diet is prudent while erythrocyte enzyme determination is in progress. Galactosemia should be excluded in any infant with septic cholestasis.

(7) Hypopituitarism may cause cholestasis. Hypoglycemia, septo-optic dysplasia, and hypothyroidism may be associated findings.

b. Perinatal infections. Cholestasis in many intrauterine viral infections is a result of hepatic necrosis; CMV, rubella, herpes, hepatitis B, enteroviruses, coxsackievirus B, and echoviruses may produce conjugated hyperbilirubinemia. Toxoplasmosis, syphilis, and bacterial infections that cause neonatal sepsis, pyelonephritis, severe enteritis, and enterocolitis may lead to cholestasis.

c. Iatrogenic disease.

(1) Total parenteral nutrition cholestasis is seen in >50% of infants with birth weights of <1000 g and in <10% of full-term infants. Prematurity, prolonged fasting, and metabolic alterations (e.g., hyperglycemia, abnormal amino acids) may be contributory.

(2) Cholestasis caused by a drug or hepatotoxin is a possibility. The clinical picture will resemble viral hepatitis.

d. Idiopathic neonatal hepatitis is a descriptive term for intrahepatic cholestasis with characteristic "giant cell hepatitis" for which no other infectious, genetic, or metabolic cause is found. With the newly discovered metabolic and genetic diseases, idiopathic neonatal hepatitis now accounts for only 10% to 20% of the intrahepatic cholestasis cases. Infants are usually male and small for gestational age, and they fail to thrive. Prominent physical findings include icterus and hepatomegaly.

21

JAUNDICE

C. CLINICAL PRESENTATION.
Jaundice, acholic stools, and dark urine are characteristic. Pruritus, lethargy, growth failure, hepatosplenomegaly, and ascites are late signs.

D. DIAGNOSTIC EVALUATION.
The Cholestasis Guideline Committee of the North American Society for Pediatric Gastroenterology, Hepatology, and Nutrition (NASPGHAN) formulated a clinical practice guideline for the diagnostic evaluation and management of cholestatic jaundice in the 2- to 8-week-old infant (**Fig. 21-8**). The American Academy of Pediatrics has endorsed these recommendations. **Table 21-4** highlights a detailed evaluation of the history and physical findings.

TABLE 21-4

HISTORY AND PHYSICAL FINDINGS TO CONSIDER FOR THE DIFFERENTIAL DIAGNOSIS OF INFANTS WITH CONJUGATED HYPERBILIRUBINEMIA

Topic	Specification Question	Implication
History	Similar problem with parents or among siblings	Occurrence in other family members implies autosomal dominant inheritance, and occurrences in sibs implies genetic disease or nongenetic recurrence pattern: e.g., α-1AT deficiency, progressive familial intrahepatic cholestasis (PFIC), Alagille syndrome, cystic fibrosis (CF)
	Consanguinity	Risk for autosomal recessive inheritance
	Maternal infection that can affect baby	TORCH infections, occasionally HBV, others
	Cholestasis of pregnancy	May be seen in PFIC
	Fetal ultrasound (yes/no; findings)	Choledochal cyst and bowel anomalies (e.g., duplication cysts) that can cause jaundice
	Past ABO or Rh disease, or Rh negative	Hemolysis
	Birth weight	SGA implies fetal involvement and weighs against biliary atresia
	Neonatal infection, including UTI, sepsis, and viral infection	Often associated with conjugated hyperbilirubinemia
	Feeding history and history of weight gain	Neonatal hepatitis can cause FTT; metabolic disease (e.g., galactosemia and hereditary fructose intolerance) can cause anorexia, FTT, and jaundice. Panhypopituitarism
	Bowel history—vomiting, stooling	Vomiting—metabolic disease, pyloric stenosis, bowel obstruction (atresia, annular pancreas); delayed stooling—CF, hypothyroidism; diarrhea—infection, metabolic disease, PFIC, CF; clay-colored stool—biliary obstruction
	Source of nutrition	Breast or formula; composition of formula; galactose-containing—galactosemia, fructose or sucrose containing—hereditary fructose intolerance

TABLE 21-4

HISTORY AND PHYSICAL FINDINGS TO CONSIDER FOR THE DIFFERENTIAL
DIAGNOSIS OF INFANTS WITH CONJUGATED HYPERBILIRUBINEMIA—cont'd

Topic	Specification Question	Implication
	Disposition	Irritable: may be associated with some metabolic disorders; "great baby, sleeps all the time, never awake," lethargic—hypothyroidism or panhypopitiuitarism
	Urine color—preferably directly observed	Dark urine—conjugated hyperbilirubinemia
	Stool color (useful to have reference such as yellow paint strip from paint dealer); preferably directly observed	Pale or clay colored; cholestasis, rule out obstruction
	Excessive bleeding	Coagulopathy; vitamin K deficiency
Physical findings	Vital signs; weight, length, OFC; weight for length	
	Global assessment of general health	
	Global assessment of nutritional status	Acute illness
	HEENT	Dysmorphic findings—Alagille syndrome, scleral icterus (qualitatively different in cholestasis versus nonconjugated jaundice), fundoscopic (intrauterine infection)
		Slit-lamp finding (Alagille syndrome, cataracts) snuffles
	Chest/heart	Evidence of pneumonia—neonatal infection
		Evidence of heart failure—congestive hepatopathy
		Murmurs or other evidence of congenital heart disease—biliary atresia, Alagille syndrome
	Abdomen	Distention
		Ascites
		Abdominal wall vasulature
		Liver size (exactly measured)
		Liver consistency
		Spleen size (below costal margin)
		Spleen consistency
		Masses
		Umbilical hernia
	Diaper exam	Dark urine—conjugated hyperbilirubinemia
		Pale or clay-colored stool—cholestasis, rule out obstruction
	Skin—bruising, petechiae, rashes	
	Neurologic—general assessment of vigor, tone, and symmetry	

From the North American Society for Pediatric Gastreoenterology, Hepatology & Nutrition Cholestasis Guideline Committee. J Pediatr Gastroenterol Nutr 39:115, 2004.

21

JAUNDICE

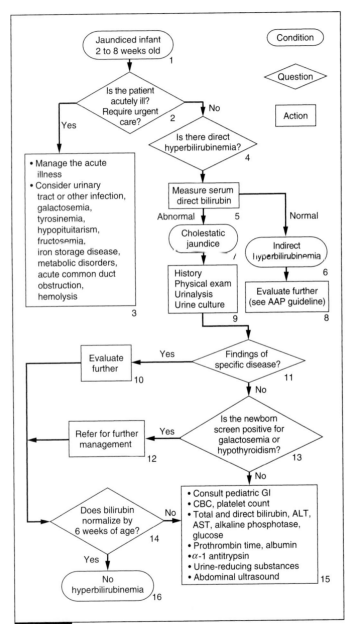

FIG. 21-8

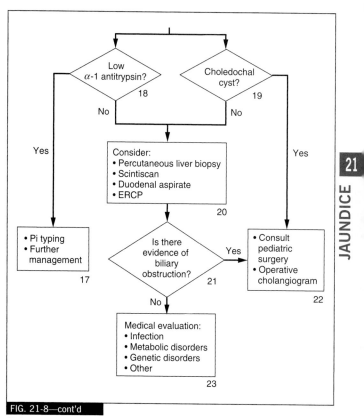

FIG. 21-8—cont'd

Cholestasis clinical practice guideline. Algorithm for a 2- to 8-week-old infant.
(From the North American Society for Pediatric Gastroenterology, Hepatology & Nutrition Cholestasis Guideline Committee. J Pediatr Gastroenterol Nutr 39:115, 2004.)

Any infant noted to be jaundiced at 2 weeks of age should be clinically evaluated for cholestasis with measurement of total and direct serum bilirubin. In an acutely ill infant, consider urinary tract or other infection. The newborn screen for galactosemia and hypothyroidism should be evaluated or repeated. Anatomic abnormality such as choledochal cyst can be diagnosed by ultrasonography. The "triangular cord" on ultrasound has high sensitivity and specificity for diagnosis of biliary atresia. Consultation with a pediatric gastroenterologist is essential for managing an infant with conjugated hyperbilirubinemia of unknown cause. A pediatric surgeon is consulted if the diagnosis of choledochal cyst or biliary atresia is entertained.

BOX 21-4

MEDICAL MANAGEMENT

Treat specific etiology

Nutrition

　Provide adequate calories

　Supplement diet with medium-chain triglycerides

　Supplement diet with fat-soluble vitamins A, D, E, and K

Pruritus and xanthoma

　Phenobarbital

　Cholestyramine

Ascites

　Low-sodium diet, 1 to 2 mEq/kg per day

　Diuretics (spironolactone preferred over furosemide unless acute diuresis is
　　required)

Liver failure, life-threatening portal hypertension, inability to provide adequate
　growth and development (consider liver transplant)

From Haber DA, Lake AM: Clin Perinatol 17:483, 1990.

E. MANAGEMENT (BOX 21-4).

Providing optimal nutrition to a cholestatic infant is difficult. Provision of medium-chain triglycerides results in better caloric intake and growth. Fat-soluble vitamins A, D, E, and K should be supplemented. Ascites and liver failure are managed by low-sodium diet and diuretics (spironolactone, 0.5 to 1 mg/kg every 8 hours by mouth; furosemide 1 to 2 mg/kg per dose by mouth or intravenously every 8 to 12 hours). Phenobarbital (3 to 10 mg/kg per day by mouth) and cholestyramine (0.25 to 0.5 mg/kg per day by mouth) are employed to promote bile flow and excretion of bile acids and cholesterol. Liver transplantation is indicated with failure to grow, evidence of liver failure, and poor quality of life. Of children with biliary atresia, 70% to 80% require liver transplantation despite clinical improvement after portoenterostomy. Thus, biliary atresia alone accounts for almost 50% of all liver transplants performed in children.

BIBLIOGRAPHY

American Academy of Pediatrics Subcommittee on Hyperbilirubinemia: Management of hyperbilirubinemia in the newborn infant 35 or more weeks of gestation. Pediatrics 114:297, 2004.

Haber BA, Lake AM: Cholestatic jaundice in the newborn. Clin Perinatol 17:483, 1990.

Kramer LI: Advancement of dermal icterus in the jaundiced newborn. Am J Dis Child 118:454, 1969.

Madan A, MacMahon JR, Stevenson DK: Neonatal hyperbilirubinemia. In Taeusch HW, Ballard RA, Gleason CA (eds): Avery's Diseases of the Newborn, 8th ed. Philadelphia, Elsevier Saunders, 2004.

Maisels MJ: Neonatal jaundice. In Avery GB, Fletcher MA, MacDonald MG (eds): Neonatology: Pathophysiology and Management of the Newborn, 5th ed. Philadelphia, Lippincott Williams & Wilkins, 1999.

North American Society for Pediatric Gastroenterology, Hepatology & Nutrition, The Cholestasis Guideline Committee: Guideline for the evaluation of cholestatic jaundice in infants. J Pediatr Gastroenterol Nutr 39:115, 2004.

Sokol RJ, Mack C, Narkewicz MR, Karrer FM: Pathogenesis and outcome of biliary atresia: Current concepts. J Pediatr Gastroenterol Nutr 37:4, 2003.

21

JAUNDICE

Infection

Timothy Townsend

FAST FACTS

Immediate Issues in the Nursery

- Prolonged rupture of membranes, chorioamnionitis, group B streptococcus colonization, prematurity, and male gender are the major risk factors associated with neonatal bacterial sepsis. These risk factors are additive such that the presence of two or three risk factors significantly increases the incidence of neonatal sepsis.
- Neutropenia along with fever in a newborn is highly suggestive of bacterial disease. Neutrophilia alone does not correlate well with neonatal sepsis.
- The white blood cell (WBC) count and differential are the best indirect indicators of bacterial infection.
- Breast-feeding is not contraindicated for any congenital infection when the mother and/or infant are receiving appropriate treatment or chemoprophylaxis. The only exception is when the mother is infected with human immunodeficiency virus (HIV) and lives in an industrialized setting (infant formula readily available and risk of viral transmission through breast milk unquantified).
- Before discharging an infant, the practitioner should know the serologic syphilis status on either the mother or the infant.

Things to Remember for Follow-up After Discharge from the Nursery

- Infants born to a mother who is positive for hepatitis B surface antigen (HBsAg+) should be retested after 9 months of life for HBsAg and anti-HBsAg to assess the efficacy of immunoprophylaxis with hepatitis B virus (HBV) vaccine and hepatitis B immunoglobulin (HBIG).
- An infant who is born to an HIV-positive mother and who has a negative initial HIV polymerase chain reaction (PCR) (done within 48 hours of delivery) should have a repeat PCR done at 2 weeks, 1 to 2 months, and 4 to 6 months.
- Late-onset GBS disease occurs from 7 days to 12 weeks after delivery and is NOT usually associated with the risk factors for early-onset disease.

Important Information for Parents

- No matter which congenital infection is present, in general no newborn should be separated from his or her mother.
- Infected neonates undergoing treatment generally do not need isolation from siblings or other children.
- In cases of neonatal infections, practitioners should discuss the short- and long-term sequelae of the specific infection involved. Emphasizing the value of early intervention services in the recovery process and identifying specialists who will assist the family with long-term monitoring and treatment of specific complications are important.

I. INTRODUCTION TO NEONATAL INFECTIONS

A. BACTERIAL AND VIRAL INFECTIONS ARE IMPORTANT CAUSES OF NEONATAL MORBIDITY AND MORTALITY.

1. Infections with varying outcomes may be caused by pathogenic bacteria or viruses acquired at different times during intrauterine and neonatal life. No agent, no matter how obscure, should be ignored as a possibility when initial probabilities do not seem to be likely.

2. Infection can occur in utero (congenital infection), at the time of delivery (natal infection), and after birth but within the neonatal period (postnatal infection).

B. THE CHOICE OF ANTIBIOTICS.

1. Universal coverage is a myth that needs to be dispelled. It is a false concept providing a false comfort, and it must not be substituted for careful observation and careful interpretation of data.

2. Initial coverage, however, is often a must. Start with the following:
   a. Coverage for those organisms that are most likely in the circumstance.
   b. Coverage for those organisms that are likely to pose the greatest threat if not treated.

3. Follow-up coverage is altered as more is learned clinically and in the laboratory.

II. BACTERIAL INFECTION AND SEPSIS

A. GENERAL.

1. Invasive bacterial infections primarily involve the bloodstream during the first month of life; meningitis is present in approximately 25% of bacteremic newborns.

2. The occurrence rate is 2 to 3:1000 live births, with a range of 1 to 10:1000 live births.

3. Sepsis is a low-incidence but high-risk problem. Accurate diagnosis is difficult because there is no definitive early diagnostic test. Therefore a large number of newborns who do not have the disease will of necessity be evaluated and treated for sepsis.

B. ETIOLOGY.

1. Group B β-hemolytic streptococcus (especially, for late-onset disease, type III) and *Escherichia coli* (K1 strains) currently account for 60% to 70% of all postnatal infections in most locations in the United States.

2. Other common pathogens include *Staphylococcus aureus, Klebsiella, Enterobacter, Serratia, Citrobacter, Pseudomonas* species, *Staphylococcus epidermidis,* α-hemolytic streptococcus, group D streptococcus (non-*Enterococcus*), *Listeria monocytogenes,* and *Enterococcus.*

3. *Streptococcus pneumoniae, Neisseria meningitidis, Haemophilus influenzae,* and groups A, C, and G streptococci are found, but much less frequently than after the postnatal period.

C. PATHOGENESIS.

1. Maternal risk factors.

a. Prolonged rupture of membranes (PROM) (>24 hours) is associated with a 1% incidence of sepsis.

b. Chorioamnionitis.

   (1) Suggested by the presence of maternal temperature >100.4° F, uterine tenderness, purulent or foul-smelling amniotic fluid or fetal tachycardia.

Note: *Epidural analgesia for labor has been associated with a 15-fold increase in the incidence of intrapartum maternal fever.*

   (2) With chorioamnionitis and PROM, the risk of sepsis increases to 3% to 5%.

c. Colonization with group B streptococcus.

   (1) Group B streptococcus is isolated from the genitourinary or gastrointestinal tract of 10% to 30% of pregnant women; colonization is persistent throughout pregnancy in 60% to 70% of these women; 40% to 70% of infants of colonized mothers become colonized, and invasive disease develops in 1 of every 50 to 75 of these infants.

   (2) Infant colonization is the result of the following:

      (a) Transplacental transmission in the presence of maternal bacteremia.

      (b) Ascending transmission through leaks in the amniotic membranes or frankly ruptured membranes.

      (c) Surface contamination during passage through the birth canal.

      (d) Intrapartum distress (meconium staining, 5-minute Apgar score <6) with aspiration of infected amniotic fluid.

2. Infant risk factors.

a. Prematurity. With PROM, gestational age <37 weeks increases the risk of sepsis 10-fold.

b. Depressed immune function in the newborn infant.

   (1) Decreased concentration of antibody to specific organisms (e.g., group B streptococcus).

   (2) Impaired neutrophil function.

   (3) Deficiency of complement, especially in low-birthweight infants.

   (4) Delayed clearance of organisms from the bloodstream.

   (5) Decreased secretory immunity.

   (6) Impaired ability to respond to capsular polysaccharide.

c. Gender. Males are 2 to 6 times more likely than females to develop sepsis.

Note: *The preceding risk factors are additive; the presence of two or three of these factors can increase the risk of neonatal sepsis up to 25 to 30 times. It is also appropriate to note that requiring personnel in the nursery to wear gowns is generally unnecessary and offers no benefit in preventing neonatal colonization.*

D. CLINICAL FEATURES.

1. Signs and symptoms of neonatal sepsis may be subtle and nonspecific. They include respiratory distress, high-pitched cry, lethargy, temperature instability (hypothermia or hyperthermia), hypotonia, vomiting, jaundice, diarrhea, abdominal distention, poor feeding, apnea, cyanotic spells, seizures, poor perfusion, petechiae, and purpura. Although any organ may be involved as part of neonatal sepsis, pneumonia and meningitis are most common. Notably, indirect hyperbilirubinemia (jaundice) in an otherwise well infant should *not* be considered an indicator of bacteremia or incipient sepsis if it is the only manifestation of the problem. Exceptions might be made in the event of late-onset jaundice or total bilirubin with >20% conjugated.

2. Fever.

a. Ten percent of full-term newborns with a temperature >37.8° C not related to environmental causes have bacterial sepsis. Among afebrile newborns, the incidence of bacterial disease is 1:10,000.

b. Risk of bacterial infection increases with height of fever; temperature >39° C is associated with a high incidence of infection.

c. Fever in the first hour of life is usually related to maternal fever.

d. Newborns with fever and bacterial disease usually, *but not always*, have other symptoms suggestive of infection.

e. Newborns should be evaluated for infection if they have fever that persists or recurs or a single episode of fever plus any other sign or symptom consistent with infection.

3. Group B streptococcal (GBS) infection .

a. Early-onset disease. Onset occurs from birth to 7 days (accounts for 80% of GBS infections of infants). All serotypes (Ia, Ib/c, Ia/c, II, III, IV, and V) are associated with infections in infants.

   (1) Risk factors include maternal colonization with group B streptococcus, bacteriuria, intrapartum fetal distress, low birth weight, prematurity, and PROM. Risk is increased with "heavy" neonatal colonization, multiple-gestation pregnancy, and history of group B streptococcal infection in a previous sibling. Recent recommendations from the Centers for Disease Control and Prevention (CDC) advocate treatment with intrapartum penicillin if the mother is colonized (determined through rectoanal and vaginal cultures at 35 to 37 weeks' gestation using selective broth media) with group B streptococcus. An alternative strategy is to not culture but to give intrapartum penicillin only to those women with the following risk factors:

      (a) Onset of labor or rupture of membranes at less than 37 weeks' gestation.

      (b) Membranes ruptured 18 or more hours.

      (c) Fever (temperature >38° C) during labor.

Note: *This strategy will miss the 25% of early-onset cases born to colonized mothers with no risk factors. All women with GBS bacteriuria during pregnancy and any*

*woman who has delivered an infant who developed GBS disease should have
intrapartum penicillin.*

    (2) GBS may cause pneumonia with or without bacteremia or
       bacteremia with or without meningitis; there is usually a sudden
       onset with fulminant course.

    (3) Clinical features include tachypnea, bradycardia, shock,
       cyanosis, apnea, pneumonia, and persistent pulmonary
       hypertension.

    (4) Laboratory findings include hypoxemia, metabolic acidosis,
       leukopenia, thrombocytopenia, and hypoglycemia.

    (5) The course is rapidly progressive; the fatality rate is 5% to 15%.

b. Late-onset disease. Onset occurs from 7 days to 8 to 12 weeks
  (accounts for 20% of GBS infections of infants).

    (1) Not usually associated with the risk factors noted with early-onset
       disease; almost always serotype III.

    (2) May cause meningitis or osteomyelitis with or without bacteremia;
       other sites of infection include omphalitis, septic arthritis,
       lymphadenitis, soft-tissue infection, breast abscess, otitis media,
       endocarditis, and pericarditis.

    (3) Usually has an insidious onset with nonspecific signs. Clinical
       features include signs and symptoms of meningitis or
       osteomyelitis (especially the right humerus). The fatality rate
       is 5% to 10%.

4. *L. monocytogenes.*

a. *L. monocytogenes* can cause a flulike illness in the mother just before
delivery; maternal blood culture may be positive.

b. The lung is the primary focus of early infection, but infection can also
result in hepatosplenomegaly, purulent conjunctivitis, skin rash, and
small granulomas on the posterior pharynx. Meningitis is present in
96% of late-onset cases.

c. Fatality rate is 40% to 80%.

E. DIFFERENTIAL DIAGNOSIS OF NEONATAL SEPSIS.

1. Metabolic disturbances.

a. Inborn errors of metabolism (e.g., urea cycle defect).

b. Hypoglycemia.

c. Electrolyte imbalance.

2. Maternal drug abuse.

3. Hemolytic disease of the newborn.

4. Congenital heart disease (e.g., hypoplastic left heart syndrome).

5. Other infections.

a. Congenital and natally acquired infections (e.g., syphilis, herpes simplex
virus [HSV], cytomegalovirus [CMV], rubella, toxoplasmosis, tuberculosis
[TB], enterovirus).

b. Disseminated fungal infection.

22

INFECTION

F. LABORATORY FINDINGS.

1. Specific diagnostic tests.

a. Isolation of bacteria from blood or cerebrospinal fluid (CSF) is the standard method to diagnose neonatal sepsis. However, the rate of proven plus highly suspected infection is undoubtedly greater than the culture-proven rate.

b. Blood culture.
   (1) Blood may be obtained by venipuncture or from a fresh umbilical artery catheter; samples of cord blood or those from an indwelling umbilical venous catheter or any type of intravascular catheter may be unreliable because of high rates of contamination.
   (2) The optimum amount of blood for culture is unclear; 1 ml is recommended, although lesser amounts may be adequate for high-grade bacteremia.
   (3) Among patients with bacteremia and without antibiotic pretreatment, the vast majority of blood cultures are positive by 48 hours. Late-growing bacteria are usually anaerobes or coagulase-negative staphylococcus or occur in newborns with antibiotic pretreatment.

c. CSF culture.
   (1) Lumbar puncture (LP) is not usually indicated in the evaluation of the full-term newborn who is considered at risk of sepsis on the basis of maternal or obstetric factors.
   (2) In infants who *develop* signs and symptoms suggestive of infection, LP is always indicated. Up to 15% of newborns with positive CSF cultures have a negative blood culture.
   (3) In interpreting CSF results, it is important to note that the CSF has a normal upper limit of 25 cells/mm^3 in the full-term newborn; however, meningitis may occur with lower cell counts. CSF glucose and protein concentrations may be difficult to interpret because of the wide range of normal values.

d. Urine culture.
   (1) May be useful in the infant with evidence of late-onset or nosocomial infection. Usually not helpful in early-onset sepsis.
   (2) Bagged specimens are unreliable; urine should be obtained by suprapubic bladder tap or, in girls, by straight in-and-out catheterization.

e. Tracheal aspirate.
   (1) Culture obtained at the time of intubation is useful in the newborn with suspected pneumonia.
   (2) A positive culture is found in half of infants who have pneumonia and a negative blood culture.

f. Detection of bacterial antigen.
   (1) The latex-particle agglutination test may be carried out in the evaluation of group B streptococcal infection.
   (2) May be applied to serum, CSF, or *concentrated* urine (obtained by suprapubic tap or in-and-out catheterization).
   (3) Sensitivity is >90%.

(4) Urine specificity is 81% to 99%; may be related to skin or urine contamination with group B streptococci or cross-reaction with other bacterial species.

Note: *A negative result does not rule out the possibility of systemic group B streptococcal infection.*

2. Nonspecific diagnostic tests.
a. White blood cell (WBC) and differential counts.
   (1) The establishment of normal reference values (see **Appendix C**) has increased the utility of these tests. Note that WBC counts can be higher in capillary than in arterial or venous samples.
   (2) Of the nonspecific tests, neutropenia is the best predictor of sepsis; neutropenia in a newborn with fever is highly suggestive of bacterial disease. Maternal hypertension, perinatal asphyxia, and intraventricular hemorrhage may also cause significant neutropenia.
   (3) Neutrophilia does not correlate well with neonatal sepsis; it may occur secondary to intrapartum maternal fever, stressful labor, or hemolytic disease of the newborn.
   (4) The ratio of immature to total neutrophils (I:T ratio) >0.2 is predictive of neonatal bacterial disease but can also be related to maternal fever and stressful labor.
   (5) Neutrophil vacuolization and toxic granulations are also suggestive of bacterial infection.

Note: *If the total neutrophil count, immature neutrophil count, and I:T ratio are normal, there is a 95% to 100% negative predictive value for sepsis.*

b. C-reactive protein (CRP).
   (1) CRP is an acute-phase globulin synthesized by the liver within 6 to 8 hours of an inflammatory stimulus; normal value is <1.6 mg/dl on days 1 to 2 and <1 mg/dl thereafter.
   (2) Sensitivity and specificity are not high enough for the CRP to be used alone as a definitive diagnostic test.
   (3) Failure to mount a CRP response may be a poor prognostic sign. Normalization of a CRP elevation may be helpful in determining response to antimicrobial therapy and duration of treatment.
c. Erythrocyte sedimentation rate (ESR).
   (1) ESR rate has been used as part of neonatal "sepsis screens."
   (2) Normal value is equal to the day of life plus 3 mm/hr up to a maximum of 15 mm/hr.
   (3) A false-positive result can occur with hemolysis; a false-negative result may be caused by disseminated intravascular coagulation (DIC).
d. Surface cultures (gastric aspirate). Gram stain and culture of surface sites are *not* useful indicators of neonatal bacterial infections; they do not distinguish the infected from the colonized infant.

22

INFECTION

386 Primary Care of the Newborn

e. Miscellaneous tests. A number of indirect tests including serum IgM, leukocyte alkaline phosphatase, fibronectin, haptoglobin, and elastase α-proteinase inhibitor levels and the limulus lysate test for endotoxin detection have been used. They are unreliable when used individually but may be helpful when used in various combinations as part of a sepsis screen. In an individual case, examination of the buffy coat smear by direct staining can be a valuable aid in the early diagnosis of sepsis.

Note: *No single test or combination of tests has proven superior to the WBC count and differential as an indirect indicator of bacterial infection. No laboratory test result should ever negate a clinical impression of sepsis.*

G. MANAGEMENT.
1. The spectrum and severity of symptoms required to prompt a sepsis workup is a matter of clinical judgment and cannot be dictated by protocol. The practitioner must rely on careful maternal and newborn history, physical examination, and laboratory findings. The goal is to identify and treat all infected infants but to avoid excessive investigation and treatment of noninfected infants. If the mother received intrapartum antibiotics for group B Streptococcus prophylaxis, clinical management of the infant may be complicated. Clinical judgment is crucial. Institution of intrapartum antibiotics as early as possible after membrane rupture may limit the risk of early-onset group B streptococcal sepsis for the infant.
2. Asymptomatic infant. The decision to treat is based on the perceived level of risk and must be considered independently for each case (**Fig. 22-1**).
3. Symptomatic infant. Clinical judgment is crucial. The burden of proof is on the practitioner to prove that there is no infection, not on the baby to prove that he or she is infected. Absence of risk factors should never dissuade one from treating a symptomatic neonate (**Fig. 22-2**).

Note: *In the asymptomatic preterm infant, treatment should be initiated with only a single obstetric or clinical risk factor.*

4. Antibiotic therapy.
a. The usual approach is to start with parenteral ampicillin (100 mg/kg per day in two divided doses daily) and gentamicin. (See **Appendix H** for dosage.) The dosing interval of gentamicin should be adjusted according to postconceptional age.
b. Monitoring the serum gentamicin levels is important; trough level should be <2 μg/ml, and peak level should be 5 to 10 μg/ml.
c. Subsequent therapy is guided by culture and sensitivity results.
   (1) Group B streptococcus: penicillin alone (preferably) and, at times, gentamicin.

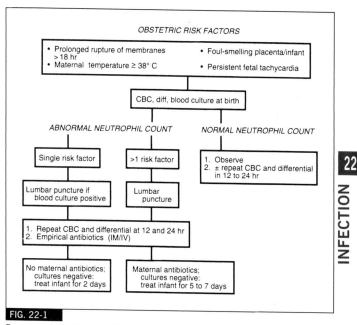

OBSTETRIC RISK FACTORS

- Prolonged rupture of membranes > 18 hr
- Maternal temperature ≥ 38° C
- Foul-smelling placenta/infant
- Persistent fetal tachycardia

CBC, diff, blood culture at birth

ABNORMAL NEUTROPHIL COUNT

Single risk factor

>1 risk factor

Lumbar puncture if blood culture positive

Lumbar puncture

1. Repeat CBC and differential at 12 and 24 hr
2. Empirical antibiotics (IM/IV)

No maternal antibiotics; cultures negative: treat infant for 2 days

Maternal antibiotics; cultures negative: treat infant for 5 to 7 days

NORMAL NEUTROPHIL COUNT

1. Observe
2. ± repeat CBC and differential in 12 to 24 hr

FIG. 22-1

Recommended approach to the diagnostic evaluation and treatment of the asymptomatic term infant with history of obstetric risk factors. *(Modified from Siegel JD: Sepsis neonatorum. In Oski FA (ed): Principles and Practice of Pediatrics. Philadelphia, JB Lippincott, 1994.)*

22

INFECTION

    (2) *L. monocytogenes:* ampicillin.

    (3) *S. aureus:* nafcillin or oxacillin (vancomycin if methicillin resistant).

    (4) *S. epidermidis:* vancomycin (need to monitor serum levels; trough level should be <10 μg/ml, peak 20 to 30 μg/ml); switch to oxacillin for susceptible organisms.

    (5) *Enterobacter, E. coli:* ampicillin plus aminoglycoside (tobramycin, gentamicin); should be guided by susceptibility pattern in individual hospital.

    (6) *Pseudomonas* species: aminoglycoside plus ticarcillin or ceftazidime.

    (7) *Enterococcus:* ampicillin plus aminoglycoside.

  d. Miscellaneous.

    (1) Appropriate cultures should be repeated after 24 to 48 hours to document sterile cultures. The usual duration of treatment is 7 to 10 days (with appropriate clinical response), but longer courses are required for meningitis, osteomyelitis, endocarditis, and septic arthritis.

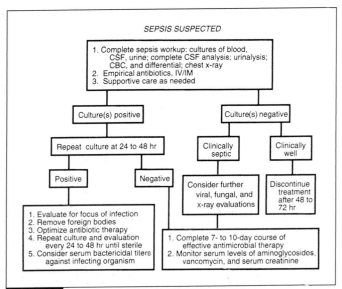

FIG. 22-2

Recommended approach to the diagnostic evaluation and treatment of the neonate with suspected sepsis. (*From Siegel JD: Sepsis neonatorum. In Oski FA (ed): Principles and Practice of Pediatrics. Philadelphia, JB Lippincott, 1994.*)

    (2) Sulfonamides and ceftriaxone displace bilirubin from albumin and should be avoided.

    (3) Chloramphenicol is no longer recommended for treatment of neonatal infection.

    (4) Third-generation cephalosporins are inactive against *Enterococcus, L. monocytogenes*, and many staphylococci.

5. **Other therapy. Granulocyte transfusions and intravenous immunoglobulin have been used in neonatal sepsis but are not recommended for routine use.**

6. **Prognosis.**

a. Depends on etiologic agent, timing of diagnosis and therapy, complications, and host factors.

b. The fatality rate is 10% to 15%, with substantial morbidity in surviving infants.

III. TORCH

A. DEFINITION.

Acronym used to focus on similarities in clinical presentation of intrauterine infections caused by toxoplasmosis (T), other (O), rubella (R),

22

INFECTION

cytomegalovirus (C), and herpes simplex virus (H). Congenital syphilis has been included by some, making the acronym TORCHES.

B. CLINICAL FEATURES ASSOCIATED WITH TORCH AGENTS (BOX 22-1).
1. Infections in newborns share common clinical findings and are clinically indistinguishable from each other.
2. Infected infants may be asymptomatic in the newborn period yet later develop disabling long-term sequelae.
3. Maternal infections are usually asymptomatic.
4. Diagnosis in the mother and newborn may require special laboratory tests.

C. DIAGNOSTIC EVALUATION.
A single TORCH titer is not a complete laboratory evaluation because there are many other agents that cause perinatal infections. The algorithm in **Fig. 22-3** gives an approach to the laboratory investigation of infants with suspected intrauterine infection.
1. The diagnosis of perinatal infection requires a synthesis of data obtained from the maternal history, the infant's physical examination, laboratory tests, and x-ray findings.
2. Despite detailed evaluation, a definite diagnosis cannot be made immediately because of the problem of passively transferred maternal IgG antibody and the technical difficulties of organism-specific IgM antibody tests.

Note: *Remember that the acronym TORCH does not go far enough. Among the perinatal infections that must often be considered and that TORCH does not include are coxsackievirus, enterovirus, hepatitis B and C, HIV, Listeria, parvovirus, and varicella.*

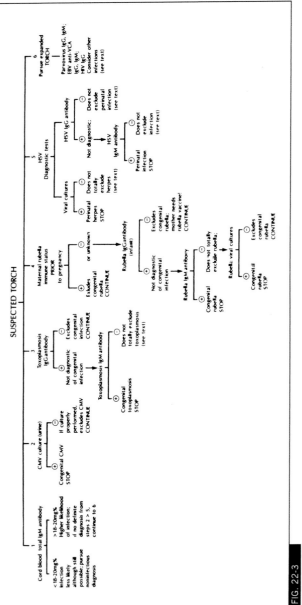

FIG. 22-3

An approach to the laboratory diagnosis of suspected TORCH infection in the neonate. EBV, Epstein-Barr virus; HIV, human immunodeficiency virus; HSV, herpes simplex virus; VCA, viral capsid antigen. *(From Kinney JS, Kumar ML* Clin Perinatol *15:727, 1988.)*

IV. VIRAL INFECTION

A. HSV.

1. **The causative agent for HSV is a DNA virus in the herpesvirus family with two antigenically and genomically distinct types.**
   a. Type 1 (HSV-1) usually involves the face and skin above the waist.
   b. Type 2 (HSV-2) involves the genitalia and skin below the waist.
   c. However, either type of virus can be found in either site.
2. **Epidemiology. The incidence of neonatal HSV infection is low; the estimated rate is approximately 1:3000 to 1:20,000 live births. The seroprevalence of HSV-2 increased 30% from 1976-1980 to 1988-1994, and now 1 in 5 persons older than the age of 12 has serologic evidence of having been infected with HSV-2.**
   a. Risk of neonatal HSV infection is highest (40% to 50%) in infants born vaginally to mothers with primary genital infection as opposed to mothers with recurrent genital infection (at most 3% to 5%).
   b. Most infants with HSV infection have been born to women without history or clinical findings of active herpetic infection during pregnancy.
3. **Transmission occurs in utero, intrapartum, or postnatally.**
   a. In utero infection is rare.
   b. Intrapartum transmission is the most common ($\approx$85% to 90% of cases) and occurs as the infant passes through the infected maternal genital tract or by ascending infection.
      (1) The incubation period is variable. Symptoms usually appear at the end of the first week of life but can appear shortly after birth or as late as 4 to 6 weeks.
      (2) HSV-2 accounts for most neonatal infections; however, 15% to 20% are caused by HSV-1.
   c. Postnatal transmission (less common) occurs from parents, hospital personnel, or an infected infant in the nursery.
4. **Clinical findings. Infants with HSV infection acquired intrapartum or postnatally can be divided into three categories:**
   a. Disease localized to skin, eye, or mouth, which has the lowest mortality rate.
   b. Encephalitis, with or without skin, eye, or mouth involvement.
   c. Disseminated infection with multiple organ system involvement (e.g., central nervous system [CNS], lung, liver, adrenals, skin, eye, mouth), which has the highest mortality and morbidity.

Note: *In utero infection results in the most severely afflicted infants; most common findings at birth: skin vesicles or skin scarring, eye disease (chorioretinitis and keratoconjunctivitis), microcephaly, or hydranencephaly.*

5. **Outcome.**
   a. Long-term prognosis after disseminated infection or encephalitis is poor. Approximately 50% of surviving children have varying degrees of

22

INFECTION

psychomotor retardation, microcephaly, hydranencephaly, porencephalic cysts, spasticity, blindness, chorioretinitis, or learning disabilities.

b. Disease localized to the skin, eye, or mouth is associated with multiple recurrences during the first 6 months of life. If there are three or more recurrences, there is a much higher risk of neurologic impairment (spastic quadriplegia, microcephaly, and blindness), which may not be apparent until 6 months to 1 year of life.

6. **Diagnostic evaluation (see Fig. 22-3).**
a. Virus isolation is the definitive method.
   (1) Obtain cultures from skin vesicles, mouth or nasopharynx, eyes, urine, and blood.
   (2) PCR is the definitive method for CSF and vitreous humor.
b. Serologic methods are not helpful because of the following:
   (1) Commonly available assays cannot distinguish between antibodies to HSV-1 and HSV-2.
   (2) The presence of passively acquired maternal IgG antibody.

7. **Treatment. Acyclovir and vidarabine are both effective; however, acyclovir is preferred.**
a. The recommended dose of acyclovir is 30 mg/kg per 24 hours in three divided intravenous doses. Some experts give high doses (45 to 60 mg/kg per day).
b. Duration of therapy has not been established; recommended minimum is 14 days.
c. Relapse of disease after therapy can occur.
d. Treat ocular infection with a topical ophthalmic drug (1% to 2% trifluridine, 1% iododeoxyuridine, or 3% vidarabine) in addition to parenteral antiviral therapy. Ophthalmologic consultation is advised.
e. The effectiveness of prophylactic antiviral therapy for exposed infants has not been determined.

8. **Prevention. Management of a pregnant mother with a history of herpes is in the province of obstetric professionals.**
a. Contact isolation is required for infants while in the nursery.
b. It is preferable to have the infant room in with his or her mother until discharge.

B. HBV.
1. **Epidemiology. HBsAg+ or HBeAg+ mothers have an 80% likelihood of transmitting the virus to their infants.**
a. Most infants will be asymptomatic, but 90% will become chronic HBV carriers if not given appropriate immunoprophylaxis.
b. Some groups of women are at particular risk for HBV infection **(Box 20-2)**.
2. **Transmission. Transplacental transmission is rare; HBV is usually transmitted during or shortly after delivery. Risk of transmission**

BOX 22-2

**U.S. PUBLIC HEALTH SERVICE'S CURRENT RECOMMENDATIONS
FOR PERINATAL SCREENING FOR HEPATITIS B SURFACE ANTIGEN**

1. Women of Asian, Pacific Island, or Alaskan Eskimo descent, whether immigrant or U.S. born
2. Women born in Haiti or sub-Saharan Africa
3. Women with histories of the following:
a. Acute or chronic liver disease
b. Work or treatment in a hemodialysis unit
c. Work or residence in an institution for the mentally retarded
d. Rejection as a blood donor
e. Blood transfusion on repeated occasions
f. Frequent occupational exposure to blood in medical and dental settings
g. Household contact with a carrier of hepatitis B virus or hemodialysis patient
h. Multiple episodes of venereal diseases
i. Percutaneous use of illicit drugs
j. Prostitution
k. Sexual partner of the above groups

From the Centers for Disease Control and Prevention: MMWR 34:313, 1985.

---

is greater if maternal infection is symptomatic or occurs late in pregnancy.

3. Clinical findings. The majority of infants are asymptomatic.
a. A small percentage (1% to 3%) are symptomatic, with jaundice and elevated liver function studies.
b. HBsAg carriers have an increased risk of developing hepatocellular carcinoma in later years.

4. Diagnosis. All pregnant women should be tested for HBsAg early in pregnancy. A positive HBsAg test result indicates current infection or the presence of a carrier state.
a. Mothers who have not received prenatal care should be tested at the time of delivery.
b. If the mother has not been tested and is not available for testing, it is essential that the infant be tested and treated appropriately.

5. Management of the infant born to an HBsAg+ mother includes immunoprophylaxis with HBV vaccine and hepatitis B immune globulin (HBIG).
a. HBIG, 0.5 ml intramuscularly, should be given as soon as possible, preferably within 12 hours.
b. If the infant is born to a high-risk mother whose HBsAg status is unknown, HBIG and vaccine should be given.
c. Administration of HBIG and HBV vaccine to an at-risk newborn is 90% effective in reducing the probability of chronic infection.

d. Regardless of maternal status, HBV vaccination should be initiated within 7 days of birth, preferably within 12 hours. Second and third doses are given 1 and 6 months after the first.
   (1) The dose is 0.5 ml intramuscularly for each vaccine product.
   (2) Infants should be tested at 9 months or later for HBsAg and anti-HBsAg. Immunoprophylaxis is not effective in 1% to 2% of cases.
e. Infants should be bathed immediately to remove maternal blood and secretions from delivery before any injections are administered. Universal precautions should be practiced. Mother and infant may room in.
f. There are no contraindications to breast-feeding for infants who have received immunoprophylaxis.
6. Preventive measures include prenatal screening of the mother and immunoprophylaxis of the infant.

C. HEPATITIS C VIRUS (HCV).
1. HCV is the most common form of non-A, non-B post-transfusion hepatitis; it is also a cause of sporadic non-A, non-B hepatitis.
2. This is an RNA virus in which infection is characterized by persistent viremia.
3. Perinatal and sexual transmission is uncommon; most cases of vertical transmission involve high-risk mothers (intravenous drug abuse, sexually transmitted diseases [STDs], coinfection with HIV, and transfusion recipient). The risk of perinatal transmission is correlated with maternal serum titer of HCV RNA and HIV coinfection.
4. Diagnostic laboratory tests.
a. Anti-HCV enzyme-linked immunosorbent assay (ELISA) and recombinant immunoblot assay (RIBA). IgG may be positive up to 18 months of age because of passive acquired maternal antibody.
b. HCV PCR is most sensitive but not readily available and is not standardized.
5. Treatment and recommendations.
a. No immunoprophylaxis is available for the prevention of perinatal disease.
b. At this time, breast-feeding is not contraindicated.

D. CYTOMEGALOVIRUS (CMV).
1. Causative agent. Human CMV is a DNA virus that belongs to the herpes virus group.
2. Epidemiology. CMV is ubiquitous and transmitted both horizontally (direct contact with virus-containing secretions, WBCs, or tissues) and vertically. Virus persists in latent form after primary infection, and reactivation can occur.
a. Three routes of vertical transmission.
   (1) Transplacental passage of maternal blood-borne virus.
   (2) At birth when descending through an infected maternal genital tract.
   (3) Postnatally by ingestion of CMV-positive breast milk.

b. Latent CMV may be carried in the WBCs and tissues of asymptomatic seropositive persons; thus recipients of seropositive blood, especially the preterm infant, are at risk.

3. Epidemiology of congenital CMV. Congenital CMV is the most common intrauterine infection (0.4% to 2.4% of all live births).

a. In the United States, 10% to 65% of childbearing-age women (depending on race and socioeconomic status) are seronegative and susceptible to primary CMV infection.

   (1) The rate of seroconversion during pregnancy is estimated to be between 1% and 2%.

   (2) Approximately 40% to 50% of pregnant women who develop primary CMV infection transmit the infection to the fetus.

b. Intrauterine infection can occur regardless of whether the mother had primary infection or reactivation during pregnancy; however, infants infected in utero during maternal reactivation are much less often affected than those exposed to maternal primary infection.

4. Clinical findings. About 95% of infected infants are asymptomatic at birth.

a. Between 10% and 20% develop mental retardation or sensorineural deafness (which is sometimes progressive).

b. Cytomegalic inclusion disease (CID), the most severe form, occurs in about 5% of infants infected in utero. Frequent findings include hepatosplenomegaly, jaundice, petechial rash/purpura, chorioretinitis, cerebral calcification, microcephaly, and sensorineural hearing loss.

c. In preterm infants, infection resulting from transfusion with CMV-seropositive blood has been associated with interstitial pneumonia.

d. Infection from the mother's virus-positive breast milk does not cause clinical disease, most likely because of the presence of passively transmitted maternal antibody; however, symptomatic disease can occur if a seronegative infant is fed CMV-positive milk from milk banks.

5. Diagnostic tests (see Fig. 22-3).

a. CMV can be isolated from urine, the pharynx, peripheral blood leukocytes, human milk, semen, cervical secretions, and other tissue and body fluids.

b. Proof of congenital infection requires positive viral cultures or a strongly positive CMV-IgM titer within 3 weeks of birth.

c. An abnormal computed tomography (CT) scan of the head in the newborn period is highly predictive of an adverse neurodevelopmental outcome in symptomatic CMV-infected neonates.

6. Treatment is supportive. However, there is evidence that a 6-week course of ganciclovir reduces the severity of hearing loss in symptomatic infants.

7. Prevention. No special precautions are recommended. Thorough hand washing after exposure to secretions is important.

a. Because approximately 1% of infants in newborn nurseries may excrete CMV and be asymptomatic, thorough hand washing should be practiced by all those in contact with infants.

22

INFECTION

b. Transmission of CMV to preterm infants via transfusion can be eliminated by the use of CMV-seronegative donors, by removal of the buffy coat, by freezing blood in glycerol before administration, or by filtration to remove the WBCs.

E. CONGENITAL RUBELLA.

1. Causative agent. An RNA virus classified as a rubivirus in the Togaviridae family.
2. Epidemiology. Humans are the source of infection. Postnatal rubella is transmitted via direct or droplet contact of respiratory secretions. The virus can be transmitted from secretions of a child with congenital rubella. Asymptomatic infection can occur. The occurrence of congenital rubella has sharply decreased as a result of routine vaccination in this country.
3. Transmission. Congenital rubella is transmitted in utero during the course of primary maternal infection; fetal infection early in pregnancy may result in teratogenesis or abortion. The risk of fetal infection and congenital anomalies decreases with increasing gestational age.
4. Clinical findings. The majority (≈68%) of neonatal infections are subclinical. Clinical findings are similar to those seen with other TORCH infections (see Box 22-1).
a. The most common abnormalities are growth retardation, cataracts, microphthalmia, glaucoma, chorioretinitis, patent ductus arteriosus, peripheral pulmonary artery stenosis, atrial or ventricular septal defects, microcephaly, mental retardation, and sensorineural deafness.
b. Infants classically have a "blueberry muffin" rash with thrombocytopenic purpura, jaundice, and hepatosplenomegaly.
5. Diagnosis (see Fig. 22-3).
a. Knowledge of maternal rubella immune status at onset of pregnancy or during previous pregnancies is the most helpful laboratory information. A positive maternal rubella test obtained late in pregnancy does not exclude rubella early in pregnancy.
b. Virus can be isolated from the throat, urine, and CSF. Infected infants shed virus in nasopharyngeal secretions and urine for years.
6. Management is supportive. Contact isolation is required for infants with congenital rubella or suspected infection.
7. Prevention. Routine prenatal or antepartum screening for rubella should be done.
a. Vaccine should be administered to susceptible women in the immediate postpartum period.
b. Breast-feeding is not contraindicated.

F. VARICELLA-ZOSTER (VZ) VIRUS.

1. Causative agent. VZ is caused by the herpesvirus that causes chicken-pox during primary infection and herpes zoster when reactivated.
a. VZ spreads by direct contact or by airborne droplet.
b. The incubation period is 14 to 16 days.

2. Clinical syndrome.

a. Maternal infection.

   (1) Infection with VZ during early pregnancy is uncommon (<5:10,000 pregnancies) and is associated with a risk of embryopathy of about 2% including hypoplastic extremities and digits, skin scarring, muscle atrophy, chorioretinitis, and cortical atrophy.

   (2) Maternal infection after the first trimester of pregnancy is associated with a lower risk to the fetus.

b. Peripartum infection.

   (1) Infants born to mothers with varicella onset within 5 days before or 2 days after delivery are exposed to the virus in the absence of maternal antibody.

   (2) Half of these infants develop varicella, with an increased risk of severe disease.

   (3) Fatality rate of neonatal varicella may be 5%.

   (4) Full-term newborn infants whose mothers develop varicella >5 days before or >2 days after delivery are not at increased risk of severe disease.

3. Diagnosis.

a. VZ infection must be suspected when there is a generalized vesicular rash, especially if there is a history of exposure to chickenpox or zoster.

b. A Tzanck smear of the vesicles may show giant cells with intranuclear inclusion bodies.

c. Viral cultures are usually positive within 3 to 4 days.

4. Treatment.

a. VZ immune globulin (VZIG) (125 units) should be given intramuscularly immediately after birth to newborns of mothers with varicella onset within 5 days before to 2 days after delivery.

b. Preterm infants (<28 weeks) who are exposed to VZ virus should receive VZIG regardless of maternal history because they may not have received maternal antibody transplacentally.

c. Acyclovir will reduce the severity of varicella and should be administered at 30 mg/kg per 24 hours in three equal doses for 7 days.

5. Prevention.

a. Infants with varicella-induced fetal malformations do not require isolation.

b. Infants exposed to maternal varicella should be isolated at birth and, if still hospitalized, until 21 or 28 days of age, depending on whether they received VZIG. Infants with acute varicella should be isolated for the duration of the vesicular rash.

c. A varicella vaccine has been licensed for routine use.

G. HIV.

1. Causative agent.

a. HIV infects many cells including T-helper lymphocytes and is the cause of acquired immunodeficiency syndrome (AIDS).

b. HIV is an RNA retrovirus that is transmitted from mother to infant transplacentally and also during birth and through breast milk.

c. The risk of perinatal infection of a child from an HIV-infected woman, in the absence of antiretroviral therapy, is estimated at 15% to 40%. With antenatal, perinatal, and postnatal antiretroviral therapies, the risk of transmission is as low as 2%.

d. The risk of transmission is increased with advanced maternal AIDS, higher viral loads, low CD4+ counts, and maternal vitamin A deficiency.

e. The incubation period of perinatally acquired AIDS is usually less than 2 years, but some infected infants do not present with symptoms until age 5 or older.

2. **Clinical syndrome. In the absence of maternal or infant antiretroviral therapy and depending on maternal CD4+ and HIV-RNA level, 10% to 15% of infants born to HIV-positive mothers demonstrate AIDS in early infancy with the following nonspecific signs:**

a. Low birthweight, failure to thrive.

b. Hepatosplenomegaly, lymphadenopathy.

c. Candidiasis.

d. Chronic diarrhea.

e. Persistent fever.

f. *Pneumocystis carinii* pneumonia (PCP).

g. Recurrent bacterial and viral infections.

3. **Approximately 15% to 20% of infants born to HIV-positive mothers present with illness later, typically with the following:**

a. Failure to thrive.

b. Lymphoid interstitial pneumonia.

c. Hepatosplenomegaly.

d. CNS abnormalities.

4. **Diagnosis.**

a. Diagnosis, although problematic, is necessary to identify the HIV-infected infant for observation, prophylaxis, and treatment.

b. All infants born to HIV-infected mothers acquire maternal IgG anti-HIV antibodies. Thus serology is not useful in determining the infant's status until about 18 months of age.

c. Advances in laboratory techniques for viral detection have made earlier diagnosis of the HIV-infected infant possible.

   (1) The sensitivity of HIV viral culture is the same as HIV-DNA and is 58% at 48 hours of life. It increases to 93% by 2 weeks and to 98% by 28 days.

   (2) The standard p24 antigen-capture assay and the immune-complex dissociated, p24 antigen-capture assay are highly specific, but the sensitivity is low; therefore, use of these assays alone is not currently recommended to exclude HIV infection.

   (3) The preferred method of diagnosing HIV infection in infants is the use of HIV PCR techniques. Culture is not routinely done.

BOX 22-3

ZIDOVUDINE REGIMEN FROM AIDS CLINICAL TRIALS GROUP PROTOCOL 076

Oral administration of 100 mg of zidovudine (ZDV) 5 times daily, initiated at 14-34 weeks of gestation and continued throughout the pregnancy.

During labor, intravenous administration of ZDV in a 1-hour loading dose of 2 mg/kg of body weight, followed by a continuous infusion of 1 mg/kg of body weight per hour until delivery.

Oral administration of ZDV to the newborn (ZDV syrup at 2 mg/kg of body weight per dose every 6 hours) for the first 6 weeks of life, beginning 8-12 hours after birth.

5. Prenatal management of HIV-infected mothers and their HIV-exposed infants. The AIDS Clinical Trials Group Protocol 076 ZDV regimen (Box 22-3) significantly reduces perinatal HIV transmission. Trials using protease inhibitors and reverse transcriptase inhibitors are under way.

6. Follow-up care of an infant born to an HIV-positive mother.

a. Infants should be followed closely. Complete blood count (CBC) and differential should be performed at birth as baseline and followed closely. PCR should be obtained within 48 hours of delivery. If positive, it should be repeated; if negative, it should be repeated at 14 days, at 1 to 2 months of age, and at 4 to 6 months.

b. PCP prophylaxis should be administered to all HIV-exposed infants in the first year of life until infection status is confirmed.

c. Once HIV infection has been confirmed in the infant, antiretroviral therapy should be started on the basis of current CDC guidelines, clinical signs and symptoms, and immune status, and PCP prophylaxis should be continued.

d. Infected infants should have serial CD4+ lymphocyte counts and determinations of viral load.

e. Studies of prophylactic intravenous immune globulin (IVIG) have shown efficacy in reduction of pyogenic infections.

f. Fever, cough, and dyspnea are common manifestations of *P. carinii* pneumonia, and this syndrome should be treated presumptively with intravenous trimethoprim-sulfamethoxazole.

g. Breast-feeding is considered by many to be contraindicated in resource-rich settings because there is an as yet unquantified risk of viral transmission through human milk; however, in underdeveloped countries, the benefit of breast-feeding is believed to outweigh any risk.

7. Expert opinion and knowledge about diagnosis and therapy are rapidly changing. It is recommended that consultation with specialists who care for HIV infection and who participate in clinical trials be undertaken.

H. ENTEROVIRUSES.

1. Causative agent. An RNA virus.

a. Viruses include 23 group A and 6 group B coxsackieviruses, 4 types of enteroviruses, and 31 echoviruses.

b. The viruses are ubiquitous and spread by the fecal–oral route. Infections are more common in summer and fall. Transmission to the newborn may be from the mother, other infants, or hospital staff.

c. The incubation period is 3 to 6 days.

2. Clinical syndromes.

a. Inapparent infection and mild febrile illness are the most common syndromes in neonates.

b. In newborn infants a sepsis-like syndrome may occur, with fever, lethargy, rash, and poor feeding. A severe septic shock syndrome with DIC has been reported.

c. Myocarditis and meningoencephalitis have been described, usually with coxsackieviruses. A severe form of hepatitis has been seen with echovirus.

3. Diagnosis.

a. Enteroviruses may be suspected on the basis of season, history of exposure, rash, and the incubation period.

b. Cultures of CSF, pharyngeal secretions, stool, and urine may yield virus.

c. PCR of CSF, nasopharyngeal secretions, or rectal swab is both sensitive and specific.

d. Because of the many different serotypes, serology usually is not helpful.

4. Treatment. There is no specific therapy for enteroviruses. Anecdotal reports of the use of human immunoglobulin to prevent spread in the nursery exist.

V. CONGENITAL TOXOPLASMOSIS

A. CAUSATIVE AGENT.
Toxoplasma gondii.

B. EPIDEMIOLOGY.
Involves a protozoan parasite that is ubiquitous and infects many warm-blooded animals, especially cats. In the United States, the estimated rate of symptomatic congenital toxoplasmosis is 1 to 4:1000 live births.

C. TRANSMISSION.
Humans become infected by ingestion of poorly cooked meats or sporulated oocysts in cat feces. Transmission from blood transfusion or organ donor can occur. The incubation period for acquired infection is 4 to 21 days. A fetus is infected by transplacental passage during maternal parasitemia.

1. Approximately 50% of infants born to mothers who seroconvert during pregnancy are infected; however, only 10% are symptomatic.

2. Prenatal diagnosis with PCR testing is rapid, safe, and accurate but not yet widely available.

D. CLINICAL FINDINGS.
Infants are frequently asymptomatic at birth. However, varying findings including maculopapular rash, generalized lymphadenopathy,

hepatosplenomegaly, thrombocytopenia, CSF pleocytosis, microcephaly, chorioretinitis, cerebral calcification, and interstitial pneumonitis may be present.

E. OUTCOME CAN BE POTENTIALLY DEVASTATING AND MAY RANGE FROM SEVERE MORBIDITY AND MORTALITY TO SUBTLE FINDINGS TO ASYMPTOMATIC.

Long-term sequelae include hydrocephalus (or microcephaly), chorioretinitis with visual difficulty, convulsions, and varying degrees of impairment of cognitive development, all as a result of intrauterine meningoencephalitis.

F. POSTNATAL DIAGNOSIS (SEE FIG. 22-3).
1. If possible, isolation of organism from placenta.
2. Fluorescent antibody tests for IgM often give false-positive results. If available, ELISA techniques to detect specific IgG and IgM are preferred; comparison with mother's serum is always necessary. There may be transplacental transfer of IgG antibodies in an uninfected neonate; in that event, these will disappear, and IgM antibodies, which are not placentally transferable, will not appear as time goes by if they are not present at birth.
3. An infectious disease consultation is recommended. Sensitivities and specificities of this group of tests make this a tricky workup.

G. TREATMENT.
1. Optimal treatment has not been established. Guidelines are shown in Box 22-4. Neurologic and developmental outcomes are significantly better for treated children compared with those who are not treated.
2. Pharmacologic treatment includes a combination of pyrimethamine and sulfadiazine or trisulfapyrimidine with folinic acid to prevent bone marrow suppression. Spiramycin should be given; however, in the United States spiramycin is available only by request to the Food and Drug Administration. CBC and platelet counts should be monitored twice weekly.
3. Corticosteroids (prednisone or methylprednisolone) should be added for patients with chorioretinitis, a high level of CSF protein, generalized infection, or jaundice.
4. Duration of therapy has not been established. An infectious disease consultation should be obtained.
5. Isolation in the nursery is not necessary.

H. PREVENTION.
Pregnant women with negative or unknown serostatus should avoid contact with cat feces or avoid cats altogether (e.g., working in gardens) and should not eat uncooked meat.

22

INFECTION

BOX 22-4

GUIDELINES FOR THE TREATMENT OF CONGENITAL TOXOPLASMOSIS

DRUGS

1. Pyrimethamine + sulfadiazine:
- Pyrimethamine: 15 mg/m^2 per day or 1 mg/kg per day (maximum daily dose is 25 mg) orally. Although the half-life of the drug is 4 to 5 days, it should be given on a daily basis unless breaking of the tablets is grossly inaccurate during preparation of the smaller doses. Then, as with small infants (e.g., when a daily dose of 3 mg is indicated), breaking of a tablet may result in a slightly higher dose, which could be administered every 2 days.
- Sulfadiazine or trisulfapyrimidines: 85 mg/kg per day by the oral route in 2 divided doses daily.
2. Spiramycin: 100 mg/kg per day by the oral route in 2 divided doses.
3. Corticosteroids (prednisone or methylprednisolone): 1.5 mg/kg per day by the oral route in 2 divided doses daily. Continue until the inflammatory process (e.g., high level of CSF protein [100 mg/dl before the age of 1 month or older], chorioretinitis) has subsided; dosage should then be tapered progressively and discontinued.
4. Folinic acid: 5 mg every 3 days (intramuscularly in young infants) during treatment with pyrimethamine. If bone-marrow toxicity occurs at this dose, increase to 10 mg every 3 days. If bone-marrow toxicity is severe, discontinue pyrimethamine until the abnormality is corrected, and then begin pyrimethamine again using 10 mg folinic acid every 3 days. In some infants, it may be necessary to administer folinic acid more frequently.

INDICATIONS

1. Overt congenital toxoplasmosis: Treatment is for 1 year in all cases. For infants in whom clinical signs of infection are present, treatment during the first 6 months is with pyrimethamine + sulfadiazine. During the following 6 months, 1 month of pyrimethamine + sulfadiazine is alternated with 1 month of spiramycin. Folinic acid should be started as soon as possible. *No treatment is usually given after 12 months of age except when there is evidence of evolution of the infection such as a flare-up of chorioretinitis.*
2. Overt congenital toxoplasmosis with evidence of inflammatory process (chorioretinitis, high level of CSF protein, generalized infection, jaundice): Treatment is as in #1 + corticosteroids.
3. Subclinical congenital Toxoplasma infection: Pyrimethamine + sulfadiazine for 6 weeks; thereafter, alternate with spiramycin. Spiramycin is given for 6 weeks, alternated with 4 weeks of pyrimethamine + sulfadiazine to complete treatment for 1 year.

BOX 22-4—Cont'd

GUIDELINES FOR THE TREATMENT OF CONGENITAL TOXOPLASMOSIS

DRUGS

4. Healthy newborn in whom serologic testing has not provided definitive results but maternal infection was proved to have been acquired during pregnancy: One course of pyrimethamine + sulfadiazine for 1 month. Consultation with appropriate authority to determine necessity for continued therapy and drug and dosage regimen. *Decision to be made on an individual basis depends on multiple factors including serologic test titers, immune load, and clinical findings.*

5. Healthy newborn born to a mother with high Sabin-Feldman dye test titer and date of maternal infection undetermined: Spiramycin for 1 month. Then regimen is as in #4. In certain cases the indication for treatment is difficult to define because of a lack of information about the pregnancy and lack of isolation attempts from the corresponding placenta.

From Remington JS, Desmonts G: Toxoplasmosis. In Remington JS, Klein JO (eds): *Infectious Diseases of the Fetus and Newborn Infant*, ed 4. Philadelphia, WB Saunders, 1995.

22

INFECTION

VI. CONGENITAL SYPHILIS

A. CAUSATIVE AGENT.

Treponema pallidum (spirochete).

B. INCIDENCE.

Once common, congenital syphilis is much less so since the penicillin era. However, there has been a significant recent increase (100-fold since 1985) as a result of poor or absent prenatal care, poverty, and drug abuse.

C. PATHOLOGIC BASIS.

Transplacental invasion of the fetus with treponemes occurs in utero and may cause abortion as early as 2 to 3 months of pregnancy; it involves septicemic spread, with potential spirochetal invasion of every body part.

Note: *Several spirochetes may be transmitted across the placenta (e.g., recent anecdotal evidence for* Borrelia burgdorferi *(Lyme disease) suggests clinically significant neurologic disease not unlike that with congenital syphilis. Other anomalies (cardiovascular, syndactyly) have also been associated.*

D. CLINICAL FINDINGS.

Half of affected infants are asymptomatic at birth. Depending on the in utero timing of the infection and the extent of spread, the clinical picture may be a combination of some or all of the following:

1. In the child with clinical disease.

a. Can be severe, even fatal.

b. Prematurity; small for gestational age (SGA).

c. Skin rash (may involve palms and soles), maculopapular or vesiculobullous.

d. Hepatomegaly, splenomegaly.

e. Jaundice.

f. Anemia (hemolytic, Coombs test result negative), thrombocytopenia, leukocytosis.

g. Persistent snuffles (nasal discharge).

h. Long-bone invasion (metaphyseal osteochondritis in the first few weeks, diaphyseal periostitis later).

   (1) Periosteal elevation.

   (2) Epiphyseal disruption (e.g., bones of the forearm).

   (3) Radiolucencies (e.g., bones of the hand).

i. Condylomata lata (particularly in moist creases).

j. Meningitis (frequent); invasion by treponemes may be unaccompanied by increased CSF cellularity or positive Venereal Disease Research Laboratory (VDRL) test result.

k. Pneumonia (infrequent).

2. In the unusual event of an infant *acquiring* syphilis on passage through the birth canal, the familiar stages of adult syphilis are possible in the absence of treatment; no manifestations, however, are noted in the immediate neonatal period.

E. DIAGNOSIS (FIG. 22-4).

1. Study neonates whose mothers are seropositive and who have the following characteristics:

a. Have untreated syphilis.

b. Were treated within 4 weeks of delivery.

c. Were treated with a drug other than penicillin.

d. Did not show a serologic response to treatment.

e. Did not have appropriate follow-up to treatment.

f. Have a treatment or diagnostic status that is in any way uncertain.

Note: *Defer discharge of any infant for whom serologic status of the infant or mother is uncertain.*

2. Serologic tests for syphilis.

a. VDRL.

b. Rapid plasma reagin (RPR). Nontreponemal screening tests; detect antibody to a cardiolipin; reported at the highest fully reactive dilution; sensitivities and specificities cannot be *fully* trusted; particularly prone to false-positive results (e.g., in the presence of autoimmune disease).

c. Treponemal tests.

   (1) Fluorescent treponemal antibody absorption test (FTA-ABS), performed on 19S fraction of serum IgM.

   (2) Microhemagglutination test for *T. pallidum* (MHA-TP); reliable but not absolute; once positive, will always be positive.

Note: *These tests are similar; to use both is redundant.*

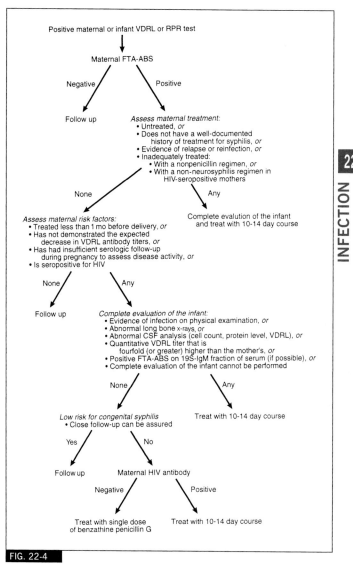

FIG. 22-4

Algorithm for management of a newborn infant born to a mother with positive nontreponemal (VDRL or RPR) test result. *(From Ikeda MK, Jenson HB: J Pediatr 117:843, 1990.)*

      (3) *T. pallidum* immobilization (TPI) test.
      (4) Treponemal tests are also positive in other spirochetal diseases
         (e.g., yaws, Lyme disease).

Note: *IgM does not cross placenta; IgM antibodies are the infant's; beware: often unreliable specificity, sensitivity about 89%.*

  d. Dark-field microscopy of available fresh discharges.
     (1) With acquired syphilis, usually possible from chancres or skin
        lesions; sensitive and specific in *experienced* hands; in congenital
        syphilis, usually possible with condylomata or vesicular lesions.
     (2) Dark-field examination of the placenta is indicated for persons at risk
        for HIV infection or for those who might not develop an immune
        response for other reasons.
  e. Direct fluorescent antibody staining of acetone-fixed exudate.

3. Guiding principles.
  a. Adequate diagnosis relies on full knowledge of the mother's disease
    status. Transmission of infection occurs almost 100% of the time during
    primary and secondary stages, usually well within 1 year of appearance
    of the chancre, but only 10% of the time during late syphilis. If the
    disease has been discovered and treated during or before pregnancy,
    approach the infant as if therapy has failed.
  b. Careful examination should be conducted for clinical findings;
    unexplained fever alone may be a clue.
  c. Perform RPR or VDRL on the baby's venous blood (do not use cord
    blood).
  d. Conclude that the infant has congenital syphilis if the titer of the
    infant's screening test equals or is greater than the mother's or if
    there is compelling clinical evidence. If there is uncertainty, obtain
    the following:
     (1) Long-bone x-rays (for periostitis or osteochondritis).
     (2) Chest x-ray (for pneumonitis).
     (3) Lumbar puncture (for CSF cell count, protein level, and
        VDRL test).
  e. If the mother has disease but the baby's workup does not suggest
    infection, watch without treatment. If the baby's screening titers are
    initially clearly lower than the mother's, repeat tests at 1- to 2-month
    intervals until negative, which is most often by 6 months. Consider for
    treatment, however, if follow-up is uncertain. Do not hesitate to seek
    consultation in the event of uncertainty.

F. TREATMENT AND SUBSEQUENT MANAGEMENT.
Newborns require treatment when there is *any* indication of active disease,
uncertainty about the mother's status or treatment history, concern about
inadequate or inappropriate maternal treatment (drugs other than

penicillin), treatment in the last 4 weeks of pregnancy, the possibility of reinfection, or the anticipation of doubtful compliance.
1. For an asymptomatic neonate who has clear CSF and nontreponemal titers greater than the mother's, give intramuscular procaine penicillin 50,000 U/kg as a single daily dose for 10 days.
2. For symptomatic or asymptomatic neonates with abnormal CSF (with or without reactive CSF VDRL, elevated cell count, or protein), give intramuscular procaine penicillin 50,000 U/kg as a single daily dose for 10 to 14 days; repeat spinal tap in 6 months and, if still positive, retreat fully.

Note: *Anticipate Jarisch-Herxheimer reaction, a temperature elevation, several hours after the first dose of penicillin; this is most often transient and does not require cessation of therapy.*

3. Repeat VDRL or RPR at 1, 2, 4, 6, and 12 months until there is a significant drop in titer; decrease should be fourfold in 3 months, eightfold in 6 months; FTA-ABS remains positive and cannot be used in follow-up.
4. Retreat if drop in titer does not occur after third repeat test, titer increases, or clinical findings persist or intensify.
5. Repeat spinal tap in 6 months if it was initially abnormal, or as needed in the event of worsening clinical findings, and every 6 months thereafter until the findings are all clear.
6. All infants with certain or uncertain diagnosis should be reported to the health department (mother and her contacts will need follow-up).

Note: *An infant successfully treated for congenital syphilis is not immune and may later contract acquired syphilis. Follow-up education and monitoring are important.*

VII. TUBERCULOSIS (CONGENITAL AND ACQUIRED)

A. DEFINITIONS.
1. Congenital TB: infection in utero.
2. Acquired TB: infection during or after delivery.

B. CAUSATIVE AGENTS.
1. *Mycobacterium tuberculosis* (most common).
2. Bovine and atypical organisms (rare).

C. INCIDENCE.
TB is rare in the newborn. Detection in early weeks suggests congenital acquisition or infection at delivery via inhalation or aspiration of infected amniotic fluid or bacilli. Women who have pulmonary TB are at risk to infect their infant after delivery.

D. PATHOLOGY.

1. Infection occurs via respiration; the breathing in of infected amniotic fluid or vaginal secretions leads to a primary complex in lungs.
2. Infection via the umbilical vein leads to a primary complex in the hepatic structures, with likelihood of miliary spread to multiple sites including the brain and serosal surfaces. Most congenital TB is the result of hematogenous spread.

E. DIAGNOSTIC CONFIRMATION.

1. Examine the placenta for tuberculous granulomas (note that their presence does not necessarily indicate disease in the infant).
2. Stain tracheal or gastric aspirates for acid-fast organisms.
3. Culture aspirates and, when indicated, bone marrow, urine, or suggestive nodes.
4. Chest x-ray (a negative x-ray does not rule out disease).
5. A Mantoux skin test (5 TU PPD) is of doubtful value but is a necessary step; a positive test result may be delayed several weeks or may never occur.
6. LP (examination and culture of CSF are necessary for appropriate assessment of the CNS).
7. Drug susceptibilities of an organism recovered from the mother should be determined. These results will help direct therapy.

F. MANAGEMENT OF THE INFANT BORN TO A MOTHER WITH TB OR INTO A TB-POSITIVE HOUSEHOLD.

1. Immediate separation at birth is controversial; it is strongly recommended by some and avoided by others. If it proves necessary, keep this period to a minimum.
2. Confirmation should be made of the presence or absence of infection in other household occupants.
3. A diagnostic workup should be done to seek out infant infection.
4. Specific clinical situations.
 a. Mother (or other household contact) with a positive tuberculin skin test reaction and no evidence of current disease.
  (1) Test infant with Mantoux test (5 TU PPD) at 4 to 6 weeks of age and at 3 to 4 months of age.
  (2) If family or mother cannot be tested immediately and situation is high risk for possible TB, consider treating infant with isoniazid (INH) (10 mg/kg per day) pending skin testing of family.
  (3) Mother should also be considered for INH preventive therapy. Breast-feeding is not contraindicated.
 b. Mother with latent disease or disease that has been treated for ≥ 2 weeks and who is considered noncontagious at delivery.
  (1) Investigate household members and extended family.
  (2) Chest x-ray and Mantoux test should be done at 4 to 6 weeks of age; if negative, repeat at 3 to 4 months of age and at 6 months.

(3) Begin INH (10 mg/kg per day). Once family has been investigated and skin test at 3 to 4 months is negative, INH can be discontinued.

(4) If mother is compliant with therapy, separation of infant and mother is not indicated. Breast-feeding is not contraindicated. However, if mother is noncompliant with therapy, Bacille Calmette-Guérin (BCG) vaccine may be considered for infant. Response to vaccine in infants may be inadequate for prevention of TB.

c. Mother with current disease and who is considered contagious at time of delivery.

(1) Infant and mother should be separated until mother begins therapy and is considered noncontagious.

(2) Management is the same as previously outlined.

d. Mother with hematogenous-spread TB.

(1) Congenital TB in the infant is possible. Infant should have Mantoux test and chest x-ray. Begin treatment immediately with INH (10 to 15 mg/kg per day), pyrazinamide (20 to 40 mg/kg per day), rifampin (10 to 20 mg/kg per day), and streptomycin (20 to 40 mg/kg per day) if diagnosis is suspected.

(2) If diagnosis is confirmed, treat with INH, rifampin, pyrazinamide, and streptomycin daily for 2 months and INH and rifampin daily for 10 months. Infectious disease consultation is necessary.

(3) If infant's chest x-ray, skin test, or clinical findings do not support diagnosis of congenital TB, infant should be separated from mother (until she is judged noncontagious) and INH (10 mg/kg per day) should be initiated until 6 months of age. If skin test is positive at 6 months of age, INH should be continued for a total of 12 months.

5. When TB or the possibility of TB is present, always make an effort to ascertain the HIV status of the mother and infant. In the event of a positive finding, act accordingly.

VIII. NEONATAL MASTITIS

A. CAUSATIVE AGENTS (IN USUAL ORDER OF FREQUENCY).

1. Staphylococci, particularly *S. aureus.*
2. *Group B streptococcus.*
3. E. coli.
4. *Pseudomonas aeruginosa.*
5. *Proteus species.*
6. Salmonella.

B. SOURCE.

Probable invasion of breast ductal system by skin flora.

C. FREQUENCY.

Unusual.

D. TIME OF ONSET.
Age 2 to 4 weeks; rarely within first week.

E. CLINICAL FINDINGS.
1. Erythema.
2. Swelling, more often firm than fluctuant.
3. Tenderness.
4. Unilateral nipple discharge (occasionally bilateral).
5. Abscess formation (uncommon).

F. DIFFERENTIAL DIAGNOSIS.
1. Milk stasis (witch's milk), hormonally induced (passive transfer from mother).
2. Hormonally induced breast development; usually bilateral, not necessarily symmetrical; absence of significant erythema or tenderness.

G. LABORATORY STUDIES.
1. If milk can be expressed.
a. Gram stain.
b. Culture and sensitivity.
c. Leukocyte count ($>10^6$/ml is significant).
2. If there is fluctuation.
a. Aspirate for smear, culture, sensitivities (incision and drainage to be performed by surgeon).
b. Blood culture.
c. CBC count.
3. If there is nipple discharge of any kind, obtain smear, culture, and sensitivities.

H. TREATMENT.
1. Pending cultures.
a. Give oxacillin, 50 mg/kg per 24 hours intravenously or intramuscularly (divided into 8-hour doses for infants >2 kg and 12-hour doses for infants <2 kg).
b. Gentamicin, 2.5 mg/kg intramuscularly every 12 hours in full-term babies.
c. Further therapy depends on results of culture, sensitivities, and clinical status.
d. For resistant *S. aureus*, use vancomycin, 15 mg/kg intravenously every 12 hours (potential nephrotoxicity and ototoxicity; as with gentamicin, requires careful monitoring of serum levels).
e. If streptococcus is cultured, begin administration of potassium penicillin G, 50,000 to 100,000 U/kg per 24 hours, divided into 12-hour doses intravenously or intramuscularly (for infants <2 kg); 50,000 to 150,000 U/kg per 24 hours, divided into 8-hour doses intravenously or intramuscularly (for infants >2 kg).
f. Hospitalization is appropriate at least until infection is clearly controlled.

IX. MATERNAL MASTITIS

A. CLINICAL FINDINGS.
1. Flulike symptoms.
2. Fever.
3. Erythematous, tender areas in one or both breasts.

B. MANAGEMENT.
1. Rest (if possible).
2. Warm compresses for 10 to 15 minutes, 3 to 4 times a day.
3. Frequent nursing, such as every $1\frac{1}{2}$ to 3 hours. This is necessary to prevent stasis and abscess development and to relieve engorgement.

Note: *Breast abscesses can develop. An obstetrician or surgeon should guide management and judgment regarding drainage and antibiotics. In the event of drainage, nursing may be temporarily interrupted on the affected breast until it is healed. The mother must continue pumping breast milk to maintain an adequate milk supply.*

X. OMPHALITIS (PRIMARY INFECTION OF THE UMBILICAL CORD)

A. CAUSATIVE AGENTS.
1. Group A streptococcus, most commonly.
2. *S. aureus.*

B. THE USUAL EXPECTATION FOR THE UMBILICAL STUMP.
(1) It dries, (2) becomes a hard, dark-brown eschar, (3) separates in about 2 weeks, and (4) epithelializes in about 3 to 4 weeks.

Note: *Ordinarily, the cord has two arteries and one vein; if there is only one artery, suspect a congenital abnormality, particularly with the kidney, but there is no extra susceptibility to infection.*

C. CLINICAL FINDINGS IN VARIOUS COMBINATIONS.
1. Erythema of varying diameters ringing cord.
2. Thickened underlying skin.
3. Purulent discharge.
4. Foul-smelling discharge.
5. Moist, fetid cord and bleeding suggest group A *Streptococcus* or *S. aureus* infection.

Note: *A palpably thickened falciform ligament (a direct route to the liver) is ominous.*

D. MAJOR CONCERNS.
1. Extension beyond immediate area of the cord.
2. Cellulitis, fasciitis of the abdominal wall.
3. Peritonitis.

22

INFECTION

4. Bacteremia/sepsis, meningitis.
5. Tetanus neonatorum.
6. Gas gangrene.
7. Ascending infection, umbilical vein to liver and portal system.
a. Portal vein thrombosis.
b. Portal hypertension.
c. Liver abscess.

E. DIFFERENTIAL DIAGNOSIS.
1. Delayed healing/umbilical granuloma (small, reddened mass; slight purulent discharge; no surrounding erythema).
a. May be the result of infection or irritation from clumps of talcum powder.
b. Silver nitrate stick application (one to several times over 2 to 3 weeks) is both diagnostic and therapeutic; failure to subside with this therapy suggests infection or other complication. Some pediatricians prefer cleansing with alcohol and sprinkling with table salt for 2 to 3 days.
2. Embryonic remnants.
a. Allantois (passage of urine through umbilicus). Methylene blue dye placed in umbilicus will be voided in urine.
b. Vitelline duct.
   (1) Passage of gas and feces through the umbilicus. Carmine red dye given orally and passed through the umbilicus confirms enteric fistula.
   (2) Mass, larger and redder than granuloma, unresponsive to silver nitrate, may be intestinal mucosa or polyp.
c. Umbilical hernia. Generally, skin is well healed.
3. Meconium-stained umbilical stump is suggestive of fetal distress and not necessarily of umbilical infection.

F. LABORATORY STUDIES.
1. Gram stain should be done of any discharge.
2. Culture and sensitivities should always be obtained when suspicious of infection.
3. CBC with differential and blood culture should be performed if there is more than a simple ring of erythema.
4. A spinal tap may be indicated, depending on the baby's clinical status.

G. THERAPY.
1. In the event of a simple ring of erythema in an otherwise clinically well child (often the case), no antibiotics are provided pending culture results (by then, erythema often will have ebbed or subsided).
2. In the event of more serious findings and until laboratory studies are available, treat promptly with the following:
a. Oxacillin, 50 mg/kg per 24 hours intravenously or intramuscularly, administered every 4 to 6 hours for infants >2 kg and every 12 hours for infants <2 kg.

b. Gentamicin, 2.5 mg/kg intramuscularly every 12 hours in term babies.

c. Adjust therapy according to culture results and clinical status; resistant *S. aureus* suggests use of vancomycin, 15 mg/kg intravenously or intramuscularly every 12 hours (potential nephrotoxicity and ototoxicity; as with gentamicin, requires careful monitoring of serum levels); clinical indication of tetanus neonatorum suggests use of potassium penicillin G.

d. Topical antibiotics are not necessary.

3. Hospitalization is indicated until the need for treatment is clarified; rehospitalization after discharge is not usually necessary in the event of a simple ring of erythema.

H. PREVENTION.

1. Topical antibiotic ointments are inappropriate.
2. Application of triple dye.
3. Alcohol wipe with diaper changes.
4. Sponge bathe with mild, nonperfumed soap; leave area dry and uncovered. Do not handle cord.

Note: *It is probably best to leave the cord alone; the more it is bothered, the longer it will hang on. There is a suggestion that some colonization speeds the process of detachment and subsequent healing. Some cords may fail to separate when expected; if the time stretches beyond 2 to 3 weeks, suspect some defect in neutrophil mobility. Do not force separation. If problem continues, neutrophil studies are in order.*

XI. CANDIDIASIS

A. CAUSATIVE AGENT.

Candida species (e.g., *C. albicans, C. pseudotropicalis, C. stellatoides, C. tropicalis, C. parapsilosis*).

B. OCCURRENCE.

Candidiasis occurs anywhere in the body (including the umbilical cord).

Note: *In a singleton delivery with membranes intact, Candida may still be found in 6% of amniotic fluids.*

C. SOURCES OF NEONATAL INFECTION.

1. Mother's vagina during delivery.
2. Intrauterine, ascending from birth canal.
3. Other person-to-person contact (it is ubiquitous).
4. Indwelling intravascular catheters; other instruments.

22

INFECTION

D. CLINICAL FINDINGS.

The incubation period is unknown; however, if lesions are present at birth or within a few hours, infection is intrauterine, ascending from the vagina; if lesions are noted after 3 to 4 days or up to a week after birth, infection occurred during delivery. Lesions localized to the mouth or skin tend to be benign, with the birth canal as the source; dissemination is more likely to follow some invasive procedure and to be nosocomial.

1. Diffuse, maculopapular, erythematous, possibly pustular rash or mucous membrane lesions may be present at birth; they can coalesce into white, cheesy, adherent patches; early lesions may be vesicular with an areola of erythema; lesions are likely to be found in warm, moist areas, particularly the diaper area.
2. Poor feeding, regurgitation, vomiting, hematemesis (esophagitis).
3. Notably, significant skin involvement is not usually accompanied by systemic (e.g., pulmonary) involvement.
4. Infants at increased risk.
   a. Very-low-birth-weight (VLBW).
   b. Other congenital infections.
   c. Abdominal surgery.
   d. Central lines (indwelling intravascular catheters).
   e. Maternal drug abuse.
   f. Prolonged use of broad-spectrum antibiotics.
   g. Immunosuppressive drugs (e.g., corticosteroids).
   h. Immunodeficiency states.
5. VLBW infants may have the following characteristics of sepsis in whole or in part:
   a. Apnea.
   b. Bradycardia.
   c. Temperature instability.
   d. Shock.
   e. Hypoglycemia; less frequently, hyperglycemia.
   f. Glycosuria.
6. No part of the body is safe (e.g., lungs, kidneys, joints, bones [often nosocomial], gastrointestinal [GI] tract [necrotizing enterocolitis], deep or subcutaneous tissues [abscesses]) as a result of penetration of minor vessels, thrombosis, or hematogenous spread. The most common sites include the following:
   a. Oral candidiasis (thrush), most often localized and benign, complicated occasionally by esophagitis and GI colonization.
   b. Skin.
   c. GI tract.

E. DIAGNOSIS IS OFTEN DIFFICULT.

With *extensive* clinical involvement, up to 35% of cases are discovered only at postmortem. The majority of the remainder are diagnosed too late for effective treatment. Laboratory tests to be considered include the following:

1. Culture: blood agar, Sabouraud medium.

Note: *Candida in any body fluid or discharge is not to be disregarded, and not to be considered a contaminant.*

2. Urinalysis: about 6% are positive; half of these are culture positive.
3. KOH preparation of skin scrapings (shows pseudomycelia, spores, pseudohyphae).
4. Gram stain of buffy coats (shows budding yeast spores).
5. Additional tests that are occasionally indicated include the following:
a. Indirect ophthalmoscopy.
b. Lung biopsy (pneumonia).
c. Echocardiography (endocarditis).
d. Renal ultrasound (positive urine).
e. Spinal tap.

Note: *CSF may show nothing in the presence of meningitis.*

f. CT (brain abscess).

F. TREATMENT.

1. Oral. Nystatin suspension, 200,000 U twice a day for 5 to 10 days. Continue until 3 days after thrush is gone.
2. Cutaneous. Nystatin ointment twice a day for 7 to 10 days; nystatin ointment with a corticosteroid should be used in severe cases. A topical or systemic antibiotic should be used if there is a secondary bacterial infection.
3. Systemic. Amphotericin B, 0.5 to 1 mg/kg intravenously; the duration of treatment is determined by the severity of illness and clinical and microbiologic response; usually approximately 4 weeks of treatment is required for disseminated candidiasis.

Note: *Infectious disease consultation for the development and implementation of an amphotericin-based management plan is strongly recommended.*

a. Caution. Side effects include cardiac arrhythmias, hypokalemia, renal toxicity, and anemia.
b. Monitor serum electrolytes, blood urea nitrogen (BUN) (discontinue with elevated BUN), and creatinine levels.
4. 5-Fluorocytosine (never give alone in infants; use only as an additional drug in severe cases); 50 to 150 mg/kg per 24 hours orally in divided doses every 6 hours. Monitor CBC and liver enzymes.
5. Meningitis. Treat as for any other systemic involvement; intrathecal amphotericin B *may* be necessary; use is controversial and should always be preceded by consultation.

6. Bladder infection. Kidney flush with amphotericin B *may* be necessary, again only after consultation.

XII. GUIDELINES FOR INFECTION CONTROL IN NURSERIES

A. ASSESSMENT.

1. Obtain mother's obstetric history from obstetrics database and delivery record.
2. Consult with labor and delivery staff about pertinent information related to the infant's need for isolation.
3. Observe infant for signs and symptoms of infectious disease during all contact with the infant.

B. INTERVENTION.

1. Universal precautions should be observed at all times by all staff of the nursery during all routine care (see section on universal precautions later in this chapter). Strict adherence to universal precautions when caring for infants and children cannot be overemphasized. Patients with known risks should be identified in accordance with hospital policy. It should be noted that caregivers who assume no identified risk and who do not comply with universal precautions place themselves, their patients, and their families at increased risk for acquiring disease.
2. For the neonate, most isolettes serve as an isolation facility and a separate room is not necessary.
3. All specimens sent to the clinical laboratory should be bagged and labeled with the appropriate type of isolation (e.g., by color-coded sticker label); individual nurseries may have different categories of isolation.
4. Contact isolation. Gowns are indicated if soiling is likely; gloves are indicated for touching infective material.
   a. Herpes simplex.
      (1) The infant with active herpes simplex should be isolated in an isolette, with gown and glove technique used.
      (2) The infant born by cesarean section to a mother with herpes without rupture of membranes before delivery requires no isolation.
      (3) The infant of a mother with active herpes lesions at the time of delivery should be identified as requiring thorough hand washing after all contact.
   b. S. aureus.
      (1) Place infant in isolette and use gown and glove precautions during all care. Careful hand washing before and after every patient contact is mandatory.
      (2) If organism is methicillin resistant, strict contact isolation is necessary.
   c. Skin infection.
   d. Colonization with gram-negative bacilli.
   e. Impetigo.

f. Conjunctivitis.

g. Gonorrhea.

5. Blood and body fluid secretions. Universal precautions are emphasized.

a. Hepatitis B and C.

(1) At-risk infants should be bathed immediately to remove maternal blood and secretions.

(2) Isolation of infants born to HBsAg+ mothers is not necessary, but their blood should be carefully handled with blood precautions.

(3) Infant may remain in bassinet.

(4) Gloves should be used for admission procedures and blood drawing.

(5) All specimens to laboratory should be labeled *blood and body secretion precautions*.

b. AIDS.

(1) Scrupulously follow universal precautions during all care.

(2) Eye protection should be worn whenever spattering of blood or body secretions is likely such as during delivery, arterial puncture, suctioning, rinsing of used surgical instruments, LP, and intubation.

6. Drainage/secretion precautions. Gowns are indicated if soiling is likely. Gloves should be used for touching infective material. Articles contaminated with infective material should be discarded or bagged and labeled before being sent for processing.

a. Syphilis.

(1) Precautions are not necessary if no lesions are present.

(2) If lesions are present, the infant should be isolated in an isolette.

b. Conjunctivitis, minor or limited abscesses, or wound infections that result in infective purulent material, drainage, or secretion require precautions.

7. Enteric isolation. Gloves are indicated if soiling is likely. Gloves are indicated for touching infective material. Hands must be washed after touching the patient or potentially contaminated articles and before taking care of another patient. Articles contaminated with infective material should be discarded or bagged and labeled before being sent for decontamination.

a. Hepatitis A. Isolation of the infant born to a mother with hepatitis A is not necessary unless the mother is jaundiced at time of delivery.

b. Necrotizing enterocolitis.

8. Strict isolation. Masks, gowns, and gloves are indicated for all persons entering the room. Hands must be washed after touching the patient or potentially contaminated articles and before taking care of another patient. Articles contaminated with infective material should be discarded or bagged and labeled before being sent for decontamination and reprocessing. Procedures for patients infected with the Varicella (chickenpox) virus include the following:

a. For a mother who reports exposure to varicella before delivery, the time of exposure and the mother's state of immunity must be

22

INFECTION

established through obstetric records and personal consultation with the mother.

b. Incubation period can range from 11 to 20 days after contact.

c. The patient can be contagious for 1 to 2 days before and 5 days after the onset of the rash.

d. An infant deemed at risk for exposure must be placed in an isolette, transported to and from the mother's room in the isolette, and given VZIG (see page 377)

e. Infants born with varicella embryopathy do not require isolation.

9. Personnel health.

a. It is generally accepted that a routine culture of personnel for staphylococcal colonization is of little value. Between 20% and 50% of personnel may be carriers at any given time. It is therefore important that the nursery and obstetric personnel assume the responsibility for reporting to their supervisors any communicable disease they might have. If appropriate, they will be excluded from working in the neonatal areas for the duration of that disease. Diseases in this category include any respiratory, skin, conjunctival, gastrointestinal, or hepatic disorders.

b. Specific disease in personnel.

(1) Herpes simplex. No essential or nonessential personnel having a herpes simplex lesion anywhere on the face or hands should be permitted to work in the nursery until the lesion is dry.

(2) Staphylococcal infection. Documented staphylococcal lesions should be handled in an acceptable and individual manner.

10. Procedures to be followed if an epidemic is suspected or proved. An epidemic of staphylococcus may be defined as two documented staphylococcus infections occurring within 2 weeks of each other including time after discharge from the nursery.

Note: *Appropriate hospital infection control officers are to be informed of the situation.*

C. PARENT TEACHING.

Parents should be taught correct isolation precautions to observe according to the disease identified.

XIII. UNIVERSAL BLOOD AND BODY FLUID PRECAUTIONS

These guidelines apply to health care workers including, but not limited to, nurses, physicians, laboratory and blood bank technologists and technicians, phlebotomists, paramedics, emergency medical technicians, housekeepers, laundry workers, and others whose work involves contact with newborns, their blood, or other body fluids or corpses. These guidelines are derived primarily from the Centers for Disease Control and Prevention (**Table 22-1**).

TABLE 22-1

UNIVERSAL PRECAUTIONS IN THE CARE OF ALL PATIENTS TO PREVENT POSSIBLE CONTAGION

Because persons of all ages and backgrounds may be sources of infection for the examiner, it is important to take proper precautions when working with blood and body fluids from all patients. Examples of sources of infection are tuberculosis, acquired immunodeficiency syndrome, or any potentially infected body fluid or discharge.

- Use gloves when the possibility exists of contact with a patient's blood or potentially infectious body secretions or excretions. **Examples:** starting intravenous lines, drawing blood, doing cardiopulmonary resuscitation (CPR) or other emergency procedures, and handling soiled linen and waste.

- Wash hands after removing gloves (do not wash gloves), and use clean gloves with each patient.

- Do not wear gloves or protective clothing when contact with the patient is unlikely to result in exposure to blood or potentially infectious body secretions or excretions. **Examples:** shaking hands, delivering supplies and medications, removing trays, and holding infants.

- Wear gown, mask, and protective eyewear in addition to gloves during procedures in which spattering of blood or body fluids may occur. **Examples:** arterial punctures, endoscopies, insertion of arterial lines, hemapheresis, and hemodialysis.

- Always be cautious when working with needles, scalpels, or other sharp instruments.

- Always dispose of needles and sharp instruments in the impervious containers readily available in health care facilities. Do not recap, clip, or bend needles or throw them in the trash.

- Use the accompanying chart as a guide in identifying precautions that should be taken in specific situations.

Procedure	Wash Hands	Guidelines Gloves	Gown	Mask	Eyewear
Talking with patients	—	—	—	—	—
Adjusting IV fluid rate or noninvasive equipment	—	—	—	—	—
Examining patient without touching blood, body fluids, mucous membranes	X	—	—	—	—
Examining patient with significant cough	X	—	—	X	—
Examining patient including contact with blood, body fluids, mucous membranes, drainage	X	X	—	—	—
Drawing blood	X	X	—	—	—

Continued

INFECTION

22

TABLE 22-1

UNIVERSAL PRECAUTIONS IN THE CARE OF ALL PATIENTS TO PREVENT POSSIBLE CONTAGION—cont'd

Procedure	Wash Hands	Gloves	Guidelines		
			Gown	Mask	Eyewear
Inserting venous access	X	X	—	—	—
Suctioning	X	X	Use gown, mask, and eyewear if bloody body fluid spattering is likely.		
Inserting body or face catheters	X	X	Use gown, mask, and eyewear if bloody body fluid spattering is likely.		
Handling soiled waste, linen, other materials	X	X	Use gown, mask, and eyewear only if waste or linen is extensively contaminated and spattering is likely.		
Intubation	X	X	X	X	X
Inserting arterial access	X	X	X	X	X
Endoscopy, bronchoscopy	X	X	X	X	X
Operative and other procedures that produce extensive spattering of blood or body fluids and are likely to soil clothes	X	X	X	X	X

Data from the Centers for Disease Control and Prevention: MMWR 36(suppl 25):3, 1987.

BIBLIOGRAPHY

A-Kader HH, Balisteri WT: Hepatitis C virus: Implications to pediatric practice. Pediatr Infect Dis J 12:853, 1993.

American Academy of Pediatrics Committee on Infectious Diseases: Chemotherapy for tuberculosis in infants and children. Pediatrics 89:161, 1992.

American Academy of Pediatrics Committee on Infectious Diseases: Hepatitis C virus infection. Pediatrics 101:481, 1998.

American Academy of Pediatrics Committee on Infectious Diseases and Committee on the Fetus and Newborn: Guidelines for prevention of group B streptococcal (GBS) infection by chemoprophylaxis. Pediatrics 90:775, 1992.

American Academy of Pediatrics and American College of Obstetricians and Gynecologists: Guidelines for Perinatal Care, 2nd ed. Elk Grove Village, Ill, AAP and ACOG, 1988.

American Academy of Pediatrics: Report of the Committee on Infectious Diseases, 24th ed. Elk Grove Village, Ill, American Academy of Pediatrics, 1997.

American College of Obstetricians and Gynecologists: Group B streptococcal infections in pregnancy. ACOG Tech Bull 170:1, 1992.

Boppana SB, Fowler KB, Yaginder V, et al: Neuroradiographic findings in the newborn period and long-term outcome in children with symptomatic congenital cytomegalovirus infection. Pediatrics 99:409, 1997.

Caralane DJ, Long AM, McKeever PA, et al: Prevention of spread of echovirus 6 in a special care baby unit. Arch Dis Child 60:674, 1985.

Centers for Disease Control and Prevention: Recommendations for protection against viral hepatitis. MMWR 34:313, 1985.

Centers for Disease Control and Prevention: Recommendations for prevention of HIV transmission in the health care setting. MMWR 36(suppl 25):3, 1987.

Centers for Disease Control and Prevention: Prevention of perinatal transmission of hepatitis B virus: Prenatal screening of all pregnant women for hepatitis B surface antigen. MMWR 37:341, 1988.

Centers for Disease Control and Prevention: Congenital syphilis in New York City, 1986-1988. MMWR 38:825, 1989.

Centers for Disease Control and Prevention: 1989 sexually transmitted diseases treatment guidelines. MMWR 38(suppl 8):5, 1989.

Centers for Disease Control and Prevention: 1994 revised classification system for human immunodeficiency virus infection in children less than 13 years of age. MMWR 43:1, 1994.

Centers for Disease Control and Prevention: Zidovudine for prevention of HIV transmission from mother to infant. MMWR 43:285, 1994.

Centers for Disease Control and Prevention: 1995 revised guidelines for prophylaxis against *Pneumocystis carinii* pneumonia for children infected with or perinatally exposed to human immunodeficiency virus. MMWR 44:RR-4, 1995.

Centers for Disease Control and Prevention: Prevention of perinatal group B streptococcal disease: A public health perspective. MMWR 45:1, 1996.

Centers for Disease Control and Prevention: Perinatal prevention of GBS disease, revised guidelines. MMWR 51: RR-11, 2002.

Centers for Disease Control and Prevention: Guidelines for the use of antiretroviral agents in pediatrics HIV infection. MMWR 7:RR-4, 1998.

Cherry JD: Enteroviruses. In Remington JS, Klein JC (eds): Infectious Diseases of the Fetus and Newborn Infant. Philadelphia, WB Saunders, 1995.

Ferrieri P: GBS infections in the newborn infant: Diagnosis and treatment. Antibiot Chemother 35:211, 1985.

Fleming DT, McQuillan GM, Johnson RE, et al: Herpes simplex virus type 2 in the United States, 1976 to 1994. N Engl J Med 337:1105, 1997.

Freij BJ, South MA, Sever JL: Maternal rubella and the congenital rubella syndrome. Clin Perinatol 15:247, 1988.

Gerber MA, Zalneraitis EL: Childhood neurologic disorders and Lyme disease during pregnancy. Pediatr Neurol 11:41, 1994.

Gerdes JS: Clinicopathologic approach to the diagnosis of neonatal sepsis. Clin Perinatol 18:361, 1991.

Gershon AA: Chickenpox, measles and mumps. In Remington JS, Klein JC (eds): Infectious Diseases of the Fetus and Newborn Infant. Philadelphia, WB Saunders, 1995.

Guidelines for the use of antiretroviral agents in pediatric HIV infection: Rockville, Md, AIDSinfo.June 25, 2003. (accessed July 6, 2004 at http://aidsinfo.nih.gov/guidelines/archive.asp.

Husson RN, Comeau AM, Hoff R: Diagnosis of human immunodeficiency virus infection in infants and children. Pediatrics 86:1, 1990.

Ikeda MK, Jenson HB: Evaluation and treatment of congenital syphilis. J Pediatr 117:843, 1990.

Kimberlin DW, Lin C, Sanchez PJ, et al: Effect of ganciclovir therapy on hearing in symptomatic congenital cytomegalovirus disease involving the central nervous system: A randomized, controlled trial. J Pediatr 143:17, 2003.

Kinney JS, Kumar ML: Should we expand the TORCH complex? A description of clinical and diagnostic aspects of selected old and new agents. Clin Perinatol 15:727, 1988.

Krasinski K, Borkowsky W: Laboratory diagnosis of HIV infection. Pediatr Clin North Am 38:17, 1991.

Lieberman E, Lang JM, Frigoletto F, et al: Epidural analgesia, intrapartum fever, and neonatal sepsis evaluation. Pediatrics 99:415, 1997.

Maisels MJ, Kringe E: Risk of sepsis with severe hyperbilirubinemia. Pediatrics 90:741, 1992.

Meyers JD: Congenital varicella in term infants: Risk reconsidered. J Infect Dis 129:215, 1974.

Miller E, Cradock-Watson JE, Ridehalgh MK: Outcome in newborn babies given antivaricella-zoster immunoglobulin after perinatal maternal infection with varicella-zoster virus. Lancet 12:371, 1989.

Modlin JF, Kinney JS: Perinatal enterovirus infections. In Aronoff SC (ed): Advances in Pediatric Infectious Disease, vol 2. St Louis, Mosby, 1987.

O'Connor EM, Sperling RS, Gelber R, et al: Reduction of maternal-infant transmission of human immunodeficiency virus type I with ZDV treatment. N Engl J Med 331:1173, 1994.

Pelke S, Ching D, Easa D, Melish ME: Gowning does not affect colonization or infection rates in a neonatal intensive care unit. Arch Pediatr Adolescent Med 148:1016, 1994.

Philip AGS, Hewitt JR: Early diagnosis of neonatal sepsis. Pediatrics 65:1036, 1980.

Pichichero MD, Todd JK: Detection of neonatal bacteremia. J Pediatr 94:958, 1979.

Pitt J: Perinatal human immunodeficiency virus infection. Clin Perinatol 18:227, 1991.

Pizzo PA, Wilfert CM: Perinatally acquired human immunodeficiency virus infection. Pediatr Infect Dis J 9:609, 1990.

Preblud SR, Alford CA: Rubella. In Remington JS, Klein JC (eds): Infectious Diseases of the Fetus and Newborn Infant. Philadelphia, WB Saunders, 1995.

Prober CG, Gershon AA: Medical management of newborns and infants born to human immunodeficiency virus seropositive mothers. Pediatr Infect Dis J 10:684, 1991.

Pylipow M, Gaddis M, Kinney JS: Selective intrapartum prophylaxis for group B *Streptococcus* colonization: Management and outcome of newborns. Pediatrics 331:631, 1994.

Remington JS, Desmonts G: Toxoplasmosis. In Remington JS, Klein JC (eds): Infectious Diseases of the Fetus and Newborn Infant. Philadelphia, WB Saunders, 1995.

Roizen N, Swisher CN, Stein MA, et al: Neurologic and developmental outcome in treated congenital toxoplasmosis. Pediatrics 95:11, 1995.

Semba RD, Miotti PG, Chiphangwi JD, et al: Maternal vitamin A deficiency and mother-to-child transmission of HIV-1. Lancet 343:1593, 1994.

Siegel JD: Sepsis neonatorum. In Oski FA (ed): Principles and Practices of Pediatrics. Philadelphia, JB Lippincott, 1990.

St. Geme JW, Murray DL, Carter J, et al: Perinatal bacterial infection after prolonged rupture of amniotic membranes: An analysis of risk and management. J Pediatr 104:608, 1984.

Stagno S: Cytomegalovirus. In Remington JS, Klein JC (eds): Infectious Diseases of the Fetus and Newborn Infant. Philadelphia, WB Saunders, 1995.

Steinhoff MC, Kinney JS: Neonatal sepsis and infections. In Reese RE, Betts RF (eds): A Practical Approach to Infectious Diseases, ed 3. Boston, Little, Brown, 1991.

Voora S, Srinivasan G, Lilien LD, et al: Fever in full-term newborns in the first four days of life. Pediatrics 69:40, 1982.

Walsh M, McIntosh K: Neonatal mastitis. Clin Pediatr (Phila) 25:395, 1986.

Whitley RJ, Nahmias AJ, Visintine AM, et al: The natural history of herpes simplex virus infection of mother and newborn. Pediatrics 66:30, 1980.

Whitley RJ, Arvin A, Prober C, et al: Predictors of morbidity and mortality in neonates with herpes simplex virus infections. N Engl J Med 324:450, 1991.

Whitley RJ: Herpes simplex virus infections. In Remington JS, Klein JC (eds): Infectious Diseases of the Fetus and Newborn Infant. Philadelphia, WB Saunders, 1990.

Yow MD: Congenital cytomegalovirus disease: A new problem. J Infect Dis 159:163, 1989.

22

INFECTION

In Utero Drug Exposure

Beryl J. Rosenstein

FAST FACTS

Immediate Issues in the Nursery

- Because in utero drug exposure often goes unrecognized, a high index of suspicion should exist in the presence of factors that are known to be associated with maternal drug use. These include: maternal infection with human immunodeficiency virus (HIV)/acquired immunodeficiency syndrome (AIDS), tuberculosis, hepatitis B and C, syphilis, and other sexually transmitted diseases; a history of multiple abortions; precipitous home delivery; placental abruption; absence of prenatal care; homelessness or unstable home; and unexplained intrauterine growth retardation (IUGR).
- Neonatal abstinence syndrome (NAS) usually appears soon after birth and reaches a peak in 4 to 5 days. The incidence decreases if the latest maternal drug use was more than 1 week before delivery. Withdrawal symptoms include irritability, restlessness, tremors, wakefulness, seizures, high-pitched cry, inability to self-quiet, yawning, sneezing, congestion, poor feeding, poor weight gain, fever, sweating, and tachypnea.
- Opioid withdrawal (with methadone being more severe than heroin) produces the most severe symptoms followed by alcohol and cocaine. Marijuana and nicotine usage is not generally associated with withdrawal symptoms. Opioids, alcohol, cocaine, and nicotine are associated with growth retardation, preterm delivery, and low Apgar scores. This is generally not true of marijuana usage, although mild growth retardation sometimes occurs.
- Infants with symptoms of withdrawal should be assessed using a neonatal abstinence scoring system. If pharmacologic treatment is indicated, the infant should demonstrate clinical stability off medication before discharge. Persistent irritability may not indicate a poor response to treatment and may continue for several months.
- Meconium is more reliable than maternal or infant urine for detecting cocaine metabolites. This type of testing, however, is not yet widely available.

Important Reminders After Discharge

- The primary components of Fetal Alcohol Syndrome (FAS) are IUGR (with microcephaly), facial dysmorphism, congenital malformations (cardiac, genitourinary, skeletal), and neurodevelopmental abnormalities (with mental retardation).
- In utero exposure to alcohol and stimulants (cocaine/amphetamines) is associated with the highest rates of persistent neurodevelopmental deficits. Studies on the severity and incidence of long-term deficits

Continued

FAST FACTS—Cont'd

from cocaine exposure are inconclusive. Persistence of microcephaly may be an important predictor of long-term developmental problems.

Helpful Information for Parents

- Alcohol, nicotine, marijuana, and cocaine readily pass into breast milk and can cause problems in the nursing infant. Cocaine is especially associated with significant morbidity and mortality, and its use is an absolute contraindication to breast-feeding.
- Consumption of alcohol and nicotine is compatible with breast-feeding. However, every effort should be made to encourage and assist cessation of smoking and moderation of alcohol intake. If more than 4 to 6 oz of wine or 12 oz of beer is to be consumed, then mothers should be advised to nurse before or at least 2 hours after alcohol intake.
- Home cardiorespiratory monitoring has not been shown to be effective in the management of in utero drug exposure, with or without symptoms, and is not recommended.

I. GENERAL CONSIDERATIONS

A. AN INCREASING NUMBER OF WOMEN OF CHILDBEARING AGE ARE USING CONTROLLED SUBSTANCES.

An estimated 10% to 15% of newborns are exposed to illicit drugs during pregnancy.

B. MOST DRUGS WITH HIGH ABUSE POTENTIAL CROSS THE PLACENTA AND TEND TO ACCUMULATE IN THE FETUS.

With drugs with high potential for abuse, dependence develops in the fetus and in the mother.

C. DRUG-EXPOSED INFANTS OFTEN GO UNRECOGNIZED AND MAY BE DISCHARGED TO HOMES WHERE THEY ARE AT INCREASED RISK OF MEDICAL AND SOCIAL PROBLEMS INCLUDING ABUSE AND NEGLECT.

D. DETECTION OF THE DRUG-EXPOSED NEWBORN REQUIRES A HIGH INDEX OF SUSPICION.

1. A comprehensive psychosocial history including specific inquiry concerning maternal drug use should be part of every obstetric and newborn evaluation.
2. However, maternal self-reporting of drug abuse is highly unreliable and maternal and newborn urine toxicology testing is a useful adjunct.
3. A positive toxicology result confirms the diagnosis of drug use, but a negative test does not rule out in utero drug exposure.

4. Drugs accumulate in meconium during the second and third trimesters and in hair during the third trimester. Metabolites of morphine, cocaine, and cannabinoids can be recovered in high concentration, and testing of hair and urine can be used to establish a profile of drug use throughout pregnancy.

Note: *Hair can test positive for in utero drug exposure for up to 3 months of age.*

5. Universal maternal toxicology screening is not recommended but may be indicated in areas with high levels of illicit drug use or in conjunction with an early discharge policy.

E. ILLICIT PRENATAL DRUG USE SHOULD BE PARTICULARLY SUSPECTED IN THE FOLLOWING SITUATIONS:
1. Maternal history of sexually transmitted diseases including HIV infection.
2. History of multiple abortions, both spontaneous and elective.
3. Unregistered or late registration for prenatal care or inadequate number of prenatal visits (these are highly predictive of prenatal substance abuse).
4. History of vague or chaotic living arrangements (e.g., homeless shelter, multiple addresses).
5. Placental abruption (cocaine, amphetamines).
6. Precipitous delivery, especially at home or under unusual circumstances.
7. Unexplained IUGR.
8. Neonatal signs and symptoms consistent with in utero drug exposure.
9. History of child neglect or abuse.
10. Hypertensive episode, severe mood swings, myocardial infarction.
11. Previous unexplained fetal demise.

F. BEING AWARE OF AND SCREENING THE MOTHER AND NEWBORN FOR OTHER PROBLEMS KNOWN TO BE SEEN IN ASSOCIATION WITH ILLICIT DRUG USE, INCLUDING THE FOLLOWING ARE IMPORTANT:
1. AIDS.
2. Tuberculosis.
3. Hepatitis B and C.
4. Syphilis.
5. Other sexually transmitted diseases.

G. HEALTH CARE WORKERS DEALING WITH DRUG-EXPOSED NEWBORNS MUST BE KNOWLEDGEABLE CONCERNING THE FOLLOWING:
1. Details of urine toxicology and meconium or hair testing procedures performed in their hospital.
2. State and local child protection reporting requirements.
3. Resources available for the treatment and support of the affected mother, newborn, and family.

II. OUTCOMES: GENERAL DRUG USE

A. RELATING SPECIFIC NEONATAL OUTCOMES TO SPECIFIC DRUG EXPOSURES BECAUSE OF MULTIPLE ASSOCIATED PROBLEMS, INCLUDING THE FOLLOWING, IS DIFFICULT:

1. Inadequate prenatal care.
2. Multiple drug use including tobacco and alcohol.
3. Poor nutrition.
4. Chaotic living conditions; physical and sexual abuse.
5. Associated infections including tuberculosis, AIDS, hepatitis B and C, and other sexually transmitted diseases.

B. MATERNAL AND NEONATAL OUTCOMES MAY VARY DEPENDING ON THE TYPE, FREQUENCY, TIMING, AND INTENSITY OF DRUG USE, BUT THERE ARE WELL-RECOGNIZED GENERIC EFFECTS OF PRENATAL DRUG USE (TABLE 23-1).

1. Maternal effects.
a. Increased rates of spontaneous abortion, stillbirth, and shortened gestation.
b. Placental abruption (cocaine, amphetamines, methamphetamine).
2. Fetal/neonatal effects.
a. Increased neonatal mortality.
b. IUGR.
c. Congenital malformations.
d. Microcephaly.
e. Intrapartum distress (meconium staining, low Apgar scores) secondary to placental insufficiency.
f. Neurobehavioral abnormalities.
g. Unexpected infant deaths, especially after in utero exposure to opiates.
h. Abnormalities of control of respiration.

III. OUTCOMES: SPECIFIC DRUG USE

A. ALCOHOL.

1. Fetal alcohol levels closely parallel those of the mother; no safe level of alcohol intake during pregnancy has been established. Advanced maternal age

TABLE 23-1

MATERNAL DRUG USE—NEWBORN OUTCOMES

	Heroin/ Methadone	Alcohol	Cocaine	Marijuana	Tobacco
Withdrawal	++	+	+	—	—
Growth retardation	+	++	+	±	++
Birth defects	—	+	+	±	—
Neurobehavioral effects	++	++	++	+	+
Perinatal mortality	↑	↑	—	—	↑
Premature birth	↑	↑	↑	—	↑
Apgar score	↓	↓	↓	±	↓

(older than 30 years) and binge drinking may significantly increase the risk of adverse neonatal outcomes.

2. Maternal effects include increased rates of spontaneous abortion and stillbirth.

3. Fetal/neonatal effects are probably dose dependent and include the following:

a. Prenatal and postnatal growth retardation (may be persistent).

b. Neonatal withdrawal syndrome (tremors, hypertonia or hypotonia, restlessness, inconsolable crying, abnormal reflexes).

c. Central nervous system (CNS) sequelae including attention-deficit disorder, mental retardation, and behavioral problems.

d. Increased incidence of congenital malformations.

e. Intrauterine distress (meconium staining, low Apgar scores).

f. Increased perinatal mortality rate.

4. Features of fetal alcohol syndrome, which affects 1:1000 live births and is one of the most common causes of mental retardation, consist of the following:

a. Severe IUGR including microcephaly.

b. Dysmorphic features (microcephaly; short palpebral fissures; ptosis; maxillary hypoplasia; long, smooth philtrum; thin vermilion border of upper lip)

c. Congenital malformations (skeletal, cardiac, genitourinary, cleft lip/palate)

d. Neurodevelopmental abnormalities including mild to profound mental retardation (average IQ = 65).

5. Treatment.

a. No specific therapy is indicated in the neonatal period.

b. Appropriate long-term follow-up of learning, developmental, and behavioral problems.

B. MARIJUANA.

1. Tetrahydrocannabinol (THC) crosses the placenta and may lead to fetal hypoxia by increasing the fetal carbon monoxide level and decreasing uterine blood flow.

2. Fetal/neonatal effects.

a. Slight shortening of gestation (average 1 week).

b. Decrease in birth weight by 100 to 150 g.

c. Transient mild neonatal neurobehavioral abnormalities (increased fine tremors and exaggerated startle, poor habituation to visual stimuli, reduced quiet sleep). At 2- and 3-year follow-ups there is no evidence of motor, cognitive, or language abnormalities.

d. There is no evidence of an increased incidence of major or minor physical anomalies.

3. No treatment is necessary for neonates exposed in utero only to marijuana.

C. NARCOTICS.

Heroin, methadone, codeine, pentazocine (Talwin), and tripelennamine (Pyribenzamine).

1. Maternal effects and common complications.
   a. Increased rates of spontaneous abortion, premature labor, premature rupture of membranes.
   b. Chorioamnionitis.
   c. Preeclampsia.
2. Fetal/neonatal effects.
   a. Increased perinatal mortality rate.
   b. IUGR including microcephaly.
   c. Intrauterine distress (meconium staining, low Apgar scores).
   d. NAS.
   e. Increased incidence of sudden unexpected death (methadone worse than heroin).

Note: *During pregnancy, medical withdrawal from opioids should occur in a perinatal unit with fetal monitoring. In general, withdrawal is not advised before 14 weeks' gestation because of the potential risk of inducing abortion and should not be performed after the 32nd week because of possible withdrawal-induced stress.*

3. NEONATAL ABSTINENCE SYNDROME (NAS)
   a. Among drug-exposed infants, 55% to 95% will exhibit some degree of NAS.
   b. Severity depends on type of drug used (methadone is worse than heroin), amount and frequency of use, maternal and infant metabolism and excretion, concomitant drug use, and timing of last use before delivery. (If >1 week has elapsed between the last maternal use and delivery, the incidence of neonatal withdrawal is low).
   c. Withdrawal symptoms usually appear soon after birth, reach a peak in 4 to 5 days, and may then occur in a subacute form for weeks to months.

Note: *The use of naloxone in the delivery room is contraindicated in infants whose mothers are known to be opioid dependent. However, in the absence of a specific history of opioid abuse, naloxone remains a reasonable option in the delivery room management of a depressed infant whose mother recently received a narcotic.*

   d. Manifestations
      (1) Irritability, restlessness, tremors, wakefulness, high-pitched cry, inability to self-quiet, abnormal sleep pattern
      (2) Myoclonus, seizures
      (3) Poor feeding, frantic sucking, increased weight loss, delay in regaining birth weight
      (4) Sneezing, yawning, vomiting, diarrhea, nasal stuffiness, fever, sweating, tachypnea

Note: *After in utero methadone exposure, onset of symptoms is usually 1 to 3 days after delivery but may be delayed up to 7 to 10 days; withdrawal may be more severe and prolonged than with heroin, and there is a higher incidence of seizures.*

There is great controversy as to whether there is any correlation between maternal methadone dose and frequency or severity of neonatal abstinence.

Note: *Buprenorphine, a synthetic opioid with a long duration of action, is now being used as a substitute for methadone in treating opioid-addicted pregnant women. Its use is associated with neonatal withdrawal of varying severity over the first 7 days. Symptoms are generally milder and of shorter duration than with methadone withdrawal, but pharmacologic treatment may be necessary.*

e. Treatment
   (1) Supportive care; quiet, comforting environment; gentle handling; swaddling (a nonoscillating waterbed has been shown to be effective).
   (2) Frequent small feedings; in infants with significant weight loss or slow weight gain, high-calorie feedings (24 calories per ounce) are indicated.
   (3) Pharmacotherapy.

Note: *Most infants can be managed without drug therapy; all of the drugs used to treat neonatal withdrawal have their own CNS effects.*

f. Indications for drug therapy.
   (1) Seizures.
   (2) Vomiting and diarrhea associated with significant weight loss.
   (3) Marked irritability and tremors that interfere with feedings and sleeping.
   (4) Fever unrelated to infection.
g. NAS scoring systems (**Fig. 23-1**) can be helpful in assessing the need for and response to drug therapy.
h. Pharmacotherapy. Diazepam, methadone, clonidine, and phenobarbital have been used, but tincture of opium (morphine) is the most frequently used drug.
   (1) Tincture of opium (10 mg/ml) is diluted 25-fold to yield a morphine equivalent of 0.4 mg/ml. The usual starting dose is 0.1 ml/kg with feedings every 4 hours as needed to control withdrawal signs and symptoms. The dose can be increased by 0.1 ml/kg per dose if the neonatal abstinence score (Finnegan score) is > 9 on two consecutive scores. Guides to adequate therapy include normal temperature curve, ability to sleep between feedings, decrease in activity, crying and motor instability, and weight gain. After stabilization (score < 9 on two consecutive scores), the dose can be decreased by 0.05 ml/kg per dose q 24 hours without altering the frequency over a 7- to 10-day period.

     The usual duration of therapy is 7 to 14 days. The infant should not be discharged home while still on medication. Some degree of irritability may persist for weeks to months and is *not* an indication for prolonged drug therapy

23

IN UTERO DRUG EXPOSURE

DATE: DAILY WEIGHT:

SYSTEM	SIGNS AND SYMPTOMS	SCORE	AM					PM			COMMENTS
	Excessive High-Pitched (other) Cry	2									
	Continuous High-Pitched (other) Cry	3									
	Sleeps <1 hour after feeding	3									
	Sleeps <2 hours after feeding	2									
	Sleeps <3 hours after feeding	1									
	Hyperactive Moro reflex	2									
	Markedly Hyperactive Moro reflex	3									
	Mild Tremors Disturbed	1									
	Moderate-Severe Tremors Disturbed	2									
	Mild Tremors Undisturbed	3									
	Moderate-Severe Tremors Undisturbed	4									
	Increased Muscle Tone	2									
	Excoriation (specific areas)	1									
	Myoclonic Jerks	3									
	Generalized Convulsions	5									
	Sweating	1									
	Fever<101 (99-100.8° F/37.2-38.2° C)	1									
	Fever>101 (38.4° C and higher)	2									
	Frequent Yawning (>3-4 times/ interval)	1									
	Mottling	1									
	Nasal Stuffiness	1									

Sneezing (>3-4 times/interval)	1	
Nasal Flaring	2	
Respiratory Rate>60/min	1	
Respiratory Rate>60/min with retractions	2	
Excessive Sucking	1	
Poor Feeding	2	
Regurgitation	2	
Projectile Vomiting	3	
Loose Stools	2	
Watery Stools	3	
TOTAL SCORE		
INITIALS OF SCORER		

Evaluator should place a check next to each sign or symptom observed at various time intervals, then add scores for total score.

FIG. 23-1

Neonatal abstinence score sheet. (From Finnegan LP: Neonatal abstinence syndrome: Assessment and pharmacology. In Rubatelli FF and Granati B, editors: Neonatal therapy: An update, New York, 1986, Excerpta Medica.)

23

IN UTERO DRUG EXPOSURE

(2) Phenobarbital may be effective for treating CNS symptoms but is not effective for the gastrointestinal manifestations of drug withdrawal. The loading dose for phenobarbital is 15 to 20 mg/kg, followed by a maintenance dose of 4 to 5 mg/kg per day, given orally at 6-hour intervals. Blood levels should be monitored (aim for a peak level of 20 to 30 mcg/ml).

(3) Paregoric use has declined because of the potentially toxic effects of its many ingredients.

i. Home cardiorespiratory monitoring is not routinely indicated.

j. There is no evidence that in utero opioid exposure leads to long-term adverse neuorocognitive effects.

D. PHENCYCLIDINE (PCP).

1. Adverse effects.

a. Increased rate of prematurity.

b. IUGR including microcephaly.

c. There may be jitteriness, tremors, high-pitched cry, irritability, nystagmus, sudden outbursts of agitation, and marked reactivity to auditory stimuli. These neurobehavioral effects represent PCP intoxication rather than drug withdrawal.

2. Treatment is supportive, using swaddling, gentle handling, and a quiet environment. Drug therapy is not usually indicated.

3. By 1 year of age, most exposed infants show normal growth and development.

E. STIMULANTS.

Cocaine, amphetamines, methamphetamine.

1. Cocaine is an illicit drug used commonly during pregnancy, often in combination with alcohol, tobacco, and other illicit drugs.

2. Pharmacology.

a. Cocaine inhibits uptake of neurotransmitters at nerve endings, leading to high circulating levels of epinephrine, norepinephrine, and dopamine.

b. High circulating catecholamine levels lead to vasoconstriction (decreased uterine blood flow, tachycardia, hypertension) and increased uterine contractility.

c. Decreased uterine blood flow leads to fetal hypoxia, which further stimulates catecholamine release.

d. Cocaine readily crosses the placenta and fetal blood-brain barrier and enters the fetal CNS.

e. Evidence indicates that cocaine exerts direct toxic effects on the fetal brain, as evidenced by the following:

(1) Abnormal neonatal electroencephalogram (EEG).

(2) Abnormal neonatal computed tomography (CT) scan.

(3) Presence of neurobehavioral abnormalities in the newborn period even when cocaine use was discontinued after the first trimester.

(4) Increased incidence of congenital cerebral anomalies.

f. Results of urine toxicology testing depend on the timing of last cocaine use in relation to testing, drug clearance rates in the mother and fetus or neonate, and the sensitivity of the drug assay. In most cases in which cocaine has been used within several days of delivery, both mother and newborn have positive results; however, in approximately 15% of cases only the mother will be positive, and in 1% to 2% only the neonate will be positive. Meconium is more reliable than maternal or neonatal urine for the detection of cocaine metabolites.

3. Maternal effects.

a. Increased rates of spontaneous abortion and stillbirth.
b. Placental abruption.
c. Shortened gestation.

4. Fetal/neonatal effects depend on the timing, frequency, duration and intensity of drug use, and concomitant drug use. There is evidence that some but not all of the adverse outcomes can be reduced if cocaine use is discontinued during the pregnancy.

a. IUGR including microcephaly. Infants usually show "catch-up" growth by 6 to 12 months, but head circumference may remain significantly smaller through 36 months. Postnatal head growth may be an important marker in predicting long-term developmental outcome.
b. Perinatal cerebral infarction; neonatal myocardial infarction.
c. Intrauterine distress (meconium staining, low Apgar scores).
d. Neonatal neurobehavioral abnormalities including abnormal sleep pattern; startles, tremors, hypertonia; poor feeding; excitability, irritability; high-pitched cry. Most of these symptoms diminish and then disappear within a few months after birth.
e. Vomiting, loose stools, sneezing.

Note: *Neurobehavioral abnormalities usually occur soon after birth and last for several days, but there may be a secondary peak of symptoms at 7 to 10 days.*

(1) Effects may be potentiated by concomitant use of other drugs (e.g., heroin).
(2) On long-term follow-up, cocaine-exposed infants may show evidence of delay in language, visual processing, reasoning, and fine-motor skills; hyperactivity; and behavioral problems; however, there is evidence that most early abnormalities improve over time. Studies on the incidence and severity of long-term neurobehavioral sequelae of in utero cocaine exposure are inconclusive.

f. Increased incidence of sudden unexpected death during infancy.
g. Increased incidence of necrotizing enterocolitis (in the absence of usual risk factors).
h. Abnormalities of control of respiration.
i. Fetal/neonatal arrhythmias (may be symptomatic and resistant to conventional therapy).

23

IN UTERO DRUG EXPOSURE

j. Increased incidence of congenital malformations (presumably secondary to fetal vascular disruption).
   (1) Intestinal atresia.
   (2) Genitourinary abnormalities. Hydronephrosis, hypospadias, Eagle-Barrett (prune-belly) syndrome.
   (3) Skeletal. Limb reduction, cranial defects.
   (4) Cardiac.
   (5) Ocular abnormalities. Strabismus, nystagmus, hypoplastic optic discs.

5. Treatment.

a. Treatment is supportive; pharmacotherapy is rarely indicated. High-calorie (24 calories per ounce) formula should be used in infants with large weight loss. Home cardiorespiratory monitoring has not been shown to be effective and is not recommended.

b. Carrying out an in-depth psychosocial evaluation of cocaine users to assess the need for drug treatment, counseling, intensive family services, protective service referral, and specialized pediatric follow-up services is important.

F. TOBACCO.

1. Effects.

a. Worldwide, maternal smoking is the leading cause of IUGR (mean reduction in birth weight of 250 g); there is a close relationship between maternal serum cotinine levels and birth weight. Passive exposure to paternal smoking also decreases birth weight.

b. Other effects of maternal smoking.
   (1) Increased rates of spontaneous abortion, placental abruption, prematurity, and perinatal mortality.

Note: *In utero tobacco exposure may double the rates of stillbirth and infant mortality.*

   (2) Intrauterine distress (meconium staining, low Apgar scores).
   (3) Neonatal neurobehavioral abnormalities (impaired habituation, orientation, consolability, orientation to sound).
   (4) Signs of nicotine toxicity (tachycardia, irritability, poor feeding).
   (5) Possible increased risk of cancer in childhood.
   (6) Increased risk for SIDS.

2. Fetal tobacco syndrome.

a. Mother smoked five cigarettes per day throughout pregnancy.

b. No evidence of maternal hypertension.

c. Evidence of symmetrical growth retardation at term without any other obvious cause of IUGR.

IV. BREAST-FEEDING

A. ALCOHOL, MARIJUANA, NICOTINE, AND COCAINE CROSS FREELY INTO BREAST MILK.

Significant morbidity and even mortality have been described in infants exposed to cocaine via breast-feeding. Moderate use of alcohol or cigarettes is compatible with breast-feeding.

B. ONGOING COCAINE USE IS AN ABSOLUTE CONTRAINDICATION TO BREAST-FEEDING.

C. WOMEN WITH A HISTORY OF SUBSTANCE ABUSE MAY BREAST-FEED IF THEY REMAIN DRUG FREE AS DEMONSTRATED BY REGULAR URINE TOXICOLOGY TESTING.

D. WOMEN ON METHADONE AND BUPRENORPHINE MAINTENANCE MAY BREAST-FEED AS LONG AS NO ILLICIT DRUG USE OCCURS.

Maintenance drugs should be taken just after breast-feeding.

BIBLIOGRAPHY

American Academy of Pediatrics Committee on Drugs: Neonatal drug withdrawal. Pediatrics 101:1079, 1998.

American Academy of Pediatrics Committee on Substance Abuse and Children With Disabilities: Fetal alcohol syndrome and alcohol-related neurodevelopmental disorders. Pediatrics 106:358, 2000.

Bauchner H, Zuckerman B: Cocaine, sudden infant death syndrome, and home monitoring. J Pediatr 117:904, 1990.

Chasnoff IJ, Hunt CE, Kleter R, et al: Prenatal cocaine exposure is associated with respiratory pattern abnormalities. Am J Dis Child 143:583, 1989.

Chiriboga CA, Brust JCM, Bateman D, Hauser WA: Dose-response effect of fetal cocaine exposure on newborn neurologic function. Pediatrics 103:79, 1999.

Dominguez R, Vila-Coro AA, Slopis JM, Bohan TP: Brain and ocular abnormalities in infants with in utero exposure to cocaine and other street drugs. Am J Dis Child 145:688, 1991.

Frank DA, Augustyn M, Knight WG, et al: Growth, development and behavior in early childhood following prenatal cocaine exposure. JAMA 285:1613, 2001.

Frassica JJ, Orva EJ, Walsh EP, Lipschultz SE: Arrhythmias in children prenatally exposed to cocaine. Arch Pediatr Adolesc Med 148:1163, 1994.

Fried PA: Marijuana use during pregnancy: Consequences for the offspring. Semin Perinatol 15:280, 1991.

Higgins S: Smoking in pregnancy. Curr Opin Obstet Gynecol 14:145, 2002.

Huestis MA, Choo RE: Drug abuse's smallest victims: In utero drug exposure. Foren Sci Internat 128:20, 2002.

Johnson K, Gerada C, Greenough A: Treatment of neonatal abstinence syndrome. Arch Dis Child Fetal Neonatal Ed 88:F2, 2003.

Jones KL: Fetal alcohol syndrome. Pediatr Rev 8:122, 1986.

Kandall SR, Gaines J, Habel L, et al: Relationship of maternal substance abuse to subsequent sudden infant death syndrome in offspring. J Pediatr 123:120, 1993.

Lacroix I, Berrebi A, Chaumerliac C, et al: Buprenorphine in pregnant opioid-dependent women: First results of a prospective study. Addiction 99:209, 2004.

Nieburg P, Marks JS, McLaren NM, et al: The fetal tobacco syndrome. JAMA 253:2998, 1985.

Osterloh JD, Lee BL: Urine drug screening in mothers and newborns. Am J Dis Child 143:791, 1989.

Ostrea EM Jr: Testing for exposure to illicit drugs and other agents in the neonate: A review of laboratory methods and the role of meconium analysis. Curr Probl Pediatr 29:41, 1999.

Ostrea EM, Chavez CJ: Perinatal problems (excluding neonatal withdrawal) in maternal drug addiction: A study of 830 cases. J Pediatr 94:292, 1979.

23

IN UTERO DRUG EXPOSURE

Rahbar F, Fomufod A, White D, Westney LS: Impact of intrauterine exposure to phencyclidine (PCP) and cocaine on neonates. J Natl Med Assoc 85:349, 1993.

Smith L, Yonekura ML, Wallace T, et al: Effects of prenatal methamphetamine exposure on fetal growth and drug withdrawal symptoms in infants born at term. J Dev Behav Pediatr 24:17, 2003.

Wachsman L, Schuetz S, Chan LS, et al: What happens to babies exposed to phencyclidine (PCP) in utero? Am J Drug Alcohol Abuse 15:31, 1989.

Wagner CL, Katikaneni LD, Cox TH, Ryan RM: The impact of prenatal drug exposure on the neonate. Obstet Gyn Clin North Am 25:169, 1998.

Wojnar-Horton RE, Kristensen JH, Yapp P, et al: Methadone distribution and excretion into breast milk of clients in a methadone maintenance programme. Br J Clin Pharmacol 44:543, 1997.

Inherited Metabolic Diseases

Ada Hamosh

FAST FACTS

Immediate Issues in the Nursery

- Metabolic disease should be considered in any newborn full-term infant who becomes acutely ill in the first 24 to 48 hours of life and has no risk factors for infection.
- An initial screen for metabolic disease should include the following:
  blood testing for pH, Pco_2, electrolytes, glucose, ammonium, complete blood cell (CBC) count with differential, aspartate aminotransferase (AST), alanine aminotransferase (ALT), total and direct bilirubin, plasma lactate, and a calculated anion gap.
  urine testing for ketones, reducing substances, ferric chloride, dinitrophenylhydrazine, and assessment of odor.
- Initial interventions should include protein restriction, caloric maintenance with glucose and lipid solutions, and assessment for hemodialysis.

Important Reminders After Discharge

- Repeat newborn metabolic screening should be considered between 1 and 2 weeks in formula-fed infants whose initial screen was done before 24 hours or in breast-fed infants whose initial screen was done before 48 hours. A final metabolic screen should be performed between 2 and 4 weeks of life.
- Infants who present with vomiting, lethargy, hypotonia, seizures, or sudden changes in feeding habits should have a detailed family history review and inquiries regarding unusual odors emanating from the body or urine.

Helpful Information for Parents

- Though many state and private laboratories may list different numbers of metabolic disorders in their screening profile, all states that use tandem mass spectrometry to screen for amino acidopathies, organic acidemias, and fatty acid oxidation defects are screening for the same analytes and therefore the same disorders. A complete listing of each state's screening protocols can be found at http://genes-r-us.uthscsa.edu/resources/newborn/state.htm.
- All states are required to test for phenylketonuria (PKU) and hypothyroidism. All other tests are optional. It is reasonable to support the use of a secondary laboratory to perform screening using tandem mass spectrometry if the birth state does not routinely test by this method and the cost is reasonable for the parents. This is especially true if there is a family history of neonatal death, male infant deaths on the maternal side, or consanguinity.
- False-positive results can occur, but confirmatory tests are accurate and can be done quickly.

I. GENERAL PRINCIPLES

A limited number of metabolic diseases cause signs and symptoms in the neonatal period. Although individually rare, collectively they represent a significant cause of neonatal morbidity and mortality. Diagnostic delay leads to irreversible central nervous system (CNS) damage or death. The classic presentation of an inborn error of metabolism is that of a normal full-term newborn who becomes acutely ill after the first 24 to 48 hours of life. The signs exhibited by a newborn with metabolic disease are indistinguishable from those seen in sepsis and in disorders of the cardiovascular system and CNS. They include poor feeding, vomiting, lethargy, hypotonia, seizures, and coma. For this reason, any neonate with no risk factors for infection (e.g., prolonged rupture of membranes, maternal fever) who is deemed sick enough to warrant a blood culture warrants an evaluation for metabolic disease.

II. INITIAL EVALUATION

A. FAMILY HISTORY.

1. Neonatal deaths in this sibship (most inborn errors of metabolism are autosomal recessive).
2. Male infant deaths on the maternal side (ornithine transcarbamylase deficiency, the most common urea cycle defect, is X-linked).
3. Consanguinity (increases the risk of autosomal recessive disorders).

B. BLOOD TESTS.

1. Venous or arterial blood gas for pH, Pco_2.
2. Serum electrolytes; calculate anion gap.
3. Serum glucose.
4. Plasma ammonium.
5. CBC count with differential.
6. Liver function tests. Serum AST and ALT, total and direct bilirubin.
7. Plasma lactate.

C. URINE TESTS.

1. Odor (patients with certain inborn errors excrete large amounts of organic acids with distinctive odors).
2. Ketones.
3. Reducing substances.
4. Ferric chloride.
5. Dinitrophenylhydrazine.

III. DIAGNOSIS

Proper and rapid diagnosis of metabolic disease is essential.

A. THERAPY IS SPECIFIC FOR EACH DISORDER.
B. IF THERAPY IS INSTITUTED EARLY, A GOOD OUTCOME IS MORE LIKELY.

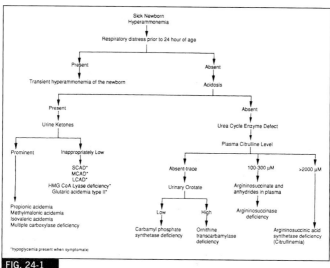

FIG. 24-1

Algorithm for the diagnosis of hyperammonemia in the newborn.

C. PROVIDE INFORMED GENETIC COUNSELING; OFTEN THERE IS A HIGH RECURRENCE RISK WITHIN A FAMILY; PRENATAL DIAGNOSIS IS POSSIBLE FOR MOST INBORN ERRORS.

D. PLASMA AMMONIUM IS ELEVATED IN SEVERAL INBORN ERRORS THAT OCCUR IN THE NEWBORN PERIOD (E.G., PRIMARY DEFECTS OF THE UREA CYCLE AND SEVERAL ORGANIC ACIDEMIAS).

An algorithm for the diagnosis of hyperammonemia of the newborn is shown in **Fig. 24-1**. Specific diagnosis of the majority of inborn errors of metabolism requires plasma amino acid analysis by quantitative column chromatography and urine organic acid analysis by gas chromatography mass spectroscopy. These studies require proper sample processing (**Table 24-1**) and should be performed only by laboratories proficient in these techniques and able to provide a rapid (1-day) result. Occasionally, skin or liver biopsy (see **Table 24-1**) may be required for diagnosis; however, presumptive therapy should begin as soon as a metabolic disorder is suspected.

IV. MANAGEMENT

A. IMMEDIATE INTERVENTIONS.

1. Discontinue protein intake.
2. Provide sufficient calories from glucose (60 kcal/kg per day) to prevent proteolysis and supplemental calories from lipid (60 kcal/kg per day).

TABLE 24-1

SAMPLE PROCESSING

Specimen	Proper Processing
Plasma: Ammonium levels rise rapidly on standing	1-3 ml in a sodium heparin (green top) tube; collect on ice and deliver immediately for analysis
Plasma: Amino acid levels change rapidly on standing and are uninterpretable after feeding	1-3 ml in a sodium heparin (green top) tube, *collected after a 4-hr fast;* deliver on ice or separate and freeze plasma for later analysis
Plasma: Carnitine	1-3 ml in a sodium heparin (green top) tube; deliver on ice or separate and freeze plasma for later analysis
Urine: Organic acids	5-10 ml; deliver on ice or freeze for later analysis
Skin biopsy: Clean a well-perfused area* with alcohol, not Betadine; use sterile technique	Immerse specimen in tissue culture medium or, if unavailable, patient's own serum; refrigerate; *do not freeze*
Liver biopsy (postmortem):† Obtain specimen as soon as possible for accurate enzyme analysis	"Flash freeze" in liquid nitrogen or on dry ice; store at -80 C for later analysis

*In a viable patient, obtain specimen from the ventral forearm.
†If at all possible, obtain specimen before death.

B. ANY INFANT IN STAGE II COMA (POOR MUSCLE TONE, FEW SPONTANEOUS MOVEMENTS, BUT RESPONSIVE TO PAINFUL STIMULI) OR WORSE IS A CANDIDATE FOR IMMEDIATE HEMODIALYSIS, FOLLOWED BY APPROPRIATE MEDICAL THERAPY.

Note: *Hemodialysis is 10 times more effective in removing small molecules than is peritoneal dialysis or arteriovenous hemofiltration. Exchange transfusion does not clear toxins that distribute in total body water and should not be considered therapy for inborn errors of metabolism.*

C. SPECIFIC THERAPY FOR HYPERAMMONEMIA.

1. Arrange for immediate hemodialysis for any patient with plasma ammonium level more than five times the upper limit of normal or with progressive encephalopathy and elevated ammonia.
2. Simultaneously perform steps listed under immediate interventions.
3. Administer a priming intravenous infusion of sodium benzoate, 250 mg/kg, sodium phenylacetate, 250 mg/kg, and arginine HCl 10% solution, 6 ml/kg, diluted in 35 ml/kg of 10% dextrose solution over 90 minutes; the same solution should then be infused over the next 24 hours (sustaining infusion).
4. Check plasma ammonium level 2 hours after completion of the priming infusion; if normal, continue maintenance infusion (cancel hemodialysis).

If elevated, start hemodialysis. If hemodialysis is still not available, start peritoneal dialysis.

Note: *These disorders are best treated by physicians experienced in the diagnosis and treatment of neonatal metabolic disease. Transporting sick patients to centers with specialized diagnostic facilities is usually advisable. Prompt transfer to a tertiary-care center equipped to perform neonatal hemodialysis may prevent CNS damage and be lifesaving.*

V. DISORDERS OF THE UREA CYCLE

A. CARBAMOYL PHOSPHATE SYNTHETASE DEFICIENCY (CPSD).

1. Signs and symptoms: vomiting, irritability, lethargy, seizures, coma.
2. Laboratory findings: respiratory alkalosis, hyperammonemia (severe), undetectable plasma citrulline, low plasma arginine, low urinary orotic acid.
3. Therapy: initial therapy as outlined in section IV, except that the arginine HCl should be reduced to 2 ml/kg in sustaining infusion. Long-term: Severe protein restriction (0.5 to 0.7 g/kg per day from natural protein, 0.5 to 0.7 g/kg per day from essential amino acids; sodium phenylbutyrate, 600 mg/kg per day; citrulline, 175 mg/kg per day).

B. ORNITHINE TRANSCARBAMYLASE DEFICIENCY (OTCD).

1. Signs and symptoms: vomiting, irritability, lethargy, seizures, coma.
2. Laboratory findings: respiratory alkalosis, hyperammonemia (severe), undetectable plasma citrulline, low plasma arginine, high urinary orotic acid.
3. Therapy: initial and long-term therapies are the same as for CPSD.

C. ARGININOSUCCINIC ACID SYNTHETASE DEFICIENCY (ASAD).

1. Signs and symptoms: vomiting, irritability, lethargy, seizures, coma.
2. Laboratory findings: respiratory alkalosis, hyperammonemia (moderate to severe), high plasma citrulline (>2000 μM), increased urinary orotate.
3. Therapy: initial, as outlined in section IV; long-term therapy includes protein restriction of 1.5 to 2 g/kg per day, sodium phenylbutyrate 600 mg/kg per day, arginine (freebase) 350 to 750 mg/kg per day.

D. ARGININOSUCCINASE DEFICIENCY.

1. Signs and symptoms: vomiting, irritability, lethargy, seizures, coma, hepatomegaly.
2. Laboratory findings: respiratory alkalosis, hyperammonemia (moderate to severe), high plasma citrulline (>100, <1000 μM), argininosuccinate and anhydrides in plasma.
3. Therapy: initial as outlined in section IV, except only intravenous arginine HCl 10% solution, 6 ml/kg or 12 g/m^2 over 90 minutes in 25 to 35 ml/kg 10% dextrose, and then repeat this infusion over the

24

INHERITED METABOLIC DISEASES

next 24 hours (i.e., no phenylacetate or benzoate required). Long-term therapy includes protein restriction to 1.5 to 2 g/kg per day, arginine (freebase) 400 to 700 mg/kg per day or 8.8 to 15.4 g/m^2 per day.

VI. DISORDERS OF AMINO ACID METABOLISM

A. MAPLE SYRUP URINE DISEASE (MSUD).

1. Etiology: branched-chain ketoacid decarboxylase deficiency.
2. Signs and symptoms: vomiting, lethargy, hypotonia alternating with spasticity, seizures, coma, maple syrup odor of sweat and urine.
3. Laboratory findings: metabolic acidosis; ketosis; usually increased anion gap; gray-green color of urine with the ferric chloride test; positive 2,4-dinitrophenylhydrazine test on urine; positive blood test for leucine by bacterial inhibition assay (included in some state newborn metabolic screens); and elevated leucine, isoleucine, and valine on plasma amino acid determination: urine organic acids positive for 2-ketoisocaproic, 2-ketoisovaleric, and 2-keto-3-methylvaleric acids.
4. Therapy: for initial therapy, eliminate natural protein from the diet, provide sufficient calories from glucose and lipid to prevent catabolism, and start hemodialysis to prevent CNS damage from leucine accumulation. Long-term therapy requires a special diet with restricted leucine, isoleucine, and valine; condition may be responsive to thiamine.

B. ISOVALERIC ACIDEMIA.

1. Etiology: isovaleryl coenzyme A (CoA) dehydrogenase deficiency.
2. Signs and symptoms: vomiting, lethargy, hypotonia, seizures, coma, "sweaty feet" odor of urine.
3. Laboratory findings: metabolic acidosis, ketosis, increased anion gap, occasional mild hyperammonemia, urine organic acids positive for isovalerylglycine and 3-hydroxyisovaleric acid.
4. Therapy: initial therapy is the same as for MSUD. If not comatose, intravenous carnitine and nasogastric glycine may be adequate treatment along with sufficient calories. Long-term therapy involves a special diet restricted in leucine and supplemental glycine to promote excretion of isovaleric acid as isovalerylglycine.

C. PROPIONIC ACIDEMIA.

1. Etiology: propionyl CoA carboxylase deficiency.
2. Signs and symptoms: vomiting, lethargy, hypotonia, seizures, coma.
3. Laboratory findings: metabolic acidosis, ketosis, elevated anion gap, neutropenia, occasional thrombocytopenia, occasional hyperammonemia (may be severe), twofold to fourfold elevation in plasma glycine; 3-hydroxypropionate and methylcitrate in urine.
4. Therapy: Initial therapy is to eliminate protein, prevent catabolism, treat acidosis (usually requires bicarbonate), and treat hyperammonemia as outlined in section IV. Long-term therapy involves a special diet

restricted in valine, threonine, methionine, and isoleucine; provide carnitine supplementation; some forms are responsive to biotin.

D. METHYLMALONIC ACIDEMIAS.

1. Etiology: methylmalonyl CoA mutase deficiency, adenosylcobalamin synthetic defect.
2. Signs and symptoms: poor feeding, vomiting, lethargy, and hypotonia; rarely, seizures and coma.
3. Laboratory findings: metabolic acidosis, ketosis, elevated anion gap, occasional hyperammonemia (may be severe), twofold to fourfold elevation in plasma glycine, methylmalonic acid in urine. Some forms also have homocystine in urine.
4. Therapy: initial therapy is the same as for propionic acidemia. Long-term therapy requires a special diet restricted in valine, threonine, methionine, and isoleucine; some forms are responsive to hydroxy-cobalamin; carnitine supplementation may be helpful.

E. MULTIPLE CARBOXYLASE DEFICIENCY.

1. Etiology: holocarboxylase synthetase deficiency.
2. Signs and symptoms: poor feeding, vomiting, lethargy, hypotonia, seizures, mild to moderate hyperammonemia, coma, urine odor of cat's urine; later, erythematous rash, alopecia, and seizures.
3. Laboratory findings: metabolic acidosis, ketosis, elevated anion gap, occasional moderate hyperammonemia, lactic acidosis, 3-methylcrotonylglycine, 3-hydroxyisovaleric acid, 3-hydroxypropionic acid, methylcitrate in urine.
4. Therapy: initial therapy as outlined in section IV, usually responsive to oral biotin (10 mg per day).

F. NONKETOTIC HYPERGLYCINEMIA.

1. Etiology: defect in the glycine cleavage system.
2. Signs and symptoms: poor feeding, seizures (burst-suppression pattern), hiccups, apnea, coma.
3. Laboratory findings: none on routine tests, threefold to fivefold increase in plasma glycine, more than 10-fold increase in cerebrospinal fluid (CSF) glycine.
4. Therapy: initial therapy is supportive. There is no consistently effective therapy, but sodium benzoate 500 to 750 mg/kg per day (orally) reduces seizures; dextromethorphan 5 to 25 mg/kg per day (orally) may be effective.

G. GLUTARIC ACIDEMIA, TYPE 1.

1. Etiology: glutaryl-CoA dehydrogenase deficiency.
2. Signs and symptoms: macrocephaly at or shortly after birth. Normal development until acute encephalopathy during a viral illness. This is

manifested by sudden onset of hypotonia, loss of head control, seizures, opisthotonus, grimacing, fisting, tongue thrusting, rigidity, and dystonia. Recovery from these basal ganglia infarcts is slow and incomplete, leading to choreoathetotic cerebral palsy (CP). Further episodes may occur with intercurrent illness.

3. Laboratory findings: hypoglycemia, metabolic acidosis, ketosis, hyperammonemia, mild elevations of liver enzymes, glutaric acid, 3-hydroxyglutaric acid, and glutaconic acid in the urine.

4. Therapy: L-carnitine glucose, insulin, and fluids during acute episodes. This disorder is detected by newborn screening using tandem mass spectrometry (see later). In those individuals, carnitine supplementation, restriction of lysine and tryptophan, and prompt initiation of intravenous glucose with any intercurrent illness to prevent decompensation has been helpful.

H. GLUTARIC ACIDEMIA, TYPE 2.

1. Etiology: electron transport flavoprotein (ETF) or ETF dehydrogenase deficiency.
2. Signs and symptoms: poor feeding, vomiting, lethargy, seizures, coma, "sweaty feet" odor to urine, hepatomegaly, may have associated anomalies (usually renal cysts).
3. Laboratory findings include severe metabolic acidosis, hypoglycemia, *no* ketosis, hyperammonemia.
4. Therapy: supportive; no effective therapy exists.

I. TYROSINEMIA.

1. Transient neonatal.
a. Etiology: unknown, probably relative deficiency of *p*-hydroxy-phenylpyruvate oxidase.
b. Signs and symptoms: poor feeding, lethargy, prolonged jaundice.
c. Laboratory findings: metabolic acidosis, hyperbilirubinemia, hypercholesterolemia, elevated tyrosine, phenylalanine, and histidine levels on plasma amino acid analysis.
d. Therapy: protein restriction to 2 g/kg per day (breast-feeding is effective).

2. Hepatorenal.
a. Etiology: fumarylacetoacetate hydrolase deficiency.
b. Signs and symptoms (not usually present until after the first week of life): failure to thrive, vomiting, diarrhea, "cabbage" odor, hepatomegaly, fever, edema, melena, epistaxis.
c. Laboratory findings: normocytic anemia, leukocytosis, occasionally thrombocytosis, hyperbilirubinemia, abnormal liver function tests, prolonged prothrombin time, hypocholesterolemia, elevated alpha-fetoprotein, elevated plasma tyrosine and methionine, hematuria, glycosuria, and generalized aminoaciduria. The presence of succinylacetone in the urine is diagnostic.
d. Therapy: special diet restricted in tyrosine, phenylalanine, and methionine; NTBC (2-(2-nitro-4-trifluorobenzoyl)-1.3-cyclohexanedione) 0.1 to

0.6 mg/kg per day is effective in 90% of patients; liver transplant is curative for the rest.

VII. DISORDERS OF CARBOHYDRATE METABOLISM

A. GALACTOSEMIA.

1. Etiology: galactose 1-phosphate uridyltransferase deficiency.
2. Signs and symptoms: poor feeding, vomiting, diarrhea, jaundice, hepatomegaly, cataracts.
3. Laboratory findings: hyperchloremic metabolic acidosis, indirect hyperbilirubinemia (early), direct hyperbilirubinemia (late), abnormal liver function tests; often associated with *Escherichia coli* sepsis; urine positive for reducing substances on Clinitest; galactose on paper chromatography of urine.
4. Therapy: discontinue galactose-containing formula (any formula with lactose), substitute a nongalactose formula (e.g., soy), supportive as needed.

B. GLYCOGEN STORAGE DISEASE, TYPES 1A, 1B.

1. Etiology: 1A: glucose-6-phosphatase deficiency; 1B: glucose-6-phosphatase translocase deficiency.
2. Signs and symptoms: hepatomegaly, seizures.
3. Laboratory findings: hypoglycemia, metabolic acidosis, ketosis, lactic acidosis, hypercholesterolemia, hypertriglyceridemia, hyperuricemia, abnormal liver function tests.
4. Therapy: long-term therapy involves frequent feeds (every 3 hours) with cornstarch and continuous enteral nightly feedings; allopurinol to treat hyperuricemia.

C. HEREDITARY FRUCTOSE INTOLERANCE.

1. Etiology: fructose 1-phosphate aldolase deficiency.
2. Signs and symptoms (require exposure to fructose, which is present in sucrose, fruit juices, Nursoy, and some oral antibiotics): vomiting, hepatomegaly, jaundice, sepsis, seizures, coma.
3. Laboratory findings: metabolic acidosis, ketosis, hypoglycemia, elevated lactate; diagnosis later confirmed by intravenous fructose tolerance test or measurement of hepatic enzyme activity.
4. Therapy: initial therapy is to discontinue fructose and supportive care; for long-term therapy, eliminate fructose and sucrose from the diet.

VIII. DISORDERS OF FATTY ACID METABOLISM

In addition to the following disorders, for each of the chain lengths there is a hydroxy-acyl-CoA dehydrogenase deficiency. Each may present with hepatic encephalopathy, cardiomyopathy/myopathy, or both. This field is rapidly growing. An acylcarnitine profile of dried blood on filter paper is diagnostic or suggestive and should always be performed when this class of disorders is considered.

A. MEDIUM-CHAIN ACYL-COA DEHYDROGENASE DEFICIENCY (MCAD).

1. Signs and symptoms: lethargy, seizures, coma, hepatomegaly, dilated cardiomyopathy, sudden infant death syndrome.
2. Laboratory findings: hypoglycemia with inappropriately low or absent urine ketones, metabolic acidosis, occasionally hyperammonemia, abnormal liver function tests, low plasma carnitine; urine organic acids show medium chain dicarboxylic acids and acylcarnitines, phenylpropionyl glycine, hexanoyl glycine, and subaryl glycine.
3. Therapy: Initial therapy is as described in section IV. If hyperammonemic, as described earlier, carnitine supplementation (100 mg/kg per day) is required. For long-term therapy, avoid prolonged fasting, add carnitine supplementation, and provide intravenous glucose infusion to prevent hypoglycemia associated with catabolism during intercurrent illness.

B. SHORT CHAIN ACYL-COA DEHYDROGENASE DEFICIENCY (SCAD).

1. Signs and symptoms are the same as for MCAD. Examination may reveal only cardiomyopathy, which can be dilated or hypertrophic.
2. Laboratory findings are the same as for MCAD, except urine organic acids show only ethylmalonic acid.
3. Therapy is the same as for MCAD.

C. VERY LONG CHAIN ACYL-COA DEHYDROGENASE DEFICIENCY (VLCAD).

1. Signs and symptoms are the same as for MCAD; hypertrophic cardiomyopathy has been described in some cases.
2. Laboratory findings are the same as for MCAD, except urine shows only dicarboxylic acids.
3. Therapy is the same as for MCAD, but a low-fat diet is recommended.

D. HYDROXYMETHYLGLUTARYL-COA LYASE DEFICIENCY (HMG).

1. Signs and symptoms are the same as for MCAD; urine has an odor similar to cat's urine.
2. Laboratory findings are the same as for MCAD, except urine shows 3-hydroxy-3-methylglutaric acid and 3-methylglutaconic acid.
3. Therapy is the same as for MCAD.

IX. CONGENITAL LACTIC ACIDOSES

A. PYRUVATE DEHYDROGENASE COMPLEX DEFICIENCY (PDH).
B. PYRUVATE CARBOXYLASE DEFICIENCY (PC).
C. DEFECTS OF THE ELECTRON TRANSPORT CHAIN (ETC).

1. Signs and symptoms may occur before 24 hours of age: hypotonia and respiratory distress from severe metabolic acidosis, apnea, coma,

- dilated cardiomyopathy; may have associated dysmorphic features; may be small for gestational age (SGA); abnormal brain imaging.
2. Laboratory findings: normoglycemic; severe metabolic acidosis caused by sharply elevated lactate, absence of other organic acids, elevated pyruvate (normal lactate/pyruvate ratio of <25) suggests PDH; decreased or normal pyruvate (increased lactate/pyruvate ratio of >35) suggests PC or ETC defects. PC deficiency type B causes lactic acidemia, citrullinemia, and hyperammonemia; ETC defects may require muscle biopsy for diagnosis.
3. Therapy: high-dose vitamin therapy may be helpful for PDH or PC; no therapy exists for ETC defects.

X. OTHER DISORDERS

Peroxisomal disorders may manifest in the newborn period with dysmorphic features and hepatomegaly (Zellweger syndrome) or with isolated neonatal seizures. Very long chain fatty acid and plasmalogen levels in whole blood (EDTA) are diagnostic or suggestive. Rarely, lysosomal storage diseases may manifest as neonatal hydrops and should be included in the differential. Smith-Lemli-Opitz syndrome (characterized by multiple congenital anomalies including ptosis, upturned nose, heart defects, cryptorchidism, and syndactyly of the second and third toes) is caused by a defect in cholesterol synthesis and can be diagnosed by measuring 7-dehydrocholesterol, which is markedly elevated in plasma. In severely affected infants, serum cholesterol is low.

XI. THE DEAD OR DYING INFANT

Any infant dying of unknown cause or of suspected metabolic disease requires a diagnosis for genetic counseling and accurate diagnosis in subsequent pregnancies. A full autopsy including x-ray skeletal survey should be performed. Specimens required for diagnosis include the following (see **Table 24-1** for proper processing):

A. BLOOD.

For assessment of plasma amino acids, plasma carnitine, and an acylcarnitine profile, obtain extra serum (clotted) and plasma (heparinized); separate and freeze; freeze the red blood cells (RBCs) separately.

B. URINE: FOR ORGANIC ACIDS, REDUCING SUBSTANCES, AND KETONES; FREEZE.
C. SKIN: FIBROBLAST CULTURE FOR ENZYMATIC ANALYSIS AND FOR DNA DIAGNOSIS.
D. LIVER: FREEZE A SPECIMEN FOR ENZYMATIC ANALYSIS.

XII. NEONATAL METABOLIC SCREENING

Every state screens for phenylketonuria and hypothyroidism, both insidious conditions that lead to preventable mental retardation. Most states also

24

INHERITED METABOLIC DISEASES

screen for the hemoglobinopathies and galactosemia. Many states screen for biotinidase deficiency (similar to multiple carboxylase deficiency, but of later onset) and congenital adrenal hyperplasia. Several states screen for cystic fibrosis (see **Chapter 26**).

As of October 2004, 21 states use tandem mass spectrometry to screen for amino acidopathies, organic acidemias, and fatty acid oxidation defects. The conditions screened by this methodology include PKU, MSUD, tyrosinemia, homocystinuria (an enzyme defect causing mental retardation, hypercoagulability, long-bone overgrowth, and ocular lens dislocation), citrullinemia, argininosuccinase deficiency, arginase deficiency, isovaleric acidemia, propionic acidemia, methylmalonic acidemias, 3-methylcrotonyl-CoA-carboxylase deficiency (a disorder ranging in phenotype from asymptomatic to mental retardation with seizures (further complicating matters, the analyte detected in infants may reflect abnormalities in the mother), MCAD, SCAD, VLCAD, LCHAD, glutaricaciduria type I, carnitine palmitoyl transferases I and II, and other known and unknown disorders. The various states and private laboratories are screening for the same analytes and therefore the same disorders, but each numbers them differently, ranging from 21 to 76 different disorders. Each laboratory using this methodology is screening for the same conditions.

Routine metabolic screening of the newborn should be performed after sufficient nutrient consumption has resulted in the accumulation of toxic metabolites, but before this accumulation has become symptomatic. The former is rarely accomplished before 24 hours of age. The initial screen should occur between 48 and 72 hours of age, except possibly in formula-fed infants, who can be screened as early as 24 hours. Repeat screening should be performed between 2 and 4 weeks of age; earlier repeat screening (1 to 2 weeks) is suggested for those breast-fed infants initially screened before 48 hours and formula-fed infants screened before 24 hours.

BIBLIOGRAPHY

Brusilow SW, Valle DL, Arn P: Symptomatic inborn errors of metabolism. In Nelson NM (ed): Current Therapy in Neonatal-Perinatal Medicine, 2nd ed. Philadelphia, BC Decker, 1989.

Burton B: Inborn errors of metabolism in infancy: A guide to diagnosis. Pediatrics 102:E69, 1998.

Fernandez J, Saudubray JM, Van den Berghe G (eds): Inborn Metabolic Diseases. Berlin, Springer-Verlag, 2000.

Pass KA, Lane PA, Fernhoff PM, et al: U.S. newborn screening system guidelines II: Follow-up of children, diagnosis, management, and evaluation. Statement of the Council of Regional Networks for Genetic Services (CORN). J Pediatr 137(4 suppl):S1, 2000.

Scriver CR, Beaudet AL, Sly WS, et al (eds): The Metabolic and Molecular Bases of Inherited Disease, 8th ed. New York, McGraw-Hill, 2001.

Wilcken B, Wiley V, Hammond J, Carpenter K: Screening newborns for inborn errors of metabolism by tandem mass spectrometry. N Engl J Med 348:2304, 2003.

Metabolism and Endocrinology

David W. Cooke

FAST FACTS

Immediate Issues in the Nursery

- Suspicion of hypoglycemia based on either symptoms or glucometer results must be confirmed by a measurement of plasma glucose that is < 45 mg/dl. Keep in mind that glucometer devices lose some accuracy in the hypoglycemic range. Also, glucose levels will decrease by 10 to 15 mg/dl for every hour the sample is left at room temperature (due to glucose metabolism by red blood cells).
- Hyperthyroidism is confirmed by levels of T_4 and T_3 that are elevated compared with age-specific normal ranges and a thyroid-stimulating hormone (TSH) that is suppressed. A history of Graves disease in the mother, either during or before the current pregnancy, and maternal hypothyroidism secondary to Hashimoto thyroiditis plus fetal tachycardia (>160 beats per minute) are indications to test for hyperthyroidism. Testing can be done from a peripheral blood sample on day 2 to 3 of life (testing earlier can be complicated by a normal neonatal surge that ceases after the first day of life).
- Any child with ambiguous genitalia should immediately undergo evaluation for an intersex condition. This evaluation should focus initially on congenital adrenal hypoplasia (CAH) and panhypopituitarism because these can result in adrenal crisis. Other infants who should be similarly evaluated include newborns with apparent male genitalia and one of the following: significant hypospadias (opening at base of penis or on perineum); bilaterally nonpalpable gonads; or any degree of hypospadias with unilateral undescended gonad. Likewise, infants with apparent female genitalia and a large clitoris (>1 cm) also warrant evaluation.

Important Reminders After Discharge

- Some infants appearing hypothyroid from the newborn screen are really euthyroid. Congenital deficiency of thyroid binding globulin (TBG) will decrease the amount of measured T_4, but the free T_4 and TSH levels will be normal (as opposed to low and elevated, respectively, if a true hypothyroid state existed). All infants with an abnormal thyroid screen (the most common presentation of congenital hypothyroidism) should have a total T_4, free T_4, and TSH drawn to confirm the diagnosis. Treatment should be initiated once these levels are drawn. Treatment can then be discontinued if all levels are in the normal range.
- Symptoms of adrenal crisis including hyperkalemia, hyponatremia, and hypovolemia generally manifest after the first week of life, though they can occur as early as the 3rd to 4th day of life. Many states

Continued

FAST FACTS—Cont'd

now routinely screen for CAH as part of their newborn screening protocol.

- Causes of late-onset hypocalcemia include hyperparathyroidism (velo-cardio-facial syndrome), vitamin D deficiency (secondary to maternal deficiency), excessive phosphate intake (commercial formulas), or mutations of calcium sensors in the kidneys (excessive urinary calcium excretion). Symptoms generally occur after 3 to 4 days of age and consist of twitching, jitteriness, tetany, or seizures.

Helpful Information for Parents

- Parents should always be alerted as to why their infants are being serially tested for hypoglycemia. Part of the discussion should include concerning symptoms and conditions that would require more intensive monitoring and therapeutic interventions.

- Congenital hyperthyroidism is mostly due to placentally transferred maternal factors. Symptoms usually subside after 3 to 12 weeks of life as the maternally derived thyroid stimulating immunoglobin is degraded.

- Once a newborn is identified as requiring evaluation for an intersex condition, the family should be informed that the child has a birth defect of the genitalia and that laboratory and radiologic studies will be necessary to determine the child's gender. The evaluation should be performed in consultation with specialists with expertise in this area. Until the evaluation is complete, the newborn should not be assigned a gender, and all medical personnel should resist any temptation to speculate what the likely gender will be on the basis of the appearance of the genitalia. If parents feel the need to assign a name, a gender-neutral name may be considered (e.g., Si(y)dney or Leslie).

GENERAL PRINCIPLES

In utero, metabolic homeostasis within the fetus is, to a great degree, under maternal and placental control. Once the umbilical cord is cut at delivery, the newborn must activate its own hormonal systems to maintain metabolic homeostasis. The two most common metabolic abnormalities in this transition period are hypoglycemia and hypocalcemia. In most cases these conditions are only transient; with minimal medical support (consisting mainly of ensuring adequate intake of glucose and calcium in feedings), the newborn achieves control of glucose and calcium levels shortly after birth. In some cases, however, hypoglycemia and hypocalcemia persist beyond the transition period after birth due to underlying hormonal or metabolic disorders that require more detailed investigation and intervention. This chapter begins with these common neonatal disorders. Other endocrine disorders that require attention in the neonatal period discussed in this chapter are: hyperglycemia, congenital hypothyroidism, congenital hyperthyroidism, and the child born with ambiguous genitalia.

I. HYPOGLYCEMIA

Fetal glucose levels, which are approximately 70% to 80% of the maternal levels, are maintained by a constant diffusion of glucose across the placenta. When this supply is interrupted at delivery, the glucose level in the newborn falls, reaching a nadir in the first 1 to 2 hours after birth. High levels of catecholamines, glucagon, growth hormone, and cortisol in the newborn activate glycogenolysis and gluconeogenesis; along with suppression of insulin secretion by the falling glucose levels, these lead to a subsequent rise in blood glucose levels. Failure of this adaptive process results in a glucose supply insufficient to meet metabolic requirements.

Hypoglycemia can be defined as a glucose level that is insufficient to meet metabolic requirements. Factors that may influence the metabolic requirements for glucose include those that increase glucose requirements (including stress and hypoxia, which lead to less efficient utilization of glucose through anaerobic glycolysis; polycythemia, through increased glucose metabolism by the increased red cell mass; hyperinsulinism, which, in addition to suppressing glycogenolysis and gluconeogenesis, suppresses ketone body formation and free fatty acid release, resulting in an increase in metabolic needs that must be met by glucose) and those that decrease glucose requirements (mainly milk feeding, due to the provision of other metabolic substrates including ingested fat and the stimulation of ketogenesis.) Thus, the glucose level that represents hypoglycemia depends on the clinical circumstances: lower glucose levels being sufficient under low-insulin, high-ketone body conditions as in a healthy breast-fed baby, compared with higher levels being necessary in the low-ketone body state present with hyperinsulinism (as in the infant of a diabetic mother). Nonetheless, it is helpful to have a glucose level that is used to guide whether intervention or investigation is warranted. For this reason, a plasma glucose level less than 45 mg/dl (2.5 mM) can be considered hypoglycemia in a newborn.

A. SCREENING.

1. Routine screening of normal term infants is not indicated.
2. Measure glucose level in at-risk infants within 1 to 2 hours after birth. Monitor glucose levels before feeds until normal levels are confirmed for 12-24 hours. Infants at risk include the following:
   a. Infants of mothers treated with β-adrenergic drugs (e.g., terbutaline), beta blockers (e.g., propranolol), oral hypoglycemics, or intravenous glucose (particularly if > 10 g/hr = 200 ml/hr of D5W fluid).
   b. Infants of insulin-dependent or gestational diabetic mothers, or of massively obese mothers.
   c. Infants who are large for gestational age (LGA; >90th percentile) [Infant of a diabetic mother; Beckwith-Wiedemann syndrome; hyperinsulinism].
   d. Infants who are small for gestational age (SGA; <10th percentile, or the smaller of discordant twins): These infants may have both transient hyperinsulinism and decreased glycogen stores contributing to their hypoglycemia.

e. Infants with significant hypoxia, perinatal distress, or Apgar scores < 5 at 5 minutes, requiring resuscitation.

f. Infants with severe erythroblastosis (cord blood hemoglobin level < 10 g/dl).

g. Infants with polycythemia.

h. Infants with exomphalos, macroglossia, and gigantism [Beckwith-Wiedemann syndrome].

i. Infants with isolated hepatomegaly [glycogen storage disease].

j. Any infant with microphallus or anterior midline defect, especially with hyperbilirubinemia [hypopituitarism].

k. Infants with a family history of neonatal hypoglycemia or unexplained death in infancy [inborn error of metabolism].

The diagnoses suggested by specific findings are noted in brackets in the previous list. Most of these conditions result in transient hypoglycemia, the exceptions being glycogen storage diseases, persistent hyperinsulinism, hypopituitarism, and inborn errors of metabolism; most cases of hypoglycemia in infants with Beckwith-Wiedemann syndrome resolve spontaneously.

3. **Glucose levels should also be monitored in infants requiring intensive care including all premature infants and those with sepsis, asphyxia, and respiratory distress.**

4. **Glucose levels should be measured in infants with symptoms consistent with hypoglycemia. The symptoms of hypoglycemia are nonspecific and, if due to hypoglycemia, should resolve with correction of the low glucose level. Symptoms of hypoglycemia in the neonate include the following:**

a. Abnormal cry.

b. Change in level of consciousness: lethargy or irritability.

c. Hypotonia or jitteriness, tremors.

d. Apnea, bradycardia, cyanosis, or tachycardia.

e. Seizures.

f. Difficulty in feeding.

g. Tachypnea.

h. Hypothermia.

5. **Measurement of glucose level. The following are important in interpreting glucose results:**

a. Whole blood glucose is approximately 15% lower than the plasma glucose. However, many glucometers used to measure glucose levels on whole blood samples are calibrated to give a result equivalent to the plasma glucose level.

b. Although treatment can be initiated for a symptomatic infant on the basis of the results measured on a glucometer, these devices are not sufficiently accurate in the hypoglycemic range for the diagnosis of hypoglycemia. Suspicion of hypoglycemia based on either symptoms or glucometer results must be confirmed by a measurement of plasma glucose.

c. Samples must be processed immediately due to red cell metabolism of glucose; glucose levels will decrease 15 to 20 mg/dl per hour in samples left at room temperature.

B. TREATMENT.

If the initial glucose level was measured by a glucometer, confirm with a laboratory-measured plasma glucose level.

1. Asymptomatic infant with plasma glucose level 25 to 45 mg/dl (1.4 to 2.5 mM):
   a. Immediately offer breast or formula feeding.
   b. Check glucose level 20 to 30 minutes after the feeding.
2. Asymptomatic infant with plasma glucose level less than 25 mg/dl (1.4 mM), asymptomatic infant who does not tolerate enteral feeding, or symptomatic infants:
   a. Parenteral glucose:
      (1) Give an intravenous bolus of glucose of 0.25 g/kg (2.5 ml/kg of 10% glucose, or 1 ml/kg of 25% glucose) over 1 to 2 minutes.
      (2) Continue the intravenous glucose at a rate of 6 to 8 mg/kg per minute (3.6 to 4.8 ml/kg/hr of 10% glucose).
      (3) Check the glucose level after 20 to 30 minutes, and then hourly until stable.
      (4) Increase intravenous glucose delivery 1 to 2 mg/kg per minute every 3 to 4 hours to maintain the plasma glucose level above 50 mg/dl (2.8 mM). An even higher glucose level should be maintained for infants with higher metabolic requirements for glucose (see earlier).
      (5) The glucose concentration and electrolyte composition of the intravenous fluid are determined by the fluid and electrolyte requirements of the infant. Glucose concentrations greater than 12.5% should be given through a centrally placed venous catheter. If glucose levels stabilize in the normal range, parenteral glucose is weaned slowly while oral feedings are advanced.
   b. Glucagon: If unable to give parenteral glucose, glucagon at a dose of 300 mcg/kg (maximum dose 1 mg) may be given subcutaneously or intramuscularly. This will increase glucose levels in infants with good glycogen stores for 2 to 3 hours, during which time intravenous access should be secured and parenteral glucose begun at 6 to 8 mg/kg per minute.
   c. Hydrocortisone (or prednisone): If the hypoglycemia persists after increasing to 12 mg/kg per minute of glucose, give hydrocortisone (5 to 10 mg/kg per day either orally or intravenously, divided in two doses) or prednisone (2 mg/kg per day orally). Measure serum cortisol and insulin before starting these medications.

C. EVALUATION.

If hypoglycemia in an infant with known risk factors for transient hypoglycemia resolves within the first week of life, no further evaluation is necessary. For other infants, investigation for an underlying cause should be initiated. This should generally be performed in consultation with specialists in endocrinology and metabolism. Glucose requirements greater

25

METABOLISM AND ENDOCRINOLOGY

than 8 mg/kg per minute are suggestive of hyperinsulinism, whereas midline defects and micropenis in a male infant suggest hypopituitarism.

II. TETANY-HYPOCALCEMIA (HYPOMAGNESEMIA)

A. DIAGNOSIS.
1. Term infants (and preterm infants > 1500 g): total calcium < 8 mg/dl (2mM) or ionized calcium < 4 mg/dl (1mM).
2. Preterm infants < 1500 g: total calcium < 7 mg/dl (1.75 mM).

B. ETIOLOGY.
1. Early neonatal hypocalcemia—occurring in the first 2 to 3 days of life.
a. Premature infants.
b. Infant of a diabetic mother.
c. Infant with birth asphyxia, perinatal stress.
d. Maternal hyperparathyroidism (previously diagnosed or unrecognized).
2. Late neonatal hypocalcemia—occurring after the first 3 days of life.
a. Hypoparathyroidism (isolated or associated with DiGeorge, CATCH-22, or other syndromes).
b. Excessive phosphate intake.
c. Vitamin D deficiency (due to maternal vitamin D deficiency).
d. Mutations of calcium sensing receptor (hypercalciuric hypocalcemia).

C. PRESENTATION.
1. Detected on screening of a high-risk infant (see early neonatal hypocalcemia mentioned previously).
2. Symptoms of hypocalcemia:
Neonatal hypocalcemia is characterized by increased neuromuscular irritability or activity—jitteriness, jerky movements of one or more limbs (twitching)—and can result in tetany or generalized convulsions. The classic signs of a high-pitched cry, facial muscle twitching when stimulated (Chvostek sign), and carpal spasm after constricting the upper arm (Trousseau sign) are seen more often in older infants but may occur in the neonate.

D. TREATMENT.
1. Once hypocalcemia is identified, the serum magnesium level should be determined. The clinical manifestations of hypomagnesemia are similar to those of hypocalcemia. In addition, hypomagnesemia can inhibit both PTH secretion and action, necessitating correction of hypomagnesemia before correcting hypocalcemia.
a. Hypomagnesemia is treated by the administration of 0.1 to 0.2 ml/kg of 50% magnesium sulfate solution (500 mg/ml) given either IV over at least 2 hours or IM. Magnesium levels should be monitored every 12 hours, with repeated doses as needed.
2. Asymptomatic infants with early-onset hypocalcemia may not require specific treatment, but treatment should be considered for infants with

total serum calcium less than 6 to 6.5 mg/dl (1.5 to 1.6 mM), particularly if there is a prolonged corrected Q-T interval on the electrocardiogram (>0.4 seconds).

3. Acute treatment for tetany and seizures.

a. 10% calcium gluconate (1 to 2 ml/kg or 9 to 18 mg/kg of elemental calcium) is given IV over 5 to 10 minutes while monitoring the heart rate for bradycardia or cardiac arrest and the infusion site for extravasation that can cause necrosis and subcutaneous calcifications. Do not infuse in an umbilical artery catheter, as this may cause arterial spasm, compromising intestinal blood flow.

b. Repeat the above dose after 10 minutes if seizures or tetany continue.

c. Follow bolus with a continuous IV infusion of calcium gluconate at a dose of 25 to 75 mg/kg per day of elemental calcium (2.25 to 6.75 ml/kg per day of 10% calcium gluconate).

d. Once calcium level is normalized, enteral calcium is begun, and IV calcium is decreased gradually over 2 to 3 days.

4. Enteral therapy may be used for asymptomatic infants or as continuing therapy once the calcium level is normalized with parenteral therapy in symptomatic infants. The enteral dose of calcium can be calculated in two ways:

a. 50 to 75 mg/kg per day of elemental calcium divided in 4 to 6 doses:

   (1) 555 to 833 mg/kg per day of calcium gluconate (5.5 to 8.3 ml/kg per day of 10% calcium gluconate)

   (2) 781 to 1171 mg/kg per day of calcium glubionate (2.2 to 3.2 ml/kg per day of 1.8 g/5 ml calcium glubionate)

b. Supplement the calcium in formula or expressed breast milk to give a calcium-to-phosphorus ratio of 4:1.

   (1) For infants with late-onset hypocalcemia due to high phosphorus intake from formula, the feedings should be changed to a low phosphorus formula (e.g., Similac PM 60/40) supplemented with additional calcium to give a 4:1 calcium-to-phosphorus ratio.

5. Hypoparathyroidism is treated with 50 to 100 ng/kg per day of calcitriol divided BID to TID (in addition to supplemental calcium, as described earlier).

III. HYPERGLYCEMIA

A. DIAGNOSIS.

There is no precise definition of hyperglycemia in the neonate. However, plasma glucose levels that exceed 180 to 200 mg/dl are clearly abnormal. Although plasma glucose levels above 150 mg/dl are probably abnormal, levels less than 200 mg/dl generally do not require treatment.

B. ETIOLOGY.

1. Iatrogenic.

Glucose requirements for infants are approximately 6 to 7 mg/kg/min. Hyperglycemia can occur in response to glucose administration that exceeds this.

25

METABOLISM AND ENDOCRINOLOGY

2. Stress-induced.

Very-low-birth-weight (<1000 g) and other critically ill infants are at risk of hyperglycemia because elevation of insulin-antagonizing factors—including catecholamines, cortisol, and cytokines—can decrease glucose utilization and lead to hyperglycemia even with normal amounts of glucose administration. Treatment with exogenous glucocorticoids can also predispose an infant to hyperglycemia. Note that the onset of hyperglycemia in a previously stable neonate may be an indicator of stress including sepsis.

3. Neonatal diabetes mellitus.

Neonatal diabetes mellitus is extremely rare. It can manifest anywhere from the first day of life to 2 to 3 months of age. The infants are typically SGA, reflecting in-utero insulin deficiency. The typical presentation is one of weight loss, dehydration, and polyuria. Hyperglycemia can be extreme (levels > 1000 mg/dl are not uncommon), while ketonemia and ketonuria are often minimal or absent. Neonatal diabetes mellitus is not caused by the autoimmune β-cell destruction as occurs in older children with type 1 diabetes (except, perhaps, for some infants at the oldest ages seen for neonatal diabetes). The specific causes for neonatal diabetes are now being elucidated:

a. Transient.

In approximately half of infants with neonatal diabetes mellitus, the requirement for treatment to maintain normal glucose levels will resolve after a period of days to months. However, in many cases hyperglycemia will recur after a number of years, typically during adolescence. This disorder is associated with loss of an imprinted region of chromosome 6q24.

b. Permanent—may be familial, although many may manifest as a sporadic case, representing new mutations.

   (1) Pancreatic agenesis.

   (2) Inactivating mutation in the gene for glucokinase, affecting glucose sensing in the β-cell.

   (3) Activating mutation in the gene for the Kir6.2 potassium channel affecting the intracellular cascade leading to insulin secretion in the β-cell.

   (4) Multisystem disorders associated with diabetes mellitus (e.g., Wolcott-Rallison).

C. TREATMENT.

1. For iatrogenic or stress-induced hyperglycemia, it is generally sufficient to decrease the rate of glucose administration.

2. For neonatal diabetes mellitus, insulin treatment is required. Insulin may also be required in stress-induced hyperglycemia in order to maintain sufficient glucose administration to provide sufficient calories for growth:

a. Intravenous insulin can be given at a rate of 0.01 to 0.1 units/kg per hour. The dose is adjusted on the basis of glucose levels measured

hourly, until glucose levels stabilize. The target glucose level should be 100 to 150 mg/dl.
b. For neonatal diabetes mellitus, treatment is generally begun with intravenous insulin. Transition to subcutaneous insulin doses and ongoing diabetes management should be done in consultation with specialists experienced with diabetes management in infants.

IV. HYPOTHYROIDISM

Congenital hypothyroidism occurs in approximately 1:3000 to 4000 live births. Because of the requirement for thyroid hormone for normal brain development, untreated congenital hypothyroidism leads to mental retardation. With prompt and appropriate treatment, however, normal development is achieved in most infants.

A. ETIOLOGY.

1. Primary hypothyroidism—(a defect at the level of the thyroid gland).
a. Thyroid dysgenesis (agenesis, hypoplasia, ectopy)—this is the most common cause of congenital hypothyroidism, accounting for the 1:3000 to 1:4000 incidence. Most are sporadic, although 2% to 5% are familial.
b. Dyshormonogenesis (a defect in the synthesis or secretion of thyroid hormone) accounts for approximately 10% of cases of congenital hypothyroidism. Autosomal recessive inheritance.
2. Central hypothyroidism (a defect at the level of the hypothalamus or pituitary). Incidence of 1:25,000 to 1:100,000. Concern for central hypothyroidism is increased in infants at higher risk of hypopituitarism such as those with midline defects (septo-optic dysplasia, cleft lip or palate) and those with signs or symptoms suggestive of other pituitary hormone deficiencies such as micropenis in male infants or hypoglycemia.
3. Transient hypothyroidism—may be caused by transplacental passage of antithyroid drugs or maternal thyroid blocking antibodies, iodine deficiency (rare in the United States), or excess (e.g., exposure of sick infants to iodine-containing antiseptics.)
4. TBG deficiency—this X-linked condition has a prevalence similar to that of thyroid dysgenesis. This is *not* a hypothyroid state: These infants (usually male) may be identified with low thyroid hormone levels on newborn screening tests. However, the low T_4 is due to the TBG deficiency; their euthyroid state is confirmed by normal free T_4 and TSH levels.
5. Hypothyroximemia of sick or premature infants. In these infants, with low total and free thyroid hormone levels and normal TSH levels, it can be difficult to determine the effect of prematurity or illness from that of central hypothyroidism; which of these infants benefit from treatment is difficult to determine.

B. SCREENING.

Screening for hypothyroidism is now routine in the United States, as well as in much of the rest of the world, although the strategy for screening differs. Knowledge of the local strategy for screening can help in interpreting both normal and abnormal results.

1. Initial T_4 assay, with TSH tested only on samples with a low T_4 level (most states in the United States use this approach).

a. This approach will identify many infants with central hypothyroidism, as well as those with primary hypothyroidism.

b. This approach will identify infants with TBG deficiency; these infants are *not* hypothyroid and so do not require treatment.

2. TSH as the screening test.

a. Will not identify infants with central hypothyroidism.

b. Some infants with congenital primary hypothyroidism have a delayed rise in TSH and will not be identified with a TSH-only screen that is done shortly after birth. Most, but not all, of these infants will be identified under protocols that require repeat testing at 1 to 2 weeks of age.

c. An infant with compensated hypothyroidism (normal T_4 but elevated TSH) will be identified by the TSH-only screen, but not by a screen that relies on an initial T_4.

C. SYMPTOMS.

Most infants with congenital hypothyroidism will be identified by newborn screen before any symptoms develop; signs and symptoms are rarely present before 6 weeks of age. However, no screening protocol is perfect, so T_4 and TSH levels should be measured in any infant with signs or symptoms of hypothyroidism: poor feeding; prolonged jaundice; lethargy; hypotonia; poor peripheral circulation; cool, mottled skin; macroglossia; large fontanels; hoarse cry; and facial edema. If the etiology is dyshormonogenesis, a goiter may exist or develop.

D. DIAGNOSIS.

1. An infant identified with an abnormal thyroid screen should have a laboratory-measured total T_4, free T_4, and TSH to confirm the diagnosis. Treatment should be initiated while awaiting the results, with treatment discontinued if the laboratory testing does not confirm the diagnosis.

2. Additional diagnostic studies (radionucleotide thyroid imaging, thyroid ultrasound) can aid in establishing the etiology of the hypothyroidism but do not affect the decision to treat; treatment should not be delayed in order to obtain these tests.

E. TREATMENT.

1. Treatment is initiated as soon as confirmatory laboratory tests are drawn.

2. L-thyroxine is begun at a dose of 10 to 15 mcg/kg/day.

3. Liquid suspensions are not reliable. L-thyroxine tablets of the correct dose are crushed and mixed with a small amount of formula or breast

milk (1 to 2 ml) and given directly to the infant (not mixed in a bottle) to ensure ingestion of the entire amount.

4. If IV thyroxine must be given, the dose is one third to one half the enteral dose; frequent monitoring is required.

V. HYPERTHYROIDISM

Hyperthyroidism occurs in approximately 2% of pregnancies complicated by maternal Graves disease. With an estimated prevalence of Graves disease of 1:500 pregnancies, approximately 1:25,000 live-born infants may have thyrotoxicosis. A history of Graves disease in the mother, either during or before the current pregnancy, and maternal hypothyroidism secondary to Hashimoto thyroiditis plus fetal tachycardia (>160 beats per minute) are indications to obtain serum T_4, T_3, and TSH levels on day 2 to 3 of life. Hyperthyroidism is confirmed by levels of T_4 and T_3 that are elevated compared with age-specific normal ranges and a TSH that is suppressed.

A. CLINICAL MANIFESTATIONS.

1. Evidence of fetal hyperthyroidism includes growth retardation, goiter (highly varying in size), advanced bone age, and craniosynostosis.
2. Neonatal manifestations may occur within 24 to 48 hours of age. However, symptoms may be delayed due to elimination of maternal antithyroid medications or thyroid-blocking antibodies from the neonatal circulation before elimination of maternal thyroid-stimulating antibodies.
3. Neonatal symptoms include irritability, flushing, tachycardia, poor feeding, failure to thrive, diarrhea, vomiting, and prolonged jaundice, as well as goiter and exophthalmos.
4. Thrombocytopenia with hepatosplenomegaly and hypoprothrombine-mia have been reported. Cardiac arrhythmia and failure may occur with severe disease.

B. THERAPY.

1. For controlling acute manifestations and tachycardia and preventing cardiac failure, give propranolol, 1 to 2 mg/kg/day in two or three divided doses.
2. If thyroid hormone levels are markedly elevated, propylthiouracil (PTU) at 5 to 10 mg/kg per day in divided doses every 8 hours or methimazole at 0.5 to 1 mg/kg/day in divided doses every 8 to 12 hours are given.
3. For thyrotoxicosis, iodides—1 to 2 drops every 8 hours of Lugol solution (50 mg/ml iodine and 100 mg/ml potassium iodide) or sodium ipodate (100 mg per day)—may be necessary and are then given for 1 to 2 weeks. Glucocorticoids may also be added to the treatment.

C. PROGNOSIS.

1. Hyperthyroidism usually subsides after 3 to 12 weeks of life as the maternally derived thyroid-stimulating immunoglobin is degraded.
2. Rare cases of persistence of the hyperthyroidism have been reported.

VI. AMBIGUOUS GENITALIA

An infant born with ambiguous genitalia is a rare event that requires careful management from both medical and social perspectives.

A. EVALUATION FOR AN INTERSEX CONDITION SHOULD BE INITIATED FOR A NEWBORN WITH CLEARLY AMBIGUOUS GENITALIA, BUT ALSO FOR NEWBORNS WITH THE FOLLOWING:

1. Apparent male genitalia, but with bilaterally nonpalpable gonads.
2. Apparent male genitalia with any degree of hypospadias (urethral opening not at the tip of the phallus) combined with even one undescended gonad.
3. Apparent male genitalia with severe hypospadias (urethral opening at the base of the phallus or on the perineum).
4. Apparent female genitalia with an inappropriately large clitoris (>1 cm of corpora in a term infant) or with any amount of posterior fusion of the labia.

B. INFANTS WITH MALE GENITALIA WITH A NORMAL-SIZED PENIS (>2.5 CM IN THE TERM INFANT) WITH HYPOSPADIAS WITH THE URETHRAL OPENING ON THE SHAFT OR GLANS OF THE PENIS OR AN INFANT WITH MALE GENITALIA WITH A NORMAL-SIZED PENIS WITH ONE NONPALPABLE GONAD DOES NOT REQUIRE EVALUATION FOR AN INTERSEX CONDITION.

The most pressing medical diagnoses to consider are hypopituitarism in the male infant with micropenis (penis < 2.5 cm in the term infant; for normal sizes for premature infants[1]) and congenital adrenal hyperplasia (CAH), as both of these situations put the infant at risk of an adrenal crisis. Although a salt-wasting crisis with hyperkalemia, hyponatremia, and hypovolemia typically presents after the first week of life, presentations as early as the 3rd or 4th day of life have been described. Therefore, it is necessary to screen newborns for CAH as it is now done routinely, for example, in Maryland.

Once a newborn is identified as requiring evaluation for an intersex condition, the family should be informed that the child has a birth defect of the genitalia and that laboratory and x-ray studies will be necessary to determine the child's gender. The evaluation should be performed in consultation with specialists in this area. Until the evaluation is complete, the newborn should not be assigned a gender, and all medical personnel should resist any temptation to speculate what the likely gender will be on the basis of the appearance of the genitalia.

REFERENCES

1. Feldman KW, Smith DW: J Pediatr 86:395, 1975.

BIBLIOGRAPHY

Beardsall K, Ogilvy-Stuart AL: Congenital hypothyroidism. Curr Pediatr 14:422, 2004.
Cornblath M et al: Controversies regarding definition of neonatal hypoglycemia: Suggested operational thresholds. Pediatrics 105:1141, 2000.

DeMarini S, Tsang RC: Disorders of calcium, phosphorus, and magnesium metabolism. In Fanaroff AA, Martin RJ (eds): Neonatal-Perinatal Medicine, 7th ed. St Louis, Mosby, 2002.

Fisher DA: Disorders of the thyroid in the newborn and infant. In Sperling MA (ed): Pediatric Endocrinology, 2nd ed. Philadelphia, WB Saunders, 2002.

Gloyn AL et al: Activating mutations in the gene encoding the ATP-sensitive potassium-channel subunit Kir6.2 and permanent neonatal diabetes. N Engl J Med 350:1838, 2004.

Haney PM: Neonatal hypoglycemia. Wellesley: UpToDate; 2002. Available at http://www.uptodate.com.

Haney PM, Stark AR: Neonatal hyperglycemia. Wellesley: UpToDate; 2004. Available at http://www.uptodate.com.

Hsu SC, Levine MA: Perinatal calcium metabolism: Physiology and pathophysiology. Semin Neonatol 9:23, 2004.

Kaefer M: Diagnosis and treatment of the undescended testicle. In Pescovitz OH, Eugster EA (eds): Pediatric Endocrinology: Mechanisms, Manifestations, and Management. Philadelphia, Lippincott Williams & Wilkins, 2004.

Kalhan SC, Parimi PS: Disorders of carbohydrate metabolism. In Fanaroff AA, Martin RJ (eds): Neonatal-Perinatal Medicine, 7th ed. St Louis, Mosby, 2002.

LaFranchi S: Clinical features and detection of congenital hypothyroidism. Wellesley: UpToDate; 2004. Available at http://www.uptodate.com.

LaFranchi S: Treatment and prognosis of congenital hypothyroidism. Wellesley: UpToDate; 2004. Available at http://www.uptodate.com.

Metz C et al: Neonatal diabetes mellitus: Chromosomal analysis in transient and permanent cases. J Pediatr 141:483, 2002.

Njolstad PR et al: Neonatal diabetes mellitus due to complete glucokinase deficiency. N Engl J Med 344:1588, 2001.

Panny SR: Letter: Notification that the Maryland Department of Health and Mental Hygiene has begun routine screening all newborns in the state for congenital adrenal hyperplasia: October 15, 2001.

Sperling MA, Menon RK: Differential diagnosis and management of neonatal hypoglycemia. Pediatr Clin N Am 51:703, 2004.

Stanley CA: Advances in diagnosis and treatment of hyperinsulinism in infants and children. J Clin Endocrinol Metab 87:4857, 2002.

Van der Kamp HJ, Noordam K, Elvers B, et al: Newborn screening for congenital adrenal hyperplasia in the Netherlands. Pediatrics 108:1320, 2001.

World Health Organization: Hypoglycemia of the newborn: Review of the literature. Geneva, World Health Organization, 1997. Available at http://www.who.int/reproductive-health/docs/hypoglycaemia_newborn.htm.

25

METABOLISM AND ENDOCRINOLOGY

Prenatal Diagnosis, Prenatal Screening, and Newborn Screening

Michael D. Cabana

I. GENERAL PRINCIPLES OF SCREENING

A. LIMITATIONS OF SCREENING AND DIAGNOSIS.

1. Although some conditions can be diagnosed before birth, the majority of birth defects and genetic conditions are *not* detected through routine prenatal diagnosis or screening.
2. Criteria for when to use screening tests.
   a. Disease is clearly defined and medically important.
   b. Natural history of the disease can be changed by a feasible intervention.
   c. Screening test is cost effective.
   d. Patient or parents have given informed consent.
3. Criteria for test effectiveness (**Fig. 26-1**).
   a. Test characteristics.
      (1) Sensitivity—how often the test is positive in the presence of the disease.
      (2) Specificity—how often the test is negative when the disease is not present.
      (3) Positive predictive value—how often the disease is present when the test is positive.
      (4) Negative predictive value—how often the disease is not present when the test is negative.
   b. Trade-offs and implications.
      (1) No test has 100% sensitivity *and* 100% specificity.
      (2) Because the purpose of screening tests is to "rule out" the presence of a disease, screening tests generally have high sensitivity (rare false negatives), but may not have high specificity (false positives).
      (3) Most screening tests must be confirmed by follow-up tests with higher specificity.
      (4) As a result, when obtaining informed consent and when discussing the results of screening tests, it is important to explain these possibilities (false negatives and false positives) to the family.

B. SCREENING AND DIAGNOSIS IN NEWBORN CARE.

1. Prenatal diagnosis: diagnoses or rules out a particular condition in the fetus.
2. Prenatal screening: identifies mothers at increased risk for having a child with the condition.
3. Newborn screening: identifies newborns at risk for having a particular condition.

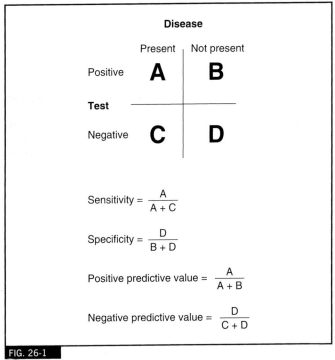

FIG. 26-1
Calculation of test characteristics for screening tests.

II. PRENATAL SCREENING

A. DEFINITION:
Tests to identify mothers at increased risk for having a child with a specific condition.

B. INDICATIONS.
1. Screening tests provide an alternative to invasive prenatal diagnosis.
2. Decreased risk to the pregnancy.
3. Should be used with deliberate caution because the tests may increase a patient's anxiety and lead to invasive prenatal testing.

C. PRENATAL SCREENING PROCEDURES.
1. Second trimester maternal serum screening. The measurement of particular chemicals in blood during second trimester allows for patient-specific risk assessment for a variety of fetal abnormalities.
a. General issues.
   (1) Standard of care in the U.S. dictates that maternal serum screening is offered to all pregnant women during the second trimester.

  (2) Results are reported as multiples of the medial (MOM; with median = 1.0).

  (3) Because normal values vary with gestational age, a common reason for false positives is inaccurate dating of the pregnancy.

b. Alpha-fetoprotein (AFP) screening.

  (1) AFP is synthesized by the fetal yolk sac, gastrointestinal tract, and liver; AFP levels are adjusted for maternal weight, race, and diabetic status.

  (2) Test administered at 15 to 18 weeks' gestation.

  (3) Elevated AFP suggestive of

   (a) Neural tube defect (spina bifida, anencephaly).

   (b) Pregnancy complications (e.g., fetal/neonatal death, preterm birth, low birth weight, and preeclampsia).

   (c) Abdominal wall or esophageal defects.

   (d) Other rare conditions.

  (4) Low AFP suggestive of

   (a) Trisomy 21; Down syndrome (average = 0.7 MOM in affected pregnancies)

   (b) Trisomy 18; Edward syndrome

c. Human chorionic gonadotropin (hCG)

  (1) hCG is a glycoprotein made by the placenta and detected in serum or urine during pregnancy

  (2) Elevated hCG suggestive of

   (a) Down syndrome (average = 2.1 MOM in affected pregnancies).

   (b) Pregnancy complications (e.g., fetal/neonatal death, preterm birth, low birth weight, and preeclampsia).

  (3) Low hCG levels suggestive of Trisomy 18.

d. Unconjugated estriol (uE3).

  (1) uE3 is a steroid hormone that is a major estrogen of pregnancy.

  (2) Low uE3 suggestive of

   (a) Down syndrome (average = 0.7 MOM in affected pregnancies)

   (b) Trisomy 18.

   (c) Smith-Lemli-Opitz syndrome.

   (d) X-linked ichthyosis.

e. Triple screen (i.e., AFP plus).

  (1) AFP, hCG, and uE3 are independent predictors of Down syndrome.

  (2) An algorithm combines information from all three tests with maternal age to estimate a patient-specific risk for Down syndrome.

  (3) Likelihood of "abnormal" triple screen increases with maternal age.

  (4) Detects approximately 60% of cases of fetal Down syndrome.

2. Prenatal Ultrasound: Variation in fetal development detected through ultrasound may suggest an underlying fetal abnormality.

a. Timing: 18 to 20 weeks.

b. Issues with interpretation.

  (1) Low sensitivity for cardiac malformations.

   (a) Only two thirds of cardiac defects are noted on routine ultrasound.

   (b) Four-chamber view of heart identifies up to 40% of major anomalies.

26

PRENATAL DIAGNOSIS, PRENATAL AND NEWBORN SCREENING

(c) High-risk pregnancies may require repeat ultrasound at 22 to 26 weeks.

(d) Family history of congenital heart disease.

(e) Maternal diabetes.

(f) Maternal use of anticonvulsants.

(2) Low specificity for many findings.

(a) "Soft signs" with unknown significance are found in up to 5% of routine ultrasounds; seen with normal healthy newborns as well.

  (i) Choroid plexus cyst.

   • Estimated 1.0% incidence in second trimester.

   • By 26 weeks' gestation, 95% are not seen again.

  (ii) Mild renal pelvic dilation (pyelectasis).

   • Estimated 0.3% to 4.5% incidence in second trimester.

   • Mild dilation of uncertain significance.

   • If significant dilation (e.g., >10 mm) increased risk of structural anomaly of kidney.

  (iii) Echogenic intracardiac foci (EIF).

   • Estimated incidence of up to 2.2% of all ultrasounds.

   • When isolated, EIF is an insensitive marker of Down syndrome.

  (iv) Single umbilical artery.

   • Estimated 1.0% incidence in all pregnancies.

   • Associated with aneuploidy, but only in the presence of other anomalies.

  (v) Mild cerebral ventricular dilatation.

(b) If multiple soft markers are found, may signify increased risk of chromosomal anomaly.

(3) Nuchal translucency.

(a) Increased thickness is associated with Down syndrome.

(b) Also associated with cardiac, renal, diaphragmatic and abdominal wall defects.

(c) Nuchal thickness >5 mm is associated with decreased overall survival.

(4) Echogenic bowel.

(a) Estimated 0.2% to 1.4% incidence in second trimester.

(b) Associated with IUGR, intra-amniotic bleeding, Down syndrome, and cystic fibrosis.

3. Carrier testing.

a. To identify parents with increased risk of having children with specific conditions.

b. Indications: It is essential to inquire about the ethnic backgrounds of both parents, with carrier testing offered if one or both members of the couple are from a high-risk ethnic group.

(1) Sickle cell anemia (African-American descent).

(2) Tay Sachs (Jewish, French-Canadian descent).

(3) Canavan disease (Jewish descent).

(4) Thalassemia (Mediterranean, Middle-Eastern, and Southeast Asian descents).

c. If both parents are identified as carriers, further fetal testing may be pursued.

d. Additional resources: The National Society of Genetic Counselors (610-872-7608 or *www.nsgc.org*).

II. PRENATAL DIAGNOSIS

A. DEFINITION:
Procedures to diagnose or rule out a particular condition in the fetus.

B. INDICATIONS:
Because prenatal diagnosis is invasive and involves risk to the fetus and mother, it is reserved for couples whose risk of having a child with a particular condition is greater than the risk associated with the diagnostic testing.

1. Any positive screening tests.
2. Maternal age >35 years at the time of delivery.
   a. Risk for a fetal chromosomal abnormality increases with advancing maternal age (**Table 26-1**).
   b. At 35 years, risk of a chromosomal abnormality is greater than the risk of amniocentesis.
3. Previous child with a genetic condition (e.g., muscular dystrophy) or birth defect (e.g., neural tube defect), or a close family member with such a condition.

TABLE 26-1

RATES (PER THOUSAND) OF CHROMOSOMAL ABNORMALITIES IN LIVE BIRTHS, BY MATERNAL AGE

Maternal Age (years)	Down Syndrome	All Abnormalities
15	1.0	2.2
20	0.5-0.7	1.9
25	0.7-0.9	2.1
30	0.9-1.2	2.6
35	2.5-3.9	5.6
36	3.2-5.0	6.7
37	4.1-6.4	8.1
38	5.2-8.1	9.5
39	6.6-10.5	12.4
40	8.5-13.7	15.8
41	10.8-17.9	20.5
42	13.8-23.4	25.5
43	17.6-30.6	32.6
44	22.5-40.0	41.8
45	28.7-52.3	53.7
46	36.6-68.3	68.9
47	46.6-89.3	89.1
48	59.5-116.8	115.0
49	75.8-152.7	149.3

From Hook EB: Rates of chromosomal abnormalities of different maternal ages. Obstet Gynecol 58:282, 1981.

26

PRENATAL DIAGNOSIS, PRENATAL AND NEWBORN SCREENING

4. History of a teratogenic exposure or maternal health condition (e.g., diabetes).
5. Ethnic descent associated with inheritable diseases.

C. PRENATAL DIAGNOSTIC PROCEDURES.

1. Chorionic villus sampling (CVS).
   a. Description: Transcervical (with a catheter) or transabdominal (with a needle) cytogenic analysis of villus tissue from the developing placenta (chorion frondosum) during the first trimester of pregnancy.
   b. Timing: First trimester, at approximately 10 weeks' gestation.
   c. Management.
      (1) If a fetal abnormality is detected, allows for earlier termination of pregnancy.
      (2) Termination during the first trimester (versus second trimester) is medically safer and is psychologically easier.
      (3) Early diagnosis may also allow for prenatal treatment in some cases (e.g., for 21-hydroxylase deficiency).
   d. Safety.
      (1) Pregnancy loss. Estimated 0.5% to 1.0% risk for miscarriage—usually due to placental injury, infection, and/or rupture of membranes.
      (2) Complications.
         (a) Vaginal bleeding may occur after CVS.
         (b) RhoGAM is given to Rh-negative unsensitized women after the procedure.
      (3) Fetal malformations:
         (a) Increased risk for transverse terminal limb defects.
         (b) Risk increases when CVS is performed earlier (less than 8 weeks' gestation).

2. Traditional amniocentesis.
   a. Description: With ultrasound guidance, a spinal needle is inserted through the maternal abdomen and uterus for withdrawal of a small amount of amniotic fluid for cytogenetic studies.
   b. Timing: 15 to 16 weeks' gestation.
   c. Safety.
      (1) Pregnancy loss: Approximately 0.5% risk for miscarriage.
      (2) Vaginal bleeding and/or leakage of amniotic fluid may occur after amniocentesis.
      (3) Infection is rare.
      (4) RhoGAM is given to Rh-negative unsensitized women after the procedure.
      (5) Fetal malformations caused by amniocentesis have been reported; however most large studies do not reveal an increased risk for fetal malformations.

3. Early amniocentesis.
   a. Description: Similar to traditional amniocentesis, except timing occurs before 15 weeks' gestation.
   b. Safety.

(1) Procedure-associated risk for miscarriage is higher than traditional amniocentesis.

(2) Early amniocentesis may increase the risk of clubfeet in the fetus.

4. Fetal Blood Sampling

a. Description: Fetal blood sample for cytogenetic analysis obtained from the umbilical or hepatic vein.

b. Indications:

(1) If a fetal anomaly is diagnosed late in pregnancy or when a mosaic result is obtained through CVS or amniocentesis.

(2) To determine hematocrit levels in fetuses at risk for anemia.

c. Timing: 18 to 20 weeks' gestation.

d. Safety: Risk of miscarriage is estimated to be 1% to 2%.

26

IV. NEWBORN SCREENING TESTS

A. SCREENING AS A "SYSTEM."

1. Screening is part of a system that includes:

a. Informed consent.

b. Obtaining screening tests in a timely manner.

c. Prompt follow-up evaluation, if needed.

d. Confirmation of diagnosis and treatment.

2. Before screening, parents have a right to informed consent—as well as a right to confidentiality regarding information from screening results.

3. Special considerations.

a. For infants discharged early (prior to 24 hours), repeat blood testing is recommended.

b. Preterm infants should have newborn screening test completed before the end of the first week of life and before any blood transfusion.

4. Before nursery discharge, all infants should have a follow-up primary care provider identified.

a. With access to the newborn screening test results.

b. Provided with contact information for the child's family.

c. Have ability to follow-up on positive or equivocal screening results.

5. Follow-up.

a. Urgent follow-up is needed for maple syrup urine disease, galactosemia, congenital adrenal hyperplasia (CAH)—all potentially fatal if not treated soon after birth.

b. Counseling and education should be provided to minimize anxiety.

c. Access to subspecialist may be required.

B. LIMITATIONS OF CURRENT SCREENING SYSTEM.

1. Newborn screening began in the early 1960s with the development of a system to easily collect and transport blood samples on filter paper (Guthrie cards) for PKU.

2. No current national standard set of newborn screening tests.

3. Each state may have different sets of screening tests (**Table 26-2**), as well as systems available for follow-up notification and services provided for treatment.

TABLE 26-2

STATE-TO-STATE VARIATION IN NEWBORN SCREENING PROGRAMS

National Newborn Screening and Genetics Resource Center

U.S. National Screening Status Report–Updated 2/14/06

The U.S. National Screening Status Report lists the status of newborn screening in the United States. The condition must be required by the state in order for a dot "•" to be added.

A circle in the brackets [•] indicates that MS/MS is used for detecting the analyte of interest.

State	PKU	CH	GAL	MSUD	HCY	BIO	SCD	CAH	CF	MS/MS Testing	OTHER
Alabama	•	•	•			•	•	•		•	
Alaska	[•]	•	•	[•]	[•]	•	•	•		•	
Arizona	•	•	•	•	•	•	•	•			
Arkansas	•	•	•			•	•	•			
California	•	•	•	C	C	•	•	•		C	
Colorado	•	•	•	C	C	•	•	•	• B	•	HIV
Connecticut	[•]	•	•	[•]	[•]	•	•	•	•	•	G6PD
District of Columbia	[•]	•	•	[•]	[•]	•	•	•		•	
Delaware	[•]	•	•	[•]	[•]	•	•	•	C	•	
Florida	•	•	•	•	•	•	•	•		•	
Georgia	•	•	•	•		•	•	•		C	TYR
Hawaii	[•]	•	•	[•]	[•]	•	•	•		•	
Idaho	[•]	•	•	[•]	[•]	•	•	•		•	
Illinois	[•]	•	•	[•]	[•]	•	•	•		•	
Indiana	[•]	•	•	[•]	[•]	•	•	•	•	•	
Iowa	[•]	•	•	[•]	[•]	•	•	•		•	
Kansas	•	•	•			•	•	•			
Kentucky	•	•	•	• A	• A	C	•	C	C		
Louisiana	•	•	•	[•]	A	•	•	•			
Maine	[•]	•	•	[•]	[•]	•	•	•		•	

State									Other
Maryland	•	•	•	•	•	•	•	[•]	
Massachusetts	•	•	•	•	A	A	•	[•]	TOXO
Michigan	•	•	•	•	C	C	•	[•]	
Minnesota	•	•	•	•	•	•	•	[•]	
Mississippi	•	•	•	•	C	C	•	•	
Missouri	C	C	B	C	C	C	•		G6PD (C)
Montana	A	A	•	A	[A]	[A]	•	•	
Nebraska	•	•	•	•	[A]	[A]	•	•	
Nevada	•	•	C	•	[•]	[•]	•	•	
New Hampshire	•	C	A	C	A	C	•	•	TOXO
New Jersey	•	•	•	•	•	•	•	•	
New Mexico	•	C	•	•	[•]	[•]	•	•	
New York	•	•	•	•	[•]	[•]	•	•	HIV
North Carolina	•	•	•	•	[•]	[•]	•	•	
North Dakota	•	•	•	•	•	•	•	[•]	
Ohio	C	•	•	•	•	•	•	[•]	
Oklahoma	•	•	•	A	•	•	•	[•]	
Oregon	C	B	C	•	[A]	[•]	•	[•]	
Pennsylvania	•	•	•	A	[A]	[•]	•	[•]	G6PD (A)
Rhode Island	A	B	•	•	[•]	[•]	•	[•]	
South Carolina	•	•	•	C	C	C	•	[•]	

Continued

26

TABLE 26-2

STATE-TO-STATE VARIATION IN NEWBORN SCREENING PROGRAMS—Cont'd

State	PKU	CH	GAL	MSUD	HCY	BIO	SCD	CAH	CF	MS/MS Testing	OTHER
South Dakota	[•]	•	•	[A]	[A]	•	A	•	B	A	
Tennessee	•	•	•	[•]	[•]	•	•	•		•	
Texas	•	•	•				•	•			
Utah	[•]	•	•	[A]	[A]		•			A	
Vermont	[•]	•	•	[•]	[•]	•	•	•		•	
Virginia	[•]	•	•	[•]	[•]	•	•	•	C	•	
Washington	[•]	•	•	[•]	[•]	•	•	•		•	
West Virginia		•	•				•	•			
Wisconsin	[•]	•	•	[•]	[•]	•	•	•	•	•	
Wyoming		•	•				•	•	•		

PKU, phenylketonuria; CH, congenital hypothyroidism; GAL, galactosemia; MSUD maple syrup urine disease; HCY, homocystinuria; BIO, biotinidase; SCD, sickle cell disease; CAH, congenital adrenal hyperplasia; CF, cystic fibrosis; MS/MS, tardem mass spectrometry; HIV, human immunodeficiency virus; G6PD, glucose-6-phosphate dehydrogenase disease; TYR, tyrosinemia; TOXO, toxoplasmosis.

A, selected populations, limited pilot programs, or by request (not mandated); B, universal testing on all babies (not mandated); C testing mandated but not yet implemented. The states are constantly revising screening requirements. It pays to be constantly aware of changes in your state. Refer on the internet to the U.S. National Screening Status Report from the National Newborn Screening and Genetics Resource Center.

4. Do not assume that children born in another state have been screened for diseases normally included in another state's current newborn screening tests.

C. SPECIFIC NEWBORN SCREENING TESTS.
1. Phenoketonuria (PKU).
a. Description: Autosomal recessive disorder characterized by inability to metabolize the amino acid phenylalanine.
b. Prevalence: 1:9000.
c. Management: On confirmation of test, phenylalanine-free infant formula should be started. Long term—dietary modification may be necessary.
d. Test must be obtained after 24 hours of age.

2. Hypothyroidism.
a. Description: Multiple etiologies; characterized by an inability to produce adequate thyroid hormone.
b. Prevalence: 1:2000.
c. Management: On confirmation of diagnosis, treatment with oral thyroid replacement hormone.
d. Test must be obtained after 24 hours of age. Test is designed only to detect early onset hypothyroidism and does not rule-out late-onset, subclinical disease beyond the newborn period.

3. Galactosemia.
a. Description: Autosomal recessive disorder. Classic form is characterized by a deficiency of galactose-1-phosphate uridyl transferase, which leads to an accumulation of galactose. Disease variants (e.g., Duarte) are associated with less severe reduction in enzymatic activity.
b. Prevalence: 1:42,000.
c. Management: Immediate exclusion of galactose from diet (including breast milk).
d. Blood transfusions may cause false negatives. Obtain test before blood transfusions.

4. Maple syrup urine disease (MSUD).
a. Description: Autosomal recessive disorder characterized by inability to metabolize branched chain amino acids. Initial signs include poor feeding and vomiting.
b. Prevalence: 1:100,000 to 1:300,000.
c. Management: Immediate treatment with infant formula that is free of branched-chain amino acids. Continued diet modification after infancy.
d. Test must be obtained after 24 hours of age.

5. Homocystinuria.
a. Description: Autosomal recessive disorder of amino acid metabolism, caused by an enzymatic defect that leads to increased levels of methionine. Infants are initially asymptomatic in the first few months of life, but later demonstrate failure to thrive, progressive mental retardation, and subluxation of the ocular lens (ectopia lentis).

b. Prevalence: 1:200,000 to 1:350,000.

c. Management: Methionine-restricted diet supplementation with cystine and medication (betaine). Some patients respond to high-dose vitamin B_6 (pyridoxine).

6. Biotinidase deficiency.

a. Description: Autosomal recessive disorder characterized by inability to synthesize biotin, a member of the vitamin B family. Deficiency results in neurologic damage.

b. Prevalence: 1:34,000.

c. Management: requires daily oral biotin supplement.

d. Blood transfusions may interfere with accuracy of test results.

7. Sickle cell disease.

a. Description: Autosomal recessive disorder characterized by changes in beta-hemoglobin chain, which leads to anemia and other sequelae including pain crises, acute chest syndrome, and compromise of splenic function.

b. Prevalence: Up to 1:600 in the African-American population.

c. Management: Patients have increased risk of infection by encapsulated bacteria. Penicillin prophylaxis is necessary as well as referral to subspecialty care.

d. Blood transfusions may interfere with accuracy of test results.

8. Congenital adrenal hyperplasia (CAH).

a. Description: Group of autosomal recessive disorders characterized by a defect in any of a series of enzymes responsible for synthesis of cortisol from cholesterol (most commonly a defect of 21-hydoxylase). Can lead to incorrect gender assignment for females, as well as adrenal crisis and death.

b. Prevalence: 1:20,000.

c. Management: Immediate referral to tertiary care center. Careful monitoring of glucose and sodium levels. Early intervention and surgical correction of ambiguous genitalia, if present.

d. False positives may be due to collection of specimen before 24 hours of age. False negatives can occur due to chronic maternal use of dexamethasone during pregnancy.

9. Medium chain acyl-CoA dehydrogenase (MCAD) deficiency.

a. Description: Autosomal recessive disorder characterized by defect in fatty acid oxidation pathway that affects ability to utilize stored fat. Episodes of hypoglycemia, hyperammonemia with low urinary ketone production during times of stress can lead to encephalopathy, liver failure, coma, and death.

b. Prevalance: 1:10,000 to 1:15,000.

c. Management: Low-fat diet and avoidance of fasting. Acute episodes treated with intravenous glucose.

10. Other tests included in some state screening programs include: toxoplasmosis, cystic fibrosis tyrosinemia, HIV, and G6PD.

BIBLIOGRAPHY

Evans MI, O'Brien JE, Dvorin E, et al: Second trimester biochemical screening. Clin Perinatol 28:289, 2001.

Hook EB: Rates of chromosomal abnormalities of different maternal ages. Obstet Gynecol 58:282, 1981.

Newborn Screening by State. National Newborn Screening and Genetics Resource Center. http://genes-r-us.uthscsa.edu/nbsdisorders.pdf. Accessed October 8, 2004.

Rochon M, Eddleman K: Controversial ultrasound findings. Obstet Gynecol Clin North Am 31:61, 2004.

Wilson JMG, Jungner G: Principles and practice of screening for disease. Geneva, World Health Organization, 1968.

26

Breast-Feeding

Judith W. Vogelhut

I. ADVANTAGES

A. LOWER RENAL SOLUTE LOAD.

B. ANTI-INFECTIVE PROPERTIES.
1. Protection against diarrhea. Bifidus factor promotes proliferation of *Lactobacillus bifidus* in infant's intestines, which discourages colonization by pathogens; secretory IgA antibodies to *Escherichia coli* continue to be produced into the second year of lactation.
2. Protection against infectious diseases, including respiratory syncytial virus (RSV), bacterial meningitis, bacteremia, urinary tract infection, and otitis media.
3. Antiviral properties.
4. Protection against necrotizing enterocolitis (NEC).
5. Promotes phagocytosis by macrophages and leukocytes.

C. ANTI-ALLERGIC PROPERTIES.
1. Decreased incidence and severity of eczema.
2. Species-specific protein; delays introduction of foreign protein.

D. BONDING.
1. Promotes special closeness between mother and baby.
2. Prolactin response increases maternal relaxation.
3. Increases maternal self-confidence.
4. Meets infant's needs for safety, security, and cuddling.

E. MAY DECREASE RATES OF SIDS, TYPE 1 AND TYPE 2 DIABETES, SOME CANCERS, OBESITY, AND ASTHMA.

II. CONTRAINDICATIONS

A. BREAST CANCER.
Mother's need for treatment takes precedence over lactation.

B. MOTHERS WHO ARE RECEIVING DIAGNOSTIC OR THERAPEUTIC RADIOACTIVE ISOTOPES OR WHO HAVE HAD EXPOSURE TO RADIOACTIVE MATERIALS (FOR AS LONG AS THERE IS RADIOACTIVITY IN THE MILK).

C. HUMAN IMMUNODEFICIENCY VIRUS (HIV) INFECTION.
It is recommended that HIV-infected women in the U.S. should not breast-feed based on the risk of transmitting the virus to the uninfected infant.

D. LIFE-THREATENING ILLNESS IN THE MOTHER.

E. GALACTOSEMIA IN THE INFANT.

F. HERPES SIMPLEX VIRUS (HSV) INFECTION.
Breast-feeding is contraindicated in the presence of active breast lesions.

G. CURRENT MATERNAL SUBSTANCE ABUSE.

H. ACTIVE UNTREATED TUBERCULOSIS IN MOTHER.
May breast-feed after at least 2 weeks of treatment.

I. TREATMENT WITH ANTI-METABOLITES OR CHEMOTHERAPEUTIC AGENTS.

Note: *Breast-feeding is **not** contraindicated in mothers who are: hepatitis B surface antigen positive; infected with hepatitis C virus; febrile (unless caused by one of the contraindications in section II); seropositive carriers of cytomegalovirus (CMV) if the infant is term.*

III. HUMAN MILK CHARACTERISTICS
A. COLOSTRUM IS PRODUCED FROM THE SECOND TRIMESTER THROUGH THE FIRST FEW POSTPARTUM DAYS;
It is yellow in appearance and has a mean energy value of 67 kcal/100ml. It contains a high concentration of immunoglobulins, especially secretory IgA.

B. TRANSITIONAL MILK
contains increasing volume, caloric content, and water-soluble vitamins; there is a decreasing concentration of immunoglobulins.

C. MATURE MILK
contains 75 kcal/100ml; it is in large part water; the fat content is most variable.
1. Foremilk is the early portion of a feeding; it is more dilute and lower in fat.
2. Hindmilk is secreted later in the feeding and has 3 to 5 times the fat content of foremilk.

IV. MANAGEMENT
A. PUT THE INFANT TO THE MOTHER'S BREAST
as soon as is feasible postpartum because early contact with the mother's breast may have an imprinting effect on mother and baby. The infant's quiet, alert state shortly after birth is conducive to nursing if mother and baby are stable.

B. ENCOURAGE ROOMING-IN.
Avoid supplemental feeding unless medically indicated; frequent nursing helps establish mother's milk supply, prevent excessive engorgement, and minimize neonatal jaundice.

C. POSITIONING.

1. Cradle position: Infant's head is in the mother's antecubital fossa, with its body rotated so that the face, chest, and abdomen are against her chest, and the infant's lower arm is behind the mother. Pillows may be needed for support; a footstool is helpful if the mother is in a chair.

2. Clutch (football) position: The infant's body is positioned on pillows to the mother's side; the infant's hips are flexed, with the back of the infant's neck supported by the mother's hand.

3. Side-lying position: The mother is positioned on her side in bed and the infant is placed on its side facing the mother. The lower breast is offered first, then mother rolls toward baby to offer upper breast or rolls to her other side to offer second breast.

D. LATCH-ON.

1. Mother supports and lifts her breast with her thumb on top and her other fingers below, staying behind the areola; mother strokes the infant's lips gently with her nipple, waits for baby to open mouth wide, and then, with nipple aimed upward toward the infant's palate, draws baby in close. The tip of the baby's nose should touch the breast; the airway can be maintained by lifting up on the breast or drawing the baby's buttocks in close.

2. Appropriate latch-on and nutritive sucking are accomplished when the infant's jaw excursions are wide, swallows are audible, and the infant's tongue is visible coming forward to the lower gum (visualized by holding down lower lip). The baby should not be pulled off the breast easily; the infant's lips are flanged outward and can be gently pulled out if necessary.

3. If baby latches on correctly and mother does not report pain, there is no need or benefit to limiting feeding time; arbitrarily doing so can limit baby's intake and promote engorgement in the mother by inadequate emptying.

4. Both breasts should be offered at each feeding, although the baby may nurse from only one. The mother should alternate the breast offered first because the baby sucks more vigorously on the first breast at each feeding. Once the milk supply is established, the mother should follow the baby's cues as to when one side is finished.

5. The infant can be removed from the breast by the mother inserting a finger into the corner of the baby's mouth between the gums to release suction.

6. The baby should be burped after each breast.

7. Avoid pacifier use.

E. ANTICIPATORY GUIDANCE.

1. It is important during prenatal and postpartum visits to identify any barriers to successful breast-feeding (**Box 27-1**).

BOX 27-1

BARRIERS TO BREAST-FEEDING

It is important to discover barriers to successful breast-feeding. There are questions which, when asked appropriately and open-ended, may help in revealing, understanding, and dealing with these barriers.

QUESTIONS TO ASK AT THE PRENATAL VISIT

How will a new baby change your life?

How are you planning to feed your baby?

Have you considered breast-feeding?

What do you know about breast-feeding?

Have you breast-fed another child? If so, how did it go?

How do most of your friends feed their babies?

Are you taking any medications?

Do you have any medical problems?

How does the baby's father feel about your breast-feeding?

May I suggest a list of books you might read about breast-feeding?

QUESTIONS TO ASK AT THE "JUST AFTER DELIVERY VISIT"

How are you planning to feed your baby?

Have you started breast-feeding yet?

Were you able to nurse in the delivery room?

Do you understand the instructions for breast-feeding?

Would you like to see a lactation consultant?

How often do you plan to nurse your baby?

Do you understand how to prevent sore nipples and breast infections?

How is the baby reacting to breast-feeding?

Are you having difficulty with the baby latching on or any other problem getting started with breast-feeding?

Do your breasts hurt or are they tender?

Are you on any medications or drugs?

Would you like to see a video about breast-feeding?

QUESTIONS TO ASK WITHIN THE FIRST WEEK AFTER DISCHARGE*

How is breast-feeding going?

Do you have any worries about it?

Are you enjoying breast-feeding?

Are you feeling tired?

Who spends a lot a time with you, and what do they think about breast-feeding?

Has your health been good since your delivery?

How long do you plan to nurse?

What contributes to that decision?

Would you like to consult a lactation specialist?

*Asking questions within the first week after discharge becomes important. It reinforces the effort of nursing at a time when many mothers may be discouraged and give it up.

Modified from Bennjamin JY, Shariat H: Contemp Pediatr 16:73, 1999.

2. Expect a full-term infant initially to nurse 8 to 12 times in 24 hours, generally 15 minutes per breast.

3. Infants usually wet at least 6 diapers in 24 hours and have at least two or three soft, yellow, seedy stools per 24-hour period; some breast-fed babies stool with each feeding initially and then less frequently after the first month. A significant variation from this pattern should be brought to the practitioner's attention.

4. In most cases, avoid supplementary bottles for the first month to allow mother and infant time to become skilled at breast-feeding, to allow for optimum milk production, and to allow time for mother's milk ejection reflex (letdown) to become conditioned.

5. Several letdowns may occur during the course of a feeding. The milk ejection reflex is characterized by slow, long sucks with frequent swallows, milk leaking from the contralateral breast, and possibly a pins-and-needles tingling in the breast. In the early postpartum period, there may be uterine cramping.

6. Infants typically experience growth spurts (milk supply lagging behind increasing demand) at 2 to 3 weeks, 6 weeks, 3 months, and 6 months. Generally, 2 to 3 days of unrestricted nursing will increase the supply enough to meet the increased demand.

7. Vitamin D supplementation is recommended and is generally dispensed as A, D, and C drops. Iron intake from breast milk is adequate for full-term infants until 4 to 6 months of age.

8. Fluoride supplementation is not needed during the first 6 months.

9. Conduct telephone follow-up with mother 48 hours after nursery discharge; the initial office or clinic visit should take place at 3 to 5 days with a second visit at 2 to 3 weeks of age. Full-term breast-fed babies most often regain their birth weight by 2 weeks.

27

BREAST-FEEDING

V. MATERNAL CONCERNS

A. FLAT OR INVERTED NIPPLES.

1. May use a breast pump briefly before offering infant the breast to increase nipple protrusion.

2. An inverted nipple may be helped by having the mother support her breast and retract her fingers toward her chest.

B. ENGORGEMENT.

1. Engorgement is a physiologic reaction caused by milk accumulation and increased vascularity.

2. Small, firm breasts are prone to more significant engorgement.

3. Frequent nursing during the colostral phase minimizes edema.

4. Areolar edema may flatten the nipple, making latch-on difficult, and causing nipple soreness.

5. Advise mother on use of warm compresses, soaks, or showers followed by gentle massage and expression of milk to soften the areola.

6. Frequent nursing maintains drainage and prevents decreased milk production from back pressure on ducts.
7. Cold compresses to breast after feeding may reduce swelling.
8. A bra should be worn for support. Avoid constricting underwires.

C. NIPPLE SORENESS.

1. Nipple soreness is best prevented by proper latch-on and positioning, alternating breast-feeding positions, and careful air drying of the breast after feedings.
2. Development of soreness is unrelated to prenatal preparation.
3. The mother should nurse first on the less-affected breast.
4. Late-onset soreness may be caused by *monilia* infection. Treatment consists of nystatin oral suspension to infant's mouth, 2 ml 4 times daily, and nystatin topically to mother's nipple and areola four times daily after feeding.
5. Remove baby gently without precipitously pulling baby off breast.
6. Baby should be held closely into mother's body. A baby who is falling away from the breast will traumatize the nipple.

D. MATERNAL DIET.

1. Mother should eat an extra 500 kcal per day.
2. Drink to quench thirst (there is no benefit to forcing fluids).
3. Limit caffeine.
4. Alcoholic beverages should be avoided. If used in moderation, breast-feeding should be avoided for 2 hours.

E. PLUGGED DUCTS.

1. Tender lump in the breast.
2. No systemic symptoms.
3. Possible factors include constricting bra, missed feedings, fatigue, or nursing multiples.
4. Treatment.
a. Moist heat before nursing.
b. Frequent feedings.
c. Remove bra if too tight.
d. Massage breast gently before and during feeding.
e. Position infant with chin toward the lump to improve drainage of affected area.
f. Watch for symptoms of mastitis.

F. MATERNAL MASTITIS.

1. Mastitis may be preceded by maternal fatigue, a plugged duct, unrelieved engorgement, or nipple trauma.
2. It is usually unilateral, and rarely bilateral. The most common organisms are *Staphylococcus aureus* and *E. coli;* rarely, *Streptococcus* can be found in bilateral mastitis.

3. The highest incidence occurs 2 to 6 weeks' postpartum.
4. Systemic symptoms may precede localized ones. Symptoms include fever, chills, malaise and body aches, nausea and vomiting, warm area on breast, tender lump or wedge in breast, or an erythematous streak.
5. Treatment.
a. Bed rest.
b. Warm compresses.
c. Frequent nursing to empty ducts.
d. Begin feedings on unaffected side if more comfortable.
e. Antibiotic therapy for 10 days (full course recommended to avoid relapse): dicloxacillin, a cephalosporin, or erythromycin.
f. Increased maternal fluid intake.
g. Remove bra and other constrictive clothing.

G. BREAST-FEEDING AND RETURNING TO WORK.

1. Assess workplace before return.
a. Privacy for pumping.
b. Adequate break time.
c. Refrigerator or cooler to store pumped milk.
d. Options concerning full-time versus part-time hours, baby brought to mother during her working hours or working from home.
2. Mother should choose a supportive babysitter and familiarize caregiver with the proper handling of breast milk.
3. Allow at least 1 month of exclusive breast-feeding before introducing artificial nipples.
4. Familiarize infant with artificial nipples 10 to 14 days before return to work.
a. Expressed breast milk may be preferred initially to ameliorate new experiences.
b. Initially, an artificial nipple may be better accepted if offered by someone other than the mother at a midday feeding rather than early morning or bedtime. Try it when the baby is drowsy rather than ravenously hungry if he or she is reluctant to take the bottle.
5. Mother should practice expressing or pumping milk and begin freezing it for later use.
6. Milk may be expressed by hand, manually-operated pump, battery-operated pump, small electric pump, or heavy-duty electric breast pump. The efficiency of the pump needed depends partly on the frequency of pumping.
7. Pump 10 to 15 minutes per breast.
8. Pump parts are washed in hot, soapy water as soon after use as possible.
9. Store milk in clean plastic bottles with lids and date the containers.
10. Milk for a healthy infant may be kept refrigerated for 72 hours, frozen in a refrigerator freezer for 1 month, and frozen at $-4°$ F for 3 to 4 months. Store away from the fan in a self-defrosting freezer; do not store in the freezer door or refrigerator door.

11. Store upright, with most recently pumped milk behind the older milk.
12. Thaw in warm water before feeding; never boil or microwave. May thaw in refrigerator and use within 24 hours. Milk that has been thawed should never be refrozen.
13. See **Box 27-2** for information on breast pumps and other paraphernalia.

BOX 27-2

BREAST PUMPS AND OTHER PARAPHERNALIA

MANUAL

Most require two hands to operate; have the advantages of being inexpensive and widely available; may be tiring.

- Kaneson
- Hollister Egnell (one-handed)
- Medela (spring express)
- White River
- Evenflo
- Gerber
- Avent

BATTERY

Approximately 4 hours' pumping time on each set of batteries; moderate pricing; convenient if not near an electric outlet.

- Gentle Expressions
- Hollister Egnell
- Medela
- Evenflo

PORTABLE ELECTRIC

Generally noisy, as are the battery pumps; one-handed operation.

- Gerber
- Mag Mag
- Evenflo
- Nurture 3 (allows double pumping)
- Medela (available for single or double pumping)

ELECTRIC PUMPS FOR PURCHASE (CLOSE TO HOSPITAL GRADE)

Expensive; probably worth it if pump is to be used over several months.

- Medela Pump in Style
- Egnell Purely Yours

HEAVY DUTY ELECTRIC PUMPS FOR RENTAL (HOSPITAL GRADE)

Expense may be disadvantage; preferable for long-term pumping; more adequate hormone stimulation; available with double-pumping kits to pump both breasts simultaneously.

- Medela Classic and portable Lactina models
- Hollister Egnell
- White River

BOX 27-2—Cont'd
BREAST PUMPS AND OTHER PARAPHERNALIA
BICYCLE HORN
Use of this pump should be discouraged; it is less expensive but can damage the breast because the amount of suction is difficult to control with the rubber bulb. Milk that goes into the bulb may be contaminated.
HAND EXPRESSION
Mothers can be taught to express milk by hand. In fact, during long-term pumping occasionally expressing by hand allows skin-to-skin contact, which may increase milk supply.
BREAST SHELLS
Hard plastic cups that can be worn inside the bra prenatally and postpartum to help alleviate flat or inverted nipples; any milk collected in the cups is to be discarded.
FEEDING TUBE DEVICE
To supplement the infant at the breast; may be useful for preterm babies, postoperatively, and with adoptive nursing.
HAND EXPRESSION FUNNEL
Catches the sprays; universal threads allow expression directly into bottle.

27

BREAST-FEEDING

VI. INFANT CONCERNS

A. JAUNDICE.

1. Jaundice may be a pathologic condition if it is visible at or before 24 hours of age.
2. Early hyperbilirubinemia may be related to infrequent feedings (<8 per 24 hours), infrequent stools, or prematurity.
3. Treatment.
   a. Early, frequent feedings.
   b. Assess infant for normal suck pattern.
   c. Augment feedings with formula if indicated; mother may need to pump her breasts to increase milk supply.
   d. Phototherapy as necessary.
4. Breast-milk (late onset) jaundice.
   a. Delayed and prolonged hyperbilirubinemia (1:200 births); usually occurs after first 3 to 5 days, peaks at approximately 2 weeks, and, if nursing continues; may persist for several weeks.
   b. Normal stooling.
   c. Cause is as yet unidentified, but may be related to glucuronyl transferase inhibitor in milk.
   d. A bilirubin level decrease of 2 mg/100 ml on discontinuing breast-feeding reassures that it is breast-milk jaundice; there will be a slight rise in the bilirubin level on resuming breast-feeding, followed by a slow, steady drop.
   e. Not a contraindication to continued nursing.

B. LOW BIRTH WEIGHT AND VERY LOW BIRTH WEIGHT.
1. Support the mother's decision to provide breast milk for infant.
2. Pumping.
   a. The mother should begin pumping as soon after delivery as possible.
   b. Use of a heavy-duty electric breast pump is preferable.
   c. Pump a total of at least 6 times in 24 hours to equal 100 minutes of pumping time.
   d. Mother can use a double-pump kit to express both breasts simultaneously.
   e. Direct nipple stimulation may improve milk ejection reflex.
   f. Allow mother 6 hours of uninterrupted rest at night.
3. Transition to breast.
   a. Infant should be held to the breast as soon as possible after stability is achieved.
   b. Any contact, even if non-nutritive, provides positive experience to help infant learn and to increase maternal milk supply.
   c. Allow sucking on finger or pacifier by the infant during gavage feedings.
   d. Feedings at breast.
      (1) Position infant with entire body supported by mother's arm.
      (2) The cross-cradle or football hold is often recommended.
   e. Lack of suck pads in cheeks and decreased muscle tone may necessitate support of infant's jaw by mother's hand while at the breast.
   f. In some cases, supplementation of breast-feeding with a feeding-tube device is helpful by decreasing the infant's exposure to artificial nipples while learning to breast-feed.
   g. A human milk fortifier may be used to supplement calories, vitamins, and minerals.
4. Discharge from the hospital.
   a. Infant may not be feeding totally at breast when discharged.
   b. Continue pumping after feeding while infant is being supplemented.
   c. Gradually decrease amount and frequency of supplements as baby's suck improves.

VII. DRUGS IN BREAST MILK
A. FACTORS TO CONSIDER.
1. **Dosage.** Determine whether drug is a single dose versus long-term use; short-acting drugs are preferable over the long-acting form.
2. Age and maturity of infant.
   a. An infant's liver can metabolize most drugs at term.
   b. Some compounds (e.g., sulfadiazine) compete for bilirubin binding sites, thus increasing the risk of kernicterus.
3. Quantity of milk consumed by the infant.
4. Experience with giving drug directly to infants: watch infant for unusual signs; weigh risk of drug versus benefit of breast-feeding.
5. Minimize effects. For most medications, schedule maternal dose just after feeding.

B. AMERICAN ACADEMY OF PEDIATRICS LIST OF DRUGS CONTRAINDICATED IN NURSING MOTHERS.
- Cyclophosphamide
- Cyclosporine
- Doxorubicin
- Methotrexate
- Amphetamine
- Cocaine
- Heroin
- Marijuana
- Phencyclidine

C. CERTAIN RADIOPHARMACEUTICALS REQUIRE TEMPORARY DISCONTINUATION OF BREAST-FEEDING.

VIII. NURSING TWINS (OR TRIPLETS)

A. BREAST-FEED AS SOON AFTER BIRTH AS POSSIBLE
if one or both babies are sufficiently stable; if both babies are unable to nurse, the mother should begin pumping within 24 hours of infants' births; if one baby is able to breast-feed, the mother can pump one breast and store the milk for the other baby.

B. POSITIONING.
Mother can breast-feed twins simultaneously to save time and increase milk production. She should start the baby that has the more efficient suck first to stimulate the milk ejection reflex, then latch on the other infant. Mother will need several pillows or a nursing pillow for support.

C. FATIGUE IS THE BIGGEST PROBLEM.
Encourage family members to arrange for help during the first 2 weeks at home, if at all possible.

D. THERE IS A HIGHER INCIDENCE OF PLUGGED DUCTS AND MASTITIS
when nursing twins or multiples secondary to increased milk production and fatigue.

E. TRIPLETS CAN BE EXCLUSIVELY BREAST-FED, OR ONE BABY EACH FEEDING MAY RECEIVE A SUPPLEMENT.
F. PROVIDE SUPPORT.
Refer mother to community resources such as peer or breast-feeding support groups or local parents of multiples; maintain telephone contact.

IX. WEANING

A. BABY-INITIATED WEANING IS IDEAL.
Weaning should be accomplished as slowly as possible.

27

BREAST-FEEDING

B. REPLACE ONE FEEDING WITH A BOTTLE OR CUP (DEPENDING ON THE AGE OF THE BABY);

Begin with midday feeding rather than early morning, naptime, or bedtime, when baby nurses for comfort as well as nutrition.

C. ALLOW A FEW DAYS FOR MILK SUPPLY TO ADJUST DOWNWARD BEFORE SUBSTITUTING ANOTHER BOTTLE OR CUP FEEDING.
D. GENERALLY, BEDTIME FEEDING IS THE LAST TO GO.
E. THERE IS A RISK OF PLUGGED DUCTS OR MASTITIS IF WEANING IS TOO RAPID.

BIBLIOGRAPHY

American Academy of Pediatrics Committee on Drugs: The transfer of drugs and other chemicals into human milk. Pediatrics 108:3,776, 2001.

American Academy of Pediatrics; Section on Breastfeeding; Breastfeeding and the use of human milk. Pediatrics115:496, 2005.

Bennjamin JY, Shariat H: Overcoming impediments to breastfeeding: How pediatricians can help. Contemp Pediatr 16:73, 1999.

Huggins K: The nursing mother's companion, ed 4, Boston, The Harvard Common Press, 1999.

LaLeche League International: The womanly art of breastfeeding, ed 4, Franklin Park, Ill, LaLeche League International, 1990.

Lawrence R: Breastfeeding: A Guide for the Medical Profession, ed 5. St. Louis, Mosby, 1999.

Riordan J, Auerbach K: Breastfeeding and Human Lactation, ed 3, Sudbury, Mass, Jones and Bartlett, 2005.

Williams-Arnold, L: Human Milk Storage for Healthy Infants and Children. Health Education Associates Inc., Sandwich, Mass, 2000.

Childbirth Education and Bonding

Henry M. Seidel

I. CHILDBIRTH EDUCATION

A. GENERAL INFORMATION.

Prenatal education, formal and informal, about childbirth education, pregnancy, labor, delivery, and the postpartum period is designed to potentiate the positive aspects of the passage to parenthood and to put the concerning aspects in context. It assumes that greater knowledge and insight in both parents or other possible caregivers help achieve goals rightly set by the individuals or couples involved. One dramatic change during recent decades involves the mother's attitude regarding analgesia during labor and delivery. The shift from a desire to sleep through it all to the wish to experience as much of it as possible has been paralleled by the development of formal approaches to education that include both mother and father or, in some instances, mother and an invited partner. Sibling involvement, depending on age, should be encouraged as much and as soon as possible.

B. BENEFITS.

1. A valid result is the documented reduced need for analgesia and anesthesia during labor and delivery; some women achieve "natural childbirth," avoiding drugs completely.
2. The subjective feeling of satisfaction most couples who participate report.
3. The support provided to the mother by the father or other partner throughout the entire experience.
4. The rapport and mutual support of all of the participants in an education group; an extension of the family.
5. The developing sense in both parents of "belonging" to the obstetric "team."
6. The sense of support for the idea of family.

C. FACILITATORS.

Maternal and newborn care are inextricably linked. If the purposes of education are to be best achieved, a combination labor, delivery, and recovery room (birthing suite) is ideal for an uncomplicated vaginal delivery. It should be set up as a comfortable, clean room with all medical and obstetric necessities readily available. The further the delivery area is from the nursery, the greater the need for support equipment at the delivery site; however, separate labor, delivery, and recovery arrangements should be available for those who wish them.

D. FAMILY-CENTERED BIRTHING.

The full involvement of everyone in the immediate family regardless of age (and some in the extended family), at home or at a freestanding birthing center, puts a huge responsibility on the professional attendant, often a nurse-midwife. Childbirth education should include responses to emergencies if this birthing option is chosen.

E. THE LAMAZE METHOD OF CHILDBIRTH EDUCATION.

Lamaze is one of the most commonly used (there are many variations) formal approaches to childbirth education in the United States. Its process and principles include the following:

1. 12 to 16 hours of classroom instruction.
2. Supplementary reading and home practice.
3. Discussions of relevant subjects.
   a. Anatomy.
   b. Physiology.
   c. Fetal growth and development.
   d. Emotional and behavioral issues, as they apply to pregnancy, labor, and delivery.
   e. Alternatives to drug-assisted labor and delivery.
   f. Issues regarding vaginal and cesarean births.
   g. Postpartum adaptations of mother and child.
   h. Advantages of and alternatives to breast-feeding.

Note: *Although most mothers in the United States breast-feed their babies for some period of time, most do not for the commonly recommended 6 months. If we agree that breast-feeding is best, a significant discussion in this regard is indicated, but it must be tempered by the life situation of the mother involved. There are alternatives when necessary.*

   i. Care of the newborn.
   j. Planned parenthood.
4. Restraint on the part of instructors to imposing their personal preferences. The method does not preach; it seeks to facilitate.
5. Recognition of varying preoccupations over time (e.g., early in pregnancy, parents tend to think about the baby; later on, about the process of labor and delivery).

F. POTENTIAL PROBLEMS

Advocates for a particular process, e.g., water births, the delivery of an infant under water, may argue for it in the face of contrary evidence by suggesting, as Elder did in 1989, that it may not be necessary to have evidence to support what some state as facts. A considerable literature on the subject avers that hospital delivery was instituted as a convenience for doctors and associated staff and for economic gain. There is no evidence to support the advantage of water birth. It falls to those of us who advise parents to be unintimidated and to insist on rigorous evaluation and resultant supportive evidence before adopting advocacy of any process. It falls to us, too, to advise accordingly. The patient, as always, may decide autonomously.

II. PARENT-INFANT BONDING
A. GENERAL INFORMATION.
The term *bonding* used in the context of the development of the primary relationship of an infant with the parents is now fixed in the jargon of baby care. Even the adopted child, deprived of some of the opportunity, is not ultimately deprived of much of the potential. There is no one event that achieves bonding or ensures it. There are *too many variables* to suggest irretrievability if some are lost or to suggest success if all are experienced.

Each parent has a separate and unique role in establishing a relationship with a new baby and, as a duo, they fulfill yet another role (see **Chapter 32**). The mother has a "sensitive" period, called by some a "primary maternal preoccupation," which develops during pregnancy and may last for a few postnatal weeks. During this time, because feelings of love are *not* necessarily instantaneous, she may be distressed if she does not feel the expected emotion. Reassurance that she will reclaim the sense of it that she may have had during pregnancy is appropriate.

The father or other partner can complement the activity of this time, providing an emotional "space" during which the mother can indulge her feelings and allow them to "flow" without undue stress. She can focus on the baby as others deal with the environment; such support helps to fortify her skills as a mother, and benefits each of them—and the baby.

During the maternal sensitive period, mother and child have a truly two-way reciprocal relationship. In a positive way their senses mesh. They entertain each other, gurgling and cooing, feeling each other's warmth. The baby cries and has needs; the parent assures and reinforces by feeding and caressing.

B. BARRIERS TO BONDING.
1. Blindness, deafness, other physical deprivations or incapacities.
2. Anxiety; "stiffness" in child and parent; maternal "projection" of negative feelings, traits, concerns onto child.
3. Drug-influenced infant (or mother).
4. Difficult labor or other maternal illness, which may make nursing more difficult.
5. Neonatal intensive care unit (NICU) placement or maternal-infant separation caused by prolonged hospital stay of one without the other.
6. Family discord.

C. FACILITATORS.
1. Fathers, too, feel better about themselves after contact with the baby; parents welcome contact *immediately* postpartum. Try to facilitate it whether delivery is vaginal or by cesarean section.

28

CHILDBIRTH EDUCATION AND BONDING

2. Placing the baby on the mother's abdomen immediately after delivery is nice to do, and some say these babies have fewer adaptive problems at home and in school in the long run. I am all for doing it, but no one has successfully isolated the many intervening variables to validate the reported long-term benefit.
3. Examine the baby in the view of or even in the arms of the mother or, if necessary, the father or other partner.
4. Encourage sucking and closeness soon after birth.
5. Try to keep the family together. Rooming-in can be very helpful and satisfying. It helps to keep the baby and the family physically and emotionally at appropriate "temperatures."
6. To the extent possible, depending on age, involve siblings as soon as it is feasible.

III. CONTINUING EDUCATION
A. GENERAL INFORMATION.
Pregnancy and delivery are the first stages in a continuing education process. The prenatal visit initiates a relationship that can be enhanced at the time of the examination of the infant in the presence of the parents. From then on, every interaction gives the chance to teach.

B. BARRIERS TO THE EDUCATIONAL RELATIONSHIP.
1. The sense of isolation many young adults feel.
2. Excessive dependency in a poorly prepared or immature parent.
3. The overworked professional.
4. Inadequate or socially disorganized family and other societal resources.

C. FACILITATORS FOR THE EDUCATIONAL RELATIONSHIP.
1. The energy and desire most new parents bring to the initial attachment to their infants.
2. The innate capacity of the newborn to adapt to the "new" environment.
3. The information gleaned from such measures as the Brazelton behavioral scale (see **Chapter 5**).
4. The telephone or e-mail, the link with the "teacher."
5. Home visits (usually by nurses) soon after hospital discharge are a marvelous opportunity to learn about the family in its many dimensions.

Note: *These facilitators do not ultimately create overdependency on the educator in most circumstances. Other variables (e.g., barriers) may. In general, increasing experience, knowledge, and insight breed self-sufficiency in parents.*

D. COUNSELING DURING THE NEWBORN PERIOD.
The following topics should be addressed in counseling new parents:
1. Feeding.
2. Voiding and stooling.
3. Skin care.

4. Cord care.
5. Safety.
6. Signs of illness.
7. Expected infant behavior (e.g., sleep pattern).
8. Clothing and other supplies.
9. Going out (e.g., excursions, visits to others, to the supermarket).
10. Involvement of others (e.g., siblings, relatives, friends, support help).
11. Develop insight to parental feelings.

Note: *The birth of twins (or more) compounds the need for attention to all details of the relationships and the needs of newborns and their parents.*

BIBLIOGRAPHY

Becker PG: Counseling families with twins: Birth to 3 years of age. Pediatr Rev 8(3):81, 1986.

Charney E: Counseling of parents around the birth of a baby. Pediatr Rev 4(6):167, 1982.

Elder: Alternative Practices: A balanced perspective. J Nurse Midwifery 34:163, 1989.

Kennell JH, Klaus MH: The perinatal paradigm: Is it time for a change? Clin Perinatal 15:80, 1988.

Klaus MH, Kennell JH: Parent-infant bonding, ed 2. St Louis, Mosby, 1982.

LaLeche League International: The womanly art of breastfeeding, ed 6, 1997.

Late M: Education campaign takes on lagging breastfeeding rates: Few babies breastfed long enough. Nation's Health 34:7, 2004.

Schroeter K: Water births: A naked emperor. Pediatrics 114: 855, 2004.

Yogman MW: Development of the father-infant relationship. In Fitzgerald HE, Lester BM, Yogman MW (eds): Theory and Research in Behavioral Pediatrics, vol 1, New York, Plenum, 1980.

28

CHILDBIRTH EDUCATION AND BONDING

Transfer to the Intensive Care Nursery

Ambadas Pathak

I. GENERAL CONSIDERATIONS

Capabilities, staffing, equipment, and patient care philosophy vary
from nursery to nursery. Hence, each nursery must develop its
own indications for transferring infants to the intensive care nursery.
In general, infants requiring frequent and close monitoring involving
placement of intravascular catheters and use of sophisticated monitors,
continuous intravenous (IV) therapy, or essentially "intensive" nursing
care require transfer to the intensive care nursery. These infants are
usually born at <34 weeks of gestation. Following are some general
recommendations, presented by category, for transfer to the intensive
care nursery.

29

A. CARDIOPULMONARY.

1. Central cyanosis requiring oxygen, associated with enlarged heart on
   chest x-ray, pallor, and hypotension: consider transposition of great
   vessels; hypoplastic left heart syndrome.
2. Respiratory distress indicated by tachypnea, retractions, flaring,
   grunting, and hypoxemia: consider respiratory distress syndrome;
   sepsis; meconium aspiration syndrome; persistent pulmonary
   hypertension; pneumothorax; diaphragmatic hernia; tracheoesophageal
   fistula.
3. Stridor at birth or soon thereafter: consider choanal atresia; micrognathia
   and glossoptosis; laryngeal web; tracheomalacia; laryngoesophageal
   defect; vascular ring compressing the trachea.

B. NEUROLOGIC.

1. Seizures: consider asphyxia; metabolic abnormalities; infection;
   intracranial hemorrhage.
2. Coma: consider metabolic abnormality; heavy maternal sedation.
3. Severe hypotonia: consider birth injury; congenital myopathy.

C. GASTROINTESTINAL (GI).

1. Abdominal distention accompanied by tenderness, absent bowel
   sounds, erythema, edema of abdominal wall, bilious vomiting, visible
   peristalsis: consider GI perforation; necrotizing enterocolitis (NEC);
   malrotation; GI obstruction.
2. Hematemesis and melena: consider swallowed maternal blood; gastric
   ulcer; volvulus; enterocolitis.
3. Congenital abnormalities: consider gastroschisis; duodenal atresia;
   omphalocele; imperforate anus.

D. GENITOURINARY.
Abdominal mass: consider hydronephrosis; multicystic kidney; dysplastic kidney; polycystic kidney; ovarian cyst; hydrometrocolpos. If the infant is otherwise stable, initial evaluation may take place in the full-term nursery.

E. HEMATOLOGIC.
1. Anemia: consider Rh or ABO isoimmunization; fetomaternal hemorrhage; internal hemorrhage.
2. Polycythemia with symptoms: consider twin-twin transfusion; small-for-gestational-age (SGA) infant; postmaturity.
3. Petechiae and purpura, especially when generalized and recurrent: consider maternal idiopathic thrombocytopenic purpura; platelet group incompatibility; bacterial and viral infections; and disseminated intravascular coagulation (DIC).
4. Hyperbilirubinemia early (within 18 hours) and rapidly progressive, needing phototherapy or exchange transfusion: consider erythroblastosis fetalis.

F. NEONATAL INFECTIONS INDICATED BY LETHARGY, TEMPERATURE INSTABILITY, RESPIRATORY DISTRESS, POOR FEEDING, PETECHIAL OR VESICULAR RASH, SCLEREMA: CONSIDER BACTERIAL AND VIRAL INFECTIONS.
G. METABOLIC.
1. Hypoglycemia, persistent: consider hyperinsulinism; Beckwith-Wiedemann syndrome.
2. Hyponatremia, profound: consider congenital adrenal hyperplasia; maternal administration of salt-free intravenous fluids.
3. Hypermagnesemia: consider tocolysis by magnesium sulfate; preeclamptic toxemia.
4. Hyperammonemia: consider inborn error of metabolism.

H. MULTIPLE CONGENITAL MALFORMATIONS.
1. Chromosomal disorders: trisomies 13, 18, and 21.
2. Pierre Robin syndrome.
3. Osteogenesis imperfecta.
4. Asphyxiating thoracic dystrophy.

I. MISCELLANEOUS.
1. Birth injury: consider diaphragmatic paralysis; cervical cord injury.
2. Severe abstinence syndrome (secondary to in utero drug exposure).
3. Apnea.

Discharge Considerations and Process

Jean S. Wheeler

I. DISCHARGE TEACHING

Note: *These guidelines are not meant to be rigid. The individual circumstances of the patient and the preferences of the practitioner mandate flexibility at all times, with the potential of addition and deletion of items.*

A. ASSESSMENT.
1. Consider past experience.
2. Evaluate knowledge base.
3. Consider common limitations after delivery.
a. Maternal sleep deprivation.
b. Physical discomfort.
c. Short hospital stay.

B. INTERVENTION.
1. Individual teaching.
2. Written instructions; handouts.
3. Videotapes.
4. Classes.

C. CONTENT.
1. Feeding.
a. Formula.
    (1) Iron fortified. Low-iron formulas should be avoided (term infants require 1 mg/kg per day of iron, assuming an average rate of absorption of 12% of dietary content; infants weighing 1500 to 2500 g require 2 mg/kg/day).
    (2) Preparation instructions (refer to illustration on can).
    (3) Thoroughly cleanse nipples and bottles before use.
    (4) 1.5 oz minimum of formula every 3 to 4 hours, increased gradually.
    (5) Additional water or juice is not recommended.
b. Breast-feeding (see **Chapter 27**).
    (1) Infant should be fed on demand every 2 to 3 hours.
    (2) Average 8 to 10 feedings every 24 hours.
    (3) Infant should feed for 10 to 15 minutes on each breast per each feeding.
    (4) Adequate rest and fluid intake by the mother are imperative.
    (5) Sore nipples indicate poor positioning.
    (6) Infant should be observed feeding by a knowledgeable caregiver to ascertain if there are proper latch, positioning, and coordinated sucking and swallowing.

30

2. Voiding and stooling.

a. Bottle-fed infants' stools are yellow-green and firm to pasty; straining is normal and not necessarily indicative of constipation.

b. Breast-fed infants' stools are bright yellow and loose; by the fourth day stooling should occur with every feeding, (a good indication of successful breast-feeding.) In the first several days after discharge, mother should notify practitioner if the infant goes longer than 24 hours without a stool or if the infant is still passing meconium by the fourth day.

c. Four to six wet diapers a day are usually indicative of adequate intake.

3. Jaundice.

a. Occurs in 50% of normal newborns and occurs more often in breast-fed infants than those who are bottle-fed.

b. Jaundice is a temporary condition and is most often not associated with disease.

c. It usually peaks at 3 to 4 days of life (when the infant is home).

d. Scleral icterus should be brought to the practitioner's attention.

e. Written as well as verbal explanation of the cause of jaundice, its significance to the infant and how to monitor for it should be given to all parents at discharge.

4. Skin.

a. Sponge bathe every day or every other day per parents' preference.

b. Tub baths must wait until after the umbilical cord remnant falls off.

c. Mild, unscented soap is preferable.

d. Shampoo scalp with each bath.

e. Lotions, oils, or powders are unnecessary.

f. Reassure parents that dry, peeling skin is expected and resolves spontaneously.

g. Diaper rash may be treated with petroleum jelly and air exposure; if persistent, parents should call practitioner.

h. Mention to parents any rash present at discharge (e.g., erythema toxicum, pustular melanosis).

i. If applicable, point out fetal scalp electrode site and instruct parents regarding signs of infection.

5. Cord care.

a. Reassure parents there is no sensation in the cord; it is not a "sore."

b. Rubbing alcohol may be applied to the cord with an alcohol-soaked cotton ball several times per day. (some controversy exists here, practitioner preference.)

c. The diaper, whether cloth or disposable, should be fastened below the cord.

d. Sponge baths are given to avoid getting the cord wet.

e. The cord will usually drop off at approximately 2 weeks.

f. Redness around the base, foul odor, or drainage from the cord should be reported to the practitioner immediately.

g. If the infant was circumcised, a petroleum jelly-impregnated gauze strip should cover the penis for 24 hours; after removing the gauze, apply petroleum jelly to the penis after each diaper change until healed, usually a few days. Parents should notify the practitioner if there is bleeding or signs of infection.

h. If a Plastibell was used after the circumcision, petroleum jelly should not be used because this could loosen the string.

6. Safety.

a. Car seats are mandatory for all car rides, including the ride home from the hospital.

b. Bottle propping is dangerous because of the risks of choking.

c. The infant should sleep on its back, not on its stomach. The side position is an alternative if necessary.

d. Infants should never be in a bed with a sleeping adult because of the risk of suffocation or falling from the bed. (There are some who may disagree with this.)

e. Avoid soft bedding, pillows, stuffed toys, plastic bags, balloons, and strings in infant's crib.

f. Pacifiers should never be placed around the infant's neck on a string or cord; strangulation may occur.

g. A plain nipple should never be used as a pacifier; the infant may aspirate it and occlude the airway.

h. Hot liquids should be avoided while handling the baby; babies burn easily.

i. Direct sunlight should be avoided; suntans are not healthy, and sunscreens contain chemicals that may not be safe for use in newborns. (Direct sunlight is not an option for treating jaundice.)

j. Smoke detectors should be installed and in working order before discharge of the baby from the hospital.

k. Cigarette smoking around the infant, both in the house and in the car, should be avoided by all members of the infant's household.

l. Keep the infant away from crowds and sick individuals for the first 4 to 5 weeks to prevent infection (e.g., excursions to the supermarket, crowded parties should not have high priority).

m. Overdressing is not necessary for a healthy, full-term baby; thermoregulatory mechanisms are usually in order by several days of age; the home does not need to be super hot, and the amount of clothing can be gauged by what is appropriate for an older child or even an adult.

n. Never leave the infant alone with a pet.

7. Expected infant behavior.

a. Hiccups are common and require no treatment.

b. Sneezing is expected and does not necessarily indicate the presence of a cold.

c. Sucking on a pacifier helps satisfy the infant's non-nutritive sucking needs and rarely leads to long-term dependency or dental problems.

d. Crying as long as 1 to $1\frac{1}{2}$ hours a day is normal in the first month. Feeding, diaper change, burping may help. Parents should hold infant and rock gently. **NEVER SHAKE A BABY.**

30

DISCHARGE CONSIDERATIONS AND PROCESS

e. There are great variations in infant sleep patterns; the cycle may be 45 to 60 minutes in the neonatal period; babies are wiser than we are—they usually get what they need; there should be reasonable quiet time, but babies often adapt to noise.

8. Signs of illness.

a. Poor feeding, cyanosis, tachypnea, irritability, lethargy, unusual skin rash, problems with the cord, vomiting, diarrhea, decreased urinary output, rectal temperature >100° F, or a change in the infant's usual behavior should be reported immediately to the practitioner.

b. Emphasize that neonatal infection is not necessarily accompanied by a fever.

D. REVIEW.

1. Questions.

a. Encourage the parents to ask questions about the baby.

b. Clarify any specific areas that are not completely understood; written instructions may be helpful.

2. Reassure new parents that many more questions will probably arise and that it is appropriate to call the practitioner.

E. FOLLOW-UP CARE.

1. Physician follow-up should be arranged before the infant's discharge.

2. Parents should be advised at the time of discharge when the baby is to return to the practitioner for the first visit.

a. Discharge before 24 hours—seen by 72 hours of age.

b. Discharge between 24 and 48 hours—seen by 96 hours of age.

c. Discharge between 48 and 72 hours—seen by 120 hours of age.

d. Low-risk for jaundice and/or discharged after 96 hours of age, 1 to 2 weeks.

3. Provide parents with the telephone number of the primary care practitioner.

4. Send newborn records to the primary care practitioner.

5. Factors influencing the time of the first pediatric visit.

a. The medical condition of the baby.

b. The length of hospital stay.

c. Experience of the mother and others caring for the baby.

d. The baby's size and gestational age. (Beware of the "large" 35- to 37-week infant.)

e. The social situation.

f. How well the baby is feeding and whether the baby is breast-feeding (a first-time breast-feeding mother should maintain close contact with the baby's practitioner and have the baby in for a weight check within the first week of life to ensure that excessive weight loss has not occurred and to provide support if commitment to nursing is wavering).

g. Risk for jaundice.

6. Home nursing visit.
a. Within 24 to 48 hours of discharge.
b. Should occur for all infants discharged at 24 hours or less.
c. Useful for breast-feeding infants. (If possible, the nurse should observe the infant nursing.)
d. To assess jaundice and obtain bilirubin in lieu of an office visit (availability and expertise of home nursing vary throughout the country).

II. SOCIAL BARRIERS TO DISCHARGE

Note: Whenever a problem is identified that may endanger an infant's safety or well-being, a social work evaluation should be requested.

A. REFERRAL.

If necessary, a referral should be made to the child protective agency in the community, and a home assessment should be completed before discharge.

B. SOME PROBLEMS THAT MAY PREVENT OR DELAY DISCHARGE.

1. Maternal history of substance abuse.
2. Present or previous history of psychiatric illness in the mother.
3. Severe illness or physical disability of the mother.
4. History of neglect or abuse of a previous child.
5. History of domestic violence.
6. Inappropriate maternal behavior or poor maternal-infant bonding.
7. Maternal homelessness or inadequate living and support arrangements.

III. PHYSICAL BARRIERS TO DISCHARGE

A. FEEDINGS.

All infants must demonstrate good breast-feeding ability or adequate formula intake before discharge.

B. PREMATURITY.

1. An infant <37 weeks of gestation or <2500 gm should be observed, if possible, for a minimum of 3 days.
2. A premature infant must demonstrate the ability to maintain a normal body temperature in an open bassinet for 24 hours (36.4° to 37° C or 97.5° to 98.6° F).
3. Jaundice in a premature infant (<37 weeks) is more likely to require treatment.

C. NEONATAL DRUG WITHDRAWAL.

1. An infant exposed to drugs in utero should be held for observation.
2. A social work evaluation should be done.
3. If symptoms occur or a urine toxicology screen on the infant is positive, a referral to child protective services should be considered. Some jurisdictions mandate referral.

30

DISCHARGE CONSIDERATIONS AND PROCESS

4. If medication is required to treat severe symptoms, the infant must be held until the medication is no longer necessary.
5. The symptomatic infant should be held until symptoms have subsided. (infants exposed to methadone may not show withdrawal for 4 to 5 days after the mother's last dose prior to the delivery.)
6. The mother should be encouraged to enter a drug treatment program.
7. Instruct mother or other caretaker regarding symptomatic and supportive care of the withdrawing infant.
8. Advise mother regarding danger of passive cocaine exposure to infant.

D. CONGENITAL ABNORMALITIES.
1. Heart murmurs believed to be pathologic should be evaluated before discharge.
2. Dislocated hips should be seen by an orthopedic specialist, an ultrasound should be obtained, and treatment begun.
3. Clubfeet should be seen and treated by an orthopedic specialist.
4. Abnormal prenatal renal ultrasound results should be evaluated before discharge.
5. Other major malformations (e.g., cleft lip/palate) may require additional time for parental education and adjustment and evaluation and coordination of services by medical subspecialists.

E. INFECTIONS.
1. Sepsis.
a. An infant at increased risk for sepsis, whether on treatment or not, should be observed a minimum of 48 hours in the hospital for signs of infection.
b. An infant born to a group B streptococcus (GBS) colonized mother, with or without intrapartum treatment, should be observed in the hospital a minimum of 48 hours (per the American Academy of Pediatrics [AAP] *Guidelines for Perinatal Care*). Discharge in 24 hours may be permitted after careful thought if (and only if) the infant is stable, pediatric follow-up is assured, there is a telephone in the home.
c. When antibiotics are started, treatment should continue in the hospital until the blood culture is negative at 48 to 72 hours.

2. Syphilis.
a. Infants with congenital syphilis or infants of mothers with syphilis who were untreated, inadequately treated, or treated in the last 4 weeks of pregnancy should receive a spinal tap and be treated for 10 days with intramuscular (IM) or intravenous (IV) penicillin administration (see **Chapter 22**).
b. The infant should be held in the hospital for completion of the penicillin course unless outpatient treatment can be arranged and compliance can be ensured.

3. Pneumonia. Infants with pneumonia should be held in the hospital for 7 to 14 days of IM or IV antibiotic administration. Home care may be an option when the infant is stable.

4. Tuberculosis; mother with positive tuberculin test (see **Chapter 22**).

F. HYPERBILIRUBINEMIA.

1. Any jaundice visible in the first 24 hours of life is abnormal and should be investigated. Initial evaluation should include a blood type and direct Coombs test, a hematocrit or hemoglobin level, and a total bilirubin level (see **Chapter 21**).

2. Healthy term newborns have developed kernicterus from nonhemolytic hyperbilirubinemia.

3. AAP Clinical Practice Guidelines on Management of Hyperbilirubinemia in the Newborn Infant 35 or More Weeks' Gestation (2004) (See **Chapter 21**).

a. Assess all infants for jaundice in a well-lit room.

b. Visual assessment of bilirubin level is often not valid.

c. Obtain a total serum bilirubin (TSB) or a transcutaneous bilirubin (TcB) on every infant who is jaundiced in the first 24 hours and consider it on infants who have risk factors for jaundice or who are jaundiced at discharge (see **Fig. 21-5**, Risk Factors for Development of Severe Hyperbilirubinemia).

d. Obtaining a bilirubin level on every newborn at the time of the metabolic screen may be considered. Interpret the bilirubin level according to the infant's age in hours. (Nonhemolytic causes.) (See Bhutani Scale, **Chapter 21**)

e. Consider Phototherapy (See **Fig. 21-6**, Guidelines for Phototherapy in Hospitalized Infants of 35 or More Weeks of Gestation).

2. Indications for phototherapy are discussed in **Chapter 21**. Home health care agencies may be able to arrange for phototherapy to be performed at home.

3. Home phototherapy is not appropriate for infants with bilirubin levels above the "optional phototherapy" range or in infants with risk factors. (AAP, 2004)

4. Infants with an elevated bilirubin level but **without hemolysis** can usually be discharged if follow-up levels can be obtained by the infant's practitioner. (AAP Bilirubin Guidelines, 2004).

IV. EARLY DISCHARGE

Is infant a candidate for early discharge (**Box 30-1**)?

GENERAL CRITERIA.

After low-risk delivery, infants may be discharged within 24 hours of birth.

1. A tentative decision should be made before delivery.

2. Discharge should be a joint plan by the obstetrician, pediatrician, and family; it should be physician directed, not insurer driven; many states have laws requiring minimum 48-hour stay after vaginal delivery.

3. Pregnancy, antepartum, intrapartum, and early postpartum periods should be uncomplicated. Any change in the status of the mother, fetus, or neonate at any stage may alter the plan.

BOX 30-1

POSTPONING NEWBORN DISCHARGE: FACTORS TO CONSIDER

MATERNAL MEDICAL FACTORS

Cesarean delivery

Abnormal labor or delivery

Medical conditions such as diabetes mellitus

Elevated temperature

Group B streptococcal colonization

Sexually transmitted disease

O or Rh-negative blood group

MATERNAL SOCIAL FACTORS

No or poor prenatal care

Substance abuse

Adolescence

Poor support system

Mental retardation or psychiatric illness

Planning adoption or foster placement

INFANT FACTORS

Preterm (≤37 weeks)

Small for gestational age

Large for gestational age

Abnormal physical examination

Vital signs, color activity, feeding

Significant congenital malformation

ABNORMAL LABORATORY FINDINGS

Hypoglycemia

Hyperbilirubinemia

Polycythemia

Anemia

Rapid plasma reagin positive

From Hurt H: Contemp Pediatr 11:76, 1994.

4. Mother should have attended prenatal education and neonatal care classes that include information on potential problems in the first 3 to 5 days of life.
5. Pediatric care after discharge must be identified.
6. The mother needs adequate support at home. Both mother and neonate should be examined in 2 to 3 days, preferably at home.

B. NEONATAL CRITERIA.

1. Single birth.
2. Uncomplicated vaginal delivery.

3. Full-term infant (38 to 42 weeks), weight appropriate for gestational age, with a normal examination by a pediatrician or nurse practitioner before discharge.
4. Uncomplicated transition.
5. Normal vital signs, stable temperature.
6. Infant demonstrates a healthy suck and swallow and has fed from breast or bottle at least twice, with coordinated suck, swallow, and breathing.
7. Infant has voided. If circumcised, no bleeding occurs for 2 hours.
8. Infant has passed stool. (If meconium has not passed by 48 hours of age, mother should be instructed to call her practitioner.)
9. No jaundice is apparent in the first 24 hours of life.
10. Laboratory tests.
   a. Maternal or cord blood test for syphilis is nonreactive.
   b. Maternal hepatitis B surface antigen is negative.
   c. Cord blood of infant should be tested for blood type and Coombs test if the mother is Rh-negative or type O.
   d. Hematocrit and blood glucose levels as clinically indicated.
   e. Metabolic screening. (If obtained at <24 hours, repeat testing should be ensured.)
   f. Hepatitis B vaccine (thimerosal-free) given or scheduled with the primary care practitioner.
11. Stable social situation.
12. Follow-up ensured.

C. MATERNAL CRITERIA.
1. Demonstrates ability with feeding technique, skin care, cord care, and temperature measurement with a thermometer.
2. Demonstrates ability to assess the infant's well-being and signs of illness.

Note: *The AAP states that it is "unlikely" the above minimum criteria and conditions can be met before 48 hours.*

D. FOLLOW-UP.
1. A home nursing or office visit should be scheduled within 24 to 48 hours to assess the following:
   a. Weight: Unclothed infant should not be more than 8% to 10% below birth weight.
   b. Feeding: Ensure infant is receiving an adequate amount; observe breast-feeding if possible.
   c. Elimination: Check frequency of urination; number and color of stools. (Is infant still passing meconium?)
   d. Jaundice. (AAP guidelines for checking bilirubin, initiating phototherapy.)
   e. Signs of illness (e.g., tachypnea, cyanosis, poor feeding, vomiting, and irritability).

30

DISCHARGE CONSIDERATIONS AND PROCESS

2. Telephone follow-up may be helpful but *should not* take the place of a visit.

V. DISCHARGE EVALUATION

A. IMPORTANCE OF EVALUATION.
Shorter postpartum hospital stays for mothers and constricted time for observation make a thorough discharge examination imperative because there is little time to observe the infant for potential problems. According to the AAP and ACOG's 2000 *Guidelines for Perinatal Care,* a newborn should be examined within 24 hours after birth and within 24 hours of discharge; therefore, many newborns will have but one physical examination.

B. GUIDANCE.
When performed in the presence of the parents, the discharge evaluation allows opportunity for providing education, answering questions, and giving anticipatory guidance.

C. NOTATIONS.
The discharge evaluation should include a complete examination, with emphasis on any points omitted or any abnormalities noted on the admission examination.

D. THE FOLLOWING AREAS SHOULD BE OF PARTICULAR NOTE:
1. General.
a. Check frequency and duration of breast-feedings; if bottle-fed, the frequency and amount of formula feedings.
b. Check number of voids and stools.
c. Compare present weight with birth weight.
d. Observe the infant's color, posture, activity, tone, and temperature.
e. Review vital signs.
2. Head.
a. Palpate fontanels and sutures.
b. Look for a cephalhematoma; may not be present at birth but may become apparent over first few days of life (increases risk of jaundice).
c. Check any caput succedaneum or cranial molding, which should be resolving.
d. Inspect any abrasions, lacerations, fetal scalp electrode site, or forceps marks, which should be healing.
e. Measure head circumference.
3. Eyes.
a. Note subconjunctival hemorrhages.
b. Look for chemical conjunctivitis, which may have resulted from eye prophylaxis (unusual with erythromycin).
c. Perform an ophthalmoscopic examination to look for red reflex, congenital cataracts, or glaucoma.

4. **Ears.**
a. Assess pinnae for normal configuration and set.
b. Check traumatic lesions such as bruises or abrasions.
c. Note preauricular tags or sinuses. (if present, hearing assessment is suggested.)
d. Check for patent canals.

5. **Nose.**
a. Check patency of nares.
b. Look for asymmetry or septal deviation, flaring.

6. **Mouth.**
a. Inspect for natal teeth, mucoid cysts, ranula, or bifid uvula.
b. Observe palate for cleft.
c. Check sucking reflex.
d. Check size and position of tongue.

7. **Neck.**
a. Examine for congenital malformations such as fistulas, cysts, lymphangiomas, or goiter.
b. Check for webbing.

8. **Chest.**
a. Count respiratory rate.
b. Observe symmetry of chest movement and ease of respirations.

9. **Heart.**
a. Note cardiac rate and rhythm.
b. Palpate point of maximum impulse.
c. Note precordium activity.
d. Auscultate for murmurs; murmurs that signify congenital heart disease are often not heard until after the first few days of life.
e. Palpate brachial and femoral pulses.

10. **Abdomen.**
a. Observe for distention.
b. Palpate for enlarged organs or masses.
c. Assess cord for bleeding or signs of infection.

11. **Genitalia.**
a. Inspect female infant for patent vagina, vaginal tags, discharge, or pseudomenses. Palpate labia for gonads.
b. Check male infant for chordee, hypospadias, undescended testes, or hydroceles; if circumcised, inspect for bleeding or infection.

12. **Skeletal.**
a. Inspect for supernumerary digits, syndactyly, metatarsus adductus, clubfoot.
b. Examine clavicles for fracture.
c. Check hips for subluxation or dislocation.
d. Inspect spine for scoliosis, sacral dimple, and/or sinus.

13. **Nervous system.**
a. Assess infant's tone and symmetry of Moro reflex.

30

DISCHARGE CONSIDERATIONS AND PROCESS

   b. Observe for tremulousness.
   c. Look for palsies of upper extremities or face.
   d. Assess suck.
14. Skin.
   a. Inspect for rashes, hemangiomas, nevi, café-au-lait marks, mongolian spots, or supernumerary nipples.
   b. Note presence and degree of any jaundice.
   E. FOLLOW-UP CONSIDERATIONS.
Any abnormality on discharge examination not requiring immediate evaluation or treatment but needing follow-up should be brought to the attention of the practitioner who will be caring for the infant.
   F. PRACTITIONER.
All newborns being discharged from the hospital should have an identified primary care practitioner to whom records should be sent.

VI. NEWBORN METABOLIC SCREENING

A. NEWBORNS IN THE UNITED STATES HAVE BEEN SCREENED FOR METABOLIC DISORDERS FOR MORE THAN 40 YEARS USING A TECHNIQUE OF BLOOD DROPS IMPREGNATED ON FILTER PAPER.

B. STATE REGULATIONS.
Because there are no federal guidelines regarding newborn metabolic screening, practitioners must be aware of regulations in their state.

C. THERE IS WIDE VARIATION FROM STATE TO STATE—
not only in which disorders are screened but also whether participation is voluntary or mandatory. (In Maryland, parental consent is required to screen the infant.)

D. NEW METHODOLOGY, TANDEM MASS SPECTROMETRY (MS/MS), NOW MAKES IT POSSIBLE TO SCREEN ENDLESS NUMBERS OF DISORDERS.
E. AS OF SPRING 2003, ABOUT ONE HALF OF STATES HAVE IMPLEMENTED MS/MS NEWBORN SCREENING OR HAVE PILOT STUDIES IN PROGRESS.
F. ORIGINAL PURPOSE OF SCREENING WAS EARLY DETECTION OF TREATABLE DISORDERS THAT WERE ASSOCIATED WITH MENTAL RETARDATION.
G. MS/MS MAKES IT POSSIBLE TO IDENTIFY MANY MORE DISORDERS, SOME TREATABLE AND SOME WITH NO KNOWN TREATMENT.

H. DISORDERS SCREENED BY MS/MS:
1. Aminoacidopathies—e.g., PKU, maple syrup urine disease, homocystinuria, tyrosinemia types I and II, etc.

2. Organic Acidemias—e.g., propionic acidemia, methylmalonic acidemia, etc.
3. Fatty Acid Oxidation Disorders—e.g., carnitine transporter defect, long chain hydroxyl acyl-CoA dehydrogenase deficiency (LCHAD), medium chain acyl-CoA dehydrogenase deficiency (MCAD), short chain acyl-CoA dehydrogenase deficiency (SCAD), etc.

I. ADVANCES IN DNA DIAGNOSTIC TESTING WILL MOST LIKELY BE USED IN NEWBORN SCREENING.
Some states are screening for cystic fibrosis (CF).
1. MS/MS looks for elevated IRT (immunoreactive trypsinogen). If IRT is elevated then DNA testing is performed.
2. DNA testing raises ethical concerns if a disease is diagnosed that has no treatment or doesn't manifest until a much later age.

J. PRESENTLY, ALL STATES SCREEN FOR PHENYLKETONURIA (PKU) AND HYPOTHYROIDISM.
It is necessary to check locally (see **Chapters 24 and 26**).

K. METABOLIC DISEASES THAT ARE SCREENED FOR IN ONE OR MORE STATES INCLUDE THE FOLLOWING:
1. Biotinidase deficiency, congenital adrenal hyperplasia, congenital hypothyroidism, cystic fibrosis, galactosemia, homocystinuria, branched-chain ketoaciduria (maple syrup urine disease), PKU, sickle cell disease, and tyrosinemia.
2. As new screening and treatment strategies become available, new tests may be added.
3. As states review their programs and populations, other tests may be deleted.

L. WHEN SHOULD SCREENING BE DONE?
1. After 24 hours of age, after feeding is well established and toxic metabolites have a chance to accumulate.
2. Screening is usually done at discharge from the hospital, preferably at 48 to 72 hours of age; a repeat test is recommended at a 2-week visit.
3. If the initial screen is obtained before 24 hours of age, a second specimen should be obtained at 1 to 2 weeks.
4. Many states have changed the cutoff for normal serum phenylalanine from 4 to 2 mg/dl because of early screening prompted by <24-hour discharge.
5. Regardless of age, a newborn screen should be obtained from all infants at discharge; missing a metabolic disorder is more likely to occur because a sample was *never* obtained rather than because it was obtained too early.

30

DISCHARGE CONSIDERATIONS AND PROCESS

VII. NEWBORN HEARING SCREENING

A. PREVALENCE OF CONGENITAL HEARING LOSS IS 1.5 TO 6/1000 LIVE BIRTHS.

B. IDENTIFICATION OF HEARING-IMPAIRED NEONATES.
1. Average age of identification is 24 to 30 months.
2. Moderate hearing losses frequently are not identified until 5 to 6 years of age.
3. Early identification is important so that interventions can be initiated that will improve speech and language acquisition.
4. Congenital cytomegalovirus (CMV) is the most common etiology of nonhereditary sensorineural hearing loss. There may now be a treatment (ganciclovir) to prevent it.
a. If an infant fails newborn hearing screening, consider screening for CMV.
b. If an infant has CMV and passes hearing screening, repeat hearing screening.
c. CMV may be added to the newborn metabolic screening in the near future.

C. UNIVERSAL NEWBORN HEARING SCREENING VERSUS SCREENING BY RISK FACTORS.
1. Screening neonates based on risk factors misses 50% of hearing-impaired neonates.
2. Universal hearing screening is recommended and is mandated by law in many states.

D. TYPE OF SCREENING.
1. Otoacoustic emissions (OAE).
2. Auditory brainstem evoked response (ABR).
3. Improvements in these technologies are making screening more efficient, cost effective, and "user friendly."

E. FOLLOW-UP HEARING SCREENING.
1. If infant fails, repeat in 3 to 4 weeks.
2. If infant passes but has risk factors, repeat within 6 months.
3. Risk factors include: Gentamicin exposure, ear anomalies—e.g., preauricular tags or sinuses, family history of congenital hearing loss, and CMV.

BIBLIOGRAPHY

American Academy of Pediatrics: Newborn screening for congenital hypothyroidism: Recommended guidelines. Pediatrics 91:1203, 1993.

American Academy of Pediatrics: Syphilis. In Pickering LK (ed): Red Book: Report of the Committee on Infectious Diseases, ed. 25. Elk Grove Village, Ill, American Academy of Pediatrics, 2000.

American Academy of Pediatrics: Hospital discharge of the high-risk neonate: Proposed guidelines. Pediatrics 102:411, 1998.

American Academy of Pediatrics Joint Committee on Infant Hearing: 1994 Position statement. Pediatrics 95:152, 1995.

American Academy of Pediatrics Subcommittee on Hyperbilirubinemia: Clinical practice guidelines: Management of Hyperbilirubinemia in the newborn infant 35 or more weeks of gestation. Pediatrics 114:297, 2004.

American Academy of Pediatrics and American College of Obstetricians and Gynecologists: Guidelines for Perinatal Care, ed 5. Elk Grove Village, Ill and Washington DC, AAP and ACOG, 2002.

Barbi M, Binda S, Caroppo S, et al, A wider role for congenital cytomegalovirus infection in sensorineural hearing loss. Pediatr Infect Dis J 2(1) 2003.

Barsky-Firkser L, Sun S: Universal newborn hearing screenings: A three-year experience. Pediatrics 99(6): 1997.

Beebe SA, Britton SA, Britton JR, et al: Neonatal mortality and length of newborn hospital stay. Pediatrics 98:321, 1996.

CDC: Prevention of perinatal group B streptococcal disease, revised guidelines from CDC, MMWR 51(RR-11):2002.

Fearing MK, Marsden D: Expanded newborn screening. Pediatr Ann 32:8, 2003.

Friedman MA, Spitzer AR: Discharge criteria for the term newborn. Pediatr Clin North Am 51 (3): 2004.

Gibson E, Cullen JA, Spinner S, et al: Infant sleep position following new AAP guidelines. Pediatrics 96:69, 1995.

Levy HL: Lessons from the past—looking to the future: Newborn screening. Pediatr Ann 32:8, 2003.

Michaels MG, Greenberg DP, Sabo DL, Wald ER: Treatment of children with congenital cytomegalovirus infection with ganciclovir. Pediatr Infect Dis J 22(6), 2003.

Rhead WJ, Irons M: The call from the newborn screening laboratory: Frustration in the afternoon. Pediatr Clin North Am 51:3, 2004.

Thilo EH, Townsend SF: Early newborn discharge: Have we gone too far? Contemp Pediatr 13:29, 1996.

Wheeler JS, Donohue PK: Newborn care after early discharge: Role of the primary care provider. Clin Rev 9:65,1992.

30

DISCHARGE CONSIDERATIONS AND PROCESS

Adoption

Patricia H. Smouse

In addition to routine neonatal care, the baby to be placed for adoption requires special considerations.

I. REASONS ADOPTION MAY BE CONSIDERED
A. YOUNG MOTHER.
B. UNWANTED PREGNANCY.
C. RAPE.
D. PARENTAL PREFERENCE.

II. TYPES OF ADOPTION
A. AGENCY ADOPTION.

Adoption occurring under the auspices of a licensed adoption agency.
1. Baby is usually discharged to an employee of the adoption agency and may then be placed in temporary foster care, allowing the birth mother some time to reconsider her decision before the baby is placed with the adoptive parents.
2. Counseling is provided to the birth mother through the adoption agency.

B. PRIVATE ADOPTION.

Adoption without involvement of a licensed adoption agency. Private adoption is usually arranged prenatally by the birth mother, adoptive family, and an attorney hired by the adoptive family.
1. Baby is discharged directly to the adoptive parents.
2. Visitation of the baby at the hospital by the adoptive family is contingent on approval by the birth mother.
3. It is essential to ensure that the birth mother is not rushed or pressured into a decision.

III. ADOPTION PROCEDURES
A. VERIFY MATERNAL DECISION TO PLACE THE BABY FOR ADOPTION.
B. BIRTH FATHER.

Ensure knowledge and consent of the adoption plan by the putative father in states that specify this requirement.

C. TERMINOLOGY.

Birth mother/birth father (those who conceived the child). Parents (parents in the adoptive family).

D. RECOGNIZE THE COMPLEX NEEDS OF THE BIRTH MOTHER AND BABY.

Involve a hospital social worker to assist with counseling of the birth mother, to explore options if prior arrangements have not been made, if the mother is ambivalent about placing the baby for adoption, to identify pertinent community resources, and to coordinate discharge according to hospital policy, and in accordance with state laws regarding adoption. Respect the birth mother's wishes for confidentiality as well as her extent of involvement with the baby. Her involvement may vary from refraining from any contact with the baby to an open arrangement in which the birth parents and adoptive parents have met prenatally and all participate in the infant's hospital course. Some involvement of the birth mother may assist her in dealing with feelings of doubt and guilt and aid in the long-term grieving process.

E. PROVIDE EMOTIONAL SUPPORT TO THE BIRTH MOTHER.
Recognize her need to discuss her feelings; despite this being a voluntary decision, she is likely to experience significant feelings of grief.

F. BIRTH MOTHER'S RIGHTS.
The birth mother has the legal right to name the baby and to sign consent for infant screening tests and procedures, including circumcision.

G. RIGHT TO MEDICAL INFORMATION.
Do not ignore the birth mother's right to medical information regarding her baby.

H. RELEASE OF MEDICAL INFORMATION.
The birth mother should sign a release of medical information for herself and her baby to the adoptive parents or agency.

I. MAKE EVERY ATTEMPT TO OBTAIN AND DOCUMENT AN EXTENSIVE FAMILY, MEDICAL, AND GENETIC HISTORY OF THE BIRTH PARENTS.
Include alcohol and other drug use as well as life style-related information that may affect the newborn later in development. Also include the history of the pregnancy and the neonatal course. Failure to obtain and document this information at this time may result in a void in the child's medical history for life.

J. PERFORM AND DOCUMENT A THOROUGH NEWBORN EXAMINATION, OBTAINING WORKUPS AND CONSULTS AS INDICATED.
K. ALL ROUTINE NEWBORN SCREENING TESTS SHOULD BE PERFORMED AND DOCUMENTED.
If maternal HIV status is unknown, testing should be done on the newborn.

IV. DISCHARGE NEEDS

A. LEGAL AUTHORIZATION OF INFANT'S DISCHARGE BY THE BIRTH MOTHER.

B. AGENCY.

If the baby is being placed with an agency, the agency should provide a copy of its license and whatever other documents the hospital requires. Picture identification of the worker picking up the baby must be verified; copies of the worker's picture identification should be placed in the medical record.

C. ADOPTIVE PARENTS.

If the baby is going directly to adoptive parents, they must provide a temporary custody order of which a true test copy remains in the medical record. Picture identification of the adoptive parents must be verified and copies placed in the chart. Some hospitals require only the birth mother's release to allow the adoptive parents to take the baby from the hospital.

D. PROVIDE ANY SPECIAL MEDICAL INSTRUCTIONS AND ROUTINE BABY CARE INFORMATION TO AGENCY WORKER OR ADOPTIVE FAMILY.

E. PROVIDE RECOMMENDATIONS REGARDING PEDIATRIC FOLLOW-UP CARE.

31

ADOPTION

BIBLIOGRAPHY

American Academy of Pediatrics and The American College of Obstetricians and Gynecologists: Guidelines for Perinatal Care, ed 5. Elk Grove Village, Ill, 2002, the Academy and the College.

American Academy of Pediatrics Committee on Early Childhood, Adoption and Dependent Care: Initial medical evaluation of an adopted child. Pediatrics 88:642, 1991.

Dewarle BK: Open adoption. Can Nurse 88:14, 1992.

McNally C: Adoption: The perinatal social worker's role in the process. Natl Assoc Perinat Social Workers 14:1, 1994.

Thaler CH: Personal communication, August 5, 1994.

The Importance of Wasting No Time

Henry M. Seidel

32

The central nervous system (CNS) of the newborn is marvelously sophisticated, a brain ready to perform with myriad neuronal connections eager to be put to constructive use. Nature and nurture have been working together since conception to bring the infant to life and, even at the very beginning, they have had a vital partner in the social context that will shape the child's experience. There is evidence that the nature of that experience, even before delivery, has a significant impact on brain development. We no longer need to be persuaded that hearing is well established early, usually by 24 to 25 weeks of gestation, or that newborns really do feel pain. Indeed, the fetus hears the mother's voice and can distinguish it from others after birth. Impressively, the sounds of classical music heard during fetal and early postnatal life are said to increase the ability to learn mathematics later on. Too much noise during gestation, however, can contribute to later deafness. The neurophysiologic ability to sense pain and to remember it is also firmly in place by the start of the third trimester. Handling and immobilization in the early hours of life can influence a baby's response to a later painful stimulus. The first breath after delivery, the "once in a lifetime event," is the logical next step for a habit established in the third month of gestation.

Thus, the full-term newborn is exquisitely sentient and well constituted for the tasks ahead. As many as 100 billion neurons, each able to produce 15,000 synapses, are ready to be influenced and firmly set by stimuli that might be healthy or noxious—an intensely realized activity from the first hours and through the first years of life. Only one half of those synapses will survive. Repeated early experiences activate synapses that, becoming permanent, more sharply define the brain's patterns. Therefore, the social context that is the baby's becomes an important player, ranking right up there with the genes. We must pay close attention to that context prenatally and in the precious hours when the new baby is in our charge in our nurseries.

Every baby is, of course, the result of a relationship between two people—a dyad. Baby makes three and that leads to three dyads, mother-baby, father-baby, and mother-father. The whole is greater than the sum of the parts, but that "whole" depends very much on the nature of the trio of dyads. This trio is the simplest construction. Each additional baby increases the number of dyads considerably, and one can imagine the complexity when the original dyad may rupture and a possible welter of new relationships develops. Still, the understanding of what may be going on in the whole of a social system requires a grasp of the issues confronting any one member in the dyad with each of the others.

Consider the original trio. Parents love their children—or do they? What was the nature of the original dyad? How does the mother take to the baby? Does nursing really please her? Does the father resent the intrusion of the child? How do the parents now feel about each other? Parental behaviors during direct interactions (e.g., feeding the child, changing a diaper, myriad other everyday events) and the content of family stories told to the child are at the foundation of an infant's developing emotional identification with parents and family. A healthy social and intellectual growth enables, in the end, a sound sense of self. There is even gathering evidence that direct responses to the incidents in everyday living resulting in maternal anxiety during the 12th to 22nd week of pregnancy could make the fetus susceptible to the later development of such disorders as attention deficit/hyperactivity syndrome. So many questions, and the answers, sometimes difficult to find, lie within each dyad.

We, who are responsible for some of the care of a newborn, must understand the plasticity of the infant's nervous system and respect that as we consider how we contribute to the baby's experience. We must educate parents about this as much as about the impressive physiologic adjustments of new life. Long ago, Leo Kanner taught me that everyone *always* needs the four "A's:" attention, affection, acceptance, and approval. The *always* is as fully relevant to the fetus and newborn as it is to any of us, and the need for the four "A's" carries the same urgency as the needs for food and water. Understanding this and assessing the availability of these four "A's" in each consideration of a dyad will go a long way to abet our effort to help each child have the best possible start in life, the "head start" that Eisenberg reminds us is as vital to our goal in care as is the physical well-being of a baby.

BIBLIOGRAPHY

American Academy of Pediatrics Committee on Environmental Health: Noise: A hazard for the fetus and newborn. Pediatrics 100:724, 1997.

Eisenberg L: Experience, brain, and behavior: The importance of a head start. N Engl J Med 340:1031, 1999.

Als H, Duffy FH, McAnulty GB, et al: Early experience alters brain function and structure. Pediatrics 113:846, 2004.

Kagan J: The role of parents in children's psychological development. Pediatrics 104:164, 1999.

Porter FL, Wolf CM, Gold J, et al: Pain and pain management in newborn infants: A survey of physicians and nurses. Pediatrics 100:626, 1997.

Porter FL, Wolf CM, Miller JP: The effect of handling and immobilization on the response to acute pain in newborn infants. Pediatrics 102:1383, 1998.

Shore R: Rethinking the Brain: New Insights into Early Development (Executive Summary). New York, Families and Work Institute, 1997.

Van den Bergh BRH, Marcoen A: Child behavior may be programmed during pregnancy. Child Dev 75:4, 2004.

Appendices

Ambadas Pathak

Appendix A

Conversion Tables and Formulas

A

TABLE A-1

TEMPERATURE EQUIVALENTS

Celsius*	Fahrenheit[†]	Celsius*	Fahrenheit[†]
34.0	93.2	38.6	101.4
34.2	93.6	38.8	101.8
34.4	93.9	39.0	102.2
34.6	94.3	39.2	102.5
34.8	94.6	39.4	102.9
35.0	95.0	39.6	103.2
35.2	95.4	39.8	103.6
35.4	95.7	40.0	104.0
35.6	96.1	40.2	104.3
35.8	96.4	40.4	104.7
36.0	96.8	40.6	105.1
36.2	97.1	40.8	105.4
36.4	97.5	41.0	105.8
36.6	97.8	41.2	106.1
36.8	98.2	41.4	106.5
37.0	98.6	41.6	106.8
37.2	98.9	41.8	107.2
37.4	99.3	42.0	107.6
37.6	99.6	42.2	108.0
37.8	100.0	42.4	108.3
38.0	100.4	42.6	108.7
38.2	100.7	42.8	109.0
38.4	101.1	43.0	109.4

Hoekelman RA, Adam HM, Nelson NM, et al: Primary Pediatric Care, 4th ed. St Louis, Mosby, 2001.
*To convert Celsius to Fahrenheit: $(9/5 \times \text{Temperature}) + 32$.
[†]To convert Fahrenheit to Celsius: $5/9 \times (\text{Temperature} - 32)$.

TABLE A-2
CONVERSION FORMULA

HEIGHT (LENGTH)

1 millimeter (mm) = 0.04 inch
1 centimeter (cm) = 0.4 inch
2.54 cm = 1 inch
1 meter (m) = 39.37 inches

WEIGHT

60 milligrams (mg) = 1 grain
28.35 grams (g) = 1 oz
454 g = 1 lb
1000 g (1 kilogram [kg]) = 2.2 lbs

MILLIGRAM-MILLIEQUIVALENT CONVERSIONS

$$mEQ/L = mg/L \times \frac{Valence}{Atomic\ weight}$$

$$mg/L = mEq/L \times \frac{Atomic\ weight}{Valence}$$

$$Equivalent\ weight = \frac{Atomic\ weight}{Valence}$$

MILLIOSMOLS

The milliequivalent (mEq) is roughly equivalent to the milliosmol (mosm), the unit of measure of osmolarity or tonicity.

Prefixes for Decimal Factors

Prefix	Symbol	Factor
mega	m	10^6
kilo	k	10^3
hecto	h	10^2
deka	da	10^1
deci	d	10^{-1}
centi	c	10^{-2}
milli	m	10^{-3}
micro	μ	10^{-6}
nano	n	10^{-9}
pico	p	10^{-12}
fento	f	10^{-15}

Hoekelman RA, Adam HM, Nelson NM, et al: Primary Pediatric Care, 4th ed. St Louis, Mosby, 2001.

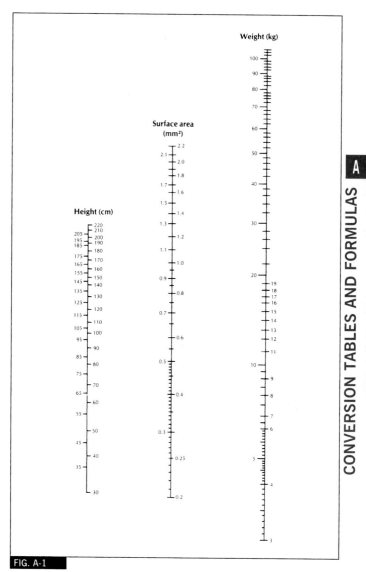

FIG. A-1

Nomogram to determine body surface area. *(From Roberson J, Shilkofski N: The Harriet Lane Handbook, 17th ed. Philadelphia, Mosby, 2005.)*

Anthropometric Charts and Tables

B

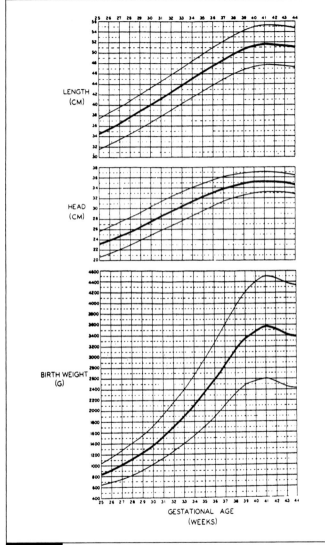

FIG. B-1

Intrauterine growth curves. *(From Usher R, McLean F: Intrauterine growth of live-born Caucasian infants at sea level: Standards obtained from measurements in seven dimensions of infants born between 25 and 44 weeks of gestation. J Pediatr 74:901, 1969.)*

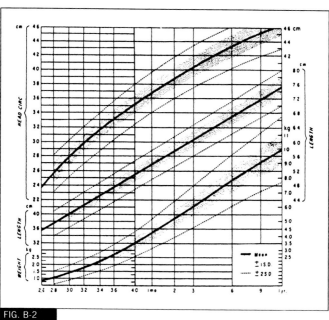

FIG. B-2

Extrauterine growth curves. *(From Babson SG, Benda GI: Growth graphics for the clinical assessment of infants of varying gestational age. J Pediatr 89:814, 1976.)*

TABLE B-1

DISTRIBUTION OF MEASUREMENTS FOR WHITE NEWBORN MALE INFANTS
(CONTROLS) BY PERCENTILES ACCORDING TO GESTATIONAL AGES

	Gestational Age (wk)					
Percentile	37	38	39	40	41	42-43
	Crown-Heel Lengths (cm)					
95	52.0	53.5	54.0	54.5	55.0	55.3
90	51.5	52.5	53.5	54.0	54.5	54.8
75	50.5	51.5	52.5	53.0	53.5	54.0
50	50.0	50.7	51.5	52.0	52.5	53.0
25	49.0	49.7	50.5	51.0	51.5	52.0
10	48.0	48.7	49.5	50.0	50.5	51.0
5	47.5	48.2	49.5	49.5	50.0	50.5
	Occipitofrontal Circumference (cm)					
95	35.5	36.0	36.4	36.8	37.2	37.4
90	35.2	35.6	35.9	36.3	36.7	37.2
75	34.6	34.9	35.3	35.7	36.0	36.2
50	34.0	34.3	34.6	34.9	35.2	35.5
25	33.4	33.7	34.0	34.3	34.7	35.0
10	32.8	33.2	33.5	33.8	34.2	34.5
5	32.4	32.7	33.1	33.4	33.8	34.2

	Gestational Age (wk)					
Percentile	37	38	39	40	41	42-43
	Birth Weights, First-born Infants (kg)					
95	3.63	3.82	3.97	4.10	4.23	4.34
90	3.50	3.70	3.86	4.00	4.13	4.24
75	3.30	3.48	3.65	3.78	3.92	4.03
50	3.10	3.27	3.43	3.57	3.70	3.82
25	2.85	3.00	3.13	3.26	3.38	3.49
10	2.70	2.84	2.96	3.08	3.18	3.28
5	2.62	2.76	2.88	3.00	3.10	3.20
	Birth Weights, Infants of Multiparas (kg)					
95	3.66	4.00	4.20	4.39	4.50	4.60
90	3.47	3.70	3.90	4.08	4.24	4.37
75	3.30	3.50	3.70	3.87	4.03	4.15
50	3.10	3.27	3.44	3.61	3.75	3.85
25	2.85	3.02	3.18	3.34	3.50	3.62
10	2.71	2.86	3.02	3.19	3.34	3.45
5	2.63	2.78	2.94	3.08	3.31	3.32

From Miller HC: Intrauterine growth retardation: An unmet challenge. AM J Dis Child 135:946,
1981.

TABLE B-2

DISTRIBUTION OF MEASUREMENTS FOR WHITE NEWBORN FEMALE INFANTS
(CONTROLS) BY PERCENTILES ACCORDING TO GESTATIONAL AGES

	Gestational Age (wk)					
Percentile	37	38	39	40	41	42-43
	Crown-Heel Lengths (cm)					
95	51.5	52.5	53.5	54.0	54.5	54.5
90	51.0	52.0	53.0	53.5	54.0	54.0
75	50.0	51.0	52.0	52.5	52.8	53.1
50	49.0	50.0	50.7	51.3	51.7	52.0
25	48.0	48.9	49.5	50.0	50.5	51.0
10	47.5	48.5	49.0	49.5	50.0	50.5
5	47.0	47.9	48.6	49.1	49.5	50.0
	Occipitofrontal Circumference (cm)					
95	35.0	35.5	35.9	36.2	36.5	36.8
90	34.5	35.0	35.4	35.7	36.1	36.3
75	33.9	34.3	34.7	35.1	35.5	35.8
50	33.2	33.6	34.1	34.5	34.8	35.2
25	32.5	32.9	33.4	33.8	34.2	34.5
10	32.0	32.4	32.8	33.2	33.6	33.9
5	31.8	32.2	32.6	32.9	33.3	33.6
	Gestational Age (wk)					
Percentile	37	38	39	40	41	42-43
	Birth Weights, First-born Infants (kg)					
95	3.44	3.72	3.90	4.03	4.12	4.20
90	3.30	3.60	3.80	3.92	4.02	4.10
75	3.17	3.38	3.57	3.70	3.82	3.94
50	3.00	3.15	3.30	3.43	3.56	3.66
25	2.79	2.93	3.07	3.18	3.29	3.37
10	2.55	2.72	2.85	2.97	3.09	3.17
5	2.46	2.61	2.76	2.89	3.01	3.10
	Birth Weights, Infants of Multiparas (kg)					
95	3.60	3.86	4.02	4.14	4.23	4.31
90	3.50	3.67	3.84	3.95	4.07	4.15
75	3.26	3.48	3.64	3.75	3.85	3.95
50	3.00	3.20	3.34	3.50	3.62	3.72
25	2.80	2.95	3.08	3.23	3.35	3.45
10	2.67	2.80	2.93	3.05	3.16	3.26
5	2.52	2.67	2.80	2.92	3.04	3.15

From Miller HC: Intrauterine growth retardation: An unmet challenge. Am J Dis Child 135:946, 1981.

B

ANTHROPOMETRIC CHARTS AND TABLES

DISTRIBUTION OF MEASUREMENTS FOR BLACK NEWBORN MALE INFANTS
(CONTROLS) BY PERCENTILES ACCORDING TO GESTATIONAL AGES

Percentile	37	38	39	40	41	42-43
			Crown-Heel Lengths (cm)			
95	51.5	52.5	53.5	54.5	54.5	54.5
90	51.0	52.0	52.7	53.5	54.0	54.0
75	50.5	51.5	52.0	52.5	53.0	53.0
50	49.5	50.0	50.5	51.0	51.5	52.0
25	48.5	49.0	49.5	50.5	50.5	51.0
10	47.5	48.0	48.5	49.0	49.5	50.0
5	47.0	47.5	48.0	48.5	49.0	49.5
			Occipitofrontal Circumference (cm)			
95	35.3	35.8	36.2	36.7	37.0	37.0
90	35.0	35.5	35.9	36.3	36.7	36.8
75	34.6	34.9	35.3	35.6	36.0	36.3
50	33.6	34.0	34.4	34.7	35.1	35.5
25	33.1	33.4	33.8	34.1	34.5	34.9
10	32.4	32.8	33.1	33.4	33.8	34.1
5	32.1	32.5	32.8	33.1	33.4	33.7
			Birth Weights (kg)			
95	3.44	3.71	3.97	4.13	4.29	4.40
90	3.38	3.62	3.84	3.97	4.10	4.15
75	3.30	3.46	3.62	3.72	3.82	3.92
50	3.08	3.18	3.30	3.40	3.50	3.60
25	2.83	2.93	3.03	3.13	3.22	3.32
10	2.63	2.73	2.82	2.90	2.99	3.08
5	2.54	2.68	2.72	2.82	2.95	3.00

From Miller HC: Intrauterine growth retardation: An unmet challenge. Am J Dis Child 135:946, 1981.

TABLE B-4

DISTRIBUTION OF MEASUREMENTS FOR BLACK NEWBORN FEMALE INFANTS
(CONTROLS) BY PERCENTILES ACCORDING TO GESTATIONAL AGES

Percentile	37	38	39	40	41	42-43
			Gestational Age (wk)			
			Crown-Heel Lengths (cm)			
95	51.0	51.7	52.5	53.3	54.0	54.0
90	50.3	51.0	51.8	52.5	53.5	53.0
75	49.5	50.5	51.0	51.5	52.0	52.5
50	49.0	49.5	50.0	50.5	51.0	51.5
25	48.0	48.5	49.0	49.5	50.0	50.5
10	47.0	47.5	48.0	48.5	49.0	49.5
5	46.5	47.0	47.5	48.0	48.5	49.0
			Occipitofrontal Circumference (cm)			
95	35.0	35.1	35.6	35.9	36.2	36.5
90	34.3	34.8	35.3	35.6	35.8	36.0
75	34.1	34.3	34.6	34.8	35.1	35.3
50	33.4	33.6	33.9	34.1	34.4	34.7
25	32.7	33.0	33.2	33.5	33.7	34.0
10	32.1	32.3	32.6	32.8	33.1	33.3
5	31.7	32.0	32.2	32.5	32.8	33.0
			Birth Weights (kg)			
95	3.44	3.65	3.83	3.97	4.00	4.15
90	3.32	3.53	3.73	3.88	3.98	4.05
75	3.14	3.32	3.48	3.60	3.73	3.85
50	2.93	3.07	3.22	3.34	3.46	3.58
25	2.70	2.83	2.95	3.08	3.03	3.32
10	2.53	2.65	2.77	2.89	3.01	3.10
5	2.43	2.54	2.65	2.77	2.89	3.01

From Miller HC: Intrauterine growth retardation: An unmet challenge. Am J Dis Child 135:946, 1981.

ANTHROPOMETRIC CHARTS AND TABLES

B

Laboratory Observations

BLOOD CHEMISTRY VALUES

ACID-BASE RESPONSE IN RESPIRATORY ACIDOSIS AND ALKALOSIS

The nomogram shown in **Fig. C-1** provides confidence bands for the normal adjustments in carbon dioxide content and pH made to acute and chronic changes in arterial P_{CO_2}.

1. Determine pH on nomogram from plotted $Paco_2$ and carbon dioxide content obtained from blood-gas measurement.
2. If pH value is not within confidence bands, alterations in carbon dioxide content and pH varies from those expected from a pure respiratory condition, and a metabolic abnormality is also present.
3. To estimate the effects of acute and chronic changes in P_{CO_2} on pH, use the following formulas:

Acute change in P_{CO_2}:

$\Delta P_{CO_2} \times 0.008 = \Delta pH$

Chronic change in P_{CO_2}:

$\Delta P_{CO_2} \times 0.003 = \Delta pH$

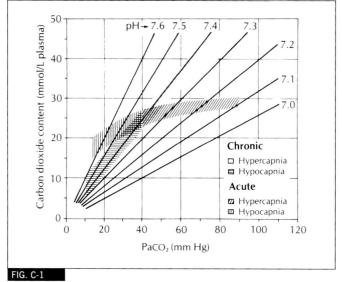

FIG. C-1

Acid-base response in respiratory acidosis and alkalosis. *(Modified from Arbus GS: An in vivo acid-base nomogram for clinical use. Can Med Assoc J 109:291, 1973.)*

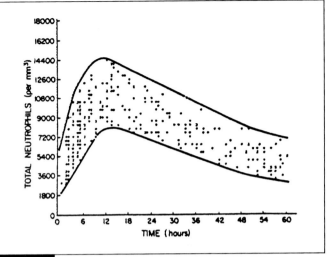

FIG. C-2

The total neutrophil count in normal infants during the first 60 hours of life. Stars represent single values; numbers represent the number of values at the same point. *(From Manroe BL et al: J Pediatr 95:89, 1979.)*

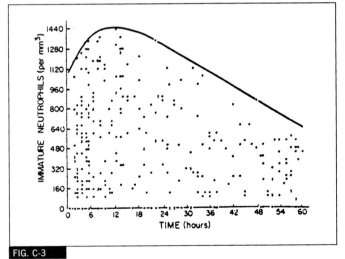

FIG. C-3

The range for immature neutrophils in normal infants during the first 60 hours of life. Stars represent single values; numbers represent the number of values at the same point. *(From Manroe BL et al: J Pediatr 95:89, 1979.)*

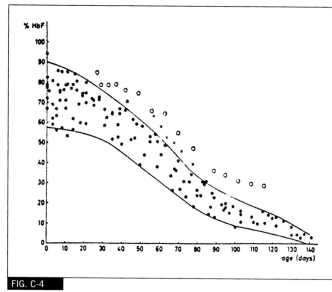

FIG. C-4

The relative concentration of HbF in infants and its variation with age. The region between the curved lines contains 120 observations in 17 normal children. *(From Garby L, Sjolin S: Acta Paediatr 51:245, 1962.)*

BOX C-1

NORMAL LABORATORY VALUES (CEREBROSPINAL FLUID)

EVALUATION OF CEREBROSPINAL FLUID

	WBC Count	Mean % PMNs
Preterm	0-25 WBCs/mm³	57%
Term	0-22 WBCs/mm³	61%
Child	0-7 WBCs/mm³	5%
GLUCOSE		
Preterm	24-63 mg/dl	1.3-3.5 mmol/L
Term	34-119 mg/dl	1.9-6.6 mmol/L
Child	40-80 mg/dl	2.2-4.4 mmol/L
CSF GLUCOSE/BLOOD GLUCOSE		
Preterm	55%-105%	
Term	44%-128%	
Child	50%	
LACTIC ACID DEHYDROGENASE		
Normal range	5-30 U/L (or about 10% of serum value)	
MYELIN BASIC PROTEIN	<4 ng/ml	
OPENING PRESSURE		
(Lateral recumbent)		
Newborn	80-110 mmH₂O	
Infant/child	<200 mmH₂O	
Respiratory variations	5-10 mmH₂O	
PROTEIN		
Preterm	65-150 mg/dl	0.65-1.5 g/L
Term	20-170 mg/dl	0.20-1.7 g/L
Child	5-40 mg/dl	0.05-0.40 g/L

CSF, Cerebrospinal fluid; PMNs, polymorphonuclear lymphocytes; WBC, white blood cell.
Modified from Oski FA: Principles and Practice of Pediatrics, 3rd ed. Philadelphia, JB Lippincott, 1999.
Roberson J, Shilkofski N: The Harriet Lane Handbook, 17th ed. Philadelphia, Mosby, 2005.

TABLE C-1
BLOOD GASES: REPRESENTATIVE VALUES IN NORMAL INFANTS AT TERM

| | Umbilical Vein | 30 min | Arterial Blood | | | | Reference |
			1-4 hr	12-24 hr	24-48 hr	96 hr	
pH	7.33	—	7.30	7.30	7.39	7.39	Reardon et al (1960)
P_{CO_2}, mm Hg	43	—	39	33	34	36	Oliver et al (1961)
HCO_3, mEq/L	21.6	—	18.8	19.5	20	21.4	Nelson et al (1962, 1963)
P_{O_2}, mm Hg	28 ± 8	—	62 ± 13.8	68	63-87		
O_2 saturation			95%	94%	94%	96%	

From Taeusch HW, Ballard RA: Avery's Diseases of the Newborn, 7th ed. Philadelphia, WB Saunders, 1998 and Bucci G et al: Biol Neonate 8:81, 1965.

LABORATORY OBSERVATIONS

TABLE C-2

ACID-BASE STATUS

Determination	Sample Source	Birth	1 hr	3 hr	24 hr	2 days	3 days
VIGOROUS TERM INFANTS, VAGINAL DELIVERY							
pH	Umbilical artery	7.26					
	Umbilical vein	7.29					
Pco_2 (mm Hg)	Arterial	54.5	38.8	38.3	33.6	34	35
	Venous	42.8					
O_2 saturation	Arterial	19.8	93.8	94.7	93.2		
	Venous	47.6					
pH	Left atrial		7.30	7.34	7.41	7.39 (Temporal artery)	7.38 (Temporal artery)
CO_2 content (mEq/L)	—	—	20.6	21.9	21.4		
PREMATURE INFANTS							
pH	Capillary (skin puncture) <1250 g				7.36	7.35	7.35
Pco_2 (mm Hg)					38	44	37
pH	>1250 g				7.39	7.39	7.38
Pco_2 (mm Hg)					38	39	38

Data from Schaffer AJ: Diseases of the Newborn, 3rd ed. Philadelphia, WB Saunders, 1971. Data from Weisbrot IM et al: J Pediatr 52:395, 1958 and Bucci G et al: Biol Neonate 8:81, 1965.

TABLE C-3

SERUM CHEMISTRIES IN TERM INFANTS

Determination	Cord		1-12 hr		12-24 hr		24-48 hr		48-72 hr	
Sodium, mEq/L*	147	(126-166)	143	(124-156)	145	(132-159)	148	(134-160)	149	(139-162)
Potassium, mEq/L	7.8	(5.6-12)	6.4	(5.3-7.3)	6.3	(5.3-8.9)	6	(5.2-7.3)	5.9	(5.0-7.7)
Chloride, mEq/L	103	(98-110)	100.7	(90-111)	103	(87-114)	102	(92-114)	103	(93-112)
Calcium, mg/dl	9.3	(8.2-11.1)	8.4	(7.3-9.2)	7.8	(6.9-9.4)	8	(6.1-9.9)	7.9	(5.9-9.7)
Phosphorus, mg/dl	5.6	(3.7-8.1)	6.1	(3.5-8.6)	5.7	(2.9-8.1)	5.9	(3-8.7)	5.8	(2.8-7.6)
Blood urea, mg/dl	29	(21-40)	27	(8-34)	33	(9-63)	32	(13-77)	31	(13-68)
Total protein, g/dl	6.1	(4.8-7.3)	6.6	(5.6-8.5)	6.6	(5.8-8.2)	6.9	(5.9-8.2)	7.2	(6.0-8.5)
Blood sugar, mg/dl	73	(45-96)	63	(40-97)	63	(42-104)	56	(30-91)	59	(40-90)
Lactic acid, mg/dl	19.5	(11-30)	14.6	(11-24)	14	(10-23)	14.3	(9-22)	13.5	(7-21)
Lactate, mmol/L†	2.3-3.0		2.0							

Modified from Taeusch HW, Ballard RA, Gleason CA (eds): Avery's Diseases of the Newborn, 8th ed. Philadelphia, WB Saunders, 2004.

*Acharya PT, Payne WW: Arch Dis Child 40:430, 1965.

†Daniel SS, Adamsons KJ, James LS: Pediatrics 37:942, 1966.

C

LABORATORY OBSERVATIONS

TABLE C-4

SELECTED CHEMISTRY VALUES IN FULL-TERM AND PRETERM INFANTS

Constituent	Preterm	Term
Ammonia (µg/100 ml)	—	90-150
Base, excess (mmol/L)	—	−10 to −2
Bicarbonate, standard (mmol/L)	18-26	20-26
Bilirubin, total (mg/dl)		
Cord	<2.8	<2.8
24 hr	1-6	2-6
48 hr	6-8	6-7
3-5 days	10-12	4-6
>1 mo	<1.5	<1.5
Bilirubin, direct (mg/dl)	<0.5	<0.5
Calcium, total (mg/dl), week 1	6-10	8.4-11.6
Ceruloplasmin (mg/dl)		1-3 mo: 5-18
		6-12 mo: 33-43
		13-36 mo: 26-55
Cholesterol (mg/dl)		
Cord		45-98
3 days-1 yr		65-175
Creatine phosphokinase (U/L)		
Day 1		44-1150
Day 4		14-97
Creatinine (mg/dl)		
Birth	Mother's level	Mother's level
10 days	1.3 ± 0.07 (mean ± SD)	1-4 day 0.3-1
1 mo	0.6 ± 0.05 (mean ± SD)	>4 day 0.2-0.4
Ferritin (µg/dl)		
Neonate		25-200
1 mo		200-600
2-5 mo		50-200
>6 mo		7-142
Gamma-glutamyl transferase (GGT) (U/L)	—	14-131
Glucose (mg/dl)		
<72 hr	20-125	30-125
>72 hr	40-125	40-125
Lactate dehydrogenase (U/L)	—	357-953
Magnesium (mg/dl)	—	1.7-2.4
Osmolality (mOsm/L)	—	275-295 (may be as low as 266)
Phosphate, alkaline (U/L) (mean ± SD)		
26-27 wk	320 ± 142	164 ± 68
28-29 wk	292 ± 87	—
30-31 wk	281 ± 85	—
32-33 wk	254 ± 72	—

TABLE C-4

SELECTED CHEMISTRY VALUES IN FULL-TERM AND PRETERM INFANTS—cont'd

Constituent	Preterm	Term
34-35 wk	236 ± 62	—
36 wk	207 ± 60	—
Phosphorus (mg/dl)		
Birth		4.5-8.7
Day 5		4.2-7.2
Month 1		4.5-6.5
SGOT/AST (aspartate amino transferase) (U/L)		24-81
SGPT/ALT (alanine amino transferase) (U/L)		10-33
Triglycerides (mg/dl)		10-140
Urea nitrogen (mg/dl)	3-25	4-12
Uric acid (mg/dl)	—	3-7.5
Vitamin A (μg/dl)	16 ± 1.0	23.9 ± 1.8
(<10 μg/dl indicates very low hepatic vitamin A stores)		
Vitamin D		
25-Hydroxycholecalciferol (ng/ml)*		20-60
1,25-Dihydroxycholecalciferol (pg/ml)*		40-90

*Serum levels affected by race, age, season, and diet.

Modified from Fanaroff AA, Martin RJ (eds): Neonatal-Perinatal Medicine: Diseases of the Fetus and Infant, 7th ed. St Louis, Mosby, 2002.

TABLE C-5

LABORATORY PARAMETERS OF ACID-BASE DISTURBANCES*

	pH	Paco$_2$	HCO$_3$ (mEq/L)	CO$_2$ Content (mEq/L)
Normal values	7.35-7.45	35-45	24-26	25-28
Disturbances				
Metabolic acidosis	↓	↓	↓	↓
Acute respiratory acidosis	↓	↑	↔	Slight ↑
Compensated respiratory acidosis	↔ or slight ↑	↑	↑	↑
Metabolic alkalosis	↑	Slight ↑	↑	↑
Acute respiratory alkalosis	↑	↓	↔	Slight ↓
Compensated respiratory alkalosis	↔ or slight ↑	↓	↓	↓

*Values obtained by arterialized capillary blood or direct arterial puncture.

From Hoekelman RA, Adam HM, Nelson NM, et al (eds): Primary Pediatric Care, 4th ed. St Louis, Mosby, 2001.

C

LABORATORY OBSERVATIONS

TABLE C-6
TRUE BLOOD SUGAR LEVELS IN NORMAL TERM AND LOW BIRTH WEIGHT INFANTS

Maternal Status	Delivery Type	Age (Hr)						
		0	0.5	1	2	4	6	24
No fluid administration	Vaginal	66	55	55	48	55	47	—
		44-84	34-90	35-89	22-73	30-71	27-78	—
Saline, IV administration	Cesarean section	64	75	76	70	60	57	54
		38-90	58-107	34-136	45-108	47-101	35-76	43-76
Glucose, IV administration	Cesarean section	109	69	66	56	58	52	68
		61-204	31-125	31-111	35-85	27-86	32-77	35-91
Glucose, IV administration	Vaginal	89	54	47	41	50	51	—
		54-163	27-98	16-82	19-71	34-80	29-80	—

From Cornblath M et al: Pediatrics 27:378, 1961.

TABLE C-7
AGE-SPECIFIC INDICES

Age	Hgb (g %) Mean (−2 SD)	Hct (%) Mean (−2 SD)	MCV (fl) Mean (−2 SD)	MCHC (g/dl RBC) Mean (−2 SD)	Reticulocytes (%)	WBC/mm³ × 1000 Mean (+2 SD)	Platelets/mm³ (× 1000) Mean (Range)
26-30 wk gestation*	13.4 (11)	41.5 (34.9)	118.2 (106.7)	37.9 (30.6)	—	4.4 (2.7)	254 (180-327)
28 wk	14.5	45	120	31	(5-10)	—	275
32 wk	15	47	118	32	(3-10)	—	290
Term† (cord)	16.5 (13.5)	51 (42)	108 (98)	33 (30)	(3-7)	18.1 (9-30)‡	290
1-3 days	18.5 (14.5)	56 (45)	108 (95)	33 (29)	(1.8-4.6)	18.9 (9.4-34)	192
2 wk	16.6 (13.4)	53 (41)	105 (88)	31.4 (28.1)		11.4 (5-20)	252

*Values are from fetal samplings.

†Under 1 mo, capillary Hgb exceeds venous: 1 hr: 3.6 gm difference; 5 days: 2.2 gm difference; 3 weeks: 1.1 gm difference.

‡Mean (95% confidence limits).

Modified from Roberson J, Shilkofski N: The Harriet Lane Handbook, 17th ed. Philadelphia, Mosby, 2005.

LABORATORY OBSERVATIONS

C

TABLE C-8
LEUKOCYTE VALUES IN TERM AND PREMATURE INFANTS (10^3 CELLS/μL)

Age (Hr)	Total White Cell Count	Neutrophils	Bands/Metas	Lymphocytes	Monocytes	Eosinophils
TERM INFANTS						
0	10.0-26	5-13	0.4-1.8	3.5-8.5	0.7-1.5	0.2-2.0
12	13.5-31	9-18	0.4-2	3.0-7	1.0-2	0.2-2.0
72	5.0-14.5	2-7	0.2-0.4	2.0-5	0.5-1	0.2-1.0
144	6.0-14.5	2-6	0.2-0.5	3.0-6	0.7-1.2	0.2-0.8
PREMATURE INFANTS						
0	5.0-19	2-9	0.2-2.4	2.5-6	0.3-1	0.1-0.7
12	5.0-21	3-11	0.2-2.4	1.5-5	0.3-1.3	0.1-1.1
72	5.0-14	3-7	0.2-0.6	1.5-4	0.3-1.2	0.2-1.1
144	5.5-17.5	2-7	0.2-0.5	2.5-7.5	0.5-1.5	0.3-1.2

From Oski FA, Naiman JL: Hematologic Problems in the Newborn, 3rd ed. Philadelphia, WB Saunders, 1982.

TABLE C-9

CHANGES IN POLYMORPHONUCLEAR NEUTROPHIL COUNT OF HEALTHY
TERM BABIES WITH AGE (CELLS/MM^3)

Postnatal Age	5th Centile	Median	95th Centile
Birth	4,120*	7,750	14,600
6 hr	6,640*	12,500	23,500
12 hr	6,640*	12,500	23,500
18 hr	6,370*	11,000	20,700
24 hr	4,830*	9,100	17,100
36 hr	3,820*	7,200	13,400
48 hr	3,080*	5,800	10,900
3 days	2,550	4,800	9,040
4 days	2,260	4,250	8,000
5 days	2,040	3,850	7,250
7 days	1,800	3,400	6,400
10 days	1,730	3,250	6,120
2 wk	1,700	3,200	6,020
3-4 wk	1,650	3,100	5,840

*About 5% of healthy preterm babies probably have a neutrophil count of < 3000 cells/mm^3 at this age.

From Gregory J, Hey E: Arch Dis Child 47:747, 1972.

TABLE C-10

THYROID FUNCTION TESTS: ROUTINE STUDIES

Test	Age	Normal	Comments
T_4 RIA (mcg/dl)	Cord	6.6-17.5	Measures total T_4 by radioimmunoassay
	1-3 days	11.0-21.5	
	1-4 wk	8.2-16.6	
	1-12 mo	7.2-15.6	
	1-5 yr	7.3-15.0	
	6-10 yr	6.4-13.3	
	11-15 yr	5.6-11.7	
	16-20 yr	4.2-11.8	
	21-50 yr	4.3-12.5	
Free T4 (ng/dl)	1-10 days	0.6-2.0	Metabolically active form; the normal range for free T_4 is very assay dependent
	>10 days	0.7-1.7	
T_3 RIA (ng/dl)	Cord	14-86	Measures T_3 by RIA
	1-3 days	100-380	
	1-4 wk	99-310	
	1-12 mo	102-264	
	1-5 yr	105-269	
	6-10 yr	94-241	
	11-15 yr	83-213	
	16-20 yr	80-210	
	21-50 yr	70-204	
TSH (mIU/ml)	Cord	<2.5-17.4	TSH surge peaks from 80-90 mIU/ml in term newborn by 30 min after birth. Values after 1 wk are within adult normal range. Elevated values suggest primary hypothyroidism, whereas suppressed values are the best indicator of hyperthyroidism.
	1-3 days	<2.5-13.3	
	1-4 wk	0.6-10.0	
	1-12 mo	0.6-6.3	
	1-15 yr	0.6-6.3	
	16-50 yr	0.2-7.6	
TBG (mg/dl)	Cord	0.7-4.7	
	1-3 days	—	
	1-4 wk	0.5-4.5	
	1-12 mo	1.6-3.6	
	1-5 yr	1.3-2.8	
	6-20 yr	1.4-2.6	
	21-50 yr	1.2-2.4	

RIA, radioimmunoassay; RU, resin uptake; T_3, triiodothyronine; T_4, thyroxine; TBG, thyroxine-binding globulin; TSH, thyroid-stimulating hormone.

From Roberson J, Shilkofski N: The Harriet Lane Handbook, 17th ed. Philadelphia, Mosby, 2005.

TABLE C-11
THYROID ANTIBODIES*

Interpretation	Antithyroglobulin	Antimicrosomal
Insignificant	<1:40	<1:400
Borderline	1:80	1:400
Significant	1:160-1:640	1:1600-1:6400
Very significant	<1:640	<1:6400

*High titers of thyroid antibodies are consistent with Hashimoto's thyroiditis.

From Siberry G, Iannone R (eds): The Harriet Lane Handbook, 15th ed. St Louis, Mosby, 2000.

TABLE C-12
SERUM T$_4$ (µG/DL) IN PRETERM AND TERM INFANTS

Age	Estimated Gestational Age (wk)				
	30-31	32-33	34-35	36-37	Term
Cord	4.5-8.5	3.3-11.7	4.3-9.1	1.9-13.1	4.6-11.8
12-72 hr	7.3-15.7	5.9-18.7	6.2-18.6	10.3-20.7	14.8-23.2
3-10 days	4.1-11.3	4.7-12.3	5.2-14.8	7.7-17.7	9.9-21.9
11-20 days	3.9-11.1	5.1-11.5	6.9-14.1	5.4-17	8.2-16.2
21-45 days	4.8-10.8	4.6-11.4	6.7-11.9	3.0-19.8	9.1-15.1
46-90 days	6.2-13	6.2-13	6.2-13	6.2-13	6.4-14

From Siberry G, Iannone R (eds): The Harriet Lane Handbook, 15th ed. St Louis, Mosby, 2000.

TABLE C-13
SERUM IMMUNOGLOBULIN LEVELS (MG/DL) IN NEWBORNS

Age	Newborn	1-3 mo
IgG	1031 ± 200	430 ± 119
	(645-1244)	(272-762)
IgA	2 ± 3	21 ± 13
	(0-11)	(6-56)
IgM	11 ± 5	30 ± 1
	(5-30)	(16-67)

From Stiehm ER, Fudenberg HH: Pediatrics 37:715, 1966.

C

LABORATORY OBSERVATIONS

TABLE C-14
ELECTROCARDIOGRAPHIC STANDARDS IN NEWBORNS

Measure	0-1		1-3		3-7		7-30	
Number of patients	189		179		181		119	
Heart rate (beats/min)	122	(99-147)	123	(97-148)	128	(100-160)	148	(114-177)
QRS axis (degrees)	135	(91-185)	134	(93-188)	133	(92-185)	108	(78-152)
P-R duration II (ms)	107	(82-138)	108	(85-132)	103	(78-130)	101	(75-128)
QRS duration V_5 (ms)	50	(26-69)	48	(27-61)	49	(26-63)	53	(27-75)
Q-T duration V_5 (ms)	290	(220-360)	280	(235-330)	272	(272-315)	258	(230-290)
P amplitude II (mV)	0.16	(0.07-0.25)	0.16	(0.05-0.25)	0.17	(0.08-0.27)	0.19	(0.09-0.29)
R amplitude V_{3R} (mV)	1.05	(0.4-1.79)	1.19	(0.52-1.95)	1.02	(0.18-1.80)	0.82	(0.3-1.5)
R amplitude V_1 (mV)	1.35	(0.65-2.37)	1.48	(0.70-2.42)	1.28	(0.5-2.15)	1.05	(0.45-1.81)
R amplitude V_5 (mV)	1	(0.25-1.85)	1.1	(0.48-1.95)	1.3	(0.48-1.95)	1.45	(0.6-2.1)
R amplitude V_6 (mV)	0.45	(0.05-0.95)	0.48	(0.05-0.95)	0.51	(0.10-1.05)	0.76	(0.26-1.35)
S amplitude V_{3R} (mV)	0.43	(0.07-1.18)	0.5	(0.05-1.2)	0.36	(0.05-0.8)	0.20	(0.05-0.64)
S amplitude V_1 (mV)	0.85	(0.1-1.85)	0.95	(0.15-1.9)	0.68	(0.1-1.5)	0.4	(0.05-0.97)
S amplitude V_5 (mV)	0.99	(0.38-1.79)	0.98	(0.2-1.59)	0.95	(0.38-1.63)	0.8	(0.24-1.38)
S amplitude V_6 (mV)	0.35	(0.02-0.79)	0.32	(0.02-0.76)	0.37	(0.02-0.8)	0.32	(0.02-0.82)
R/S amplitude V_{3R}	1.5	(0.2-4.8)	1.6	(0.2-4.2)	1.8	(0.2-5.8)	1.9	(0.2-2.5)
R/S amplitude V_1	2.2	(0.4-7)	2	(0.4-5.4)	2.8	(0.05-7.2)	2.9	(1.1-6.3)
R/S amplitude V_5	0.7	(0-7)	1	(0-5)	1.5	(0-5)	2	(0.5-1)
R/S amplitude V_6	2	(0-8)	3	(0-9)	2	(0-8)	4	(0-9)
Mean (5% and 95% values)								

Age in Days

From Davignon A, et al: Pediatr Cardiol 1:123, 1979-1980.

Procedures*

I. VENIPUNCTURE

A. HEEL OR FINGER STICK (FIG. D-1).

1. Warm extremity to provide optimal blood flow and more accurate samples. To prevent burns, do not use a warming towel that is warmer than 40°C.
2. Lance either the lateral or medial side of the heel; avoid the heel pad. For digital artery sampling, use the lateral surface of the distal phalanx of second, third, or fourth finger.
3. Use a 2.5-mm lancet or an Autolet for optimal skin penetration.
4. Wipe away the first drop of blood with dry gauze. Alcohol used in cleansing skin may produce hemolysis.
5. Massage (but do not squeeze) finger or heel.
6. Samples may be inaccurate if patient is poorly perfused or polycythemic.

B. EXTERNAL JUGULAR PUNCTURE. USED FOR BLOOD SAMPLING IN PATIENTS WITH INADEQUATE PERIPHERAL VASCULAR ACCESS OR DURING RESUSCITATION.

1. Restrain infant securely (**Fig. D-2**).
2. Extend neck and turn head slightly to one side. This accentuates the posterior margin of contralateral sternocleidomastoid muscle. This may be facilitated by positioning the infant so that its head falls over the side of the table or by placing a rolled towel under the infant's shoulders.
3. Prepare the area carefully with povidone-iodine and 70% alcohol.
4. To distend the external jugular vein, occlude its most proximal segment or provoke child to cry. The vein runs from the angle of the mandible to the posterior border of the lower third of the sternocleidomastoid muscle.
5. While continually providing negative suction on the syringe, insert the needle at about a 30-degree angle to the skin. Continue as with any peripheral venipuncture.

Note: *Hematoma, pneumothorax, and infection can be complications.*

C. FEMORAL PUNCTURE. FOR VENOUS OR ARTERIAL BLOOD SAMPLING OF PATIENTS WITH INADEQUATE VASCULAR ACCESS OR DURING RESUSCITATION.

*Modified from Siberry G, Iannone R (eds): The Harriet Lane Handbook, ed 15. St Louis, Mosby, 2000.

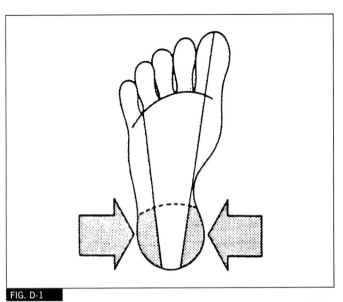

FIG. D-1

Recommended sites (*shaded areas*) for warmed heel puncture. *(From Blumenfeld TA, Turi GK, Blanc WA: Lancet 1:230, 1979.)*

Careful skin preparation is needed to prevent septic arthritis. Femoral puncture is particularly hazardous in neonates and is not usually recommended or appropriate in this age group. Avoid femoral punctures in children who are thrombocytopenic, have coagulation disorders, or are scheduled for cardiac catheterization.

1. Have an assistant hold the child securely, with the hips flexed and abducted (in a frog-leg position).
2. Prepare area as for blood culture with povidone-iodine and 70% alcohol.
3. Locate the femoral pulse, then insert the needle 2.0 cm distal to the inguinal ligament and 0.5 cm medial to the femoral pulse.
4. Insert the needle slowly at a 30-degree angle to the skin to a depth of approximately 0.5 to 0.75 cm. Continually aspirate while maneuvering the needle until blood is obtained.
5. Withdraw the needle and apply direct pressure to the puncture site for a minimum of 5 minutes.

D. INTERNAL JUGULAR PUNCTURE.

1. Securely restrain the infant.
2. Extend the infant's neck and turn the head slightly to one side. This accentuates the posterior margin of the sternocleidomastoid muscle.

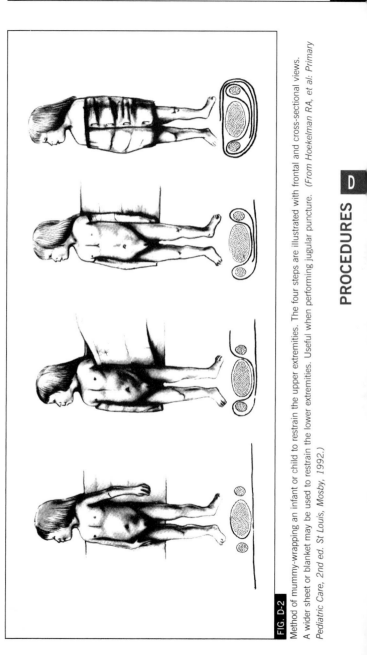

FIG. D-2

Method of mummy-wrapping an infant or child to restrain the upper extremities. The four steps are illustrated with frontal and cross-sectional views. A wider sheet or blanket may be used to restrain the lower extremities. Useful when performing jugular puncture. *(From Hoekelman RA, et al: Primary Pediatric Care, 2nd ed. St Louis, Mosby, 1992.)*

PROCEDURES

D

This may be facilitated by positioning the infant so that its head falls over the side of the table or by placing a rolled towel under the infant's shoulders.
3. Prepare the area as for blood culture with povidone-iodine and 70% alcohol.
4. Insert the needle just deep to and behind the posterior margin of the sternocleidomastoid muscle, approximately halfway between its origin and insertion. Advance the needle under the muscle, parallel to the skin surface, and in the direction of the suprasternal notch. Advance for a distance equal to the width of the sternocleidomastoid muscle.
5. While exerting suction, slowly withdraw needle until blood is withdrawn.
6. After obtaining blood, hold child upright and apply pressure to the puncture site.

II. UMBILICAL ARTERY CATHETERIZATION

Umbilical artery catheterization is used to obtain vascular access and monitor blood pressure and blood gas levels in critically ill neonates.

A. CATHETER PLACEMENT.
1. Restrain infant. Prepare and drape umbilical cord and adjacent skin using sterile technique. Place sterile drapes sparingly to expose infant to the radiant warmer.
2. Determine the length of catheter to be inserted for either high (T6 to T9) or low (L3 to L4) position. Place marker (sterile bandage or tape) on catheter at desired length.
3. Flush catheter with sterile saline solution before insertion.
4. Place sterile umbilical tape around base of cord. Cut through cord horizontally approximately 1.5 to 2.0 cm from skin; tighten umbilical tape to prevent bleeding.
5. Identify the large, thin-walled umbilical vein and smaller, thick-walled arteries. Use one tip of open curved iris forceps to gently probe and dilate one artery. Then gently probe with both points of closed forceps and dilate artery by allowing forceps to open gently.
6. Grasp catheter 1 cm from tip with toothless forceps and insert catheter into the lumen of the artery. Gently advance catheter to desired distance. DO NOT FORCE. If resistance is encountered, try loosening umbilical tape, applying steady gentle pressure, or manipulating the angle of the umbilical cord to the skin.
7. Secure the catheter with both a suture through the cord and marker tape and a tape bridge. Confirm the position of the catheter tip by x-ray.
8. Look for complications of catheter placement, such as blanching or cyanosis of the lower extremities, ischemia, perforation, thrombosis, embolism, and infection.

B. CATHETER POSITION. Umbilical artery catheters may be placed in either of two positions: Low-line position, between lumbar vertebrae 3 and 4, or high-line position, between thoracic vertebrae 6 and 9. The length of catheter required to achieve either position may be determined using a standardized graph or a regression formula. Catheter length is about one third the crown-heel length.

1. Graphic representation.
a. Determine the shoulder-umbilical length by measuring the *perpendicular* line dropped from the tip of the shoulder to the level of the umbilicus. Note that a diagonal measurement will be inaccurate.
b. Use the graph on the next page to determine the catheter length to be inserted for either a high or low line **(Fig. D-3)**. For a low line, the tip of the catheter should lie just above the aortic bifurcation (avoid the renal artery orifice, around L2). With a high line the tip should be above the diaphragm. Add length for the height of the umbilical stump.

2. Birth weight (BW) regression formula.
a. High line: Umbilical artery (UA) catheter length (cm) = $(3 \times BW \text{ [kg]}) + 9$
b. Low line: UA catheter length (cm) $\approx BW \text{ (kg)} + 7$

Note: *Formula may not be appropriate for infants who are small for gestational age (SGA) or large for gestational age (LGA).*

III. UMBILICAL VEIN CATHETERIZATION

Umbilical vein catheterization is used to obtain vascular access in critically ill neonates.

A. CATHETER PLACEMENT.
1. After restraining the infant, clean, drape, and cut the umbilical stump as for umbilical artery catheterization.
2. Determine the length of the catheter needed to place the catheter tip in the inferior vena cava above the level of the ductus venosus or hepatic veins. Place a marker (sterile bandage or tape) on the catheter at desired length.
3. Flush the catheter with sterile saline solution before insertion.
4. Isolate a thin-walled umbilical vein; clear thrombi with forceps, and insert catheter. Gently advance catheter to desired distance. DO NOT FORCE. If resistance is encountered, try loosening umbilical tape, applying steady gentle pressure, or manipulating the angle of the umbilical cord to the skin.
5. Secure the catheter as described for the umbilical artery catheter. Confirm the position of the catheter tip by x-ray.

D

PROCEDURES

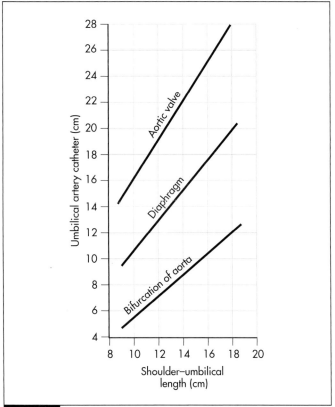

Umbilical artery catheter length. *(From Siberry G, Iannone R (eds): The Harriet Lane Handbook, 15th ed. St Louis, Mosby, 2000.)*

Note: *Hemorrhage, infection, air embolism, and arrhythmias are possible complications.*

B. CATHETER POSITION. The umbilical catheter should be placed in the inferior vena cava above the level of the ductus venosus and the hepatic veins. The length of the catheter necessary to achieve this position can be determined using the graph or regression formula.

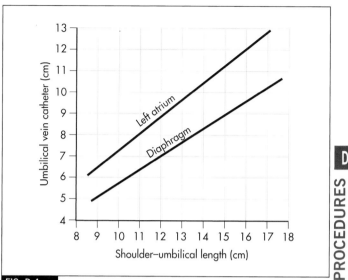

FIG. D-4

Umbilical vein catheter length. *(From Siberry G, Iannone R (eds): The Harriet Lane Handbook, 15th ed., St Louis, Mosby, 2000.)*

D

PROCEDURES

1. Graphic representation.
a. Determine the shoulder-umbilical length by measuring the perpendicular line dropped from the tip of the shoulder to the level of the umbilicus. Note that a diagonal measurement will be inaccurate.
b. Using **Fig. D-4**, determine the catheter length needed to place the tip between the diaphragm and left atrium. Add length for the height of the umbilical stump.
2. Birth weight regression formula: UV catheter length (cm) $\times$ (0.5 $\times$ UA catheter length [cm]) $+1$. Formula may not be appropriate for SGA or LGA infants.

IV. NEONATAL EXCHANGE TRANSFUSION

See **Chapter 19** for volume calculations.

Note: *Complete blood count, reticulocyte count, peripheral smear, bilirubin, Ca, glucose, total protein, infant blood type, and Coombs test should be performed on preexchange samples of blood because they are no longer of diagnostic value on postexchange blood. If indicated, also save preexchange blood for serologic or chromosomal studies.*

A. SENSITIZED CELLS OR HYPERBILIRUBINEMIA.

1. Crossmatch donor blood against maternal serum for first exchange and against postexchange blood for subsequent exchanges.
2. Use type O-negative (low titer) blood; may use infant's type if there is no chance of maternal-infant incompatibility. Blood should be stored at room temperature, either fresh or up to 48 hours old, and anticoagulated with ACD or CPD unless infant is acidotic or hypocalcemic.
3. Infant should be NPO during and at least 4 hours after exchange. Empty the infant's stomach if it was fed within 4 hours of procedure.
4. Follow infant's vital signs and temperature closely; have resuscitation equipment ready.
5. Prepare and drape patient for sterile procedure.
6. Insert umbilical artery and vein catheters as described. During the exchange, blood is removed through the umbilical artery catheter and infused through the venous catheter. If unable to pass an arterial catheter, use a single venous catheter.
7. Prewarm blood in quality-controlled blood warmer if available; do not improvise with a water bath.
8. Exchange 15-ml increments in vigorous full-term infants, smaller volumes for smaller, less stable infants. Do not allow cells in donor unit to sediment.
9. Withdraw and infuse blood at rate of 2 to 3 ml/kg per minute to avoid mechanical trauma to patient and donor cells.
10. Give 1 to 2 ml of intravenous (IV) 10% calcium gluconate solution slowly for ECG evidence of hypocalcemia. Flush tubing with NaCl before and after calcium infusion. Observe for bradycardia during infusion.
11. To complete the double-blood volume exchange, transfuse 160 ml/kg for a full-term infant and 160 to 200 ml/kg for a preterm infant.
12. Send the last aliquot withdrawn for Hct, smear, glucose, bilirubin, potassium, Ca^{++}, and type and crossmatch.

B. ANEMIC HEART FAILURE.
Have O-negative concentrated red blood cells (RBCs) in the delivery room. Perform a partial exchange with packed RBCs to correct anemia and failure (30 to 50 ml/kg). Allow infant to stabilize if possible before attempting a full two-volume exchange.

C. COMPLICATIONS.

1. Cardiovascular. Thromboemboli or air emboli, thromboses, dysrhythmias, volume overload, and cardiorespiratory arrest.
2. Metabolic. Hyperkalemia, hypernatremia, hypocalcemia, hypoglycemia, and acidosis.
3. Hematologic. Thrombocytopenia, disseminated intravascular coagulation (DIC), overheparinization (may use 10 μg protamine for each unit of heparin in donor unit), and transfusion reaction.

4. Infectious. Hepatitis, HIV, and bacteremia.
5. Mechanical. Injury to donor cells (especially from overheating), vascular or cardiac perforation, and blood loss.

V. CHEST TUBE PLACEMENT

Chest tube placement is used for evacuation of pneumothorax, hemothorax, chylothorax, large pleural effusion, or empyema for diagnostic and/or therapeutic purpose.

A. TECHNIQUE.

1. Position the infant with the affected side up. Preferably, chest tubes are placed in the third or fourth intercostal space in the midaxillary line, avoiding breast tissue.
2. If necessary, temporarily decompress the pneumothorax by inserting a "butterfly" or angiocath in the same location in the ipsilateral anterior second intercostal space.
3. After cleaning and anesthetizing the area locally with 0.5% lidocaine, make a 0.5-cm incision directly over the rib below the desired interspace. Insert a small curved hemostat to bluntly dissect a track over the superior margin of the rib through the intercostal muscles and into the pleural cavity.
4. Place a clamp 0.5 to 1.0 cm from the tip of the chest tube and pass through the previously punctured space into the pleural cavity. Angle the tube anteriorly and superiorly and insert it the desired distance.
5. Secure tube to chest wall with suture through skin incision and then around tube. Cover incision with petroleum gauze and a sterile dressing.
6. Connect the chest tube to 15- to 20-cm water suction for decompression via one-way valve. Confirm position and function with chest x-ray.

B. COMPLICATIONS. LUNG PERFORATION, HEMORRHAGE, SCARRING, AND TUBE MALPOSITION.

VI. LUMBAR PUNCTURE

Lumbar puncture (LP) facilitates examination of the spinal fluid for suspected infections.

A. PRECAUTIONS.

1. Increased intracranial pressure. Before LP, perform funduscopic examination. The presence of papilledema, retinal hemorrhage, or clinical suspicion of increased intracranial pressure may be contraindications to the procedure. A sudden drop in intraspinal pressure by rapid release of cerebrospinal fluid (CSF) may cause fatal herniation. If LP is to be performed, proceed with extreme caution.
2. Bleeding diathesis. A platelet count of $\geq 50,000/mm^3$ is desirable before LP. Correct any clotting factor deficiencies.

3. Overlying skin infection. May result in inoculation of CSF with organisms.

B. TECHNIQUE.

1. Apply a eutectic mixture of local anesthetics (EMLA).
2. Position the child in either the sitting position or lateral recumbent position with hips, knees, and neck flexed. Ensure that a small infant's cardiorespiratory status is not compromised by positioning.
3. Locate the desired interspace (either L3-L4 or L4-L5) by drawing a line between the top of the iliac crests.
4. Clean the skin with povidone-iodine and 70% alcohol. Drape conservatively so as to be able to monitor the infant. Use a spinal needle with a stylet. (Epidermoid tumors from introduced epithelial tissue have been reported.)
5. Anesthetize overlying skin with 0.5% lidocaine.
6. Puncture skin in the midline just below the palpated spinous process, angling slightly cephalad. Advance several millimeters at a time and withdraw stylet frequently to check for CSF flow. In small infants, one may not feel a change in resistance or "pop" as the dura is penetrated.
7. If resistance is met, withdraw needle to the skin surface and redirect angle slightly.
8. Send CSF sample for appropriate studies: cultures, glucose, protein, cell count and differential, antigen detection tests, VDRL.

VII. THORACENTESIS

Thoracentesis is done to obtain diagnosis or relief of an abnormal collection of fluid within the pleural space.

A. TECHNIQUE.

1. Ideally, perform procedure with the patient sitting and with an assistant standing in front to support the patient.
2. Select the interspace to be tapped on the basis of dullness to percussion and the level of effusion on the erect chest x-ray. Ultrasound examination can help clarify location of the effusion if there is confusion as to its exact location. In the event of a small effusion, the patient may be tilted laterally toward the affected side to maximize the yield.
3. Clean and drape the chest.
4. Use a local anesthetic to infiltrate the skin, the underlying tissue, and the pleura in the interspace above the rib.
5. Attach a large-bore needle or intravenous catheter attached to a three-way stopcock and syringe. With needle bevel down, insert needle directly on the rib below the desired interspace, and "walk" the needle over the superior edge of the rib. Gradually advance the needle; a "pop" is felt on entering the pleural space. Advance the catheter 2 to 3 mm and remove the stylet.

6. Attach a syringe with a stopcock to the hub of the catheter and slowly withdraw the desired volume of fluid.
7. At the end of the procedure, withdraw the needle or catheter and place an occlusive dressing over the thoracentesis site.
8. Obtain a follow-up chest x-ray after thoracentesis to rule out pneumothorax.
9. Send pleural fluid for routine laboratory studies.

VIII. URINARY BLADDER CATHETERIZATION

Bladder catheterization is used to obtain urine for culture when a urinary tract infection or sepsis is suspected.

A. TECHNIQUE.

1. Prepare the urethral opening using sterile technique.
2. In the male, apply gentle traction to the penis in a caudal direction to straighten the urethra.
3. Gently insert a lubricated catheter into the urethra. Slowly advance the catheter until resistance is met at the external sphincter. Continued pressure will overcome this resistance and the catheter will enter the bladder. In the female, only a few centimeters of advancement is required to reach the bladder.
4. Carefully remove the catheter once the specimen is obtained.

Note: *Trauma to the urethra or bladder, vaginal catheterization, and infection are possible.*

IX. SUPRAPUBIC BLADDER ASPIRATION

Avoid this procedure in children with genitourinary tract anomalies.

A. TECHNIQUE.

1. The infant's diaper should be dry, and the infant should not have voided in the 30 to 60 minutes before the procedure. Anterior rectal pressure in females or gentle penile pressure in males may be used to prevent urination during the procedure.
2. Restrain the infant in the supine, frog-leg position. Clean the lower abdomen suprapubic area with povidone-iodine and 70% alcohol.
3. The site for puncture is 1 to 2 cm above the symphysis pubis in the midline. Use a syringe with a 22-gauge 1-inch needle and puncture at 10 to 20 degrees to the perpendicular, aiming slightly caudad.
4. Exert suction gently as the needle is advanced until urine enters syringe. The needle should not be advanced more than 2.5 cm. Aspirate the urine with gentle suction.

Note: *Hematuria (usually microscopic), intestinal perforation, abdominal wall infection, and bleeding are possible.*

D

PROCEDURES

Breast Milk and Chemicals

TRANSFER OF DRUGS AND OTHER CHEMICALS INTO HUMAN MILK*†

This section provides lists of the pharmacologic or chemical agents transferred into human milk and their possible effects on the infant or on lactation, if known (**Tables E-1 to E-7**). The fact that a pharmacologic or chemical agent does not appear in the tables is not meant to imply that it is not transferred into human milk or that it does not affect the infant but indicates that there are no reports in the literature. These tables should assist the physician in counseling a nursing mother regarding breast-feeding when the mother has a condition for which a drug is medically indicated.

E

The following should be considered when prescribing drug therapy for lactating women:

1. Is the drug therapy really necessary? Consultation between the pediatrician and the mother's physician can be most useful.
2. Use the safest drug (e.g., acetaminophen rather than aspirin for oral analgesia).
3. If there is a possibility that a drug may present a risk to the infant (e.g., phenytoin, phenobarbital), consideration should be given to measurement of blood concentrations in the nursing infant.
4. Drug exposure to the nursing infant may be minimized by having the mother take the medication just after completing a breast-feeding or just before the infant has his or her lengthy sleep period.

Data have been obtained from a search of the medical literature. Because methodologies used to quantitate drugs in milk continue to improve, this current information will require continuous updating.

Physicians who encounter adverse effects in infants fed drug-contaminated human milk are urged to document these effects in a communication to the American Academy of Pediatrics (AAP) Committee on Drugs and the U.S. Food and Drug Administration (http://www.fda.gov/medwatch/index.html). Such communication should include the generic and brand names of the drug, the maternal dose and mode of administration, the concentrations of the drug in milk and maternal and infant blood in relation to time of ingestion, the age of the infant, and the method used for laboratory identification. Such reports may significantly increase the pediatric community's knowledge regarding drug transfer into human milk and the potential or actual risk to the infant.

Acknowledgment

The Committee on Drugs would like to thank Linda Watson for her work in reference identification, document retrieval, and manuscript preparation.

Committee on Drugs, 2000-2001

Robert M. Ward, MD, Chairperson
Brian A. Bates, MD
William E. Benitz, MD
David J. Burchfield, MD
John C. Ring, MD
Richard P. Walls, MD, PhD
Philip D. Walson, MD

Liaisons

John Alexander, MD
U.S. Food and Drug Administration Alternate
Donald R. Bennett, MD, PhD
American Medical Association/United States Pharmacopeia
Therese Cvetkovich, MD
U.S. Food and Drug Administration
Owen R. Hagino, MD
American Academy of Child and Adolescent Psychiatry
Stuart M. MacLeod, MD, PhD
Canadian Paediatric Society
Siddika Mithani, MD
Bureau of Pharmaceutical Assessment Health Protection Branch, Canada
Joseph Mulinare, MD, MSPH
Centers for Disease Control and Prevention
Laura E. Riley, MD
American College of Obstetricians and Gynecologists
Sumner J. Yaffe, MD
National Institutes of Health

Section Liaisons

Charles J. Coté, MD
Section on Anesthesiology
Eli O. Meltzer, MD
Section on Allergy and Immunology

Consultant

Cheston M. Berlin, Jr, MD

Staff

Raymond J. Koteras, MHA

*From the American Academy of Pediatrics Committee on Drugs: The transfer of drugs and other chemicals into human milk, Pediatrics 108:776, 2001.
†The recommendations in this statement do not indicate an exclusive course of treatment or serve as a standard of medical care. Variations, taking into account individual circumstances, may be appropriate.

TABLE E-1

CYTOTOXIC DRUGS THAT MAY INTERFERE WITH CELLULAR METABOLISM OF THE NURSING INFANT

Drug	Reason for Concern, Reported Sign or Symptom in Infant, or Effect on Lactation
Cyclophosphamide	Possible immune suppression; unknown effect on growth or association with carcinogenesis; neutropenia
Cyclosporine	Possible immune suppression; unknown effect on growth or association with carcinogenesis
Doxorubicin*	Possible immune suppression; unknown effect on growth or association with carcinogenesis
Methotrexate	Possible immune suppression; unknown effect on growth or association with carcinogenesis; neutropenia

*Drug is concentrated in human milk

TABLE E-2

DRUGS OF ABUSE FOR WHICH ADVERSE EFFECTS ON THE INFANT DURING BREAST-FEEDING HAVE BEEN REPORTED*

Drug	Reported Effect or Reasons for Concern
Amphetamine[†]	Irritability, poor sleeping pattern
Cocaine	Cocaine intoxication: irritability, vomiting, diarrhea, tremulousness, seizures
Heroin	Tremors, restlessness, vomiting, poor feeding
Marijuana	Only one report in literature; no effect mentioned; very long half-life for some components
Phencyclidine	Potent hallucinogen

*The Committee on Drugs strongly believes that nursing mothers should not ingest drugs of abuse because they are hazardous to the nursing infant and to the health of the mother.
[†]Drug is concentrated in human milk.

TABLE E-3

RADIOACTIVE COMPOUNDS THAT REQUIRE TEMPORARY CESSATION OF BREAST-FEEDING*

Compound	Recommended Time for Cessation of Breast-feeding
Copper 64 (^{64}Cu)	Radioactivity in milk present at 50 h
Gallium 67 (^{67}Ga)	Radioactivity in milk present for 2 wk
Indium 111 (^{111}In)	Very small amount present at 20 h
Iodine 123 (^{123}I)	Radioactivity in milk present up to 36 h
Iodine 125 (^{125}I)	Radioactivity in milk present for 12 d
Iodine 131 (^{131}I)	Radioactivity in milk present 2-14 d, depending on study
Iodine^{131}	If used for treatment of thyroid cancer, high radioactivity may prolong exposure to infant
Radioactive sodium	Radioactivity in milk present 96 h
Technetium 99m (^{99m}Tc), ^{99m}Tc macroaggregates, ^{99m}Tc O$_4$	Radioactivity in milk present 15 h to 3 d

*Consult nuclear medicine physician before performing diagnostic study so that radionuclide that has the shortest excretion time in breast milk can be used. Before study, the mother should pump her breast and store enough milk in the freezer for feeding the infant; after study, the mother should pump her breast to maintain milk production but discard all milk pumped for the required time that radioactivity is present in milk. Milk samples can be screened by radiology departments for radioactivity before resumption of nursing.

E

BREAST MILK AND CHEMICALS

TABLE E-4

DRUGS FOR WHICH THE EFFECT ON NURSING INFANTS IS UNKNOWN BUT MAY BE OF CONCERN*

Drug	Reported or Possible Effect
Antianxiety	
Alprazolam	None
Diazepam	None
Lorazepam	None
Midazolam	—
Perphenazine	None
Prazepam[†]	None
Quazepam	None
Temazepam	—
Antidepressants	
Amitriptyline	None
Amoxapine	None
Bupropion	None
Clomipramine	None
Desipramine	None
Dothiepin	None
Doxepin	None
Fluoxetine	Colic, irritability, feeding and sleep disorders, slow weight gain
Fluvoxamine	—
Imipramine	None
Nortriptyline	None
Paroxetine	None
Sertraline[†]	None
Trazodone	None
Antipsychotic	
Chlorpromazine	Galactorrhea in mother; drowsiness and lethargy in infant; decline in developmental scores
Chlorprothixene	None
Clozapine[†]	None
Haloperidol	Decline in developmental scores
Mesoridazine	None
Trifluoperazine	None
OTHERS	
Amiodarone	Possible hypothyroidism
Chloramphenicol	Possible idiosyncratic bone marrow suppression
Clofazimine	Potential for transfer of high percentage of maternal dose; possible increase in skin pigmentation
Lamotrigine	Potential therapeutic serum concentrations in infant
Metoclopramide[†]	None described; dopaminergic blocking agent
Metronidazole	In vitro mutagen; may discontinue breast-feeding for 12-24 hr to allow excretion of dose when single-dose therapy given to mother
Tinidazole	See metronidazole

*Psychotropic drugs, the compounds listed under antianxiety, antidepressant, and antipsychotic categories, are of special concern when given to nursing mothers for long periods. Although there are very few case reports of adverse effects in breast-feeding infants, these drugs do appear in human milk and, thus, could conceivably alter short-term and long-term central nervous system function.
[†]Drug is concentrated in human milk relative to simultaneous maternal plasma concentrations.

TABLE E-5

DRUGS THAT HAVE BEEN ASSOCIATED WITH SIGNIFICANT EFFECTS ON SOME NURSING INFANTS AND SHOULD BE GIVEN TO NURSING MOTHERS WITH CAUTION*

Drug	Reported Effect
Acebutolol	Hypotension; bradycardia; tachypnea
5-Aminosalicylic acid	Diarrhea (one case)
Atenolol	Cyanosis; bradycardia
Bromocriptine	Suppresses lactation; may be hazardous to the mother
Aspirin (salicylates)	Metabolic acidosis (one case)
Clemastine	Drowsiness, irritability, refusal to feed, high-pitched cry, neck stiffness (one case)
Ergotamine	Vomiting, diarrhea, convulsions (doses used in migraine medications)
Lithium	One-third to one-half therapeutic blood concentration in infants
Phenindione	Anticoagulant: increased prothrombin and partial thromboplastin times in one infant; not used in the United States
Phenobarbital	Sedation; infantile spasms after weaning from milk containing phenobarbital, methemoglobinemia (one case)
Primidone	Sedation, feeding problems
Sulfasalazine (salicylazosulfapyridine)	Bloody diarrhea (one case)

*Blood concentration in the infant may be of clinical importance.

TABLE E-6

MATERNAL MEDICATIONS USUALLY COMPATIBLE WITH BREAST-FEEDING*

Drug	Reported Sign or Symptom in Infant or Effect on Lactation
Acetaminophen	None
Acetazolamide	None
Acitretin	—
Acyclovir†	None
Alcohol (ethanol)	With large amounts, drowsiness, diaphoresis, deep sleep, weakness, decrease in linear growth, abnormal weight gain; maternal ingestion of 1 g/kg daily decreases milk ejection reflex
Allopurinol	—
Amoxicillin	None
Antimony	—
Atropine	None
Azapropazone (apazone)	—
Aztreonam	None
B₁ (thiamin)	None
B₆ (pyridoxine)	None
B₁₂	None
Baclofen	None
Barbiturate	**See Table E-5**
Bendroflumethiazide	Suppresses lactation

Continued

BREAST MILK AND CHEMICALS   **E**

TABLE E-6

MATERNAL MEDICATIONS USUALLY COMPATIBLE WITH BREAST-FEEDING*—cont'd

Drug	Reported Sign or Symptom in Infant or Effect on Lactation
Bishydroxycoumarin (dicumarol)	None
Bromide	Rash, weakness, absence of cry with maternal intake of 5.4 g/day
Butorphanol	None
Caffeine	Irritability, poor sleeping pattern, excreted slowly; no effect with moderate intake of caffeinated beverages (2-3 cups/day)
Captopril	None
Carbamazepine	None
Carbetocin	None
Carbimazole	Goiter
Cascara	None
Cefadroxil	None
Cefazolin	None
Cefotaxime	None
Cefoxitin	None
Cefprozil	—
Ceftazidime	None
Ceftriaxone	None
Chloral hydrate	Sleepiness
Chloroform	None
Chloroquine	None
Chlorothiazide	None
Chlorthalidone	Excreted slowly
Cimetidine†	None
Ciprofloxacin	None
Cisapride	None
Cisplatin	Not found in milk
Clindamycin	None
Clogestone	None
Codeine	None
Colchicine	—
Contraceptive pill with estrogen/progesterone	Rare breast enlargement; decreases in milk production and protein content (not confirmed in several studies)
Cycloserine	None
D (vitamine)	None; follow up infant's serum calcium level if mother receives pharmacologic doses
Danthron	Increased bowel activity
Dapsone	None; sulfonamide detected in infant's urine
Dexbrompheniramine maleate with d-isoephedrine	Crying, poor sleeping patterns, irritability
Diatrizoate	None
Digoxin	None
Diltiazem	None
Dipyrone	None
Disopyramide	None

TABLE E-6

MATERNAL MEDICATIONS USUALLY COMPATIBLE WITH BREAST-FEEDING*—cont'd

Drug	Reported Sign or Symptom in Infant or Effect on Lactation
Domperidone	None
Dyphylline†	None
Enalapril	—
Erythromycin†	None
Estradiol	Withdrawal, vaginal bleeding
Ethambutol	None
Ethanol (cf. alcohol)	—
Ethosuximide	None, drug appears in infant serum
Fentanyl	—
Fexofenadine	None
Flecainide	—
Fleroxacin	One 400-mg dose given to nursing mothers; infants not given breast milk for 48 hr
Fluconazole	None
Flufenamic acid	None
Fluorescein	—
Folic acid	None
Gadopentetic (Gadolinium)	None
Gentamicin	None
Gold salts	None
Halothane	None
Hydralazine	None
Hydrochlorothiazide	
Hydroxychloroquine†	None
Ibuprofen	None
Indomethacin	Seizure (one case)
Iodides	May affect thyroid activity; see iodine
Iodine	Goiter
Iodine (povidone-iodine, e.g., in a vaginal douche)	Elevated iodine levels in breast milk, odor of iodine on infant's skin
Iohexol	None
Iopanoic acid	None
Isoniazid	None; acetyl (hepatotoxic) metabolite secreted but no hepatotoxicity reported in infants
Interferon-α	—
Ivermectin	None
K₁ (vitamin)	None
Kanamycin	None
Ketoconazole	None
Ketorolac	—
Labetalol	None
Levonorgestrel	—
Levothyroxine	None
Lidocaine	None
Loperamide	—
Loratadine	None

E

BREAST MILK AND CHEMICALS

Continued

TABLE E-6

MATERNAL MEDICATIONS USUALLY COMPATIBLE WITH BREAST-FEEDING*—cont'd

Drug	Reported Sign or Symptom in Infant or Effect on Lactation
Magnesium sulfate	None
Medroxyprogesterone	None
Mefenamic acid	None
Meperidine	None
Methadone	None
Methimazole (active metabolite of carbimazole)	None
Methohexital	None
Methyldopa	None
Methyprylon	Drowsiness
Metoprolol†	None
Metrizamide	None
Metrizoate	None
Mexiletine	None
Minoxidil	None
Morphine	None: infant may have measurable blood concentration
Moxalactam	None
Nadolol†	None
Nalidixic acid	Hemolysis in infant with glucose-6-phosphate dehydrogenase (G6PD) deficiency
Naproxen	—
Nefopam	None
Nifedipine	—
Nitrofurantoin	Hemolysis in infant with G6PD deficiency
Norethynodrel	None
Norsteroids	None
Noscapine	None
Ofloxacin	None
Oxprenolol	None
Phenylbutazone	None
Phenytoin	Methemoglobinemia (one case)
Piroxicam	None
Prednisolone	None
Prednisone	None
Procainamide	None
Progesterone	None
Propoxyphene	None
Propranolol	None
Propylthiouracil	None
Pseudoephedrine†	None
Pyridostigmine	None

TABLE E-6

MATERNAL MEDICATIONS USUALLY COMPATIBLE WITH BREAST-FEEDING*—cont'd

Drug	Reported Sign or Symptom in Infant or Effect on Lactation
Pyrimethamine	None
Quinidine	None
Quinine	None
Riboflavin	None
Rifampin	None
Scopolamine	—
Secobarbital	None
Senna	None
Sotalol	—
Spironolactone	None
Streptomycin	None
Sulbactam	None
Sulfapyridine	Caution in infant with jaundice or G6PD deficiency and ill, stressed, or premature infant; appears in infant's milk
Sulfisoxazole	Caution in infant with jaundice or G6PD deficiency and ill, stressed, or premature infant; appears in infant's milk
Sumatriptan	None
Suprofen	None
Terbutaline	None
Terfenadine	None
Tetracycline	None; negligible absorption by infant
Theophylline	Irritability
Thiopental	None
Thiouracil	None mentioned; drug not used in the United States
Ticarcillin	None
Timolol	None
Tolbutamide	Possible jaundice
Tolmetin	None
Trimethoprim/ sulfamethoxazole	None
Triprolidine	None
Valproic acid	None
Verapamil	None
Warfarin	None
Zolpidem	None

*Drugs listed have been reported in the literature as having the effects listed or no effect. The word "none" means that no observable change was seen in the nursing infant while the mother was ingesting the compound. Dashes indicate no mention of clinical effect on the infant. It is emphasized that many of the literature citations concern single case reports or small series of infants.
†Drug is concentrated in human milk.

E

BREAST MILK AND CHEMICALS

Composition of Nutritional Products

TABLE F-1	
COMMON CALORIC SUPPLEMENTS	
Component	**Calories**
PROTEIN	
Casec	3.7 kcal/g (0.9 g protein)
	17 kcal/tbsp (4 g protein)
CARBOHYDRATE	
Polycose	Powder: 3.8 kcal/g
	8 kcal/tsp
	Liquid: 2 kcal/ml, 10 kcal/tsp
FAT	
MCT oil[†]	7.7 kcal/ml
Vegetable oil	8.3 kcal/ml

*Use these caloric supplements when you want to increase protein or when you have reached the maximum concentration tolerated and wish to further increase caloric density.

[†]MCT oil is unnecessary unless there is fat malabsorption.

Roberson J, Shilkofski N: The Harriet Lane Handbook, 17th ed. Elsevier Mosby, Philadelphia, 2005.

TABLE F-2
INFANT FORMULA ANALYSIS (PER LITER)

Formula	kcal/ml (kcal/oz)	Protein g (% kcal)	Carbohydrate g (% kcal)	Fat g (% kcal)	Na (mEq)	K (mEq)	Ca (mg)	P (mg)	Fe (mg)	Osmolality (mOsm/kg water)	Suggested Uses
Alimentum (Ross)	0.67 (20)	19 (11) Casein hydrolysate L-Cystine, L-Tyr, L-Trp	69 (41) Sucrose 67% Modified tapioca starch	37 (48) MCT oil (33%) Safflower oil (39%) Soy oil (28%)	13	20	708	506	12	370	Infants with food allergies, protein, or fat malabsorption
America's Store Brand (Wyeth Nutritionals)	0.67 (20)	14.6 (9) Nonfat milk Whey protein concentrate	71 (42) Lactose	35 (47) Oleo oil Coconut oil HO safflower + sunflower oil Soy oil	6.5	14	425	284	12	—	Infants with normal GI tract
America's Store Brand for older Infants (Wyeth Nutritionals)	0.68 (20)	22 (13) Cow's milk protein	69 (40) Lactose Corn syrup solids	37 (48) Oleo Coconut oil HO Soy	9.6	21.5	816	571	12	280	Infants 4.6 mo and older with normal GI tract
America's Store Brand Soy (Wyeth	0.67 (20)	18 (11) Soy protein isolate	69 (41) Corn syrup solids	35 (47) Palm olein HO safflower	6.5	14	608	425	12	—	Infants with allergy to cow's milk,

Nutritionals)	L-Methionine	Sucrose	or HO sunflower Coconut oil Soy oil							lactose malabsorption galactosemia
Enfacare with iron (Mead Johnson)	0.74 (22)	21 (11) Nonfat milk · Demineralized whey	79 (43) Maltodextrin · Lactose · Citrates	39 (46) HO sunflower oil · Soy oil · MCT oil · Coconut oil	11	20	890	490	13	230	Infants with conditions such as prematurity
Enfamil AR (Mead Johnson)	0.67 (20)	16.8 (10) Nonfat milk	74 (44) Lactose (57%) Rice starch (30%) Maltodextrins (13%)	34 (46) Palm olein (45%) Soy oil (20%) Coconut oil (20%) HO sunflower oil (15%)	12	19	530	360	12	240	When a thickened feeding is desired (should not be concentrated >24 kcal/oz)
Enfamil with Iron [low iron] (Mead Johnson)	0.67 (20)	14 (9) Nonfat milk · Demineralized whey	73 (44) Lactose	36 (48) Palm olein (45%) Soy oil (20%) Coconut oil (20%) HO sunflower oil (15%)	8	19	530	360	12 [5]	300	Infants with normal GI tract

COMPOSITION OF NUTRITIONAL PRODUCTS F

Continued

TABLE F-2
INFANT FORMULA ANALYSIS (PER LITER)—cont'd

Formula	kcal/ml (kcal/oz)	Protein g (% kcal)	Carbohydrate g (% kcal)	Fat g (% kcal)	Na (mEq)	K (mEq)	Ca (mg)	P (mg)	Fe (mg)	Osmolality (mOsm/kg water)	Suggested Uses
Enfamil with Iron 24 [low iron] (Mead Johnson)	0.8 (24)	17 (9) Nonfat milk whey	88 (43) Lactose	43 (48) Palm olein (45%) Soy oil (20%) HO sunflower oil (15%) Coconut oil (20%)	10	23	630	430	15 [6]	360	Infants with normal GI tract requiring additional calories
Enfamil Lactofree (Mead Johnson)	0.67 (20)	14 (9) Milk protein isolate	74 (43) Corn syrup solids	36 (48) Palm olein (45%) Soy oil (20%) Coconut oil (20%) HO sunflower oil (15%)	9	19	550	370	12	200	Infants with lactose malabsorption
Enfamil Premature Formula 20 [w/Fe] (Mead Johnson)	0.67 (20)	20 (12) Demineralized whey Nonfat milk	75 (44) Corn syrup solids Lactose	35 (44) MCT oil (40%) Soy oil Coconut oil	11	18	1120	560	1.7 [12]	260	Preterm infants

Enfamil Premature Formula 24 [w/Fe] (Mead Johnson)	0.8 (24)	24 (12) Demineralized whey Nonfat milk	9 (44) Corn syrup solids Lactose	41 (44) MCT oil (40%) Soy oil Coconut oil	14	21	1340	670	2 [15]	310	Preterm infants
Evaporated milk formula*	0.67 (20)	27 (16) Cow's milk	72 (43) Lactose Corn syrup	31 (41) Butterfat	21	32	1066	832	0.8	—	Infants with normal GI tract; need vitamin C and iron supplements
Isomil (Ross)	0.67 (20)	17 (10) Soy protein isolate Methionine	70 (41) Corn syrup Sucrose	37 (49) Soy oil (30%) Coconut oil (30%) HO safflower oil (40%)	13	19	709	507	12	200	Infants with allergy to cow's milk, lactose malabsorption, galactosemia
Isomil DF (Ross)	0.67 (20)	18 (11) Soy protein isolate Methionine	68 (40) Corn syrup Sucrose Soy fiber	37 (49) Soy oil (60%) Coconut oil (40%)	13	19	709	507	12	240	Short-term management of diarrhea; contains fiber

*13 oz evaporated whole milk, 19 oz water, 2 tbsp corn syrup.

COMPOSITION OF NUTRITIONAL PRODUCTS

F

Continued

TABLE F-2
INFANT FORMULA ANALYSIS (PER LITER)—cont'd

Formula	kcal/ml (kcal/oz)	Protein g (% kcal)	Carbohydrate g (% kcal)	Fat g (% kcal)	Na (mEq)	K (mEq)	Ca (mg)	P (mg)	Fe (mg)	Osmolality (mOsm/kg water)	Suggested Uses
MJ3232A (Mead Johnson)	0.42 (12.7)	19 (18) Casein hydrolysate L-Cystine, L-Tyr, L-Trp	28 (27) Tapioca starch CHO selected by physician	28 (55) MCT oil (85%) Corn oil (15%)	13	19	640	430	13	250	Infants with severe CHO intolerance (CHO must be added)
Neocate (SHS North America)	0.69 (21)	20 (12) Free amino acids	78 (47) Corn syrup solids	30 (41) Safflower oil Coconut oil Soy oil	11	26	837	628	12	375	Infants with severe food allergies
Nestlé Carnation Alsoy (Nestlé)	0.67 (20)	21 (11) L-Methionine Soy protein isolate	68 (44) Sucrose Maltodextrin	36 (45) Palm olein (47%) Soy oil (26%) Coconut oil (21%) HO safflower oil (6%)	10	20	702	413	13	270	Infants with allergy to cow's milk, lactose malabsorption, galactosemia
Nestlé Carnation Follow-up (Nestlé)	0.67 (20)	18 (10) Nonfat milk	89 (53) Corn syrup Lactose	28 (37) Palm olein (47%) Soy oil (26%) Coconut oil (21%)	11	23	811	603	13	326	Infants 4-12 mo with normal GI tract

HO safflower oil (6%)

Product (Manufacturer)	kcal/mL (kcal/oz)	Protein g (%) / source	Carbohydrate g (%) / source	Fat g (%) / source							Indications
Nestlé Carnation Follow-up Soy (Nestlé)	0.67 (20)	21 (12) Soy protein isolate Methionine	81 (48) Maltodextrin Sucrose	29 (40) Palm olein (47%) Soy oil (26%) Coconut oil (21%) HO safflower oil (6%)	12	20	905	603	13	200	Infants 4-12 mo with allergy to cow's milk, lactose malabsorption, galactosemia
Nestlé Carnation Good Start (Nestlé)	0.67 (20)	16 (10) Partially hydrolyzed whey	74 (44) Lactose Maltodextrins	35 (46) Palm olein (47%) Soy oil (26%) Coconut oil (21%) HO safflower oil (6%)	7	17	429	241	10	300	Infants with normal GI tract
Nutramigen (Mead Johnson)	0.67 (20)	19 (11) Casein hydrolysate L-Cystine, L-Tyr, L-Trp	75 (44) Corn syrup solids Modified cornstarch	34 (45) Palm olein (45%) Soy oil (20%) Coconut oil (20%) HO sunflower oil (15%)	14	19	640	430	12	320	Infants with food allergies

COMPOSITION OF NUTRITIONAL PRODUCTS

F

Continued

TABLE F-2
INFANT FORMULA ANALYSIS (PER LITER)—cont'd

Formula	kcal/ml (kcal/oz)	Protein g (% kcal)	Carbohydrate g (% kcal)	Fat g (% kcal)	Na (mEq)	K (mEq)	Ca (mg)	P (mg)	Fe (mg)	Osmolality (mOsm/kg water)	Suggested Uses
Portagen (Mead Johnson)	0.67 (20)	24 (14) Na caseinate	78 (46) Corn syrup solids Sucrose	32 (40) MCT oil (86%) Corn oil (14%)	16	22	640	470	13	230	Infants with fat malabsorption, intestinal lymphatic obstruction, chylothorax
Pregestimil (Mead Johnson)	0.67 (20)	19 (11) Casein hydrolysate L-Cystine, L-Tyr, L-Trp	69 (41) Corn syrup solids (60%) Modified cornstarch (20%) Dextrose (20%)	38 (48) MCT oil (55%) Corn oil (10%) Soy oil (25%) HO safflower oil (10%)	11	19	766	500	12	320	Infants with food allergies, protein or fat malabsorption
ProSobee (Mead Johnson)	0.67 (20)	17 (10) L-Methionine Soy protein isolate	73 (42) Corn syrup solids	37 (48) Palm olein (45%) Soy oil (20%) Coconut oil (20%) HO sunflower oil (15%)	10	21	710	560	12	200	Infants with allergy to cow's milk, lactose malabsorption, galactosemia

RCF* (Ross) [w/Fe]	0.4 (12)	20 (20) Soy isolate	— Selected by physician	36 (80) Soy oil Coconut oil	13	19	709	507	12	*	Infants with severe CHO intolerance (CHO must be added) Modified for ketogenic diet
Similac with Iron [low iron] (Ross)	0.67 (20)	14 (8) Nonfat milk Whey protein	73 (43) Lactose	36 (49) Soy oil (30%) Coconut oil (30%) HO safflower oil (40%)	7	18	527	284	12 [5]	300	Infants with normal GI tract
Similac with Iron 24 (Ross)	0.8 (24)	22 (11) Nonfat milk	85 (42) Lactose	42 (47) Soy oil (60%) Coconut oil (40%)	12	27	726	565	15	380	Infants with normal GI tract requiring additional calories
Similac Lactose Free (Ross)	0.67 (20)	14.5 (9) Milk protein isolate	72.3 (43) Corn syrup solids (55%) Sucrose (45%)	36.5 (49) Soy oil (60%) Coconut oil (40%)	9	18	568	378	12	200	Infants with lactose malabsorption

Continued

COMPOSITION OF NUTRITIONAL PRODUCTS

F

TABLE F-2
INFANT FORMULA ANALYSIS (PER LITER)—cont'd

Formula	kcal/ml (kcal/oz)	Protein g (% kcal)	Carbohydrate g (% kcal)	Fat g (% kcal)	Na (mEq)	K (mEq)	Ca (mg)	P (mg)	Fe (mg)	Osmolality (mOsm/kg water)	Suggested Uses
Similac Neosure (Ross)	0.73 (22)	19 (10) Nonfat milk Whey protein concentrate	77 (41) Lactose (50%) Maltodextrins (50%)	41 (49) MCT oil (25%) Soy oil (45%) Coconut oil (30%)	11	27	784	463	13	250	Preterm infants, after hospital discharge, until good catch-up growth
Similac PM 60/40 (Ross)	0.67 (20)	15 (9) Whey protein concentrate Na caseinate	69 (41) Lactose	38 (50) Soy oil (12%) Coconut oil (38%) Corn oil (50%)	7	15	378	189	5	280	Infants who require lower calcium and phophorus levels
Similac Special Care 20 [w/Fe] (Ross)	0.67 (20)	18 (11) Nonfat milk Whey protein concentrate	72 (42) Corn syrup solids (50%) Lactose (50%)	37 (49) MCT oil (50%) Soy oil (30%) Coconut oil (20%)	13	22	1216	676	[12] 2.5	235	Preterm infants
Similac Special Care 24 [w/Fe] (Ross)	0.8 (24)	22 (11) Nonfat milk Whey protein concentrate	86 (42) Corn syrup solids (50%) Lactose (50%)	44 (49) MCT oil (50%) Soy oil (30%) Coconut oil (20%)	15	27	1452	806	[15] 3	280	Preterm infants

*Available as concentrated liquid. Nutrient values vary depending on amount of added carbohydrate (CHO) and water. A total of 12 fl oz of concentrated liquid with 15 g CHO and 12 fl oz water yields 20 kcal/fl oz formula with 68 g CHO/L.
For most current information, refer to formula websites or labels.
Roberson J, Shilkofski N: The Harriet Lane Handbook, 17th ed., Elsevier Mosby, Philadelphia, 2005.

TABLE F-3
HUMAN MILK AND FORTIFIERS ANALYSIS (PER LITER)

Formula	kcal/ml (kcal/oz)	Protein g (% kcal)	Carbohydrate g (% kcal)	Fat g (% kcal)	Na (mEq)	K (mEq)	Ca (mg)	P (mg)	Fe (mg)	Osmolality (mOsm/kg water)	Suggested Uses
Human milk* (mature)	0.69 (20)	10 (6) Human milk protein	72 (42) Lactose	39 (54) Human milk fat	7	13	280	147	0.4	286	Infants
Human milk* (Preterm)	0.67 (20)	14 (8) Human milk protein	66 (40) Lactose	39 (52) Human milk fat	11	15	248	128	1.2	290	Preterm infants
Enfamil Human Milk Fortifier (per packet) (Mead Johnson)	3.5 kcal per packet (–)	0.3 (29) Whey protein isolate Na casinate	0.26 (30) Corn syrup solids	0.16 (42) From caseinate	0.12	0.13	23	11	0.36	—	Fortifier for preterm human milk
Similac Human Milk Fortifier (Ross) per packet	3.5 kcal per packet	0.25 (29) Whey protein concentrate Nonfat milk	0.45 (51) Corn syrup solids	0.09 (23) MCT oil	0.16	0.4	29	17	0.09	—	Fortifier for preterm human milk
Similac Natural Care Human Milk Fortifier (Ross)	0.8 (24)	22 (11) Nonfat milk Whey protein concentrate	86 (42) Corn syrup solids (50%) Lactose (50%)	44 (47) MCT oil (50%) Soy oil (30%) Coconut oil (20%)	15	26.6	1694	935	3	280	Fortifier for preterm human milk

Continued

F

COMPOSITION OF NUTRITIONAL PRODUCTS

TABLE F-3

HUMAN MILK AND FORTIFIERS ANALYSIS (PER LITER)—cont'd

Product										
Preterm Human Milk + Enfamil Human Milk Fortifier (1 ptk/25 ml)	0.79 (24)	27 (13) Human milk protein Whey protein concentrate Na caseinate	82 (42) Lactose Corn syrup solids	41 (46) Human milk fat	165	18	1140	590	15	410	Preterm infants
Preterm Human Milk + Similac Human Milk Fortifier (1 packet/25 ml)	0.79 (24)	23 (12) Nonfat milk Whey protein concentrate Human milk protein	82 (42) Lactose Corn syrup solids	41 (47) MCT oil Human milk fat	17	30	1380	776	4.6	385	Preterm infants
Preterm Human Milk + Similac Natural Care 75:25 ratio	0.7 (21)	16 (9) Human milk protein Nonfat milk Whey protein concentrate	71 (40) Lactose Corn syrup solids	40 (51) Human milk fat MCT oil Soy oil Coconut oil	12	18	610	330	1.65	288	Preterm infants
Preterm Human Milk + Similac Natural Care 50:50 ratio	0.74 (22)	18 (10) Human milk protein Nonfat milk Whey protein concentrate	71 (40) Lactose Corn syrup solids	41 (50) Human milk fat MCT oil Soy oil Coconut oil	13	21	971	531	2.1	285	Preterm infants

From Ross Products Division, Abbott Laboratories, Inc.

*Composition of human milk varies with maternal diet, stage of lactation, within feedings, diurnally, and among mothers.

Roberson J, Shilkofski N: The Harriet Lane Handbook, 17th ed., Elsevier Mosby, Philadelphia, 2005.

Physical Observations

NEUTRAL THERMAL ENVIRONMENTAL TEMPERATURES

For healthy naked infant in an incubator of moderate humidity (50% saturation). Range shown is that needed to maintain normal body temperature without increasing heat production or evaporation loss by more than 25% **(Fig. G-1)**.

G

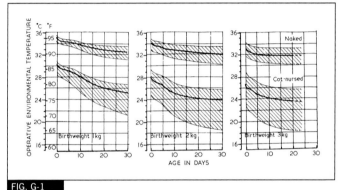

FIG. G-1

Range of temperature to provide neutral environmental conditions for baby lying either dressed in cot or naked on warm mattress in draft-free surroundings of moderate humidity (50% saturation) when mean radiant temperature is same as air temperature. Hatched area shows neutral temperature range for healthy babies weighing 1 kg, 2 kg, or 3 kg at birth. Approximately 1° C should be added to these operative temperatures to derive appropriate neutral air temperature for a single-walled incubator when room temperature is less than 27° C (80° F) and more if room temperature is much less than this. *(From Hey F, Katz G: Arch Dis Child 45:328, 1970.)*

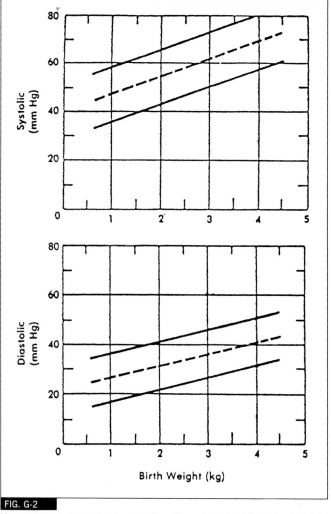

FIG. G-2

Linear regression *(broken lines)* and 95% confidence limits *(solid lines)* of systolic *(top)* and diastolic *(bottom)* aortic blood pressures and birth weights in 61 healthy newborn infants during the first 12 hours after birth. For systolic pressure, $y = 7.13x + 40.45$; $r = 0.79$. For diastolic pressure, $y = 4.81x + 22.18$; $r = 0.71$. For both, $n = 413$ and $P < .001$. *(From Versmold HT, et al: Pediatrics 67:607, 1981.)*

TABLE G-1

TIME OF FIRST VOID AND FIRST STOOL IN 500 INFANTS

Hours	395 Full-Term Infants		80 Preterm Infants		25 Post-term Infants	
	No. of Infants	Cumulative %	No. of Infants	Cumulative %	No. of Infants	Cumulative %
First void						
In delivery room	51	12.9	17	21.2	3	12
1-8	151	51.1	50	83.7	4	38
9-16	158	91.1	12	98.7	14	84
17-24	35	100	1	100	4	100
>24	0	—	0	—	0	—
First stool						
In delivery room	66	16.7	4	5	8	32
1-8	169	59.5	22	32.5	9	68
9-16	125	91.1	25	63.8	5	88
17-24	29	98.5	10	76.3	3	100
24-48	6*	100	18†	98.8	0	—
>48	0	—	1‡	100	0	—

From Clark DA: Pediatrics 60:457, 1977.

*At 25, 26, 27, 28, 33, and 37 hours.

†Five stooled more than 36 hours after birth at 38, 39, 40, 42, and 47 hours.

‡At 59 hours.

PHYSICAL OBSERVATIONS

G

TABLE G-2

ENDOTRACHEAL TUBE SIZE

| Infant Weight (gm) | Endotracheal Tube Diameter | |
	Inside	Outside
<1000	2.5 mm	12F
1000-1500	3 mm	14F
1500-2200	3.5 mm	16F
≥2200	4 mm	18F

From Avery GB, Fletcher MA, MacDonald MG (eds): Neonatology, 5th ed. Philadelphia, Lippincott Williams & Wilkins, 1999.

TABLE G-3

DEPTH OF INSERTION OF AN OROTRACHEAL TUBE FROM THE LIPS OF A PREMATURE INFANT

Infant Weight (kg)	Depth of Insertion (cm)
1	7
2	8
3	9
4	10

Modified from Avery GB, Fletcher MA, MacDonald MG (eds): Neonatology, 5th ed. Philadelphia, Lippincott Williams & Wilkins, 1999.

Neonatal Pharmacology

The differences in drug disposition for newborns when compared with adults are due to the underdevelopment of those organ systems affecting drug absorption, distribution, metabolism, and excretion **(Table H-1)**. For these reasons, a neonate cannot be considered a small adult. There is considerable immaturity.

DRUG DOSES FOR NEONATES

Abbreviations:

ALT, alanine aminotransferase
AST, aspartate aminotransferase
bid, twice a day
BUN, blood urea nitrogen
CBC, complete blood count
CNS, central nervous system
CSF, cerebrospinal fluid
ECG, electrocardiogram
ET, endotracheal
GI, gastrointestinal
Hct, hematocrit
HIV, human immunodeficiency virus
ID, intradermal
IHSS, idiopathic hypertrophic subaortic stenosis
IM, intramuscular
IT, intratracheal
IV, intravenous
LFT, liver function test
PCA (postconceptional age in weeks) = gestational age (weeks) + postnatal age (weeks)
PNA, Postnatal age (days)
PO, by mouth
PR, by rectum
PRN, as needed
PSVT, paroxysmal supraventricular tachycardia
PTT, partial thromboplastin time
PVC, premature ventricular contraction
qd, every day
qid, four times a day
qod, every other day
RDA, recommended dietary allowance
RDS, respiratory distress syndrome
RSV, respiratory syncytial virus
SC, subcutaneous
SGOT, serum glutamic-oxaloacetic transaminase
TIBC, total iron binding content
TSH, thyroid-stimulating hormone

H

TABLE H-1

GENERAL CHARACTERISTICS OF THE PHARMACOKINETIC PROCESS IN NEONATES AS COMPARED WITH ADULTS

Characteristic	Relative to Adult	Age Until Adult Level Reached	Pharmacokinetic Effect	Example Drug
ABSORPTION				
Peroral				
pH	Lower acid output	3 mo	↓ Bioavailability of acid drug	Phenobarbital
GI motility	Gastric emptying time is 6-8 hr at birth	6-8 mo	Unpredictable bioavailability	Digoxin
GI contents	Decreased amounts of bile acid pools and pancreatic enzymes; underdeveloped bacterial flora	About 1 yr	↓ Bioavailability of fat-soluble drug	Vitamin E
Intramuscular	Low vascular perfusion, delay	?		
Percutaneous	Increased, especially in preterm infants	Months	↑ Absorption	Lindane/Kwell (contraindicated—have caused seizures)
DISTRIBUTION				
% Body water	High extracellular and total body water rapidly changes in first year	About 12 yr	↑ Volume of distribution	Aminoglycosides
% Fat	Full-term birth at 12%-16%; increases from 5-10 yr of age followed by a decrease	About 17 yr		

NEONATAL PHARMACOLOGY H

Plasma proteins	Lower total protein, albumin, and α-1 acid glycoprotein; Higher unconjugated bilirubin and free fatty acids	Gradual changes over first year; Gradual changes over first year	↑ Volume of distribution and free drug concentration	Phenytoin, lidocaine
Blood-brain barrier	Immature barrier caused by incomplete myelination	?	↑ CSF penetration	Aminoglycosides
METABOLISM				
P-450 enzyme	Lower at birth, isoenzyme specific	2 wk-6 mo	↑ Elimination $T_{1/2}$	Phenobarbital
Glucuronidation	Lower at birth	3-4 yr	Minor metabolite	Acetaminophen
Sulphation	At adult level		Major metabolite	Acetaminophen
Glycine conjugation	At adult level			
Overall capacity	Further impaired by prematurity or disease			
ELIMINATION				
Glomerular filtration	Lower, especially in premature infants	About 6 mo	↑ Elimination $T_{1/2}$	Aminoglycosides
Tubular secretion	Lower	About 6 mo	↑ Elimination $T_{1/2}$	Penicillins

Modified from Pelkon O: Curr Opin Pediatr 2:220, 1990; Misap RL, Hill MR, Szefler SL: In Evans WE (ed): Applied pharmacokinetics, 3rd ed., Spokane, Wash, Applied Therapeutics, 1992.

Table H-2, prepared in large part by Dr. Carlton K.K. Lee, contains both generic and trade names, information on how drugs are supplied, and their usual dose and route of administration. Brief remarks regarding side effects, drug interactions, precautions, effect on breast-feeding, and other relevant factors are included.

Note in the "How Supplied" column that the unit quantity in which a drug is supplied is listed in parentheses after the drug concentration. Suspension formulations marked by an asterisk are not commercially available and must be extemporaneously compounded by a pharmacist. References for these formulations and for the contents of the formulary are provided at the end of this section of the appendix. Drug dilutions may be necessary to enhance the accuracy of dose delivery for certain drugs. **Check with your respective pharmacy for specific dosage forms and concentrations available at your institution.**

TABLE H-2

DRUG DOSES FOR NEONATES

Drug	How Supplied	Dose and Route	Remarks
Acetaminophen (Tylenol, Tempra, Panadol, and others)	Infant drops: 80 mg/0.8 ml Elixir: 160 mg/5 ml Child solution/suspension: 160 mg/5 ml Suppository: 80, 120 mg	10-15 mg/kg/dose PO/PR q6-8 hr Some advocate loading dose of 20-25 mg/kg/dose for PO or 30 mg/kg/dose for PR.	Delayed hepatotoxicity occurs in overdose. Avoid use in suspected G6PD deficiency. Some preparations contain alcohol and/or phenylalanine. Breast-feeding: compatible.
Acetazolamide (Diamox)	Suspension*: 25, or 50 mg/ml Injection: 500 mg/5 ml Contains 2.05 mEq Na$^+$ per 500 mg drug	IV/PO: 5 mg/kg/24 hr ÷ q8h, increase as required to 25 mg/kg/24 hr *For hydrocephalus (IV/PO):* Day 1: 25 mg/kg/24 hr ÷ q8h Day 2: 50 mg/kg/24 hr ÷ q8h Day 3: 75 mg/kg/24 hr ÷ q8h Day 4 and greater: 100 mg/kg/24 hr ÷ q8h	Contraindicated in hepatic failure, severe renal failure, and hypersensitivity to sulfonamides. Paresthesias, polyuria, drowsiness, GI irritation, transient hypokalemia, reduced urate excretion, and metabolic acidosis may occur with long-term therapy. Avoid IM administration because injectable product has a high pH. Bicarbonate replacement therapy may be required, especially during long-term use (see citrate or sodium bicarbonate). Breast-feeding: compatible.

Continued

NEONATAL PHARMACOLOGY **H**

TABLE H-2

DRUG DOSES FOR NEONATES—cont'd

Drug	How Supplied	Dose and Route	Remarks
Acyclovir (Zovirax)	Suspension 200 mg/5 ml Injection in powder (with sodium): 500, 1000 mg Injection in solution (with sodium): 25, 50 mg/ml Contains 4.2 mEq Na⁺ per 1 gm drug Ointment: 5% (15 g) Cream: 5% (2 g)	*Neonatal (HSV & HSV encephalitis):* <35 wk PCA: 40 mg/kg/24 hr ÷ q12hr IV × 14-21 days. ≥35 wk PCA: 60 mg/kg/24 hr ÷ Q8hr IV × 14-21 days. Topical use, apply ointment 5-6 times a day for 7 days *Varicella zoster: Immunocompromised or immunocompetent host IV:*1500 mg/m²/24 hr ÷ q8hr for 7-10 days *Immunocompetent host PO:* 80 mg/kg/24hr ÷ qid for 5 days; begin immediately after signs or symptoms	Can cause renal impairment. Adequate hydration is essential to prevent renal tubular crystallization. Encephalopathic reactions have been reported. May cause nausea, vomiting, diarrhea, headache, dizziness, arthralgia, fatigue, rash, insomnia, fever. Infuse IV dose over 1 hr at a concentration ≤ 7 mg/ml. Adjust dose in renal impairment. Breast-feeding: compatible.
Adenosine (Adenocard)	Injection: 3 mg/ml (2, 4 ml)	*For PSVT:* 0.05 mg/kg IV push; if not effective within 2 minutes, increase dose by 0.05 mg/kg increments every 2 minutes to a **maximum** of 0.25 mg/kg/dose	$T_{1/2}$ < 10 seconds; may precipitate bronchoconstriction. Side effects include facial flushing, headache, shortness of breath, dyspnea, nausea, and chest pain. **Contraindicated** in second-and third-degree AV block. Theophylline and caffeine may antagonize its effect. Breast-feeding: safety not established.
Albumin, human (Normal serum albumin)	Injection: 5% (50 mg/ml), 25% (250 mg/ml); both contain 130-160 mEq Na⁺/L	*Hypoproteinemia:* IV, 0.5-1 gm/kg/dose over 2-4 hr; repeat every 1-2 days or as calculated to replace ongoing losses.	Fever, chills, rash, tachycardia, and hypervolemia may occur. **Contraindicated** in severe CHF or anemia. Use with **caution** in hypervolemia. 5% concentration generally

Alprostadil
(PGE$_1$,
Prostaglandin E$_1$,
Prostin VR)

Injection: 500 μg/ml
Contains dehydrated alcohol

Hypovolemia: IV 0.5 gm/kg/dose,
repeat prn; usually infused
over 0.5-1 hr (faster rates
may be clinically necessary)
(**maximum** dose: 6 gm/kg/24 hr)
Initial: 0.05-0.1 μg/kg/min; advance
to 0.2 μg/kg/min if necessary
Maintenance: When increase in PO$_2$
is noted, decrease immediately to
lowest effective dose;
doses >0.4 μg/kg/min not likely
to produce additional benefit

used; 25% concentration is generally reserved
for fluid- and sodium-restricted patients.
Dilutions of the 25% product should be
made with D5W or NS. Breast-feeding: safety
not established.
For palliation only: Continuous vital sign
monitoring is essential. May cause apnea,
fever, seizures, flushing, bradycardia,
hypotension, diarrhea, gastric outlet
obstruction, and reversible cortical
proliferation of long bones (with
prolonged use). Decreases platelet aggregation.
Breast-feeding: safety not established.

Amikacin sulfate
(Amikin)

Injection:
50 or 250 mg/ml

See following chart

Ototoxicity, nephrotoxicity, rash, fever,
eosinophilia, and headache may occur.
Monitor levels.
**Therapeutic levels: peak, 20-30 mg/L; trough,
5-10 mg/L.** Recommended serum sampling
time at steady-state; trough within 30 minutes
before the third consecutive dose and peak
30-60 minutes after the administration of the
third consecutive dose. Adjust dose with renal
impairment. Ototoxic effects are synergistic
with furosemide. Administer dose at least 2 hr
before or after penicillins and cephalosporins
(may blunt serum concentration). Breast-
feeding: Use with caution.

NEONATAL PHARMACOLOGY H

Continued

TABLE H-2

DRUG DOSES FOR NEONATES—cont'd

Drug	How Supplied			Dose and Route	Remarks

AMIKACIN SULFATE

Postconceptional Age (wk)	Postnatal Age (days)	Dose (mg/kg/dose)	Interval (hr)
≤29†	0-7	18	48
	8-28	15	36
	>28	15	24
30-33	0-7	18	36
	>7	15	24
≥34	0-7	15	24
	>7	15	12-18

Monitoring serum levels is essential, especially in infants. Side effects: restlessness, GI upset, seizures, arrhythmias.

Drug	How Supplied	Dose and Route	Remarks
Aminophylline (Aminophyllin and various other brand names)	Injection (IV): 25 mg/ml (79% theophylline) Oral liquid: 105 mg/5 ml (240 ml) (86% theophylline) **Note:** Pharmacy may dilute IV and oral dosage forms to enhance accuracy of smaller doses	IV loading: 6 mg/kg IV over 20 min (each 1.2-mg/kg dose raises the serum theophylline concentration 2 mg/L) IV maintenance (continuous IV drip): Neonates, 0.2 mg/kg/hr *Neonatal apnea:* Loading dose IV or PO, 5-6 mg/kg; maintenance dose IV or PO, 1-2 mg/kg/dose q6-8h	**Therapeutic level: For neonatal apnea, 6-13 mg/L; for bronchospasm 10-20 mg/L.** Recommended guidelines for obtaining levels: IV bolus: 30 min after infusion IV continuous; 12-24 hr after initiation of infusion *PO liquid (peak):* 1 hr after dose *PO liquid (trough):* Just before dose. Ideally, obtain levels after achievement of steady-state (1-6 days). However, levels may be obtained before steady-state to assess safety. Drug interactions: Increased levels with erythromycin, cimetidine; decreased levels with phenobarbital, rifampin, phenytoin.

Drug	Preparations	Dosage	Notes
Amoxicillin (Amoxil, Larotid, Trimox, and others)	Drops: 50 mg/ml (15, 30 ml) Suspension: 125, 250 mg/5ml (80, 100, 125, 150 ml)	PO: 20-40 mg/kg/24 hr ÷ q8h	**NOTE:** Several oral liquid preparations are dye free. Consult with pharmacist if it is an issue. Breast-feeding: compatible. Similar to ampicillin. May cause abdominal cramps, cutaneous reactions, diarrhea, hypersensitivity reactions, interstitial nephritis, pancytopenia, pseudomembranous colitis, and urticaria. Adjust dose in renal failure. Breast-feeding: compatible.
Amoxicillin-clavulanic Acid (Augmentin)	Suspension: 125, 250 mg/5ml (31.25 and 62.5 mg clavulanate/5 ml) (75, 100, 150 ml); or 200, 400 mg/5ml (28.5 and 57 mg clavulanate/5ml) (50, 75, 100 ml) Contains 0.63 mEq K⁺ per 125 mg clavulanate	Dosage based on amoxicillin component *Children* < 3 mo: 30 mg/kg/24 hr ÷ bid PO (recommended dosage form is 125 mg/5 ml suspension)	See amoxicillin for side effects. Diarrhea primarily caused by clavulanic acid. Reduce dose in renal failure. 200, 400 mg/5 ml concentrations and Augmentin ES-600 (600 mg/5 ml) contain phenylalanine and should not be used by phenylketonurics. Breast-feeding: compatible.
Amphotericin B (Fungizone)	Injection: 50 mg Cream: 3% (20 gm) Lotion: 3% (30 ml)	Topical: Apply to affected area bid-qid IV: Mix with D₅W to a concentration of 0.1 mg/ml (peripheral administration) or 0.25 mg/ml (central line only), pH >4.2; infuse over 2-6 hr	Fever, chills, nausea, and vomiting are common side effects. Monitor renal, electrolytes, and hematologic status closely. Hypokalemia (may cause digoxin toxicity—if receiving both drugs), hypomagnesemia, renal tubular acidosis, renal failure, acute hepatic failure,

*Or significant asphyxia, PDA, indomethacin use, poor cardiac output, reduced renal function.

NEONATAL PHARMACOLOGY H

Continued

TABLE H-2

DRUG DOSES FOR NEONATES—cont'd

Drug	How Supplied	Dose and Route	Remarks
Amphotericin B (Fungizone)—cont'd	Suspension: 125, 250 mg/5 ml (100, 150, 200 ml)	Optional test dose: 0.1 mg/kg/dose IV up to a **maximum** of 1 mg infused over 2 hr (followed by remaining initial dose) Initial dose: 0.25-0.5 mg/kg/dose Increment: Increase as tolerated by 0.25-0.5 mg/kg/24 hr qd or qod **Maximum dose:** 1.5 mg/kg/24 hr	and phlebitis may occur. Drug is incompatible in normal saline. A more concentrated solution of 0.25 mg/ml can be used for fluid-restricted patients but must be administered only through a central line. Breast-feeding: safety not established.
Ampicillin (Omnipen, Polycillin, Principen, and others)	Injection: 125, 250, 500 mg, 1 gm, 2 gm Contains 3 mEq Na⁺/gm drug	IV or IM: 50 mg/kg/dose	Same side effects as penicillin, with cross-reactivity. Rash is commonly seen at 5-10 days. May cause interstitial nephritis. Adjust dose in renal failure. Breast-feeding: Use with caution (adverse effects are rare, three potential problems exist for nursing infants: bowel flora modification, allergic response, and interference of culture results for fever workup).

For Ampicillin, dosing table:

PCA	PNA	Interval (hr)
≤29	≤28	12
≤29	>28	8
30-36	≤14	12
30-36	>14	8
37-44	≤7	12
37-44	>7	8
≥45	All	6

For meningitis and group B streptococcal sepsis use 100 mg/kg/dose with the same guidelines as above.

Drug	How Supplied	Dose and Route	Remarks
Ampicillin/Sulbactam (Unasyn)	Injection: 1.5 g = ampicillin 1 g + sulbactam 0.5 g 3 g = ampicillin 2 g + sulbactam 1 g Contains 5 mEq Na⁺ per 1.5 g drug combination	Dosage based on ampicillin component: Infant >1 month: Mild/moderate infections: 100-150 mg/kg/24 hr ÷ q6hr IM/IV Meningitis/severe infections: 200-300 mg/kg/24 hr ÷ q6hr IM/IV	Similar spectrum of antibacterial activity to ampicillin with the added coverage of beta-lactamase-producing organisms. Adjust dose in renal failure. Similar CSF distribution and side effects to ampicillin. Breast-feeding: safety not established.

Atropine sulfate

Injection: 0.05, 0.1, 0.3, 0.4, 0.5, 0.8, 1 mg/ml

Cardiopulmonary resuscitation: IV, IM, SC: 0.01-0.03 mg/kg/dose; repeat q10-15 min prn (may give via ET tube at 2-3 times the above doses)

Minimum single dose 0.1 mg
Maximum single dose 0.5 mg

Hyperthermia, tachycardia, urinary retention, constipation, and dry mouth may occur. Administer via endotracheal tube in the presence of bradycardia.
Caution with patients sensitive to sulfate. Breast-feeding: compatible.

Aztreonam
(Azactam)

Injection: 0.5, 1, 2 gm
Contains approximately 780 mg L-Arginine per 1 gm of drug

Neonates (IV/IM): 30 mg/kg/dose:
<1.2 kg and 0-4 wk age: q12 hr
1.2-2 kg and 0-7 days: q12 hr
1.2-2 kg and >7 days: q8 hr
>2 kg and 0-7 days: q8 hr
>2 kg and >7 days: q6 hr

Low cross-allergenicity between aztreonam and other beta-lactams. May cause thrombophlebitis, eosinophilia, and liver enzyme elevation. Good CNS penetration. Adjust dose in renal failure. Breast-feeding: compatible.

Bacitracin
(Ak-Tracin)

Ophthalmic ointment:
1% or 500 U/gm (3.5, 3.75 gm)

Ophthalmic: Apply a ¼ to ½ inch ribbon to the conjunctival sac qid

Ophthalmic ointment may cause blurred vision. Rash and allergic reactions may occur. Patients sensitive to neomycin may also be sensitive to bacitracin. Breast-feeding: safety not established.

Beractant
(Survanta)

Suspension: 25 mg/ml (4, 8 ml); each ml contains 0.5-0.75 mg triglycerides, 1.4-3.5 mg free fatty acids and <1 mg protein (bovine source)

Prophylactic therapy: 4 ml/kg/dose intratracheally as soon as possible; up to four doses may be given at intervals no shorter than q6h during the first 48 hr of life.

Rescue therapy: 4 ml/kg/dose intratracheally, immediately after the diagnosis of RDS; may repeat dose as needed q6hr to **maximum** of 4 total doses

All doses are administered intratracheally. If the suspension settles during storage, gently swirl the contents—**do not shake.** Each dose is divided into four 1 ml/kg aliquots; administer 1 ml/kg in each of four different positions (slight downward inclination with head turned to the right, head turned to the left; slight upward inclination with head turned to the right, head turned to the left). Transient bradycardia, O_2 desaturation, pallor, vasoconstriction, hypotension, endotracheal tube blockage, hypercarbia, hypercapnia, apnea, and hypertension.

Continued

NEONATAL PHARMACOLOGY **H**

TABLE H-2
DRUG DOSES FOR NEONATES—cont'd

Drug	How Supplied	Dose and Route	Remarks
Caffeine citrate	Injection: 20 mg/ml (citrate salt) = 10 mg/ml caffeine base (3 ml) Oral liquid: 20 mg/ml (citrate salt) = 10 mg/ml caffeine base	**Doses based on caffeine citrate salt:** *Neonatal apnea:* Loading dose (IV, PO), 10-20 mg/kg/dose × 1; maintenance dose (IV, PO), 5-10 mg/kg/dose qd, first dose 24 hr after load	**Therapeutic levels for apnea: 5-25 mg/L.** Steady-state is typically achieved in 3 weeks of continuous dosing. Levels obtained prior to steady-state are useful for preventing toxicity. Cardiovascular, neurologic, or GI toxicities occur when levels are > 50 mg/L. **Avoid caffeine benzoate, may cause kernicterus.** Breast-feeding: compatible.
Calcium carbonate (40% calcium)	Suspension: 1250 mg/5 ml Powder: 454 gm Each gm of salt contains 20 mEq = 400 mg of elemental calcium	**Dosage based on calcium carbonate salt:** *Neonatal hypocalcemia:* 125-375 mg/kg/24 hr PO ÷ q4-6h **Maximum dose 2500 mg/24 hr**	Administer each dose with meals or with lots of fluid. May cause constipation, hypophosphatemia, hypomagnesemia, and vomiting. May reduce absorption of iron. Some products may contain a trace amount of sodium. Breast-feeding: safety not established.
Calcium chloride (27% calcium)	Injection: 100 mg/ml 10% (1.36 mEq Ca^{++}/ml); each gm of salt contains 13.6 mEq = 270 mg of elemental calcium	**Doses based on calcium chloride salt:** *Maintenance/hypocalcemia:* 200-300 mg/kg/24 hr PO as 2% solution ÷ q6h *For cardiac arrest:* IV, 20 mg/kg/dose (0.2 ml/kg/dose) q10 min	May cause GI irritation, phlebitis. Use intravenously with **extreme caution.** Acidifying effect; give only 2-3 days, then change to another Ca^+ salt. Treat IV infiltrate with hyaluronidase. **Maximum IV administration rates:** IV Push: **DO NOT EXCEED** 100 mg/min IV Infusion: **DO NOT EXCEED** 45-90 mg/kg/hr with a **maximum concentration** of 20 mg/ml. Breast-feeding: safety not established.

Calcium glubionate
(Neocalglucon)
(6.4% calcium)

Syrup: 1.8 gm/5 ml; each 5 ml contains 5.8 mEq = 115 mg of elemental calcium

Doses based on calcium glubionate salt:
Neonatal hypocalcemia:
1200 mg/kg/24 hr PO ÷ q4-6hr
Maintenance: 600-2000 mg/kg/24 hr PO ÷ qid (**maximum dose 9 gm/24 hr)**

Administer before feeding for best absorption. Absorption inhibited by phosphate load. High osmotic load of syrup (20% sucrose) may cause diarrhea. Breast-feeding: safety not established.

Calcium gluceptate
(8.2% calcium)

Injection: 220 mg/ml (22%) (0.9 mEq Ca/ml); each gm of salt contains 4.1 mEq = 82 mg of elemental calcium

Doses based on calcium gluceptate salt:
Hypocalcemia: 200-500 mg/kg/24 hr IV ÷ q6hr
For cardiac arrest: IV, 110 mg/kg/dose (=0.5 ml/kg/dose) IV q10 min

See calcium gluconate
Maximum IV administration rates:
IV push: **DO NOT EXCEED** 100 mg/min
IV infusion: **DO NOT EXCEED**
150-300 mg/kg/hr with a **maximum concentration** of 55 mg/ml
Breast-feeding: safety not established.

Calcium gluconate
(9% calcium)

Injection: 100 mg/ml (10%); each gm of salt contains 4.8 mEq = 90 mg of elemental calcium

Doses based on calcium gluconate salt:
Maintenance/hypocalcemia: IV 200-800 mg/kg/24 hr ÷ q6hr; PO, 400-800 mg/kg/24 hr ÷ q 6 hr
For cardiac arrest: IV, 100 mg/kg/dose (= 1 ml/kg/dose) q 10 min

If given by IV route, administer slowly and watch for bradycardia, hypotension, and extravasation. May produce arrhythmias in digitalized patients. Precipitates with bicarbonates. Tissue necrosis may result from infiltrates. **Do not use scalp vein.**
Maximum IV administration rates:
IV push: **DO NOT EXCEED** 100/mg/min
IV infusion: **DO NOT EXCEED** 120-240 mg/kg/hr with **maximum concentration** of 50 mg/ml
Breast-feeding: safety not established.

Calfactant
(Infasurf)

Intratracheal suspension: 35 mg/ml (3, 6 ml); each ml contains 26 mg

Prophylactic therapy:
3 ml/kg/dose intratracheally as soon as possible; up to a total of

All doses administered intratracheally. If suspension settles during storage, gently swirl the contents—**do not shake.** Manufacturer

Continued

NEONATAL PHARMACOLOGY

TABLE H-2

DRUG DOSES FOR NEONATES—cont'd

Drug	How Supplied	Dose and Route	Remarks
Calfactant (Infasurf)—cont'd	phosphatidylcholine and 0.26 mg of surfactant protein B. (bovine source)	three doses may be given q12hr *Rescue therapy:* 3 ml/kg/dose intratracheally immediately after the diagnosis of RDS. May repeat doses as needed q12hr to a **maximum** of three total doses.	recommends administration through a side-port adapter into the endotracheal tube with two attendants (one to instill drug and another to monitor and position patient). Each dose is divided into two 1.5 ml/kg aliquots; give 1.5 ml/kg in each of two different positions (infant positioned to the right or left side dependent). Administration is made while ventilation is continued over 20-30 breaths each aliquot, with small bursts timed only during the inspiratory cycles. A pause followed by evaluation of the respiratory status and repositioning should separate the two aliquots. Common adverse effects include cyanosis, airway obstruction, bradycardia, reflux of surfactant into the ET tube, requirement for manual ventilation, and reintubation.
Captopril (Capoten)	Suspension:* 0.75, 1 mg/ml Tablets: 12.5, 25, 50, 100 mg	0.1-0.4 mg/kg/24 hr PO ÷ q6-8 hr **Maximum:** 6 mg/kg/24 hr	Adjust with renal failure. May cause rash, coughing, proteinuria, neutropenia, and hypotension. Known to decrease aldosterone and increase renin production. Breast-feeding: compatible.
Cefazolin (Ancef, Zolicef) (first generation)	Injection: 0.5, 1, 5, 10 gm (contains 2.1 mEq Na+ per 1 gm of drug)	<7 days (IV or IM): 40 mg/kg/ 24 hr ÷ q12hr ≥7 days (IM or IV): ≤2 kg, 40 mg/kg/24 hr ÷ q12 hr	Use caution in penicillin-allergic patients and reduce dose in renal failure. May cause phlebitis, leukopenia, thrombocytopenia, elevated liver enzymes,

Cefepime (Maxipime) (fourth generation)	Injection: 0.5, 1, 2 gm (contains 725 mg L-arginine per 1 gm drug)	>2 kg, 60 mg/kg/24 hr ÷ q8hr
		>2 mo (IV or IM): 100 mg/kg/24 hr ÷ q 12 hr; Use 150 mg/kg/24 hr ÷ q 8 hr for meningitis or serious infections
Cefotaxime (Claforan) (third generation)	Injection: 0.5, 1, 2, 10 gm (contains 2.2 mEq Na+ per 1 gm of drug)	<1 wk (IV or IM): 100-150 mg/kg/24 hr ÷ q12 hr
		1-4 wk (IV or IM): 150-200 mg/kg/24 hr ÷ q8hr
Ceftazidime (Fortaz, Tazidime, Tazicef, Ceptaz [arginine salt]) (third generation)	Injection: 0.5, 1, 2 gm (contains 2.3 mEq Na+ per 1 gm of drug) (Ceptaz contains 349 mg L-arginine per 1 gm of drug)	IM or IV (< 2kg): <7 days, 100 mg/kg/24 hr ÷ q12hr ≥7 days, 150 mg/kg/24hr ÷ q8hr IM or IV (≥2 kg): <7 days, 100-150 mg/kg/24 hr ÷ q8-12 hr ≥7 days, 150 mg/kg/24 hr ÷ q8hr

false-positive urine reducing substance. Breast-feeding: compatible.

Use with caution in penicillin-allergic patients and reduce dose in renal failure. Good activity against *P. aeruginosa* and other Gram-negative bacteria plus most Gram positives (*S.aureus*). May cause thrombophlebitis, gastrointestinal discomfort, transient increases in liver enzymes, false-positive urine reducing substance (Clinitest) and Coombs test. Breast-feeding: compatible.

Use with **caution** in penicillin-allergic patients and reduce dose in renal failure. Toxicities similar to other cephalosporins; allergy, neutropenia, thrombocytopenia, eosinophilia, positive Coombs test, elevated BUN, creatinine, and liver enzymes. Breast-feeding: compatible.

Use with **caution** in penicillin-allergic patients and reduce dose in renal failure. Good *Pseudomonas* coverage and CSF penetration. Breast-feeding: compatible.

Continued

NEONATAL PHARMACOLOGY H

TABLE H-2

DRUG DOSES FOR NEONATES—cont'd

Drug	How Supplied	Dose and Route	Remarks
Ceftizoxime (Cefizox) (third generation)	Injection: 0.5, 1, 2, gm (contains 2.6 mEq Na⁺ per 1 gm drug)	100–200 mg/kg/24 hr IV/IM ÷ q6-8 hr	Use with **caution** in penicillin-allergic patients. May cause transient elevation of liver enzymes and diarrhea. Good CNS penetration. Reduce dose in renal failure. Breast-feeding: compatible.
Ceftriaxone (Rocephin) (third generation)	Injection: 0.25, 0.5, 1, 2, 10 gm (contains 3.6 mEq Na⁺ per 1 gm drug)	IV or IM (<2 kg): 50 mg/kg/dose q24hr IV or IM (≥2 kg): <7 days, 50 mg/kg/dose q24hr ≥7 days, 75 mg/kg/dose q24hr *Uncomplicated gonococcal Ophthalmia:* 50 mg/kg × 1 **Maximum dose** 125 mg/dose	Use with **caution** in penicillin-allergic patients. May cause diarrhea, increased hepatic enzymes, reversible cholelithiasis, sludging in gallbladder. Use with **caution** in neonates at risk for hyperbilirubinemia. Breast-feeding: compatible.
Cefuroxime (Zinacef), (second generation)	Injection: 0.75, 1.5, 7.5 gm (contains 2.4 mEq Na⁺ per 1 gm drug)	IM or IV: 20–60 mg/kg/24hr ÷ q12hr	Use with **caution** in penicillin-allergic patients and reduce dose in renal failure. May cause thrombophlebitis at infusion site. Other toxicities are those of other cephalosporins. Not recommended for meningitis. Breast-feeding: compatible.
Chloral hydrate (Aquachloral suppretes and others)	Syrup: 250 mg/5 ml, 500 mg/5 ml Suppository: 324 mg	PO or PR: *Sedative:* 25-50 mg/kg/24 hr ÷ q6-8hr *Hypnotic:* 50 mg/kg as a single dose	Gastric irritation (dilute PO doses); **caution** with hepatic, renal, cardiac, or pulmonary disease. **Caution** when using with furosemide and anticoagulants. Accumulation of major metabolites may occur with chronic administration. Breast-feeding: compatible.

Drug	Formulations	Dosage	Comments
Chloramphenicol (Chloromycetin)	Injection: (as sodium succinate): 1 gm (contains 2.25 mEq Na$^+$ per 1 gm drug)	Loading dose (all ages): IV 20 mg/kg Neonates: <2 kg: IV 25 mg/kg/24 hr qd ≥2 kg: <7 days: IV 25 mg/kg/24 hr qd; ≥7 days: IV 50 mg/kg/24 hr ÷ q12 hr **NOTE:** Initiate maintenance therapy beginning **12 hr after loading dose**	Dose recommendations are only guidelines for therapy; monitoring of blood levels is essential in neonates and infants. Drug is poorly absorbed by IM route. Follow hematologic status for dose-related or idiosyncratic marrow suppression. Gray baby syndrome may be seen with levels >50 mg/L. Concomitant use of rifampin may lower serum levels. Chloramphenicol may increase phenytoin levels. **Therapeutic levels: 15-25 mg/L.** IV route preferred because of the lack of an oral liquid dosage form and wide variations in plasma levels with PO route. Breast-feeding: unknown with concerns.
Chlorothiazide (Diuril, Diurigen)	Suspension: 250 mg/5 ml (237 ml) Injection: 500 mg (20 ml) (contains 5 mEq Na$^+$ per 1 gm of drug)	PO/IV: 10-20 mg/kg/dose q12hr	Use with **caution** in liver and severe renal disease. May cause hyperbilirubinemia, hypokalemia, alkalosis, hyperglycemia, hyperuricemia, hypomagnesemia, blood dyscrasias, pancreatitis. Avoid IM administration. Breast-feeding: compatible.
Cimetidine (Tagamet)	Syrup: 300 mg/5 ml: contains 2.8% alcohol Injection: 150 mg/ml	5-20 mg/kg/24 hr IM/PO/IV ÷ q6-12 hr	May cause diarrhea, rash, and elevated liver function tests. Inhibits cytochrome P450 oxidative system to increase serum levels of theophylline, phenytoin, lidocaine, and diazepam. Reduce dose in renal failure. Breast-feeding: compatible.

Continued

NEONATAL PHARMACOLOGY

H

TABLE H-2

DRUG DOSES FOR NEONATES—cont'd

Drug	How Supplied	Dose and Route	Remarks
Citrate: Sodium citrate and citric acid (Bicitra, Cytra-2)	Each ml contains 1 mEq Na^+ and 1 mEq HCO_3^- equivalent	Dosing based on citrate: PO: 2-3 mEq/kg/24 hr ÷ tid-qid	Adjust dose to maintain urine pH. 1 mEq of citrate is equivalent to 1 mEq HCO_3^-—provided patient has normal liver function. Bicitra is preferred over Polycitra (1 ml = 1 mEq Na and K and 2 mEq citrate) and Polycitra-K (1 ml = 2 mEq K and citrate) because of hidden amounts of potassium. Breast-feeding: safety not established.
Clindamycin (Cleocin)	Oral liquid (as palmitate): 75 mg/5 ml (100 ml) Injection: 150 mg/ml (contains 9.45 mg/ml benzyl alcohol)	<2 kg (IV, IM): <7 days: 10 mg/kg/24 hr ÷ q12h ≥7 days: 15 mg/kg/24 hr ÷ q8h ≥2 kg (IV, IM): <7 days, 15 mg/kg/24 hr ÷ q8h; ≥7 days, 20 mg/kg/24 hr ÷ q6h Full term (IV, IM): 20-30 mg/kg/24 hr ÷ q6h	Not indicated in meningitis. Use with caution in hepatic insufficiency. Pseudomembranous colitis may occur up to several weeks after cessation of therapy but generally is uncommon in pediatric patients. May cause diarrhea, rash, Stevens-Johnson syndrome, granulocytopenia, thrombocytopenia, or sterile abscess at injection site. Breast-feeding: compatible.
Clotrimazole (Lotrimin, Mycelex)	Cream: 1% (15, 30, 45, 90 gm) Topical solution: 1% (10, 30 ml) Lotion: 1% (30 ml)	Topical: Apply to affected skin area bid	May cause erythema, blistering, or urticaria where applied. Avoid contact with eyes. Breast-feeding: safety not established.
Cortisone			See hydrocortisone, dexamethasone, methylprednisolone, prednisone.

Cyclopentolate (Cyclogyl)	Ophthalmic solution: 0.5%, 1%, 2% (2, 5, 15 ml)	1 drop of 0.5% solution in each eye 10-30 min before examination; apply pressure over nasolacrimal sac for at least 2 min to minimize absorption	Do not use in narrow-angle glaucoma. Onset of action: 15-60 min. May cause burning sensation, tachycardia, loss of visual accommodation. Breast-feeding: safety not established.
Dexamethasone (Decadron, Hexadrol)	Elixir: 0.5 mg/5 ml (100 ml) (some preparations contain 5% alcohol) Oral solution: 0.1, 1 mg/ml (30 ml) (some preparations contain 30% alcohol) Injection: (as sodium phosphate salt): 4, 10, 20, 24 mg/ml (some preparations may contain benzyl alcohol or methyl/propyl parbens)	*Airway edema:* 0.5 – 2 mg/kg/24 hr IV/IM ÷ Q6h (begin 24 hr before extubation and continue for 4-6 doses postextubation) *Croup:* 0.6 mg/kg/dose PO/IV/IM × 1 (use sodium phosphate injection)	See hydrocortisone. Not recommended for systemic therapy in the treatment of chronic lung disease in very low birth weight infants due to increased risk of adverse events (Pediatrics 109: 330, 2002). Dexamethasone acetate salt for injection is used IM in adults. Breast-feeding: Unknown with concerns.
Diazepam (Valium)	Oral solution: 1, 5 mg/ml 19% alcohol Injection: 5 mg/ml contains 40% propylene glycol, 10% alcohol, and 1.5% benzyl alcohol	PO, IV, IM: *Sedative:* 0.02-03 mg/kg/dose q6-8h slow IV push *Seizure:* 0.3-0.75 mg/kg/dose	Diluted injection may precipitate. IM absorption is poor. Respiratory depression and hypotension may occur. IV administration rate: No faster than 2 mg/min. Breast-feeding: unknown with concerns.

Continued

NEONATAL PHARMACOLOGY H

TABLE H-2

DRUG DOSES FOR NEONATES—cont'd

Drug	How Supplied	Dose and Route	Remarks
Diazoxide (Proglycem)	Suspension: 50 mg/ml (30 ml); contains 7.25% alcohol	*Hyperinsulinemic hypoglycemia:* 8-15 mg/kg/24 hr PO ÷ q8-12 hr	Hypoglycemia should be treated initially with IV glucose; diazoxide should be used only if refractory to glucose infusion. May cause sodium and fluid retention, rash, hyperuricemia, and arrhythmias. Hyperglycemic effect with PO administration occurs within 1 hr with a duration of 8 hr. Breast-feeding: safety not established.
Didanosine (ddI, Videx)	Oral pediatric powder (for 10 mg/ml solution); 2, 4 gm	Neonates and infants <3 months: 100 mg/m²/24 hr PO ÷ q12h	May cause diarrhea, abdominal pain, peripheral neuropathy (dose related), electrolyte abnormalities, hyperuricemia, increased liver enzymes, rash, and pancreatitis. Administer all doses on an empty stomach. Impairs absorption of drugs requiring an acidic environment (e.g., ketoconazole); see www.aidsinfo.nih.gov/ guidelines for additional information. Breast-feeding: unknown with concerns.
Digoxin (Lanoxin)	Pediatric injection: 100 μg/ml (1 ml) Injection: 250 μg/ml (2 ml) (both injection products may contain propylene glycol and alcohol) Elixir: 50 μg/ml (60 ml); (may contain 10% alcohol)	Total digitalizing dose, PO: Preterm: 10 μg/kg × 1 followed by 5 μg/kg q8-18h × 2 Term: 15 μg/kg × 1, followed by 7.5 μg/kg q8-18h × 2; IV: Preterm: 7.5 μg/kg × 1, followed by 3.75 μg/kg q8-18h × 1 Term: 10 μg/kg × 1, followed by 5 μg/kg q8-18h × 2	*IV route for acute digitalization:* administer IV over 5-10 min. **NOTE:** Two different IV strengths. Adverse effects include arrhythmias, bradycardia, nausea, and vomiting. Should not be given in conjunction with calcium because this may potentiate bradycardia. Therapeutic levels are generally 0.5-2 ng/ml. However, neonates may require higher levels because of the serum assay's inability to differentiate maternal digoxin-like substances.

Antiarrhythmic doses may be higher than these (for CHF). IV dose is about 75% of PO dose. Digoxin toxicity may occur when taking amphotericin B (because of hypokalemia). **Antidote:** Digoxin Immune Fab. Breast-feeding: compatible.

Daily maintenance doses (begin 12 hr after last digitalizing dose),
PO:

Preterm: 5 µg/kg/24 hr divided bid
Term: 8-10 µg/kg/24 hr divided bid
IV:

Preterm: 3-4 µg/kg/24 hr divided bid;
Term: 6-8 µg/kg/24 hr divided bid

Digoxin immune FAB Injection: 38 mg/vial
(Digibind)

First, determine total body digoxin load (TBL):

TBL (mg) = serum digoxin level (ng/ml) × 5.6 × wt (kg) ÷ 1000, or

TBL (mg) = mg digoxin ingested × 0.8

Then calculate digoxin immune Fab dose

Dose in number of digoxin immune Fab vials: # vials = TBL ÷ 0.5

Infuse IV over 15-30 min (through 0.22 micron filter)

Contraindicated if hypersensitive to sheep products or if renal or cardiac failure.
May cause severe hypokalemia, decreased cardiac output, rash, edema. Breast-feeding: safety not established.

Dihydrotachysterol Solution: 0.2 mg/ml (20 ml)
(DHT, DHT Intensol) (20% alcohol)
1 mg = 120,000 I.U. of vitamin D_2

Hypoparathyroidism: PO:
0.05-0.1 mg/dose qd

Monitor serum Ca^{++} and PO_4. Toxicities include hypercalcemia and hypervitaminosis D. More potent than vitamin D_2 but more rapidly inactivated (half-life is hours vs. weeks). Titrate dose with patient response. Oral Ca^{++} supplementation may be required. Activated by 25-hydroxlation in liver; does not require 1-hydroxylation in kidney. Breast-feeding: safety not established.

NEONATAL PHARMACOLOGY H

Continued

TABLE H-2

DRUG DOSES FOR NEONATES—cont'd

Drug	How Supplied	Dose and Route	Remarks
Diphenhydramine (Benadryl)	Elixir/liquid/syrup: 12.5 mg/5 ml (120 ml); may contain up to 5.6% alcohol Injection: 50 mg/ml	PO or IV: 5 mg/kg/24hr ÷ q6h *For anaphylaxis:* 1-2 mg/kg IV slowly	Sedation, hypotension, paradoxical excitement, nausea, vomiting, dry mucous membranes may occur. Breast-feeding: unknown with concerns.
Dobutamine (Dobutrex)	Injection: 12.5 mg/ml (contains sulfites)	IV: 2.5-15 µg/kg/min **Maximum recommended dose:** 40 µg/kg/min To prepare infusion: 6 × wt (kg) × desired dose (µg/kg/min) ÷ IV infusion rate (ml/hr) = mg of drug to be added to 100 ml compatible IV fluid	Monitor blood pressure and vital signs. Contraindicated in IHSS. Tachycardia, arrhythmias (PVCs), and hypertension may occasionally occur (especially at higher infusion rates). Correct hypovolemic states before use. **Avoid extravasation** (phentolamine is the antidote). Breast-feeding: safety not established.
Dopamine (Inotropin)	Injection: 40, 80, 160 mg/ml	Low-dose IV: 2-5 µg/kg/min increases renal blood flow with minimal effects on heart rate and cardiac output Intermediate-dose IV: 5-15 µg/kg/min increases renal blood flow, heart rate, cardiac contractility, cardiac output High-dose IV: >20 µg/kg/min alpha-adrenergic effects prominent; decreases renal perfusion **Maximum recommended dose** 20-50 µg/kg/min To prepare infusion: Same as for dobutamine	Extravasation may lead to necrosis (phentolamine is the antidote). High dose may constrict renal arteries. Tachyarrhythmias, ectopic beats, hypertension, vasoconstriction, and vomiting may occur. Do not use in pheochromocytoma, tachyarrhythmias, or hypovolemia. Breast-feeding: safety not established.

Doxapram (Dopram)	Injection: 20 mg/ml (20 ml) (contains 0.9% benzyl alcohol)	*Methylxanthine refractory neonatal apnea:* Load with 2.5-3 mg/kg over 15-30 min followed by a continuous infusion of 1 mg/kg/hr titrated to the lowest responsive dose **Maximum dose** 2.5 mg/kg/hr	Hypertension occurs with higher doses (>1.5 mg.kg/hr). May also cause tachycardia, arrhythmias, seizures, hyperreflexia, hyponatremia, abdominal distention, and sweating. Avoid extravasation. Breast-feeding: safety not established.
EMLA (eutectic mixture of lidocaine and prilocaine)	Cream: Lidocaine 2.5% + procaine 2.5%: 5-gm kit (with dressings); 30-gm tube Topical anesthetic disk: Lidocaine 2.5% + prilocaine 2.5%: 1 gm (box of 2s or 10s)	*Circumcision:* 1 gm/dose × 1. Apply one third of dose to lower abdomen, then extend penis upward and gently press against abdomen. Apply remainder of dose to Tegaderm dressing and place over the penis. Tape dressing over abdomen so that the cream surrounds the penis. Leave in place for 60-80 minutes, remove dressing, and wipe off cream. (Based on Taddio et al: N Engl J Med 336:1197, 1997).	Use with caution in patients with G6PD deficiency and in patients with renal and hepatic impairment. Prilocaine has been associated with methemoglobinemia. Should not be used with methemoglobin-inducing agents (e.g., sulfa drugs, acetaminophen, nitrofurantoin, nitroglycerin, nitroprusside, phenobarbital, phenytoin). Breast-feeding: safety not established.
Enalaprilat (Vasotec IV)	Injection: 1.25 mg/ml (contains 0.9% benzyl alcohol)	IV: 5-10 µg/kg/dose over 5 min q8-24 hr (intervals determined by blood pressure measurements)	Enalapril is its oral dosage form and is a pro-drug that must be converted to the active Enalaprilat. Side effects include nausea, coughing, diarrhea, headache, hypotension, and hypersensitivity. Reduce dosage in patients with renal impairment. Breast-feeding: compatible.

Continued

NEONATAL PHARMACOLOGY **H**

TABLE H-2

DRUG DOSES FOR NEONATES—cont'd

Drug	How Supplied	Dose and Route	Remarks
Epinephrine (Adrenaline)	Injection: 1:1000 (aqueous) as 1 mg/ml (1,30 ml) 1:10,000 (aqueous) prefilled syringes as 0.1 mg/ml (10 ml)	*Resuscitation (IV, ET, IM):* 1:10,000, 0.1-0.3 ml/kg (0.01-0.03 mg/kg) q3-5 min *Hypotension (IV drip):* 0.1-1 µg/kg/min To prepare infusion: same as for dobutamine	May produce tachycardia, arrhythmias, hypertension, vomiting. Necrosis may occur at site of repeated local injections. ET doses should be diluted with normal saline to a total volume of 1-2 ml before administration. Follow with several positive pressure ventilations. Breast-feeding: safety not established.
Ergocalciferol (Calciferol, Drisdol, Vitamin D₂)	Oral drops: 8000 IU/ml (60 ml) Injection: 500,000 IU/ml 40 IU = 1 µg	*Dietary supplementation (PO):* 400 IU qd	Monitor serum Ca⁺⁺, PO₄, and alkaline phosphatase. Serum Ca⁺⁺ and PO₄ product should be <70 mg/dl. Vitamin D₂ must be activated by hydroxylation in liver and kidney. Breast-feeding: unknown with concerns.
Erythromycin (Erythrocin, Pediamycin, and others)	Ophthalmic ointment: 0.5% (1, 3.5 gm) Suspension: Erythromycin estolate, 125 mg/5 ml, 250 mg/5 ml; erythromycin succinate, 100 mg/2.5 ml (50-ml drops), 200 mg/5 ml, 400 mg/5 ml	*Ophthalmic:* Apply ½-inch ribbon to affected eye bid-qid PO: Weight <2000 gm: 0-7 days: 20 mg/kg/24 hr ÷ q12h >7 days: 30 mg/kg/24 hr ÷ q8h Weight ≥ 2000 gm: 0-7 days: 20 mg/kg/24 hr ÷ q12 h >7 days: 40 mg/kg/24 hr ÷ q8h	Candidiasis (oral, perianal), stomatitis, irritability caused by esophageal irritation, and epigastric discomfort may occur. Allergic reaction is rare. Hypertrophic pyloric stenosis in neonates receiving prophylactic therapy for pertussis and life-threatening episodes of ventricular tachycardia associated with prolonged QTc interval have been reported. To prevent cross-infection and ensure sterility, never share the use of an ophthalmic ointment tube among multiple patients (all tubes must be individualized). Interacts with theophylline (aminophylline) by increasing theophylline levels. Breast-feeding: compatible.

Drug	Preparations	Dose	Comments
Epoetin Alfa (Erythropoietin, Epogen, Procrit)	Injection: 2,000, 3,000, 4,000, 10,000, 20,000, 40,000 U/ml; multidose vials contain 1% benzyl alcohol	*Anemia of prematurity:* 25-100 U/kg/dose SC 3x per week; alternatively, 200-400 U/kg/dose IV/SC 3x per week for 2-6 weeks: (total dose per week is 600-1400 U/kg)	Evaluate serum iron, ferritin, TIBC before therapy. Iron supplementation recommended during therapy unless iron stores are already in excess. Monitor Hct, blood pressure, clotting times, platelets, BUN, serum creatinine. Peak effect in 2-3 weeks. Reduce dose when target Hct is reached or when Hct increases > 4 points in any 2-week period. May cause hypertension, seizures, hypersensitivity reactions, edema. Breast-feeding: safety not established.
Fentanyl (Sublimaze)	Injection: 50 µg/ml	IM or IV: 1-2 µg/kg/dose q30-60 min prn; may be used as a continuous IV infusion; start with 1 µg/kg/hr, then titrate to effect (usual range 1-3 µg/kg/hr)	Onset of action 1-2 min with a peak action of about 10 min. As with other opiates, respiratory depression occurs and may persist beyond the period of analgesia. Give IV dose over 3-5 min; rapid infusion may cause respiratory depression via severe muscular rigidity. Naloxone is the antagonist. Reduce dose in renal impairment. Breast-feeding: compatible.
Ferrous sulfate (Feosol, Fer-In-Sol, iron preparations, and others)	Ferrous sulfate (20% elemental Fe) Drops (Fer-In-Sol): 75 mg (15 mg Fe) /0.6 ml (50 ml); 125 mg (25 mg Fe)/1 ml (50 ml) Elixir (Feosol): 220 mg (44 mg Fe)/5 ml (5% alcohol)	*Prophylaxis:* 1-2 mg elemental Fe/kg/24hr ÷ qd-bid PO *Iron-deficiency anemia:* 3-6 mg elemental Fe/kg/24 hr ÷ qd-bid PO	Iron preparations are variably absorbed. Vitamin C enhances absorption, whereas antacids decrease absorption. May cause nausea, constipation, black tarry stool, lethargy, hypotension, and GI upset. Breast-feeding: safety not established.

Continued

NEONATAL PHARMACOLOGY H

TABLE H-2

DRUG DOSES FOR NEONATES—cont'd

Drug	How Supplied	Dose and Route	Remarks
Fluconazole (Diflucan)	Injection: 2 mg/ml (100, 200 ml); each 1 mg of drug contains 4.5 mEq Na Oral suspension: 10 mg/ml (35 ml), 40 mg/ml (35 ml)	Loading dose: 12 mg/kg IV/PO Maintenance dose: 6 mg/kg IV/PO with the following dosing intervals (see following table)	May cause nausea, headache, rash, vomiting, abdominal pain, hepatitis, cholestasis, and diarrhea. Neutropenia, agranulocytosis, and thrombocytopenia have been reported. Inhibits CYP 450 2C9/10 and CYP 450 3A3/4 (weak inhibitor) drug metabolizing enzymes. May increase effects, toxicity, or levels of cyclosporin, midazolam, phenytoin, rifabutin, tacrolimus, theophylline, warfarin, oral hypoglycemics, and AZT. Rifampin increases fluconazole metabolism. Adjust dose in renal failure. Breast-feeding: compatible.

Postconceptional Age (wk)	Postnatal Age (days)	Dosing Interval (hr) and time (hr) to start 1st maintenance dose after load
≤29	0-14	72
	>14	48
30-36	0-14	48
	>14	24
37-44	0-7	48
	>7	24
>45	all ages	24

Drug	How Supplied	Dose and Route	Remarks
Flucytosine (Ancobon, 5-FC, 5-Fluorocytosine)	Oral liquid*: 10 mg/ml	PO: 20-40 mg/kg/dose q6h	Common side effects include nausea, vomiting, diarrhea, rash, CNS disturbance, anemia, leukopenia, and thrombocytopenia. Monitor CBC, BUN, serum creatinine, alkaline phosphatase, AST, and ALT. Reduce dose in renal impairment. **Therapeutic levels: 25-100 mg/L.** Breast-feeding: unknown with concerns.

| **Folic Acid** (Folvite and others) | Oral solution*: 50 µg/ml, 1 mg/ml Injection: 5 mg/ml; contains 1.5% benzyl alcohol | *Folic acid deficiency:* 15 µg/kg/dose qd PO, IM, IV, SC **Maximum dose** 50 µg/24 hr RDA: Necnates-6 mo, 25-35µg qd PO | Normal levels: Serum >5 ng/ml, RBC 150-200 ng/ml. May mask hematologic effects of vitamin B_{12} deficiency but not prevent progression of neurologic abnormalities. Breast-feeding: compatible. |
| **Fosphenytoin** (Cerebyx) | Injection: 50 mg phenytoin equivalent (PE) (75 mg fosphenytoin)/1 ml (2, 10 ml; each 1 mg PE provides 0.0037 mmol of phosphate) | **All doses are expressed as phenytoin sodium equivalents (PE):** See phenytoin and use the conversion of 1 mg phenytoin = 1 mg PE | **All doses should be prescribed and dispensed in terms of mg phenytoin sodium equivalents (PE) to avoid medication errors.** Fosphenytoin is a prodrug of phenytoin and needs to be metabolized to the active phenytoin. Safety in pediatrics has not been fully established. Use with **caution** in patients with porphyria. Consider amounts of formaldehyde (metabolic by-product in trace amounts) and phosphates delivered by fosphenytoin. May cause hypokalemia (with rapid IV administration), dizziness, ataxia, rash, exfoliative dermatitis, nystagmus, diplopia, and tinnitus. Avoid abrupt withdrawal of drug. Monitor blood pressure and ECG during IV loading dose administration. **Maximum IV infusion rate:** 3 mg PE/kg/min. IM administration may be given via one or two separate sites. |

Continued

*Indicates suspensions not commercially available; must be extemporaneously compounded by a pharmacist. See references.

H

NEONATAL PHARMACOLOGY

TABLE H-2

DRUG DOSES FOR NEONATES—cont'd

Drug	How Supplied	Dose and Route	Remarks
Fosphenytoin (Cerebyx)—cont'd			**Therapeutic levels: 10-20 mg/L (free and bound phenytoin) OR 1-2 mg/L (free only).** Recommended peak serum sampling times in adults (may be different for newborns): 4 hours after IM dose or 2 hours after IV dose. See phenytoin for drug interactions. Breast-feeding: compatible.
Furosemide (Lasix and others)	Injection: 10 mg/ml Oral liquid: 10 mg/ml (contains 11.5% alcohol) 8 mg/ml (contains 0.2% alcohol)	IM, IV: 0.5-2 mg/kg/dose q12-24 hr **IV maximum** 2 mg/kg/dose PO: 1-4 mg/kg/dose q12-24 h, **PO maximum** 6 mg/kg/dose	Half-life is prolonged in premature infants. Can cause alkalosis, hypocalcemia, hypochloremia, hyponatremia, hypokalemia, and increased calcium excretion. Potential ototoxicity with aminoglycosides. Breast-feeding: safety not established.
Gentamicin (Garamycin and others)	Injection: 10, 40 mg/ml Ophthalmic ointment: 0.3% (3.5gm) Ophthalmic drops: 0.3% (5 ml) Topical ointment: 0.1% (15 gm) Topical cream: 0.1% (15 gm)	Parenteral (IM or IV): (see following table)	Monitor levels (peak and trough), monitor renal status; may cause proximal tubule dysfunction. Watch for ototoxicity. **Therapeutic levels: 5-10 mg/L (peak); <2 mg/L (trough).** Peak levels of 8-10 mg/L have been recommended in pulmonary infections, neutropenia, osteomyelitis, and sepsis. Recommended serum sampling time at steady-state: trough within 30 minutes before the third consecutive dose and peak 30-60 minutes

GENTAMICIN

Postconceptional Age (wk)	Postnatal Age (days)	Dose (mg/kg/dose)	Interval (hr)	
≤29‡	0-7	5	48	after the third dose. Eliminated more quickly in patients with cystic fibrosis, burns, or neutropenia. Neonatal doses are the same for gentamicin and tobramycin, but amikacin dose is about three times higher. Avoid physical contact with penicillin and cephalosporins (may blunt serum concentration). Breast-feeding: use with caution.
	8-28	4	36	
	>28	4	24	
30-33	0-7	4.5	36	
	>7	4	24	
≥34	0-7	4	24	
	>7	4	12-18	

Glucagon HCl (GlucaGen)

Injection: 1 mg/vial (1 U = 1 mg)

For hypoglycemia: <20 kg: (IM, SC, IV), 0.02-0.03 mg/kg/dose up to 0.5 mg q20 min PRN

Onset of action: IM: 8-10 min; IV: 1 min. Duration of action: IM: 12-27 min, IV: 9-17 min. Noted to have cardiostimulatory effect at high doses even in the presence of beta-blockade. Do **not** delay starting glucose infusion while awaiting effect of glucagon. May cause nausea, vomiting, and tachycardia. Breast-feeding: safety not established.

Heparin sodium

Lock flush solution (porcine-based): 1, 10, 100 U/ml
Injection: 1000, 2000, 2500, 5000, 7500, 10,000, 20,000, 40,000 U/ml;

Initial: IV 75 U/kg bolus
Maintenance IV: 28 U/kg/hr as constant infusion, or 50-100 U/kg/dose q4h
Heparin flush: Peripheral IV, 1-2 ml of 10 U/ml solution q4h; central lines, 2-3 ml of 100 U/ml solution q24h

Adjust dose to give clotting time of 20-30 min or PTT of 1.5-2.5 times control value before dose. PTT is best measured 6-8 hr after initiation or change in dose.
Toxicities: Bleeding, allergy, alopecia, and thrombocytopenia. **Antidote:** Protamine sulfate (1 mg per 100 U heparin in previous 4 h).

‡Or significant asphyxia, PDA, indomethacin use, poor cardiac output, reduced renal function.

NEONATAL PHARMACOLOGY H

Continued

TABLE H-2

DRUG DOSES FOR NEONATES—cont'd

Drug	How Supplied	Dose and Route	Remarks
	Some products may be preservative free or contain benzyl alcohol 120 U = approximately 1 mg		**NOTE:** Central line heparin flush dosage may be heparinizing; if so, use less heparin. A preservative-free flush product is preferred. Breast-feeding: compatible.
Hepatitis B immune globulin (Bayhep-B H-BIG)	Injection: 1, 4, 5 ml Injection (prefilled syringe): 0.5 ml Some preparations may contain thimerosal	*Positive maternal HBsAg:* IM 0.5 ml within 12 hours after birth *Percutaneous inoculation:* IM, 0.06 ml/kg/dose × 1 within 24 hr of exposure	Local pain at injection site, urticaria, angioedema. Anaphylaxis is rare. Breast-feeding: safety not established.
Hepatitis B vaccine (Recombivax HB, Engerix-B)	Injection: Engerix-B 20 µg/ml (0.5-, 1-, 10-ml vials and 0.5-, 1-ml prefilled syringes); Recombivax HB, 10 µg/ml (0.5-, 1-, 3-ml vials and 0.5-, 1-ml prefilled syringes); 40 µg/ml (1-ml vials) Some preparations may contain thimerosal	*Positive maternal HbsAg:* IM, Engerix-B 10 µg (0.5ml) or Recombivax HB 5 µg (0.5 ml) at birth (within 12 hr), 1 mo, and 6 mo of age (total 3 doses) **NOTE:** HBIG × 1 should also be administered at birth. *Negative maternal HbsAg:* IM, Engerix-B 10 µg (0.5 ml) or Recombivax HB 2.5 µg (0.25 ml) or 0.5 ml of Recombivax HB pediatric formulation (2.5 µg/0.5 ml) at 0-2 days, 1-2 mo after first dose, and 6-18 mo of age (total 3 doses)	Local reactions at the injection site, allergic reactions, or neuropathic effects may occur. **NOTE:** Recombivax HB is available in 2 different concentrations (10 and 40 µg/ml). Breast-feeding: safety not established.

Hyaluronidase (Amphadase, Vitrase)	Injection: (Amphadase): 150 U/ml (1 ml), bovine source containing thimerosal Powder for injection (Vitrase): 6200 U; ovine source (pharmacy can make a 15-U/ml dilution)	*Extravasation:* Dilute drug to 15 U/ml; give 1 ml (15 U) by injecting 5 separate injections of 0.2 ml (3 U) at borders of extravasation site SC or ID using 25- or 26-gauge needle	**Contraindicated** in dopamine and α-agonist extravasation. May cause urticaria. Administer as early as possible (minutes to 1 hour) after IV extravasation. Patients receiving large amounts of salicylates, cortisone, ACTH, estrogens or antihistamines may decrease the effects of hyaluronidase (use larger doses).
Hydralazine (Apresoline)	Oral liquid*: 1.25, 2, 4, mg/ml Injection: 20 mg/ml Some dosage forms may contain tartazines or sulfite	PO: 0.25-1 mg/kg/dose q6-8h IV/IM: 0.15 mg/kg/dose q6h; increase as needed in 0.1 mg/kg increments up to **maximum** of 2 mg/kg/dose q6h	Use with caution in severe renal disease (reduce dose in renal impairment) and cardiac disease. May cause lupus-like syndrome (reversible), cardiovascular, neurologic, GI, hematologic, and dermatologic reactions. May cause reflex tachycardia. Breast-feeding: compatible.
Hydrochlorothiazide (Hydro-Par, Esidrix, Oretic, Hydrodiuril)	Oral solution: 50 mg/5 ml	PO: 1-2 mg/kg/dose q12h	See Chlorothiazide. May cause fluid and electrolyte imbalances, hyperuricemia. Administration with feeding seems to improve absorption. Do not use in patients with renal or hepatic failure. Breast-feeding: compatible.

Continued

NEONATAL PHARMACOLOGY H

*Indicates suspensions not commercially available; must be extemporaneously compounded by a pharmacist. See references.

DRUG DOSES FOR NEONATES—cont'd

Drug	How Supplied	Dose and Route	Remarks
Hydrocortisone (Solu-cortef and others)	Oral suspension (cypionate salt): 10 mg/5 ml (120 ml) Injection (sodium succinate): 100, 250, 500, 1000 mg Injection (sodium phosphate): 50 mg/ml; contains sulfites and parabens	*Physiologic replacement (PO):* 15-25 mg/m²/24 hr or 1 mg/kg/24 hr ÷ tid *Congenital adrenal hyperplasia (maintenance therapy):* 15-24 mg/m²/24 hr PO ÷ tid *Treatment of pressor- and volume-resistant hypotension:* 20-40 mg/m²/24 hr IV PO ÷ bid-tid	Treatment of more than 7-10 days requires gradual dosage reduction to avoid adrenal insufficiency, immunosuppression, hyperglycemia, growth delay, leukocytosis, and gastric irritation. Breast-feeding: unknown with concerns.
Imipenem-Cilastatin (Primaxin)	Injection: 250, 500, 750 mg; contains 3.2 mEq Na per 1 gm drug	<1 wk: 50 mg/kg/24 hr IV ÷ q12h 1-4 wk: 50-75 mg/kg/24 hr IV ÷ q8h 4 wk-3 mo: 100 mg/kg/24 hr IV ÷ q6h	Administer IV over 30-60 minutes. May cause pruritus, GI symptoms, seizures, hypotension, elevated LFTs, blood dyscrasias, and penicillin allergy. Reduce dose in renal impairment. Breast-feeding: safety not established.
Immune globulin	IM preparation (Bay Gam): 150-180 mg/ml (2, 10 ml) IV preparation for reconstitution: Gammagard S/D, Gammar-P IV, Iveegam, Panglobulin, Polygam S/D: 1, 2.5, 5, 6, 10, 12 gm per vial IV preparation in solution: Gamunex, Gamimune-N, Venoglobulin S: 50, 100 mg/ml (5%, 10%)	*Primary immunodeficiency:* 300-400 mg/kg/dose IV every month or more frequently *Idiopathic thrombocytopenic purpura:* 1 gm/kg/dose IV qd for 1-2 days IV administration guidelines vary among products; check respective package inserts for initial and **maximum** infusion rates	May cause tenderness, erythema, and induration at injection site. Rare hypersensitivity reaction, especially when given rapidly. Gamimune-N contains maltose and may cause an osmotic diuresis. **Contraindicated** in IgA deficiency except Gammagard or Polygam. IV preparations containing sucrose should not be infused at a rate > 3 mg/kg/min to decrease risk of renal dysfunction. Delay immunizations after IVIG administration. Breast-feeding: safety not established.

Indomethacin
(Indocin IV)

Injection: 1 mg

Closure of ductus arteriosus:
Infuse intravenously over 20-30 min

Age	#1	#2	#3
<48hr	0.2	0.1	0.1
2-7	0.2	0.2	0.2
>7	0.2	0.25	0.25

Infants < 1500 gm 0.1-0.2 mg/kg q24 hr may be given for an additional 3-5 days

Maintenance dose regimens have been recommended to improve overall efficacy of PDA closure. In neonates, monitor renal and hepatic function before and during use. **Contraindicated** in neonates with BUN ≥ 30 mg/dl, creatinine ≥ 1.8 mg/dl, active bleeding, coagulation defects, and necrotizing enterocolitis. Keep urine output > 0.6 ml/kg/hr. IV is the preferred route of administration for treatment of PDA. Reductions in cerebral blood flow have been associated with rapid infusions (<5 min). May decrease platelet aggregation and cause GI distress (ulcer, nausea, diarrhea), headache, and blood dyscrasias. Breast-feeding: compatible.

Insulin
(regular)

Injection: many preparations at concentrations of 40, 100, 500 U/ml
Diluted concentrations of 1 U/ml or 10 U/ml may be necessary

Hyperglycemia: IV infusion, 0.01-0.1 U/kg/hr; SC (intermittent doses), 0.1-0.2 U/kg/dose q6-12h

Only regular insulin for injection may be administered intravenously. For hyperkalemia, administer glucose 0.5 gm/kg with 0.3 U insulin/per gm of glucose over 2 hr. Lower dosage may be required for patients in renal compromise. Breast-feeding: safety not established.

Isoniazid
(INH, Nydrazid, Laniazid)

Syrup: 50 mg/5 ml
Injection: 100 mg/ml

Tuberculosis (prophylaxis): PO, 10 mg/kg/24hr qd or 20-40 mg/kg/dose PO twice weekly (after 1 mo of daily therapy) for total of 12 mo

Should not be used alone for treatment. Peripheral neuropathy, optic neuritis, seizures, encephalopathy, psychosis, and hepatic side effects may occur with higher doses and in combination with rifampin.

Continued

NEONATAL PHARMACOLOGY   H

TABLE H-2

DRUG DOSES FOR NEONATES—cont'd

Drug	How Supplied	Dose and Route	Remarks
Isoniazid (INH, Nydrazid, Laniazid)—cont'd		*Tuberculosis (treatment):* PO, 10-15 mg/kg/24 hr qd or 20-30 mg/kg/dose twice-weekly (after 1 mo of daily therapy) additional drugs are necessary in complicated disease	Follow LFTs monthly. Diarrhea has been associated with use of syrup dosage form. Supplemental pyridoxine (1-2 mg/kg/24 hr) is recommended. Inhibits hepatic microsomal enzymes to increase serum levels of diazepam, phenytoin. May be given IM when oral therapy is not possible. Breast-feeding: compatible.
Isoproterenol (Isuprel)	Prefilled syringes, inj: 0.02 mg/ml (10 ml) Injections: 200 mg/ml (1, 5 ml); Contains sulfites	Initial: 0.05-0.1 µg/kg/min; increase by 0.1 µg/kg/min q5-10 min until desired effect or when heart rate > 180-200 beats/min **Maximum** dose 2 µg/kg/min Prepare infusion as for dobutamine	Use with care in CHF, ischemia, or aortic stenosis. May precipitate arrhythmias when used in combination with epinephrine. Patients should be monitored for arrhythmias, hypertension, and myocardial ischemia. Tachycardia, nervousness, restlessness, flushing of the face or skin, nausea, vomiting, and hypoglycemia may occur. Breast-feeding: safety not established.
Lamivudine (Epivir, 3TC)	Oral solution: 10 mg/ml (**NOTE:** Epivir-HBV is another oral liquid dosage form indicated for hepatitis B and comes in a 5-mg/ml concentration)	HIV: 2 mg/kg/dose PO bid	May be administered with food. May cause fatigue, nausea, diarrhea, skin rash, pancreatitis, and abdominal pain. Concomitant use with co-trimoxazole may result in the increase of lamivudine levels. Adjust dose in renal impairment. See www.aidsinfo.nih.gov/ guidelines for additional information. Breast-feeding: unknown with concerns.

NEONATAL PHARMACOLOGY   H

Lidocaine (Xylocaine L-M-X) and others	Injection: 0.5, 1, 1.5, 2, 4, 10, 20% (1% sol = 10 mg/ml) Some preparations may be combined with epinephrine Cream topical: (L-M-X) 4% (5, 15, 30 gm)	*Antiarrhythmic:* IV, 1 mg/kg infused over 5-10 min; may be repeated q10 min 5 times prn; infusion dose 10-50 µg/kg/min (see dobutamine for infusion preparation) *Circumcision:* 1 gm of cream placed around the shaft of the penis covered with plastic wrap for 20 min. Perform circumcision within 5-10 min.	May cause hypotension, seizures, asystole, and respiratory arrest. Decrease dose in presence of hepatic or renal failure. Transient erythema has been reported with use in circumcision. **Contraindicated** in Stokes-Adams attacks, sinoatrial, atrioventricular, or intraventricular block. Monitor blood levels **(therapeutic range 1.5-5 mg/L). Toxicity** may occur at levels > 5 mg/L for neonates. Breast-feeding: compatible.
Linezolid (Zyvox)	Oral suspension: 100 mg/5 ml (150 ml); contains phenylalanine and sodium benzoate Injection: 2 mg/ml (100, 200, 300 ml)	<7days old: 10 mg/kg/dose IV/PO q12 hr; if response is suboptimal, increase dose to 10 mg/kg/dose q8 hr ≥7 days old: 10 mg/kg/dose IV/PO q8 hr	Most common side effects include diarrhea, headache, and nausea. Anemia, leukopenia, pancytopenia, thrombocytopenia may occur in patients at risk for myelosuppression and who receive regimens > 2 wk. Complete blood count monitoring is recommended in these individuals. Use caution when using adrenergic (epinephrine, pseudoephedrine) agents; may increase blood pressure. Oral suspension product must be gently mixed by inverting the bottle 3-5 times before each use (do not shake). Breast-feeding: safety not established.
Lorazepam (Ativan)	Injection: 2, 4, mg/ml (each contains 2% benzyl alcohol and propylene glycol)	IV: 0.05-0.1 mg/kg infused over 2-5 min	Limited data in newborns. May cause respiratory depression, especially in combination with other sedatives. Onset of action: 1-5 min. Duration of action: 3-24 hr. Breast-feeding: unknown with concerns.

Continued

TABLE H-2
DRUG DOSES FOR NEONATES—cont'd

Drug	How Supplied	Dose and Route	Remarks
Magnesium sulfate (9.9% magnesium)	Injection: 100 mg/ml (0.8 mEq/ml), 125 mg/ml (1 mEq/ml)	*Hypomagnesemia:* IV, 50-100 mg/kg/dose q8-12 hr as needed **Maximum dose** 1 gm/24 hr	When given IV, beware of hypotension, respiratory depression, and hypermagnesemia. Calcium gluconate (IV) should be available as antidote. Use with **caution** in patients with renal insufficiency and with digoxin. Breast-feeding: compatible.
Meropenem (Merrem)	Injection: 0.5, 1 gm Each 1 gm drug contains 3.92 mEq Na	20 mg/kg/dose IV using the following dosage interval: <7 days old: q 12 hr ≥7 days old: 1.2-2 kg: q 12 hr; >2 kg: q 8 hr	**Contraindicated** in patients sensitive to carbapenems or with a history of anaphylaxis to beta-lactam antibiotics. Drug penetrates well into the CSF. May cause diarrhea, rash, nausea, vomiting, oral moniliasis, glossitis, pain and irritation at the IV injection site, and headache. Adjust dose in renal impairment. Breast-feeding: safety not established.
Methylene blue	Injection: 10 mg/ml (1%)	*Methemoglobinemia:* IV, 1-2 mg/kg/dose over 5 min; may be repeated in 1 hr if necessary	Use **cautiously** in patients with G6PD deficiency or renal insufficiency. May cause nausea, vomiting, diaphoresis, and abdominal pain. Causes blue-green discoloration of urine. Breast-feeding: safety not established.
Methylprednisolone (Medrol, Solu-Medrol, Depo-Medrol)	Injection: sodium succinate (Solu-Medrol) 40, 125, 500, 1000, 2000 mg; dilutions may be required to ensure accuracy of dose delivery; consult pharmacist	*Anti-inflammatory/immunosuppressive* IV, IM: 0.5-1.7 mg/kg/24 hr or 5-25 mg/m²/24 hr ÷ q6-12 hr	Hydrocortisone preferred for physiologic replacement. Less mineralocorticoid effect than hydrocortisone. Intravenous product may contain benzyl alcohol. Dose of methylprednisolone: one sixth dose of cortisone. Acetate salt form of the drug is used for intramuscular, intra-articular, and intralesional injection in adults. Breast-feeding: unknown with concerns.

Drug		
Metoclopramide (Reglan)	Syrup: 1 mg/ml; may contain sodium benzoate Injection: 5 mg/ml *Gastroesophageal reflux PO, IV:* 0.05–0.1 mg/kg/dose tid qid	May cause extrapyramidal symptoms, especially at higher doses (give diphenhydramine as remedy). Use with **caution** in patients with history of seizures. Reduce dosage in renal-compromised patients. Breast-feeding: unknown with concerns.
Metronidazole (Flagyl)	Suspension*: 100 mg/5 ml or 50 mg/ml Injection: 500 mg or 5 mg/ml ready to use (contains 28 mEq Na per 1 gm of drug) *Anaerobic infection:* Loading dose (IV) 15 mg/kg; maintenance dose 7.5 mg/kg (initiate 1 dosing interval after loading)	Nausea, diarrhea, urticaria, dry mouth, leukopenia, vertigo, and peripheral neuropathy may occur. Candidiasis may worsen. Potentiates anticoagulants. IV infusion must be given slowly over 1 hr. Initial drug of choice for antibiotic-associated pseudomembranous colitis over oral vancomycin. Adjust dosage for liver and renal compromise. Breast-feeding: unknown with concerns.

PCA	PNA	Interval (hr)
≤29	0–28	48
≤29	>28	24
30–36	0–14	24
30–36	>14	12
37–44	0–7	24
37–44	>7	12
≥45	All	8

Drug		
Morphine sulfate (Various)	Injection: 0.5, 1, 2, 4, 5, 8, 10, 15, 25 mg/ml Oral solution: 2, 4, 20 mg/ml *Analgesia/tetralogy spells:* IV, IM, SC, 0.05–0.2 mg/kg/dose q4 hr prn Continuous IV: 0.01–0.02 mg/kg/hr; begin with lower dose and titrate to effect *Opiate withdrawal:* PO, 0.08–0.2 mg/dose q3–4 hr prn	PO dose is approximately 6 times IV/IM dose. Respiratory depression reversible with naloxone. May cause nausea, vomiting, constipation, hypotension, bradycardia, increased intracranial pressure, miosis, and biliary or urinary tract spasm. Breast-feeding: use with caution.

Continued

NEONATAL PHARMACOLOGY

H

*Indicates suspensions not commercially available; must be extemporaneously compounded by a pharmacist. See references.

TABLE H-2

DRUG DOSES FOR NEONATES—cont'd

Drug	How Supplied	Dose and Route	Remarks
Mupirocin (Bactroban)	Ointment: 2% (15, 22, 30 g); contains polyethylene glycol Cream: 2% (15, 30 g); contains benzyl alcohol Nasal ointment: 2% (1g), as calcium salt	Topical: Apply small amount TID to affected area for 5-14 days. Intranasal: Apply small amount intranasally 2-4 times/24 hr for 5-14 days	**Avoid** contact with the eyes. Do not use topical ointment preparation on open wounds due to concern of systemic absorption of polyethylene glycol. May cause minor local irritation. If clinical response is not apparent in 3-5 days with topical use, re-evaluate infection. Intranasal administration may be used to eliminate carriage of S. aureus, including MRSA.
Nafcillin (Unipen, Nallpen)	Injection: 0.5, 1, 2, 4 gm (contains 2.9 mEq Na⁺ per 1 gm of drug)	IV: 25 mg/kg/dose <table><tr><td>Weight (kg)</td><td>PNA</td><td>Interval (hr)</td></tr><tr><td><2</td><td>≤7</td><td>12</td></tr><tr><td><2</td><td>>7</td><td>8</td></tr><tr><td>≥2</td><td>≤7</td><td>8</td></tr><tr><td>≥2</td><td>>7</td><td>6</td></tr></table>Severe infections: ≤7 days, 100 mg/kg/24 hr ÷ q8-12 hr >7 days, 150-200 mg/kg/24 hr ÷ q6-8 hr	Allergic cross-sensitivity with penicillin. CSF penetration is poor unless meninges are inflamed. High incidence of phlebitis with IV route of administration. Reduce dose in renal insufficiency. Breast-feeding: use with caution.
Naloxone (Narcan)	Injection: 0.4 mg/ml (1 ml); 1 mg/ml (2 ml) Neonatal injection: 0.02 mg/ml (2 ml)	Opiate intoxication: IV, IM, SC, 0.1-0.2 mg/kg/dose; may repeat every 2-3 min prn Continuous infusion: 0.01 mg/kg/hr; titrate to effect	Does not cause respiratory depression. Short duration of action may necessitate multiple doses. Use with **caution** in patients with cardiac disease. Tachycardia, hypertension, tremors, and seizures are possible. Administration to an infant of a drug-addicted mother may result in seizures and withdrawal

Neomycin sulfate (Mycifradin Neo-fradin)	Oral suspension: 125 mg/5 ml; contains parabens	Premature and full-term infants: PO, 50 mg/kg/24 hr ÷ q6hr

symptoms. Breast-feeding: safety not established.

Follow for renal toxicity or ototoxicity.

Contraindicated in ulcerative bowel disease or intestinal obstruction. Oral absorption is limited, but levels may accumulate. Consider dosage reduction in renal failure. Breast-feeding: safety not established.

Neostigmine (Prostigmin and others)	Injection: 0.25, 0.5, 1 mg/ml (methylsulfate); may contain parabens or phenol	*Myasthenia gravis:* Diagnosis, 0.04 mg/kg × 1 IM with atropine 0.011 mg/kg/dose IV immediately before neostigmine. Treatment, 0.01-0.04 mg/kg/dose q2-3hr prn IM/IV/SC *For reversal of nondepolarizing neuromuscular blockade:* IV, 0.025-0.1 mg/kg/dose with atropine or glycopyrrolate to prevent severe vagal reaction.

Titrate for each patient, but avoid excessive cholinergic effects. **Caution** in asthmatics. **Contraindicated** in patients with GI and urinary obstruction. May cause cholinergic crisis, bronchospasm, salivation, nausea, vomiting, diarrhea, miosis, diaphoresis, lacrimation, bradycardia, hypotension, fatigue, confusion, respiratory depression, and seizures. Reduce dose in renal impairment. **Antidote:** Atropine 0.01-0.04 mg/kg/dose IV. Breast-feeding: safety not established.

Nevirapine (NVP, Viramune)	Suspension: 10 mg/ml (240 ml); contains parabens	*Prevention of HIV perinatal transmission:* Maternal antenatal dose: 200 mg × 1 at the onset of labor Neonatal postpartum dose: 2 mg/kg/dose × 1 within 72 hr of birth

May be administered with food. Use with **caution** in hepatic or renal dysfunction. May cause skin rash (may be life-threatening), sedation, headache, and GI discomfort.

Discontinue therapy if a severe rash or rash with fever, blistering, oral lesions, conjunctivitis, and muscle aches occur. Drug induces the

Continued

NEONATAL PHARMACOLOGY

H

TABLE H-2

DRUG DOSES FOR NEONATES—cont'd

Drug	How Supplied	Dose and Route	Remarks
Nevirapine (NVP, Viramune)—cont'd			CYP 450 3A4 drug- metabolizing isoenzyme to cause an autoinduction of its own metabolism within the first 2-4 wk of continuous therapy. Cimetidine, erythromycin, ketoconazole can increase serum levels of nevirapine. See www.aidsinfo.nih.gov/ guidelines for additional information. Breast-feeding: unknown with concerns.
Nystatin (Mycostatin, Nilstat, and others)	Oral suspension: 100,000 U/ml Topical powder, ointment, cream: 100,000 U/gm (15, 30 gm)	Oral: preterm infants: 0.5 ml (50,000 U) to each side of mouth qid; term infants: 1 ml (100,000 U) to each side of mouth qid; Topical: Apply bid-tid	May produce local irritation, diarrhea, and GI symptoms. Treat until 48-72 hr after resolution of symptoms. Systemic absorption is poor through mucous membranes, intact skin, and GI tract. Breast-feeding: compatible.
Oxacillin (Various generic brands)	Oral solution: 250 mg/5 ml Injection: 0.5, 1, 2 gm (contains 2.8-3.1 mEq Na per 1 gm drug)	IV or IM: 25-50 mg/kg/dose PCA / PNA / Interval (hr): ≤29 / 0-28 / 12 ≤29 / >28 / 8 30-36 / 0-14 / 12 30-36 / >14 / 8 37-44 / 0-7 / 12 37-44 / >7 / 8 ≥45 / All / 6	Rash, diarrhea, nausea, vomiting, epigastric discomfort or fullness, and SGOT elevation may occur. PO administration is not recommended. Use higher dosage for meningitis. Reduce dose in renal failure. Breast-feeding: use with caution.
Palivizumab (Synagis)	Injection: 100 mg/ml (0.5, 1ml)	RSV prophylaxis for one of the following conditions: 1. ≤2 yr with chronic lung disease	RSV season is typically November through April in the northern hemisphere but may begin earlier or persist later in certain communities.

	2. Premature infant (≤28 wk gestation) <12 mo of age 3. Premature infant (29-32 wk gestation) <6 mo of age 4. Hemodynamically significant cyanotic and acyanotic congenital heart disease Dose: 15 mg/kg/dose IM monthly just before and during RSV season	Use with **caution** in patients with thrombocytopenia or any coagulation disorder because of IM route. May cause rhinitis, rash, pain, increased liver enzymes, pharyngitis, cough, wheeze, diarrhea, vomiting, conjunctivitis, and anemia.
Pancuronium bromide (various generic brands)	Injection: 1, 2 mg/ml (contains 1% benzyl alcohol)	Initial: 0.02 mg/kg/dose IV Maintenance: 0.05-0.1 mg/kg/dose IV q 0.5-4 hr prn	Must be prepared to intubate within 2 min of induction. Drug effect accentuated by hypothermia, acidosis, neonatal age, decreased renal function, halothane, succinylcholine, hypokalemia, and aminoglycoside antibiotics. May cause tachycardia, mild salivation, and rash. Reduce dose in severe renal failure. **Antidote:** neostigmine (with atropine or glycopyrrolate). Breast-feeding: safety not established.
Paregoric (camphorated opium tincture)	Camphorated tincture: 2 mg/5 ml (0.4 mg morphine/ml) (some preparations contain up to 45% alcohol and benzoic acid or camphor)	*Opiate withdrawal:* Initial, 0.08-0.12 mg (morphine equivalent) (0.2-0.3 ml) per dose q3-4 hr; increment, 0.05 ml/dose until symptoms abate (rare to exceed 0.28 mg or 0.7 ml/dose) **Maximum dose** 0.4-0.8 (morphine equivalent) mg/kg/24 hr or 1-2 ml/kg/24 hr	Same side effects as morphine (e.g., constipation, lethargy). After symptoms are controlled for several days, dose is gradually decreased over 2-4 wk (e.g., by 10% every 2-3 days). **NOTE: Deodorized opium tincture contains 10 mg morphine/ml and is 25 times stronger than the camphorated product.** Breast-feeding: use with caution.

Continued

NEONATAL PHARMACOLOGY H

TABLE H-2

DRUG DOSES FOR NEONATES—cont'd

Drug	How Supplied	Dose and Route	Remarks
Penicillin G preparations— benzathine (Permapen, Bicillin L-A)	Injection: 600,000 U/ml (contains parabens and providone)	*Congenital syphilis* (asymptomatic infants born to mothers with syphilis): 50,000 U/kg × 1	Provides sustained levels for 2-4 weeks. Do not administer IV. Use with **caution** in patients with renal or cardiac impairment and seizure disorders. Breast-feeding: use with caution.
Penicillin G Preparations— Potassium and Sodium (Pfizerpen and others)	Potassium: injection, 1, 5, 20 million units (contains 1.7 mEq of K$^+$ and 0.3 mEq of Na$^+$ per 1 million units of drug) Sodium: injection, 5 million units (contains 2 mEq of Na$^+$ per 1 million units of drug)	IV or IM: ≤7 days, <2 kg, 50,000-100,000 U/kg/24 hr ÷ q12hr; ≥2 kg, 75,000-150,000 U/kg/ 24 hr ÷ q8hr. >7 days, <2 kg, 75,000-150,000 U/kg/ 24 hr ÷ q8hr, ≥2 kg, 100,000-200,000 U/kg/ 24 hr ÷ q6hr *Group B streptococcal meningitis:* IV/IM: ≤7 days: 250,000-400,000 U/kg/ 24 hr ÷ q8hr >7 days: 450,000 U/kg/24 hr ÷ q6hr	1 mg = approximately 1600 units. Side effects: anaphylaxis, hemolytic anemia, interstitial nephritis. Half-life may be prolonged by concurrent use of probenecid. Reduce dose in renal impairment. For meningitis, use higher daily dose at shorter dosing intervals. Use for 10-14 days in congenital syphilis. Breast-feeding: use with caution.
Penicillin G Preparations— Procaine (Wycillin and others)	Injection: 600,000 U/ml (contains 120 mg procaine per 300,000 U) (may contain parabens, phenol, povidone and formaldehyde)	*Congenital syphilis:* IM, 50,000 U/kg/dose q24hr × 10-14 days	Provides sustained levels for 2-4 days. May cause sterile abscess at injection site. Contains 120 mg procaine per 300,000 U; this may cause allergic reactions, CNS stimulation or seizures. Use with **caution** in neonates. Do not use IV. Breast-feeding: use with caution.
Phenobarbital (Luminal	Elixir: 20 mg/5 ml (contains 13.5% alcohol)	*For seizures:* Loading dose, IV, 20 mg/kg over 10 min; up to an additional	IV administration may cause respiratory arrest or hypotension. **Contraindicated** in patients

and others)

Injection: 30, 60, 65, 130 mg/ml (some products may contain alcohol, benzyl alcohol, and propylene glycol)

5 mg/kg until seizure control up to total dose of 40 mg/kg is reached; maintenance, 3-5 mg/kg/24 hr ÷ q12hr IV, IM, PO

Chronic anticonvulsant: Initial, 2-4 mg/kg/24 hr ÷ qd-bid × 2 weeks, followed by maintenance, 5 mg/kg/24 hr ÷ qd-bid

with hepatic or renal disease and porphyria. **Therapeutic levels: 15-40 mg/L.** Recommended serum sampling time at steady-state; trough level obtained within 30 minutes before the next scheduled dose after 10-14 days of continuous dosing. However, levels may be obtained before steady-state to assess safety. Induces liver enzymes, thus decreases blood levels of many drugs (e.g., warfarin). Reduce dose in renal failure. **IV push not to exceed 1 mg/kg/min.** Breast-feeding: use with caution.

Phenytoin (Dilantin and others)

Injection: 50 mg/ml (2, 5 ml); contains alcohol and propylene glycol
Oral suspension: 125 mg/5 ml (240 ml); contains ≤0.6% alcohol

Status epilepticus: IV, loading dose, 15-20 mg/kg, infused at a rate <0.5 mg/kg/min; PO, IV, maintenance, 4-8 mg/kg/24 hr qd-bid; flush IV with saline before and after dose
Antiarrhythmic: IV 1.25 mg/kg over 5-10 min (or <0.5 mg/kg/min); repeat up to 15 mg/kg

Therapeutic blood level monitoring: 10-20 mg/L of free and bound phenytoin (probably lower at 6-14 mg/L because of reduced protein binding in neonates) OR 1-2 mg/L (free only). Recommended serum sampling times: trough levels (PO/IV) within 30 min before next scheduled dose; peak or post-load level (IV) 1 hr after end of IV infusion. For routine monitoring, measure trough. Do **not** administer intramuscularly. Oral absorption is reduced in neonates. IV infusion requires sufficient dilution (<5 mg/ml) with 0.9% NaCl solution. Start IV administration soon after dilution so that precipitation of the drug is avoided. An experienced person should supervise. Breast-feeding: compatible.

Continued

NEONATAL PHARMACOLOGY H

TABLE H-2
DRUG DOSES FOR NEONATES—cont'd

Drug	How Supplied	Dose and Route	Remarks
Phosphorus supplements (sodium and potassium = Neutra-Phos); (potassium = Neutra-Phos-K); sodium phosphate; potassium phosphate	Oral dosage forms (to be reconstituted in 75 ml H₂O per capsule or packet); Na⁺ and K⁺ phosphate (Neutra-Phos), caps, powder, 7 mEq Na, 7 mEq K, 250 mg (8 mM) P; K phosphate (Neutra-Phos-K), caps, powder, 14.25 mEq K, 250 mg (8 mM) P Injection: Na, 94 mg (3 mM) P + 4 mEq Na/ml; K, 94 mg (3 mM) P + 4.4 mEq K/ml Conversion: 31 mg P =1 mM P	PO: 31-46.5 mg (1-1.5 mM) phosphorus/kg/24 hr ÷ bid; consider the additional cations (Na⁺ or K⁺) in each dosage form	May cause tetany, hyperphosphatemia, hyperkalemia, hypocalcemia. PO dosing may cause nausea, vomiting, abdominal pain, or diarrhea. Use with **caution** in patients with renal impairment. Breast-feeding: safety not established.
Phytonadione	See vitamin K1		
Piperacillin (Pipracil)	Injection: 2, 3 gm (contains 1.85 mEq Na per 1 gm of drug)	IM or IV: 50-100 mg/kg/dose | PCA	PNA	Interval (hr)
---	---	---
≤ 29	0-28	12
≤ 29	> 28	8
30-36	0-14	12
30-36	> 14	8
37-44	0-7	12
37-44	> 7	8
≥ 45	All	6		Similar to penicillin. Adjust dosage in renal impairment. May falsely lower aminoglycoside serum level results if the drugs are infused close to one another; allow a minimum of 2 hr between infusions to prevent this interaction. Breast-feeding: use with caution.

Piperacillin/ Tazobactam (Zosyn)	8:1 ratio of piperacillin to tazobactam: Inj. powder: 2 gm piperacillin and 0.25 gm tazobactam; 3 gm piperacillin and 0.375 gm tazobactam; 4 gm piperacillin and 0.5 gm tazobactam	**All doses based on piperacillin component** Infants <6 mo: 150-300 mg/kg/24 hr IV ÷ q6-8 hr	Tazobactam is a beta-lactamase inhibitor, thus extending the spectrum of piperacillin. Like other penicillins, CSF penetration occurs only with inflamed meninges. See Piperacillin and Penicillin Preparations—Aqueous Potassium and Penicillin Sodium for additional comments. Adjust dose in renal impairment. Breast-feeding: use with caution.
Poractant alfa (Curosurf)	Intratracheal susp: 80 mg/ml (1.5, 3 ml); contains 0.3 mg surfactant protein B per each 1 ml (porcine source)	*Prophylactic therapy:* 2.5 ml/kg/dose intratracheally as soon as possible; up to 2 subsequent 1.25 ml/kg/doses may be given at 12-hr intervals for a **maximum** total dose of 5 ml/kg. *Rescue therapy:* 2.5 ml/kg/dose intratracheally, immediately following the diagnosis of RDS. May administer 1.25 ml/kg/dose q12 hr for 2 doses as needed up to a **maximum** total dose of 5 ml/kg.	All doses are administered intratracheally via 5F feeding catheter. Drug should be slowly warmed to room temperature and gently turned upside-down for uniform suspension (do not shake) before administration. Each dose is divided into 2 aliquots, with each aliquot administered into one of the two main bronchi by positioning the infant with either the right or left side dependent. After the first aliquot is administered, remove the catheter from the ET tube and manually ventilate the infant with 100% oxygen at a rate of 40-60 breaths/min for 1 min. When the infant is stable, reposition the infant and administer the second dose. Then remove the catheter without flushing. Transient episodes of bradycardia, decreased oxygen saturation, reflux of surfactant into the ET tube, and airway obstruction have occurred during dose administration.

Continued

NEONATAL PHARMACOLOGY

H

TABLE H-2
DRUG DOSES FOR NEONATES—cont'd

Drug	How Supplied	Dose and Route	Remarks
Prednisone (various)	Solution: 5 mg/5 ml (may contain alcohol)	*Anti-inflammatory or immunosuppressive:* 0.5-2 mg/kg/24 hr ÷ q 6-12 hr	See Hydrocortisone. Prednisone must be converted in the liver to methylprednisolone. Breast-feeding: compatible.
Procainamide (Procanbid and others)	Injection: 500 mg/ml Suspension*: 5, 50, 100 mg/ml	IV: Initial, 1 mg/kg infused over 5 minutes q5-10 min prn to a **maximum** of 15 mg/kg (100 mg total **maximum**); maintenance, 20-50 µg/kg/min (see dobutamine for infusion preparation/calculations)	**Contraindicated** in myasthenia gravis, complete heart block, systemic lupus erythematosus, torsades de pointes. Asystole, myocardial depression, anorexia, vomiting, nausea, rash, and lupus-like syndrome may occur. Blood level monitoring is helpful. **Therapeutic range: procainamide, 3-10 mg/L; N-acetyl procainamide (NAPA), 5-30 mg/L.** Monitor IV use closely, along with blood pressure and ECG readings. Administer at a rate of < 20 mg/min to avoid severe hypotension. Adjust dose in renal failures. Breast-feeding: compatible.
Propranolol (Inderal)	Injection: 1 mg/ml Solution: 4, 8 mg/ml Concentrated solution: 80 mg/ml	*Arrhythmias:* Initial dose, IV, 0.01-0.2 mg/kg infused over 10 min to a **maximum** of 1 mg/dose (may repeat q6 hr prn); maintenance/non-emergent dose, PO, 0.05-0.25 mg/kg/dose q6 hr *Tetralogy spells:* Acute, IV, 0.15-0.25 mg/kg/dose over 10 min (may repeat in 15 min × 1); maintenance dose, PO, 1-2 mg/kg/dose q6 hr	**Contraindicated** in asthma and heart block. Use with **caution** in presence of obstructive lung disease, heart failure, or renal or hepatic disease. May cause hypoglycemia, hypotension, nausea, vomiting, depression, weakness, bronchospasm, and heart block. Concurrent use with barbiturates, indomethacin, or rifampin may cause decreased activity of propranolol. Concurrent use with cimetidine, hydralazine, chlorpromazine, or verapamil may lead to

Propylthiouracil (PTU)	Tablets: 50 mg Oral suspension*: 5 mg/ml	PO: 5-10 mg/kg/24 hr ÷ q 8 hr	increased activity of propranolol. IV and PO doses are not bioequivalent. Administer IV doses over 10 min. Breast-feeding: compatible.
		May cause blood dyscrasia, fever, liver disease, dermatitis, urticaria, malaise, and CNS stimulation or depression. Dosage may be adjusted to maintain normal T_3, T_4, and TSH levels. Falsely elevates prothrombin time. Reduce dose in renal impairment. Breast-feeding: compatible.
Prostaglandin E	See Alprostadil	
Protamine sulfate	Injection: 10 mg/ml (5, 25 ml)	*Heparin antidote:* 1 mg will neutralize approximately 100 U of heparin; for IV heparin, base dose on amount received in previous 2 hr; <30 min (IV) 1 mg/100 U heparin; 30-60 min (IV), 0.5-0.75 mg/100 U heparin; >120 min (IV), 0.25-0.375 mg/100 U heparin **Maximum dose** IV, 50 mg with rate not to exceed 5 mg/min	Dosage depends on route of administration and time elapsed since heparin dose. Can cause hypotension, bradycardia, dyspnea, and anaphylaxis. Rarely, heparin rebound has occurred. Breast-feeding: safety not established.
Pyridoxine (Vitamin B₆)	Injection: 100 mg/ml Tablets: 25, 50, 100 mg	*Pyridoxine-dependent seizures:* Diagnostic dose, IV/IM, 50-100 mg × 1; maintenance dose, PO, 50-100 mg qd	May be given IV, IM, or SC when oral administration is not feasible. Sedation may occur. Breast-feeding: compatible.

Continued

NEONATAL PHARMACOLOGY

*Indicates suspensions not commercially available; must be extemporaneously compounded by a pharmacist. See references.

TABLE H-2

DRUG DOSES FOR NEONATES—cont'd

Drug	How Supplied	Dose and Route	Remarks
Pyrimethamine (Daraprim)	Tablets: 25 mg Suspension*: 2 mg/ml	*Congenital toxoplasmosis* (administer with sulfadiazine): PO, loading dose, 2 mg/kg/24 hr ÷ q12 hr × 2 days Maintenance 1 mg/kg/24 hr PO-qd × 2-6 months, then 1 mg/kg/24 hr 3 × per week to complete 12 mo of therapy	Blood dyscrasias, glossitis, leukopenia, folic acid deficiency, rash, or seizures may occur. Folinic acid supplementation (5 mg every 3 days) is recommended so that hematologic complications are avoided. For additional information on congenital toxoplasmosis see Clin Infect Dis 18:38, 1994. Breast-feeding: compatible.
Ranitine (Zantac)	Injection: 25 mg/ml Syrup: 15 mg/ml; contains 7.5% alcohol and parabens	PO: 2-4 mg/kg/24 hr ÷ q8-12 hr IV: 2 mg/kg/24 hr ÷ q6-8 hr IV continuous infusion: Administer daily IV dosage over 24 hours (may be added to parenteral nutrition solutions)	GI disturbance, malaise, sedation, arthralgia, and hepatotoxicity may occur. Data limited in neonates. Adjust dose in renal failure. Breast-feeding: compatible.
Rifampin (Rimactane, Rifadin)	Oral suspension*: 10, 15, 25 mg/ml Injection: 600 mg	*Tuberculosis* (use with Isoniazid): IV/PO, 10-20 mg/kg/24 hr ÷ q12-24 hr or 10-20 mg/kg/dose twice weekly; twice weekly therapy may be used after 1-2 mo of daily therapy (CDC recommendations) *Meningitis prophylaxis*: (<1 mo): *Neisseria meningitides*, PO, 10 mg/kg/24 hr ÷ q12h × 2 days; *Haemophilus influenzae*, PO, 10 mg/kg/24 hr qd × 4 days	Causes red discoloration of body secretions (urine, saliva, and tears). Induces hepatic microsomal enzymes; may need increased doses of digoxin, phenytoin, theophylline, etc. Use with **caution** in liver disease. May cause GI irritation, allergy, headache, fatigue, ataxia, confusion, fever, hepatitis, blood dyscrasia, and elevated BUN and uric acid. Reduce dose in renal failure. Food ingestion delays absorption. IV dose is similar to PO dose. Breast-feeding: compatible.

Sodium bicarbonate	Injection: 8.4% (1 mEq/ml) 50 ml Prefilled syringes: 4.2% (0.5 mEq/ml), 8.4% (1 mEq/ml), 10 ml (1 mEq bicarbonate provides 1 mEq Na$^+$)	*Resuscitation:* IV, 1-2 mEq/kg/dose (using 4.2% strength) infuse slowly only if infant is ventilated adequately *Correction of metabolic acidosis:* HCO_3^- (mEq) = 0.3 × wt (kg) × base deficit (mEq/L)	NaHCO$_3$ comes in 8.4% and 4.2% strengths. Use 4.2% for peripheral line administration because of a lower osmolarity of 900 mOsm/L. The 8.4% strength (1800 mOsm/L) is hyperosmolar and may cause tissue necrosis. The 8.4% solution should be diluted 1:1 with preservative-free sterile water. Metabolic alkalosis, hypernatremia, hypokalemia, hypocalcemia, edema, and tissue necrosis (during extravasation) may occur. Breast-feeding: safety not established.
Sodium polystyrene sulfonate (Kayexalate, SPS, Kionex)	Powder: 454 gm (1 tsp = 3.5 gm) Suspension: 15 gm/60 ml (contains 21.5 ml sorbitol and 65 mEq Na per 60 ml) Contains 4.1 mEq Na$^+$ per 1 gm of drug	*Practical exchange ratio:* 1 mEq K per 1 gm resin Calculate dose according to desired exchange; usual dose: 1 gm/kg/dose PO q6 hr or q2-6 hr rectally **NOTE:** Suspension may be given PO or PR	1 mEq Na is delivered for each mEq K removed. Use cautiously in presence of renal failure. **Do not** administer with antacids or laxatives containing magnesium or aluminum. May cause hypokalemia, hypomagnesemia, hypocalcemia, and systemic alkalosis. Breast-feeding: compatible.
Spironolactone (Aldactone)	Suspension:* 1, 2, 5, 25 mg/ml	PO: 1-3 mg/kg/24 hr ÷ bid	**Contraindicated** in patients with acute renal failure. May potentiate ganglionic blocking agents and other antihypertensives. May cause GI distress, rash, and hyperkalemia. Breast-feeding: compatible.

Continued

*Indicates suspensions not commercially available; must be extemporaneously compounded by a pharmacist. See references.

NEONATAL PHARMACOLOGY

H

TABLE H-2

DRUG DOSES FOR NEONATES—cont'd

Drug	How Supplied	Dose and Route	Remarks
Streptomycin sulfate	Injection: 400 mg/ml (2.5 ml)	Administer by IM route only: Newborns, 10-20 mg/kg/dose q24 hr; infants, 20-30 mg/kg/24 hr ÷ q12 hr	Adjust dose in presence of renal insufficiency. Follow auditory status. May cause CNS depression or other neurologic problems, myocarditis, serum sickness, nephrotoxicity, and ototoxicity. **Therapeutic levels: peak 15-40 mg/L, trough <5 mg/L.** Recommended serum sampling time at steady-state: trough within 30 minutes before the third consecutive dose and peak 30-60 minutes after the third dose. Therapeutic levels are not achieved in CSF. For tuberculosis, use in conjunction with other antituberculosis drugs. Breast-feeding: compatible.
Sulfadiazine	Suspension:* 100 mg/ml	*Congenital toxoplasmosis*: (Administer with pyrimethamine and folinic acid) PO, 100 mg/kg/24 hr ÷ bid for 12 mo	**Contraindicated** in porphyria and hypersensitivity to sulfonamides. Use **caution** in infants < 2 mo because of risk of hyperbilirubinemia and in hepatic or renal dysfunction. May cause crystalluria (keep output high and alkaline), fever, rash, hepatitis, lupus-like syndrome, vasculitis, or bone marrow depression. For additional information on congenital toxoplasmosis, see Clin Infec Dis 18:38, 1994. Breast-feeding: use with caution.

Surfactant, pulmonary

See Beractant (Survanta), calfactant (Infasurf), or poractant alfa (Curosurf)

Theophylline

See Aminophylline

Ticarcillin
(Ticar)

Injection: 3, 20 gm
(contains .5-6.5 mEq
Na$^+$ per 1 gm of drug)

IV: 75 mg/kg/dose

Weight (kg)	PNA	Interval (hr)
<2	0-7	12
<2	>7	8
≥2	0-7	8
≥2	>7	6

May cause inhibition of platelet aggregation, bleeding diathesis, hypernatremia, hypocalcemia, allergy, rash, or increased SGOT. **Do not mix** with aminoglycoside in same solution. Reduce dosage in renal failure. Breast-feeding: compatible.

Tobramycin
(Nebcin, Tobrex, and others)

Injection: 10, 40 mg/ml;
(may contain phenol and bisulfites)
Ophthalmic ointment (Tobrex): 0.3% (3.5 gm)
Ophthalmic solution (Tobrex): 0.3% (5 ml)

Neonates (IV or IM): See gentamicin
Ophthalmic: Apply thin ribbon of ointment to affected eye bid-tid or 1-2 drops of solution to affected eye q4 hr

Therapeutic levels: peak 5-10 mg/L, trough: <2 mg/L. Recommended serum sampling times at steady-state: trough within 30 minutes before the third consecutive dose and peak 30-60 minutes after the third dose. Ototoxicity, nephrotoxicity, myelotoxicity, and allergic reaction may occur. Ototoxic effects are synergistic with furosemide. Higher doses may be necessary in patients with cystic fibrosis, burns, osteomyelitis, or neutropenia. Adjust dose in renal impairment. Breast-feeding: use with caution.

Continued

*Indicates suspensions not commercially available; must be extemporaneously compounded by a pharmacist. See references.

NEONATAL PHARMACOLOGY

H

TABLE H-2

DRUG DOSES FOR NEONATES—cont'd

Drug	How Supplied	Dose and Route			Remarks

Drug	How Supplied	Dose and Route	Remarks
Vancomycin (Vancocin)	Injection: 500, 1000 mg Oral solution: 1, 10 gm (reconstitute to 500 mg/6 ml)	IV: 10-15 mg/kg/dose Give 15 mg/kg/dose if CNS is involved For colitis: PO, 10 mg/kg/dose q6h	Ototoxicity, nephrotoxicity, allergy may occur. "Red man" syndrome associated with rapid IV infusion. Infuse over 60 min; may be infused over 120 min if 60 min not tolerated. Adjust dose in renal failure. **NOTE:** Diphenhydramine is used to treat "red man" syndrome. Although the monitoring of serum levels is controversial, the following guidelines are recommended. **Therapeutic levels: peak 25-40 mg/L, trough 5-10 mg/L.** Recommended serum sampling time at steady-state: trough within 30 minutes before the third to fifth consecutive dose and peak 60 minutes after the third to fifth dose. The IV dosage form may be given orally as a more cost-effective alternative. Metronidazole (PO) is the drug of choice for colitis caused by *Clostridium difficile*. Breast-feeding: safety not established.
Varicella-zoster immune globulin (VZIG)	1 vial = 125 U (≈1.25 ml), 625 U (≈6.25 ml); contains 10%-18% globulin and may contain thimerosal	Weight 10 kg or less: 125 U IM 10.1-20 kg: 250 U IM; administer dose within 96 hr postexposure	**Contraindicated** in severe thrombocytopenia because of IM injection. May induce anaphylactic reactions in IgA-deficient individuals. Interferes with immune response to live virus vaccines such as measles, mumps, and rubella; defer administration of live vaccines 5 months after VZIG dose. Local discomfort at

For the Vancomycin Dose and Route column, the IV dosing table:

PNA	Weight (kg)	Interval (hr)
<7	<1.2	24
<7	1.2-2	12-18
<7	>2	8-12
≥7	<1.2	24
≥7	1.2-2	8-12
≥7	>2	8

Verapamil
(Isoptin, Calan)

Injection: 2.5 mg/ml

IV: 0.1-1.2 mg/kg (**maximum dose 5 mg**) infused over 2 min; if response is inadequate, repeat in 30 min × 1

injection site may occur. **Do not** administer intravenously because systemic reactions could occur. Breast-feeding: safety not established.

Contraindicated in cardiogenic shock, severe CHF, sick sinus syndrome, or third-degree atrioventricular block and during treatment with beta blockers. Monitor ECG during infusion. Bradycardia, atrioventricular block, asystole, hypotension, and apnea may occur. Have calcium and isoproterenol ready to reverse hypotension and bradycardia. Breast-feeding: compatible.

Vitamin A
(Aquasol)

Injection: 50,000 IU/ml (2 ml)

Prophylactic therapy for children at risk for deficiency: 100,000 IU q4-6 mo PO
Daily dietary supplement: Infants up to 1 yr (PO), 1250 IU qd

Avoid toxicity. Adverse effects seen with high doses include irritability, drowsiness, increased intracranial pressure, erythema, vomiting, diarrhea, papilledema, and visual disturbances. May increase adverse effects of warfarin. Breast-feeding: safety not established.

Vitamin D₂

See Ergocalciferol

Vitamin E
(Aquasol E)

Oral drops: 50 IU/ml (12 ml)
1 IU = 1 mg of di-alphatocopherol acetate

Vitamin E deficiency:
PO 25-50 IU/24 hr
RDA:
Premature infant (<3 mo): 25 IU/24 hr
Infant (<6 mo): 3 IU/24 hr
Infant (6-12 mo): 4 IU/24 hr

Nausea, diarrhea, and intestinal cramps may occur. Breast-feeding: safety not established.

Continued

NEONATAL PHARMACOLOGY H

TABLE H-2
DRUG DOSES FOR NEONATES—cont'd

Drug	How Supplied	Dose and Route	Remarks
Vitamin K₁ (Aqua-Mephyton, Konakion, Phytonadione, Mephyton)	Tablets: 5 mg Injection: 2, 10 mg/ml (contains benzyl alcohol)	*Neonatal hemorrhagic disease:* Prophylaxis, 0.5-1 mg/dose IM, SC, or IV × 1; treatment, 1-2 mg/dose/24 hr IM, SC, or IV *Oral anticoagulant overdose:* Infants (IM, SC, or IV) 0.5-2 mg/dose *Vitamin K deficiency:* Infants (IM or IV), 1-2 mg/dose × 1; PO: 2.5-5 mg/24 hr	Follow PT/PTT. Use with **caution** in presence of severe hepatic disease. Large doses (>25 mg) in newborn may cause hyperbilirubinemia. **IV injection rate not to exceed 3 mg/m²/min or 1 mg/min.** IV dose may cause flushing, dizziness, hypotension, or anaphylaxis. **IV administration is indicated only when other routes of administration are not feasible.** Breast-feeding: compatible.
Zidovudine (AZT, Azidothymidine, Retrovir)	Syrup: 50 mg/5 ml; contains 0.2% sodium benzoate Injection: 10 mg/ml	*Prevention of HIV maternal transfer:* PO, 2 mg/kg/dose q6 hr × 6 wk; IV, 1.5 mg/kg/dose q6 hr × 6 wk; Initiate first dose (PO or IV) within 8-12 hr after birth; IV administration over 1 hr with a concentration ≤4 mg/ml	Side effects include anemia, granulocytopenia, nausea, and headache. Use with **caution** in renal or hepatic impairment. Drug interactions: acyclovir, ganciclovir, and drugs inhibiting glucuronidation enhance toxic effects of AZT. **Do not administer IM.** See N Engl J Med 331:1173, 1994 for entire dosing protocol (antenatal and postnatal). Breast-feeding: unknown with concerns.

REFERENCES

American Academy of Pediatrics Committee on Infectious Diseases: 2003 Redbook. Elk Grove, Ill, the Academy, 2003.

Committee on Drugs: The transfer of drugs and other chemicals into human milk. Pediatrics 108:776-789, 2001.

Jew RK, Mullen RJ, Soo-Hoo W: Extemporaneous Formulations. Bethesda, MD, American Society of Health System Pharmacists, Inc., 2003.

McEveyt G, McQuarrie GM (eds): Drug Information 2003. Bethesda, MD, American Hospital Formulary Service, 2003.

Micromedex Healthcare Series Electronic Drug Information. Thomson Micromedex, Greenwood Village, CO, Thomson Healthcare.

Nelson JD: Pocketbook of Pediatric Antimicrobial Therapy, 15th ed. Baltimore, Williams & Wilkins, 2002-2003.

Pagliaro LA, Pagliaro AM (eds): Problems in Pediatric Drug Therapy, 3rd ed. Hamilton, Ill, Drug Intelligence Publications, Inc., 1995.

Robertson J, Shilkofski N (eds): The Harriet Lane Handbook, 17th ed. Philadelphia, Elsevier Mosby, 2005.

Taketomo CK, Hodding JH, Kraus DM (eds): Pediatric Dosage Handbook, 11th ed. Hudson, OH, Lexicomp, 2004.

Yaffe S, Aranda J: Pediatric Pharmacology, 2nd ed. Philadelphia, WB Saunders, 1992.

Young TE, Mangum OB: Neofax 2003: A manual of drugs used in neonatal care, 16th ed. Columbus, OH, Acorn Publishing, 2003.

H

NEONATAL PHARMACOLOGY

Index

Note: Page numbers followed by f indicate figures; t, tables; b, boxes.

INDEX

INDEX